CLINICAL REFRACTION

by

Irvin M. Borish, O.D., D.O.S., LL.D., D.Sc.

College of Optometry

Indiana University

Third Edition

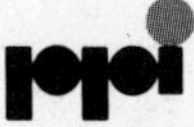

The Professional Press, Inc.

COMPLETELY REVISED

ISBN-0-87873-008-7
Library of Congress Catalog Card Number: 70-132836

Published by The Professional Press, Inc.
101 East Ontario Street, Chicago, Illinois 60611

Printed in the U.S.A.

Table of Contents

Section I—Refractive Status of the Eye

Section II—Preliminary and Adjunct Examination

12. TONOMETRY 457

13. OPHTHALMOSCOPY 501

14. FIELD CHARTING 527

15. COLOR VISION TESTING 585

Section III—Refraction

19. SUBJECTIVE TESTING 715

20. PHOROMETRY 805

Section IV—Analysis and Prescription

27. ABSORPTION LENSES 1115

28. BIFOCALS, MULTIFOCALS, AND PROGRESSIVE ADDITION LENSES 1133

Section V—Monocularity and Strabismus

29. STRABISMUS/DEFINITION, DEVELOPMENT AND CLASSIFICATION 1175

ABBREVIATIONS

Since certain journals appear repeatedly among the references, they have been coded by means of abbreviations in order to save space. These are as follows:

American Journal of Ophthalmology	AJOph
American Journal of Optometry and Archives of the American Academy of Optometry	AAAO or AJOpt
American Journal of Physiological Optics	AJPhys Opt
Archives of Ophthalmology	Arch Oph
British Journal of Ophthalmology	BJOph
British Journal of Physiological Optics	BJPhys Opt
Eye, Ear, Nose, and Throat Monthly	EENT
International Ophthalmology Clinics	IOC
Investigative Ophthalmology	InvOph
Journal of the American Medical Association	JAMA
Journal of the American Optometric Association	JAOA
Journal of the Optical Society of America	JOSA or J Opt Soc Am
Ophthalmic Optician	OphOpt
Optical Journal and Review of Optometry	OJRO
Optical Developments	Opt Dev
Optician	Opt
Optometric Weekly	Opt Weekly
Optometric World	Opt World
Transactions of American Academy of Ophthalmology	Trans Am Acad Oph

In addition, foreign countries and states are abbreviated by common appellations, as N.Y. for New York, International as Int., Vision as Vis., Society as Soc., and similar terms abbreviated by readily recognizable appelations.

References in foreign languages and those specifically so cited are secondary references. Titles preceded by an asterisk are not specifically cited as references in the text, but are given by the author as part of the bibliographic material utilized.

CLINICAL REFRACTION

THIRD EDITION

19 Subjective Testing

I. INTRODUCTION

A. The subjective test is an attempt to determine the refractive status of the eye by the use of subjective criteria, usually in the form of responses from the patient to changes in lens power before the eyes, descriptive of relative variations in the appearance of some form of test chart. Since the refractive status is reflected in either a spherical lens which corresponds to the theoretical over-all error of refraction, a cylindrical lens which corresponds to the astigmatism, or a combination of both, the criteria employed are usually those having to do with the combination of lenses which appear to give the patient the maximum visual acuity.

1. However, since the determination of this acuity is made by the patient, and since the concept of the "sharpest" vision may be influenced by factors other than the elements involved in a focus of the smallest blur circle upon the retina, the subjective finding may not always accurately reflect the purely refractive status of the eye. Intelligence, interpretation, past experience, habits of accustomed retinal images, inability to discriminate small differences, and other similar non-refractive influences, plus certain refractive influences yet to be mentioned, may disturb the proximity of the subjective finding to the refractive status actually existing.

B. Generally, the smaller the circle of least confusion and the closer it is to the retina, the sharper the visual acuity. Bearing in mind the influences which may obviate this rule, the climax of subjective refraction may be stated as depending upon a criterion which is expressed as:

1. The *strongest plus* lens or the *weakest minus* lens which grants the patient the *maximum* possible acuity of vision.

a. Since the hyperope may have the principal focus behind his eye and may move it to the retina by virtue of his accommodation, a number of plus powers up to the one actually determining his refractive status may result in maximum acuity. Likewise, a number of minus powers beyond the power actually expressing the status of the myope will place the focus of the myopic eye beyond the retina, from where the accommodation may move it to the retina. Since negative accommodation is not conceded beyond the static state, too little minus or too much plus will place the focus for either before the retina, from which position the accommodation cannot move it towards the retina and in which position acuity must be less than when the focus is upon the retina. Consequently, only the maximum plus lens or weakest minus lens, respectively, will keep the focus beyond the vagaries of accommodation and still permit it to fall upon the retina with corresponding maximum acuity.

(1) If the plus is weakened or the minus strengthened beyond this point, no actual improvement in acuity can take place; accommodation merely restores the image to the retina and frequently reduces slightly the size of the image so that the patient may report that while he cannot see a better line than he did before, the line he was reading seems smaller. This reduction in size may also be interpreted as the letters looking more intense. Such a report, if accompanied by the report of reduction in size, should not be interpreted to indicate an improvement in vision since it is a good indication of when the stopping point has been passed.

C. Since, to determine the proper power, the accommodation must be controlled so that the static refraction of the eye can be found, classic procedure accents the necessity for holding the accommodation passive and various means for doing so have been developed. This is basically an outgrowth of the concept that asthenopia was primarily due to the excessive use of accommodation and that relaxation of the total accommodative effort was required to provide relief. Of recent years, clinical experience tends to indicate that while accommodative effort may produce asthenopia, the total relaxation of accommodation may neither be required, or even desirable, nor necessarily possible and that the tendency to force plus power upon the subject may involve potentially new sources of asthenopia not previously implicated.

1. The average young hyperope, with good amplitude of accommodation, appears to establish a relatively habitual accommodative response, which might be interpreted as hypertonicity of the ciliary muscle. While this hypertonicity may be relaxed by artificial means during the testing procedures and an estimate of the total hyperopia determined, quite frequently an attempt to wear the full plus correction results only in blurred acuity and discomfort due to the re-institution of some of the habitual accommodative response. While persistence with the correction may rehabituate the patient so that the full lens is ultimately worn, actual experience indicates that the patient in the meanwhile finds the blur intolerable and usually discards the correction. A partial correction will be worn with clear vision and with relief of the asthenopia. As time goes on, the patient will accept such additional power as further onset of discomfort necessitates until such time as the total correction is finally accepted with readiness and absence of blur. The files of most practitioners reveal numerous records of young hyperopes who have successively, at intervals of two or three years, accepted more plus power and who gained relief of asthenopic symptoms with each successive change until their recurrence demanded an increase in the correction. Such individuals accepted the increase in plus with alacrity when they were ready for it, despite the relative latent and manifest amounts of their hyperopia or severity of their symptoms.

a. A few cases do exhibit a reluctance to accept the full correction and gain but little relief from a partial correction. However, such cases are readily detected by other indications in the routine examination.

D. Nevertheless, some basic point of reference must be assumed for the determination of the refractive status of the eye. The term refractive status means the power of the eye with accommodation at rest. Obviously, astigmatism may be concealed or varied by accommodative action, and in most cases the visual acuity does reflect with reasonable accuracy the relative relation of the focus and retina. However, the basic pattern of subjective determination of the refractive status has depended upon some method of controlling the accommodation and upon successive reports of visual acuity to relative changes of the lens powers.

1. Where the error is merely a spherical one, the responses to alterations of acuity are sufficient. But where astigmatism exists, the possibility of securing good acuity with only a partial or no correction of the astigmatism is very prevalent.

2. Consequently, the determination of the refractive status of the eye depends upon two forms of correction: first, most important and most difficult, the location and correction of astigmatism, if any; and second, the determination of the precise sphere which actually represents the refractive status.

E. Cycloplegia

1. As a precise measurement of both the spherical and astigmatic refraction depends upon inactive accommodation, various methods of insuring the stability of the accommodation are advocated. The most emphatic of these is the use of cycloplegia.

2. Advantages and Disadvantages.

a. The chief advantage of using cycloplegia is that accommodation is fixed in an inactive state, spasms of accommodation are relaxed, and convergent strabismus due to overactive accommodation may also be relaxed. Extremely small pupils are dilated.

b. However, optometrists oppose the use of cycloplegics for refraction, and a large proportion of medical refractionists prefer not to use them for various and numerous reasons. Among these is the fact that the eye is presented under totally abnormal circumstances with not merely the functional accommodation paralyzed, but in some instances the normal ciliary tonicity; if milder cycloplegia is used, the amount of ciliary paralysis is often indeterminate and varies both with the individual and the particular cycloplegic used; the aberrational effects of a dilated pupil are often not considered in the final results; recognition of accommodative anomalies is confused; glaucomatous reactions may be incited; and the ultimate correction is either arbitrarily calculated or a manifest re-examination is required anyway.

(1) Tait and Sinn (1936), in a study of the effect of homatropine upon the ciliary tissues, found 21% of the cases in which the tonus was inhibited and 9% in which it was increased by cycloplegia. The effects bore no relation to the amplitude of accommodation and were not reliably predictable.

(2) O'Brien and Bannon (1949), in a comparison of results under cycloplegia with those found without it, revealed that almost 75% of all cases agreed within an experimental or clinical allowance of ± 0.50 D., approximately 24% revealed greater plus power under cycloplegia; and 1.3% revealed less plus power under cycloplegia. Cylindrical corrections agreed in both axis (5°) and power (0.25 D.) in 80 to 85% of the cases. As might be expected, young hyperopes (under age 10) predominated among those showing more plus under cycloplegia. This tendency of younger hyperopes showing the greatest difference was also found by Bothman (1932) who noted a difference of from 0.39 D. to 0.88 D. more plus with the cycloplegic. Adults showed the least difference.

(3) Shlaifer (1949) likewise reported in a long study of various kinds of cycloplegics that the results were unpredictable both as to effect upon tonicity or extent of accommodative inhibition. Kurtz found results varying little from O'Brien and Bannon's. Seigneur found in a study of 1000 army cases that the hyperopes revealed more plus under cycloplegia (of 308: 110 same, 8 less plus, 190 more plus) but that myopes likewise revealed more minus under cycloplegia (of 410: 285 same, 103 more minus, 22 less minus). In cases of astigmia, cycloplegia was found of little ultimate benefit. Other studies (Bannon, 1947, and Garbus, 1949) revealed, similarly, the

curious paradox of substantially large numbers of myopes accepting more minus under cycloplegia than without it or of very few, if any, cases of pseudo-myopia revealed by its use.

(4) Morris (1950), in a comparative study of pre-cycloplegic, cycloplegic, and post-cycloplegic refraction, found that hyperopes usually revealed one diopter less plus acceptance without a cycloplegia than with, while myopes revealed the very same error either way. Astigmatism varied occasionally by 0.50 D. with a 15° difference in axis, but usually also resulted in identical findings.

(5) One hundred and twenty-two young Army applicants (Rengstorff, 1966) revealed a mean dioptric difference of +0.37 D. in 41% of the cases and of –0.36 D. in 48% of the cases in favor of cycloplegia; 37.6% revealed less than 0.25 D. in either direction.

3. Brickley and Ogle (1953) commented that cycloplegia actually does eliminate the residual accommodation, but the variance in findings is due to (1) the fact that the conjugate point on the retina is 0.50 D. proximal to infinity, (2) the depth of focus, and (3) the blur is not recognized in large test-type letter targets.

4. While authoritative opinion is sharply divided, the question of its use among medical refractionists appears to be a matter of personal technique and choice. Unfortunately, the reliance upon the cycloplegic frequently resulted in a hasty or careless technique for the subjective refraction (Beach, 1948), in which the examiner either placed overdue reliance upon his objectively determined findings, or failed to develop a consistent procedure adaptable to a subsequent manifest (non-cycloplegic) retest.

5. A subjective routine done under cycloplegia often is not so much a routine as a matter of trial and error. Since accommodation is paralyzed, the focus of the eye may be located either in front of or behind the retina. Astigmatic foci may lie both behind, both in front, or one in front and one behind the retina. While the retinoscopy usually indicates the course to be followed, the refractionist may find himself at different times using minus or plus lenses and cylinders, varying his procedure with each case. The methods used for cycloplegic subjectives are, of course, scarcely practicable for the manifest routine with accommodation active.

F. Fogging Technique

1. The most perfect non-cycloplegic control of the accommodation for subjective testing is gained by the use of the "fogging" technique. This consists of insuring that the foci of both principal meridians lie in front of the retina and is usually accomplished, in the hyperope, by a plus lens stronger than the maximum correction of either meridian, or in the myope, by a minus lens weaker than the minimum correction of either meridian. The fogging technique has the advantage of being consistent for either cycloplegic or non-cycloplegic routine; of employing a consistent cylinder, always minus, which corresponds to the interpretation of the astigmatic charts; and of proceeding in an orderly fashion from one step to the next despite the nature of the refractive error. The method has the advantage of providing a correction within the tolerable limits of wearability, of correcting all but the most incorrigible accommodative effort (Bannon, 1947), and of determining the refractive status under reasonably habitual physiologic circumstances.

a. The usual technique consists of two phases – one monocular and one binocular. The monocular technique also consists of two aspects: first, the determination of the cylindrical power and axis and second, the determination of the final spherical power. The binocular consists of equalization, or binocular balance, and the final binocular Rx for the best or chosen acuity (Hebbard).

II. TYPES OF ASTIGMATIC CHARTS

A. Since the determination and correction of the ametropia is the first and most difficult aspect of the subjective routine, a variety of procedures has been developed for this purpose. Most of these are related to the instrumentation and the chart used. These methods may be divided into the following categories:

1. *Fixed Clock or Sunburst Dials (Figure XIX-l)*

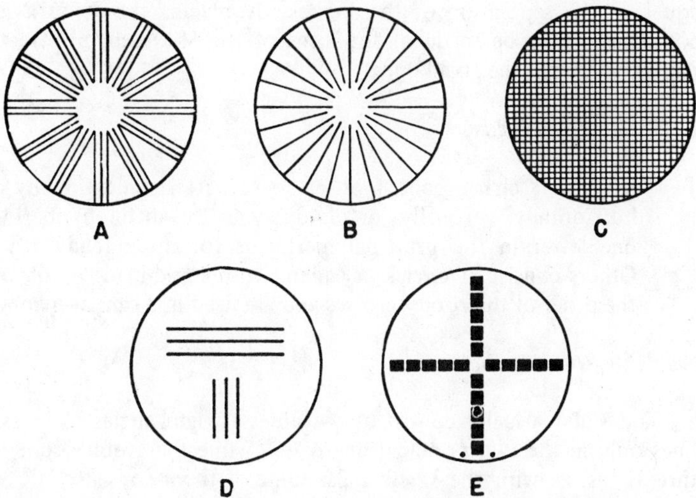

Figure XIX-1. Types of dials used in testing astigmatism. (A) Three lines per spoke clock dial. (B) Sunburst dial. (C) Rotary grid. (D) Rotary T. (E) Broken line rotary cross.

a. These dials consist of spokes radiating from an unmarked center.

(1) *The clock dial* introduced by John Green in 1868 consisted of twelve radiations at angular intervals of 30°, each radiation usually consisting of three separate lines spaced to be distinguishable at an acuity of 20/25 or 20/30. Some clock dials have only single line spokes, although these are usually associated with the sunburst dial.

(2) *The sunburst dial* usually consists of single spokes radiating at 10° intervals. Some of these encompass only half a circle while others complete a full circle.

(a) *The Lancaster dial* consists of black lines on a light background.

(b) *The Friedenwald dial* consists of black lines with a white border on a gray background.

[1] *The Guth dial* also uses a gray background.

(c) *The Eastman dial* consists of fine lines upon a background of finer lines one-third the width of the target lines and paralleling the radial lines. Black and white areas are equal. The lines discontinue at the center to avoid a black area at the intersection. The background lines are subliminal and below the threshold at 20 feet creating a gray, uniform effect. In astigmatism, the radial lines fade into the background rather than blur. They become invisible with less astigmatic error. Brecker, Lewis, and Eastman (1959) found the invisibility a better end point than the "more or less blur" criteria of ordinary charts.

(d) Some dials were composed of dotted lines (Sheard, 1923) and others of dashes or several lines per meridian. The principles were similar with variations to attempt to emphasize the difference between the best and poorest meridian and abet the blurring or fading of the weakest meridian into the background.

to emphasize the difference between the best and poorest meridian and abet the blurring or fading of the weakest meridian into the background.

b. Some fixed dials contain a movable section which can be rotated above the fixed spokes. This section usually consists of a V figure with its apex at the center and bisecting an angle equal to the separation of the spokes. By placing the V on a selected spoke, additional comparison may be made of the arms of the V which, in effect, constitutes new spokes halfway between the fixed ones.

c. *Patterns and Grids*

(1) Some charts consist of letters or patterns individually made up of lines running horizontally, vertically, or obliquely in the different meridians. These present some one letter in the principal meridians for more ready recognition than the others. Others consist of circles or squares with a grid made up of lines crossing each other on the order of the rotary crosses and are used in a similar manner.

2. *Movable or Rotating Dials*

a. These dials usually consist of two lines at right angles or crossing each other to present lines only in the two principal meridians. While the average spoke consists of either one or three lines, as with the fixed dials, some of them consist of dots or oblongs spaced to be distinguishable at a visual acuity corresponding to 20/30.

b. *Arrowhead dials.*

(1) Among the ingenious movable dials developed are those in which a rotatable cross contains an arrowhead-like figure at the end of or adjacent to one of the lines of the cross (Figure XIX-2). These are usually formed by two lines set at either a 45°, 30°, or 15° angle to the line they adjoin or accompany and thereby represent meridians corresponding to those positions to either side of the meridian towards which the line itself is directed. Since the darkest and faintest lines in astigmatism lie at right angles to each other, and lines between vary in blackness according to their angular distance from the two principal meridians, the two arrowhead spurs or arms would be equally black only if the lines of the cross were precisely on the principal meridians. If the lines were slightly off the principal meridians, one arm of the arrowhead would be blacker than the other, and the true meridian would be located when the cross was moved until the two arms of the arrow were equally black.

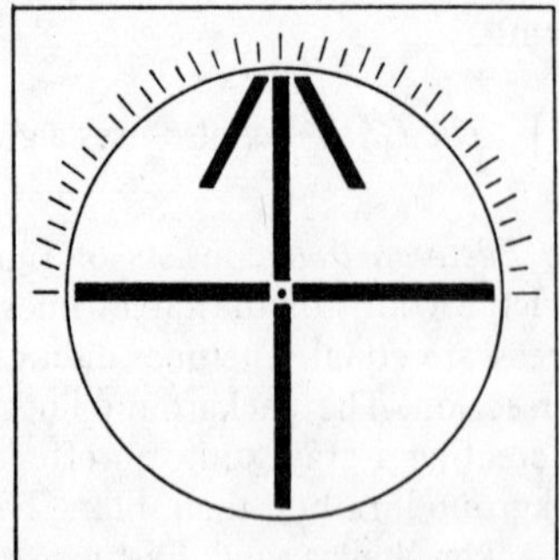

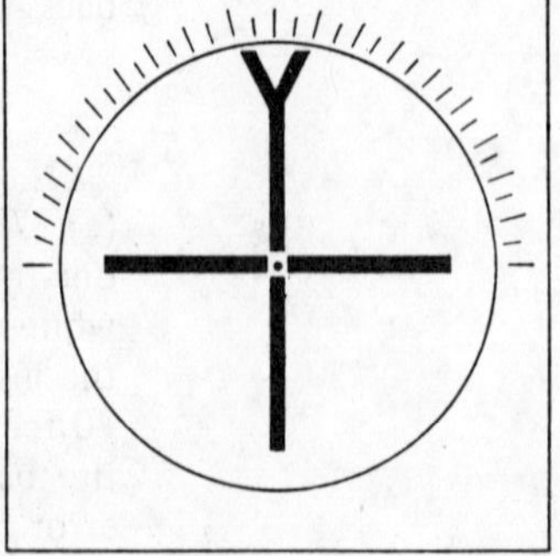

Figure XIX-2. Types of Rotary Arrowhead Charts. A. Lebensohn's astigmometer, utilizing adjacent arrowhead with apex pointing out, B. Inverted arrowhead chart, with apex pointing in.

(a) *The Crisp chart* consists of a cross with a single bisector line placed 45° from the arms of the cross. When this bisector is on the true meridian, the cross is equally black in both directions. It follows a similar principle to the arrowhead chart.

(b) *Lebensohn's Astigmometer* chart is an arrowhead chart consisting of two crossing lines with an inverted V forming an angle of 60° with one line as an arrowhead pointing to one of a ring of numbers around the chart. When the chart is rotated so that the prongs of the inverted V forming an arrowhead are equally distinct, the line bisecting the V is on one principal meridian. If one wing of the arrow is darker and the eye is fogged, the line is rotated away from the darker wing until both are equal, and the new position is the correct axis. Minus cylinders are added at right angles to the darker line until the cross is equally distinct. The Lebensohn chart can be used for the Crisp-Stine test which will be discussed later (Figure XIX-2).

[1] Stine believed that the arrowhead should be at a 90° rather than a 60° angle because of the influences of obliquely crossed cylinders.

c. *Other rotating dials*

(1) *The Elleman dial* consists of five sets of dual parallel lines, 5 to 6 mm. wide each, and 8 mm. apart. Each set is separated from the others by 72°.

(a) Each set bisects an opposite pair providing a visual angular difference of only 36°. At any position of the dial, one set of lines is within 18° of the true axis.

(b) The most distinct set is noted and the true axis is found by rotating the dial until the two opposite sets are alike.

(c) Cylinder is added at right angles to the darkest line until all lines are equally clear. The cylinder power is then over-corrected and the blur to equal extents of the adjacent lines is observed.

(d) The dial is rotated 5°. If all lines blur equally, the power is correct.

[1] If the lines nearer the original arm are darker, more cylinder is needed.

[2] If the lines farther away from the original arm are darker, less cylinder is needed.

(e) If two arms are equally dark, the true axis lies between them. If three are equally dark, two of them are opposite the best line, which represents the axis.

(2) *The Robinson-Cohen dial* (Figure XIX-1) consists of two broken lines at right angles to each other made up of black dashes upon a red background. One line is identified by two black dots at one end of it. The red background aids in locating the proper fog position since the red rays are the least refrangible, and if the red rays of both meridians are in front of the retina or on it, accommodation should be fully relaxed.

(a) If the approximate axis is unknown, the chart is rotated to present the lines in various meridians until both appear equally distinct. At this point, the true axis lies 45° between the lines. The lines are moved to that position 45° away, where one is seen blacker than the other, and the indicator gives the axis meridian of the line with the two dots. Minus cylinder is added at right angles to the blacker line until both are equal.

(b) The correction of the astigmatism may be further checked by adding a +0.25 or +0.50 sphere before an eye in which the lines have been apparently equalized. If, under the added fog, one of the lines now becomes more distinct than the other, the astigmatism has not been fully corrected (Tour, 1965).

(3) *The Raubitschek dial (Ioskiascopy test of Pascal)*

(a) Raubitschek varied the arrowhead dial by forming a V-like target of two parabolic arcs so designed that some portion of one of the arcs lies in almost every meridian of the protractor. The two lines, known as wings, begin as closely spaced parallel lines in the same meridian and end as parallel lines, but widely separated, in the same meridian after turning away from each other through a 90° angle (Figure XIX-3). The point of the arrow is directed towards a protractor scale surrounding the chart. One section of one wing will correspond to the major meridian of any existing astigmatism. The angle of the wings is such that a shadow or dark part on the wing will travel faster when the dial is rotated to approach the true axis. Thus, the shadow moves as fast at the last critical 10° as at the previous 80°.

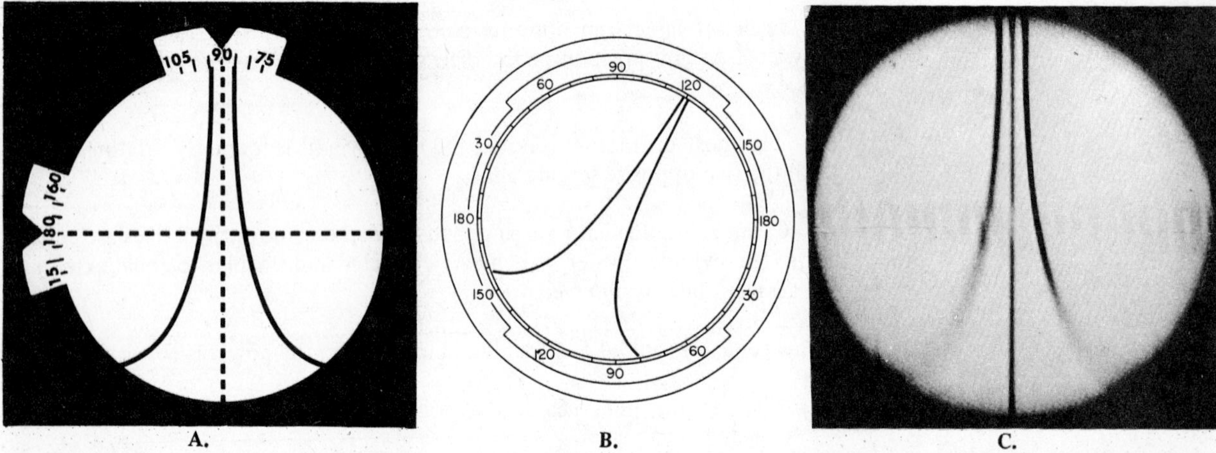

Figure XIX-3. Raubitschek Dial. A. adaptation to paraboline, showing axis scale and pointers. B. original Raubitschek Dial. C. appearance of wings when off true axis.

(b) *To find the axis:*

[1] The retinoscopic sphere is fogged by a +0.50 D. sphere with no cylinder before the eye.
[2] If astigmatism exists, one wing has a relatively dark area called the shadow.
[3] If the chart is rotated, the shadow moves along the wing to the portion parallel to the major meridian.

[a] The change is gradual if the movement is away from the major meridian and rapid if towards the major meridian.

[4] The chart is rotated until the tips of both wings show equally distinct and lengthy shadows.

[a] The dial is always rotated towards the less distinct tip in order to find the end point.

[5] The minus correcting cylinder axis lies 90° from the tip position.

(c) *To find the power:*

[1] *Raubitschek's method*

[a] Use the principle of obliquely crossed cylinders. A known cylinder is introduced at a known angle to the true axis. The tips are no longer equal. The angles through which the chart must again be rotated indicate the true power according to the following table:

[b] **TABLE XIX-1 – ESKRIDGE TABLE**

Correction Cylinder	**Target Rotation in Degrees from Major Meridian When Lens Power Indicated is Placed Axis 40 Degrees from True Minus Axis**					
	–.50 Cyl	**–1.00 Cyl**	**–1.50**	**–2.00**	**–2.50**	**–3.00**
–.25	27.82					
–.50	20.00	27.81				
–.75	15.24	23.42	27.81			
–1.00	12.14	20.00	24.76			
–1.25	10.11	17.34	22.18	25.48		
–1.50	8.62	15.24	20.00	23.42		
–1.75	7.50	13.56	18.16	21.60	24.21	
–2.00	6.64	12.19	16.58	20.00	22.66	
–2.25		11.06	15.24	18.59	21.26	
–2.50			14.08	17.34	20.00	
–2.75			13.07	16.23	18.86	21.05
–3.00			12.19	15.24	17.82	20.00
–3.25				14.35	16.88	19.04
–3.50				13.56	16.02	18.15
–3.75					15.24	17.34
–4.00					14.52	16.58
–4.25						15.88
–4.50						15.24
–4.75						14.64
–5.00						14.08

Example: If tips align at 155° and axis is at 65°. Remove fogging lens, place a –1.00 D. cyl at 115°. Shadow is not equal and rotation until they are equal, extends to 17° from original axis. –1.25 D. is true cylinder.

[2] *The Pascal-Raubitschek method*

[a] Fog the patient with a +0.50 sphere.

[b] Place the tips of the arrow in two positions 90° apart. If alike in both, there is no astigmatism.

[c] If one wing shows a blacker or larger shadow, rotate towards the less distinct wing until both are equal. The protractor reveals the principal meridian.

[i] If the correct axis is passed, the shadow will leap from one wing to the other.

[ii] At the incorrect axis, one wing will show a longer shadow than the other.

[d] After a principal meridian is found, place the tips 35° from that position (called the rotation angle).

[e] Place a cylinder of known power 20° from the true axis (known as the test angle) in the interval of the rotation angle.

[i] For example, if the axis is 90 and the rotation angle is at 145°, place a cylinder at 110°, not at 70°.

[ii] If both tips are equal, the power is correct.

[iii] If the wing nearer the true axis is darker, the cylinder is too weak.

[iv] If the wing farther from the true axis is darker, the cylinder is too strong.

[v] Increase or decrease the cylinder power until the wings reverse at the next addition or are equal.

[f] For most cases, the 35° as the rotation angle is sufficient, and 20° as the test angle is satisfactory, but for very high cylinders, a 40° rotation angle with a 10° test angle can be used.

[i] To find the rotation and test angle, the following formula is supplied:

$$\frac{90 - \text{test angle}}{2} = \text{the rotation angle.}$$

[3] *Heath's method (1959):*

[a] Rotate the tips of the arrow 20 or 30° away from the true principal meridian.

[b] Add cylinder at the originally indicated axis until both wing tips are equally shadowed.

[c] The amount equalizing the tips is the proper cylinder.

(4) *The Paraboline chart (Bannon, 1958)*

(a) The Paraboline chart consists of the Raubitschek arrow with a broken-line cross intersecting it so that when the arrow is directed at one principal meridian, the broken lines lie in the major meridians for direct contrast. A sunburst dial with a movable pointer is on the same slide.

(b) The patient is fogged +0.50 D. and directed towards the lines of the sunburst dial. The pointer is located at the darker lines.

(c) The slide is moved to expose the Raubitschek arrow.

(d) The principal meridian is located by equalizing the shadows on the wings as in prior descriptions.

[1] The dashed line which bisects the wing tips should stand out more sharply than the line at right angles.

[2] Minus cylinder is added in the meridian of the faintest dashed line until the lines are equally clear.

(e) Another method of checking the power of the cylinder with the Raubitschek chart is to rotate the wings a complete 90° so that very widely separated portions of the arrow are darker. As a wider portion of the target is blurred, less error in judging the quality of the tips will be induced.

(5) *The Raubitschek arrow test*

(a) The original dial was modified by Raubitschek by aligning the two black lines which formed the original wings with a white border on a grey background printed on a rotating disc. The unfocused portions of the lines would thereby, merge with the background.

(b) The front disc has a slit with a radial sighting wire longitudinally bisecting it along the meridian opposite that of the point of the arrow. Through this slit a portion of the back disc, upon which the front one rotates, is visible. The back disc consists of a series of black curving lines which are drawn over a system of blue parallel arcs. The intersections of these bear figures representing dioptric powers.

(c) The axis is found by the usual equalization of the wing tips. Both the front and back discs rotate together for this purpose.

(d) An approximate minus cylinder is placed at either 10°, 20°, or 30° from the true axis. The different blue lines seen through the slit each correspond to the 10°, or 20°, or 30° positions, respectively.

(e) As the wings are no longer equal, only the front disc with the arrow is rotated until the wing tips are equal again. The back disc is held constant.

[1] If the cylinder is placed 10° off the axis, the blue line corresponding to the 10° off position is followed in the slit until it leads to the intersection of the radial sighting wire in the slit and a black curve at a black figure, the latter giving the true power. If the cylinder had been placed either 20° or 30° off axis, the blue line corresponding to either the 20° or 30° position would have been used. If the cylinder was placed at, for example, 20° and the 20° blue line did not show in the slit, the front disc would be held constant and the back one rotated until the 20° line did show. The thickest curved lines bear figures representing diopters. A quarter and a half diopter curves consist of thinner lines placed between them.

(f) The black curves are constructed on the formula:

$$A = C \times \frac{\text{Sin } (C - 2\phi)}{\text{Sin } (\phi - \theta)}$$

in which A is the amount of the astigmatism, C is the power in diopters of the inserted cylinder, , ϕ is the guide angle, θ is the angle of the 10°, 20°, or 30° used between the axis chosen and the real axis.

[1] For plus cylinders, ϕ the guide angle, is included between the axis of the cylinder and the direction of the arrow point when the shadows are equal.

[a] For example, if the tips of the arrow were equal at an 85° position, a plus cylinder would be placed at 65° (θ = 20°). If the results then showed them eaual again at 115°, then ϕ would be 115° –65° or 50°.

[2] For a minus cylinder, the guide angle is placed between the axis of the cylinder and a perpendicular to the arrow point where the shadows are equal.

[a] For example, if the tips of the arrow are equal at 85°, a minus cylinder would be placed at 65° (θequals 20°). If the results again showed the arrow equal at 115°, ϕ will be 115 – 90 + 65 = 50°.

(6) *Marano's chart* (1958, 1959, 1962), (Figure XIX-4).

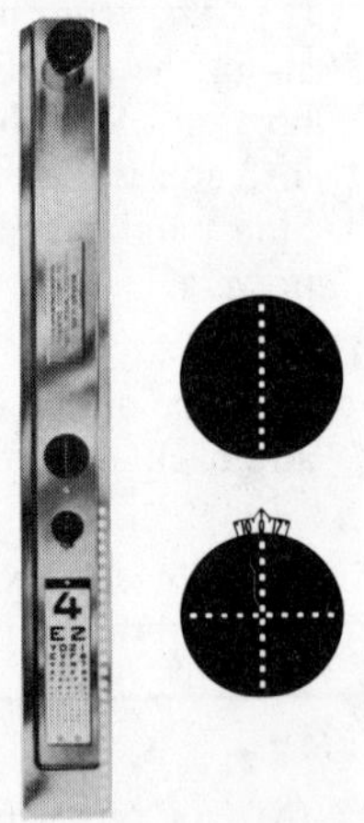

Figure XIX-4. Marano Chart.

(a) This chart is based on the fact that color unification takes place in astigmatism and saturation and linearity modify it. The slide consists of one chart with a single line made up of rectangles of alternate red and green on a black background. These two complementary colors, if mixed, will make up an apparently white color. Another slide consists of a cross made up of similar rectangles which if mixed will produce the same effect. Under actual test, the dashes or colored squares will fuse to produce either an orange line, a white line, a yellowish-orange line, or a yellow line, depending on the subject.

(b) The technique consists of the following:

[1] The patient is unfogged to the best acuity at the maximum plus with only spheres before the eye.

[2] The single line is rotated. If no astigmatism exists, the lines will show red, green, or a constant color in every position. If astigmatism exists, it will appear a brilliant yellow in the position of the axis, or as noted above, sometimes white, yellowish-orange, or orange, due to the overlap of the astigmatic bundles of the two complementary colors. At the position at which the yellow line appears, the axis is indicated on a numerical dial.

[3] The chart is then moved to the cross lines, which also consist of colored rectangles which are registered with the single line. Minus cylinder is added until the yellow lines revert to a red/green and both lines look alike.

[4] The test must be made in a dark room or with the screen in a shadow box and with an illuminized reflecting screen.

[5] The full chart also contains an acuity chart and a dial indicator on the slide. The acuity chart registers from 20/400 to 20/20. There are four 20/20 lines in an order of decreasing visibility.

[6] Schuman (1964) tested the chart against the cross cylinder and other chart methods, such as the Robinson-Cohen, and found a very high correlation of results. It is claimed that the technique is valid even with red/green anomalous patients. Even if color visibility is very poor, the patient is able to tell if one line is thinner or more solid or brighter.

III. THE PROPER AMOUNT OF FOG

A. If a lens is placed before the eye so that both principal meridians are located in front of the retina, the vision will be blurred in accordance with the power of the lens. Since accommodation will be maximally relaxed, no means of placing either the focus of one of the meridians or the circle of least confusion on the retina will be available. As the power of the lens is reduced, the meridian closest to the retina will begin to approximate the retina, and one set of spokes will become visible and successively more dominant. At a certain point, one meridian will focus on the retina and the other will focus in front of it by the interval of Sturm. At this point one meridian will be most clear in comparison to the other. This is known as the *point of greatest contrast* (Figure XIX-5).

1. If a subsequent reduction in the fogging lens is made, the meridian on the retina will be moved slightly behind it if accommodation remains inactive while the one in front will be moved still closer to the retina. While the former will actually be less clear than it was at the position of retinal focus, the latter will be clearer than it was, and the actual contrast between the two will be reduced. Also, the position of the retina will more closely approximate that of the circle of least confusion and the visual acuity may be sharper on a letter chart than before.

2. If accommodation becomes active and restores the weaker meridian to the retina, the two principal meridians will occupy the same positions which they did when the weaker meridian was first placed on the retina, and while the contrast will not diminish, it will also not increase with subsequent reductions in the power of the fogging lenses.

B. The optimum position for measuring the astigmatism would be at the point of greatest contrast, at which point, the fogging lens itself would actually correspond to the sphere of the correction. Since this point would only be determinable upon the basis of the patient's response, and since an error in judgment of the various extents of contrast would be most likely, this point is actually seldom used for fear that the fogging power may be reduced beyond the point of control of accommodation. Also, since the radiations of most astigmatic charts are based upon a 20/30 visual angle, reduction to this point would make most meridians, in small amounts of error, almost equally visible. The proper place for stopping the unfogging procedure to test for astigmatism is, therefore, at a point safely short of exposing the accommodation to action, yet close enough to the visibility of the spokes to provide critical contrast without passing the critical angle of the spokes themselves.

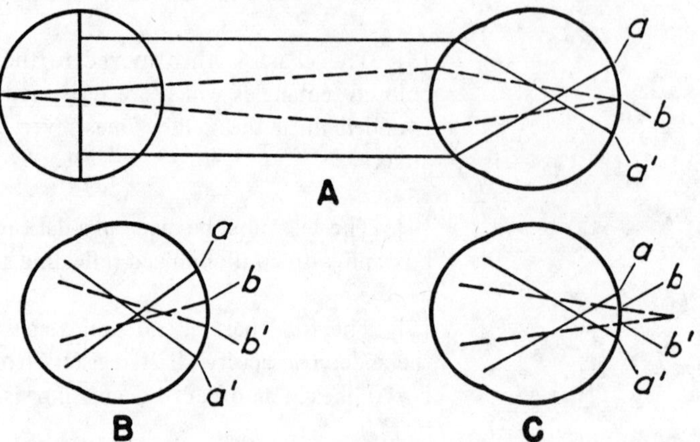

Figure XIX-5. Illustrating point of greatest contrast. (A) Point of greatest contrast, with one meridian on the retina. (B) Too much fog, both meridians in front of retina. (C) Too little fog, approaching circle of least confusion. Accommodative action would restore meridians to positions in (A). aa′ diameter of blur circle of strongest meridian; bb′ diameter of blur circles of weakest meridian.

C. Methods of determining the proper amount of fog.

1. An emmetropic or hyperopic eye will not be under fog without lenses before the eye. A myopic eye will be fogged, but usually more than is required.

2. The simplest method of securing a starting point for the fogging lens is to use the retinoscopy spherical correction, after the total has been transposed to minus cylinders, plus the value of the working distance. This will usually provide from 1.50 to 2.00 D. of fog more than is required.

   a. If the patient is started without any lens, a plus lens of 2.00 D. may be placed before the eye. This should blur the vision beyond 20/100. If it does not, additional plus may be added.

   b. If the patient is unable to see 20/40 to begin with, he may suffer from either myopia or absolute hyperopia. If the former, minus will have to be added. The addition of minus should improve the vision.

   c. If an absolute hyperope, addition of minus will make the vision worse and plus will be required. This plus may at first improve the acuity, but sufficient plus should be added to again blur the vision.

   d. If the acuity is quite poor and neither plus nor minus lenses improves it, the condition may be one of amblyopia and the subjective determination therefore more difficult.

3. Since the routine follows that of retinoscopy, the patient is usually properly seated and the

refractor properly adjusted. Ordinarily, the eye with the lesser error or better entrance acuity is refracted first, although any standard procedure, such as first right eye and then the left eye, may be habitually used. The eye not under test must be occluded.

4. The plus lens is reduced, keeping, thereby, the accommodation relaxed until the proper point for the detection of astigmatism is reached. (In myopia the minus is increased to the same point.)

a. If a *letter chart* is used, the fogging lens is reduced until the 20/40 line can barely be seen. The patient is then referred to the astigmatic chart.

(1) If a very high degree of astigmatism exists, the patient may not be able to secure the required acuity by spherical lenses alone. In such instances, when the best possible acuity has been reached with minimum reduction of the plus fogging lens, the patient should be referred to the astigmatic chart with that lens before the eye.

(2) Many practitioners prefer to unfog upon a *clock dial.* Since the three lines per spoke dial require acuity of approximately 20/30 to distinguish the three lines, the unfogging stopping point is determined by the maximum plus through which the patient can barely distinguish the three lines in any spoke. This procedure is preferable in mixed astigmatism.

b. If a *sunburst* or clock dial of single lines per spoke is used, the stopping place is the point where any one of the lines appears fairly distinct.

c. In using a *rotary dial,* the unfogging stopping point is based upon the same considerations as in using the other dials. Since, however, only two meridians are presented at any time, this necessitates rotation of the dial throughout the different meridians with each lens change. Consequently, unless a previous clue indicating the location of the principal meridians is available, the rotary dial is cumbersome at this stage of the proceedings.

(1) The axis indicated by the retinoscopy or ophthalmometry is frequently used for this purpose and generally works fairly well, although frequently it requires minor modification.

(2) Where a line made up of dashes constitutes the arms of the cross, the recognition of one of the lines as broken is an ideal stopping place. However, the lighter line rather than the darker one will ordinarily be recognized as the broken line.

5. Hebbard suggests that a +1.50 D. sphere be placed before the eye, and that the patient's attention be called to the set of lines on the chart. If most of the lines are clear, or even if one set is exceptionally clear, +0.25 D. spheres can be added in steps until that line starts to blur. If all of the lines are too blurred to detect a more distinct line, –0.25 D. steps can be applied until one set seems more distinct, although still slightly blurred. If all the lines appear equally blurred at the same time through either procedure, no astigmatism exists.

a. Hebbard also suggests beginning the subjective technique with the Skiametry findings in place where it is assumed that they are quite reliable. In such a case, a +0.75 D. sphere is placed over the skiametric correction, which should reduce the acuity to 20/25 or less. If it does not, more plus is required. Either a total clock dial or a rotating cross may be used in this technique, but if the rotating cross is used, it is aligned with the axes of the cylinders as found by retinoscopy. If a clock dial, attention is called only to those lines which coincide with or are 90° from the axis of the cylinder found by the retinoscope.

IV. DETERMINATION OF THE AXIS

A. After the proper stopping point for the unfogging procedure has been determined, according to any of the above methods, the patient is asked to determine whether any one single or group of lines appear in better focus than the others.

1. Where a rotary dial is used, the question need only refer to the two arms of the cross.

B. With Clock or Sunburst Dial

1. In high amounts of astigmatism, the better focused line will be confined to one or two spokes. In lower amounts of astigmatism, there may be a group of spokes which appear almost equally focused.

a. In such instances, the patient is asked to distinguish the blackest or most prominent of the group, or if this is impossible, to select the center spoke of the black or prominent group.

2. If one line can be selected, the axis of the correcting minus cylinder lies 90° from the meridian of the line.

a. A simple designation is that of indicating the spokes in concordance with the hours of a clock (if the spokes are 30° apart) such as 12 to 6 for the vertical spoke or 3 to 9 for the horizontal spoke. The smaller of the two numerals indicating the darker line is then multiplied by 30 to secure the axis of the correcting minus cylinder. For example, if the darker line were 2 to 8, the axis of the minus cylinder would be 60; if 5 to 11, the axis would be 150.

3. Since a gap of from 30 to 10° exists between spokes and since the actual astigmatic axis may lie between the spokes, the axis should be refined further before correction is attempted.

a. Usually the patient is asked to compare the relative blackness of the two spokes on either side of the one noticed as the blackest or center one. If both are equally black, the original spoke indicates the principal meridian. If one is blacker than the other, the principal meridian lies somewhat in the direction of the blacker of the two.

(1) For example, if 2 to 8 were the original blacker spoke, the patient would be asked to determine whether 1 to 7 or 3 to 9 were the blacker. If 3 to 9 were blacker than 1 to 7, the principal meridian lies between 2 to 8 and 3 to 9.

(2) Since 2 to 8 had been blacker than 3 to 9, the meridian lies closer to the position of 2 to 8. As the difference between them is 30°, and as they would have appeared equally black if the meridian had fallen exactly between them, it is probably about 10° from 2 to 8 in the direction of 3 to 9. The axis of the correcting cylinder would be placed in the 70th rather than the 60th meridian.

(3) The same procedure is employed for sunburst dials except that since the spokes are closer together, one of them is more likely to fall at the precise meridian position.

b. The V indicator, previously mentioned, is also used in conjunction with the sunburst or clock dial. The apex of the V is placed precisely on the darkest spoke and the patient asked to contrast the darkness of the two arms of the V. If both are equally black, the original spoke represents the principal meridian, but if one arm is darker than the other, the principal meridian lies between the original spoke and the darker arm.

4. If no spokes appear blacker or all seem equally blurred, no astigmatism is indicated.

C. Arrowhead Dials

1. If a previous concept of the axis exists from other tests, the cross is presented in the assumed meridians. If not, the cross is rotated until a contrast is found. (Note technique in previous section for Lebensohn and Raubitschek dials.) The line with the wings of the arrowhead is placed in the meridian in which it appears, the blacker of the two lines making up the cross. The wings of the arrowhead are compared for relative blackness. If equally black, the cross lies in the principal meridians. If one wing is blacker, the cross is rotated until the two wings are equal.

a. Pascal (1952) notes that if the chart is one in which the V of the arrowhead has its apex adjacent to the end of the line of the cross, the chart is rotated away from the black limb of the arrowhead, but if it is one which lies on either side of the line of the cross, as in the Lebensohn chart, the chart is rotated towards the blacker line. This might be simplified to include any eventuality by stating that where the apex of the arrow points towards the center of the chart, turn away from the blacker wing, and where the apex points towards the rim of the chart, turn towards the blacker wing.

D. With the Rotary Cross

1. The rotary cross is presented with the two arms in the approximate principal meridians. If one arm appears blacker than the other, the precise position of the principal meridian is checked in one of two ways.

a. The patient is directed to pick out the position in which the blacker line appears at its blackest while the operator slowly rotates the cross in both directions from the first position. The place at which it appears blackest indicates the principal meridian.

b. The operator rotates the cross until the patient reports that both arms seem equally black or clear. Since this can only occur, in the presence of astigmatism, when the arms are at equal distances to either side of the principal meridians, the principal meridians can be located at a point 45° from the position of either one of the arms, when reported equal.

(1) An additional clue is provided by those types of rotary crosses which have the arms made up of dashes or by the grid type of charts. When the lines of the cross or grid are not precisely on axis, the dashes will appear oriented at an angle to the direction of the line, or the intersections of the grid will appear in a step-like formation rather than perfectly continuous.

2. As with the other charts, when the arms of the cross or lines of the grid are placed in the principal meridians, the axis of the correcting cylinder is placed perpendicular to the meridian of the darkest arm or lines.

3. If over a –0.75 D. cylinder is needed, it may be advisable to add a +0.25 D. sphere for each –0.50 cylinder above that amount in order to keep the entire bundle of rays in the vitreous. Another method may be to add just enough plus before each addition of cylinder to keep the better line slightly blurred (Hebbard).

V. CORRECTING THE ASTIGMATISM

A. Once the principal meridians have been determined and the axis of the correcting minus cylinder located, the correction consists simply of increasing the power of the minus cylinder until the contrasted lines appear equally black.

1. *Sturm's interval* is collapsed in the direction of the posterior focal line with minus cylinder until coincidence with the circle of least confusion is reached.

B. Usually, the power of the cylinder is increased beyond that point until a reversal occurs, and the previously lighter lines now appear the blacker. This provides a range which indicates the patient's subjective acceptance of cylindrical correction. However, the weakest cylinder which actually equalizes the lines is noted as the correction, since the others may be merely the placement of one meridian behind the retina which permits accommodation to restore the astigmatic cone to the position of retinal interception of the circle of least confusion.

1. If increase of the cylinder does not produce a reversal point or if the original blacker lines reappear as blacker, the astigmatism may be irregular, and the weakest cylinder which equalizes the two most closely represents the correction.

C. Frequently, as the correction is increased towards the point of equality on the clock or other dials, the darkest lines shift to another position, or the steps of the grid or dash line cross reappear. This indicates that the axis is not precisely located, and the axis of the correcting cylinder must be altered to a new position. The shift of the lines in small amounts of astigmatism may be as much as 45°. If a change in power of the cylinder produces a shift in excess of that, or reverses the lines, then the amount added is too great.

1. If the shift is as much as 45°, a small rotation of the axis may restore the original dark lines. However, if such a rotation does not do so, it is advisable to shift the axis to a new position perpendicular to the new blackest lines.

D. Where the point of equality is approached, and the chart suddenly indicates the lines of both principal meridians as blacker than the lines of meridians in between, the astigmia is probably irregular.

E. Where reliance for the correction of astigmia is placed upon the tests described, the thorough practitioner usually uses both a clock or sundial and a rotary T or cross. The initial general positions of the principal meridians are located by means of the first and refined as much as possible. The cross or T is placed in the positions indicated by the clock dial, and the axis is further refined. The power is usually also determined on the cross or T.

1. Many practitioners also employ the retinoscopy findings instead of the clock dial in conjunction with the cross or T chart. The latter is placed in the meridional positions of the retinoscopy indication, with the working distance lens before the eye. The working distance is reduced until one arm appears black. The subsequent procedure for checking the axis and power described above is then followed. It must be repeated that if the retinoscopy employed plus cylinders, the total correction must first be transposed to one employing minus cylinders and the cylindrical element removed before the working distance is reduced.

a. If the retinoscopic technique that Hebbard mentioned is used, in which the retinoscopic correction with a fogging lens is employed with either a clock dial or with a cross, the patient's attention is called to comparison of the lines paralleling or at right angles to the astigmatic meridians. If the retinoscopic cylinder is correct, both these meridians will appear equal. If the lines parallel to the axis of the correcting cylinder are blacker, the cylinder lens has over-corrected the error. If the lines at right angles to the axis are more prominent, the cylinder lens is too weak.

(1) If both lines appear equally black, a –0.25 D. cylinder may be added to see if the line parallel to the axis of that cylinder becomes blacker. Or, the original cylinder may be reduced by 0.25 D. to see if the line perpendicular to the axis becomes blacker.

b. This technique assumes, of course, that the original axis found by the retinoscope is precise. If that axis is incorrect, the combination of oblique cylinders may present widely disparate lines as darker.

c. Carter (1966-67) comments that the axis error is significant only by virtue of the resultant power error which it produces. From his graph, the following approximate table of the relationship of induced power error and axis error is presented:

(1) **TABLE XIX-2.**

Correction Cylinder	Approximate Degrees of Axis Error Producing Indicated Power Error:		
	0.12 D.	**0.25 D.**	**0.50 D.**
0.50 D.	7	12	25
1.00	4	6+	12
2.00	2	4	8
3.00	1½	2½	5
4.00	1¼	2¼	4
5.00	1	2+	3½
6.00	¾	2	3

2. Whenever the power is determined on the T or cross chart, the patient finds it simpler because the confusion of the intermediate lines is removed. However, the shifts in the meridians mentioned earlier cannot be detected unless all meridians are checked with each change of power. Consequently, the most thorough procedure may utilize the clock dial for the determination of the position of fog and for the preliminary location of the principal meridians, the cross or T for precise location of the axis, and then the dial again for power.

VI. CHECKING CYLINDER UNDER FOG

A. The dial may be completely blurred by an increase of the fogging lens and the fog slowly reduced while the patient notes whether the various lines appear at the same time and with equal distinctness.

B. The T or cross chart may be presented with a crossed cylinder. This device consists of a lens of effective power of minus, 0.12, 0.25, 0.37, 0.50, or any selected power in one meridian, and an effective plus power of the same amount in the other. The common powers are –0.37 comb. +0.75, so that one meridian is effectively a –0.37 while the other at right angles is a +0.37. The handle is mounted at a position between the two meridians. By rotating the handle, the lens spins to present first the minus effect and then the plus effect in the same meridians. The crossed cylinder is placed so that the axis of the plus power coincides with the axis of the correcting cylinder, and the patient is directed to note the appearance of the T or cross. One arm should appear blacker. The device is now rotated so that the minus power axis coincides with the correcting cylinder axis. The lines perpendicular to those which previously appeared blacker should appear blacker now. If the reversal does not occur, but the lines appear more nearly equal when the minus axis coincides with the axis of the minus correcting cylinder, more power is needed; if they are more nearly equal when the plus axis coincides with the minus correcting cylinder axis, less power is needed.

C. Other methods of checking the correction are those employing the use of the crossed cylinders upon the letter chart, and that employing the use of the rotating cylinder upon a sunburst dial. These will be discussed in separate sections, since they require the determination of the spherical correction before their employment.

VII. DETERMINING THE SPHERE

A. Assuming that the astigmatism has been adequately corrected, the subjective procedure then requires the introduction of a letter test chart.

B. The fogging lens is then increased until the acuity is poorer than 20/60. The fog is slowly reduced until the 20/60 line can be read and its amount noted. Further reduction should improve the acuity until the best possible line can be read with the maximum plus or weakest minus lens. This lens represents the spherical element of the correction.

1. Approximately 1.00 D. should be required to bring the acuity from 20/60 to 20/20. If accommodation becomes active, the reduction will definitely exceed this amount, indicating action of the accommodation.

a. The actual amount cannot be limited to so precise a value because the aberrations of the eye do not permit selection of a fine focus but of the circle of least confusion. The hyperfocal curve, described in the chapter on acuity, may vary somewhat with each individual and present a change in the size of the circles which may not correspond to the changes in lens power. Thus, one lens may result in little change in blur circle size and the next so marked a change as to improve acuity by more than one line. Ordinarily, however, a change in lens power should produce a noticeable change in acuity, and where poor acuity appears stationary with successive changes, spasticity may be suspected.

2. Reduction beyond the lens which places the focus upon the retina will result ordinarily in the restoration of the focus to the retina by action of the accommodation. Since this does not refine the focus the acuity is not actually improved.

a. Some techniques call for the unfogging procedure to be halted when an arbitrary standard of acuity such as 20/20 is reached. Since the acuity represents the actual resolving power of the eye, and since addition of lenses which do not alter the actual size of the focal circles will not affect this resolving power, it cannot be predicated that the true refractive status of the eye has been ascertained by any lens short of that which permits the finest focus and discrimination permissible by the optics and anatomy of the particular eye under test. Stopping short of the maximum acuity attainable may serve a diagnostic purpose, but it does not determine the refractive status. Going beyond the point at which accommodation is not permitted to become active likewise does not determine the refractive status. Hence, the dictum: the maximum plus or least minus power which permits the maximum acuity possible for that eye.

3. The approximate sphere may be determined at this stage by procedures utilizing features of special equipment. The most available special device for determining the sphere at this stage are the Voerhoff circles found on the Robinson-Cohen slide.

a. These consist of two pairs of double circles, each double circle consisting of one circle within a larger circle. The width of the lines comprising the circles are of two different dimensions, one pair being of approximately 20/30 and the other pair of 20/60 acuity.

b. The duochrome filter permits one of a pair of equally sized circles to be presented upon a red background and the other upon a green background.

c. The patient reports when the reduction of plus power or fog permits both circles of the same size to be equally distinctive as seen in the two colors, or if equality is impossible, the circle in the green to be more distinct than that in the red.

4. Usually, if the cylinder is reasonably close to the proper amount and axis position, it will be found that the lens which permits the circles to appear equally black will also record normal or maximum vision.

VIII. CHECKING THE SPHERE (Monocular)

A. As discussed in the chapter on Visual Acuity, the ordinary test chart presents too great a step from one line to the next when the lines of smaller letters are reached. Consequently, a lens may actually make an improvement in acuity, but one that is insufficient to permit the patient to read the subsequent line. This is particularly true when the final sphere has been practically reached. The patient may read the 20/20 line without being able to read more than one or two letters of the 20/15 line. While a subsequent reduction in spherical power may be reported as making the letters blacker or the chart brighter, no further letters may be read. Since the danger of accommodative action is present and may make the letters appear more distinct by slightly reducing their size and concentrating the light in a smaller image, the average refractionist hesitates to accept such a report as truly indicative of better acuity. Even when the patient is enabled to read one or two additional letters, some hesitancy is required, since the pattern of improvement may not follow the range of visibility of the respective letters as determined and noted in the chapter on Visual Acuity. The patient may read a difficult letter in the next line, report that the next lens makes the line better, and then read a more visible letter while miscalling the one previously read.

1. The Clason Projector permits refinement of the spherical element of the prescription upon the basis of the best acuity for successive lens changes without other procedure.

a. The movable lens system of the instrument permits the same letter to be altered in size continuously within the limits of the ordinary chart's shift from one row or line to the next.

b. When the line of best acuity has been reached, the letters may be reduced in size until they are invisible and then increased to the bare limit of recognition. The position of the lens system can be noted.

c. With successive changes in lens power, the procedure is repeated – always from invisibility towards visibility, and the lens system position read from the indicator until the point is reached where further reduction of the fog does not result in recognition of a smaller projection of the letters. The maximum plus lens which permits the letter to be recognized at the irreducible size position represents the best sphere.

(1) Since the same row of letters is used, the line may be filtered by a selector so that only a few letters at a time are presented, or the same letters singly in varying order, to prevent memorization or mere familiarity influencing the result.

B. To determine the actual refractive status upon the basis of vision is actually to determine improvement by comparison on the patient's part of the relative blur of a set of letters at successive stages. This is particularly true when the critical point at which improvement no longer moves the vision to a successive line of test-types is reached. As Allen (1950) points out, Hofstetter found that to determine a blur on a given size letter might require as much as ± 1.00 D. addition on test letters and to determine one on the Verhoeff rings might require ± 0.50 D. (Fry). Consequently, more discriminating methods may be required for the final precise determination. Two such methods are the use of minimal illumination for letters of the same size and the duochrome or bichrome check test.

1. *Minimal Illumination*

a. In the chapter on Visual Acuity, mention is made of the technique of Ferree and Rand for evaluating acuity upon the basis of the relative intensity required to view a letter of minimum size. This principle may be utilized in checking the power of the sphere by first determining the best row of letters visible under ordinary illumination of the chart and halting at the point where further alteration of the sphere does not improve acuity to the next line.

b. At that point the gradations of letter size between the line read and the next smaller line may exceed the relative improvement which subsequent changes of lens power can produce. A different criterion, that of minimum visibility, is then introduced.

(1) The chart is dimmed until the line previously read is no longer readable. This may be done by closing the diaphragm or turning the rheostat.

(2) The illumination is increased from the point of invisibility to the point of first

visibility and the position of the diaphragm or rheostat is noted.

(3) The illumination is again decreased to invisibility and the lens power altered by one step.

(4) The reading of the diaphragm or rheostat is again noted when visibility is restored and compared to the reading of the previous lens.

(5) The procedure is repeated so long as a change in lens indicates visibility of the same row of letters with less illumination than the previous lens; the alteration of the intensity of illumination is always from invisibility to visibility.

(a) Luckiesh and Moss (1941 and 1942) in developing a device known as the Visibility Meter, which employs an absorption wedge, have found that with their device the visibility of a fixed target varies with variations from the proper or best refraction in either the direction of too much fog or too little fog. Since their apparatus operates under special conditions, the application of this determinant to ordinary testing conditions at the usual test distances cannot be predicated, but it seems appropriate to consider that the maximum plus or least minus which enables the patient to read a given line of letters under the lowest possible intensity of illumination represents the most precise estimate of the refractive status.

2. *Duochrome or Bichrome Refraction (Figure XIX-6)*

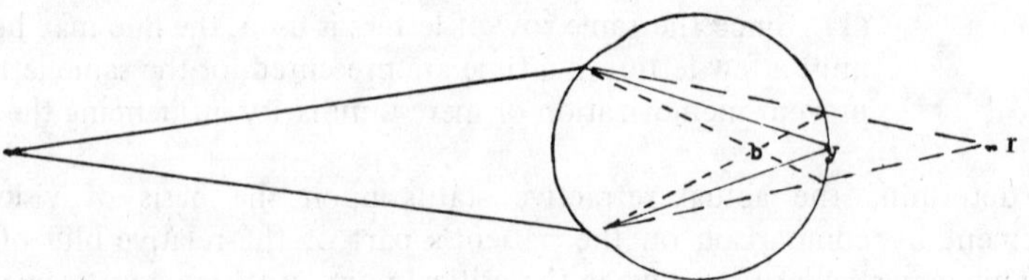

Figure XIX-6. Illustrating the chromatic aberration of the eye in relation to the duochrome test. *b* focus of blue rays; *y* focus of yellow rays; *r* focus of red rays. With *y* on the retina, the blur circles of *b* and *r* are equal. If *y* is moved forward by additional plus lens, the blur circle of *r* is smaller than that of *b*, as *b* is moved farther from the retina and *r* closer. If *y* is moved back of the retina by too little plus, the reverse holds true.

a. While the chromatic aberration of the eye has been recognized as a factor in caustic focus produced by spherical aberration, it is only comparatively recently that practical applications of this feature to the determination of the refractive status of the eye have been made. Since it has been fairly well established that the eye has its greatest sensibility to yellow light, it has been predicated that the average patient accepts as his position of maximum acuity that focus of the caustic which places the smallest yellow blur circle upon the retina (Pech, 1933). However, the difference in the size of the blur circles may be rather small, particularly if the eye has a long focal length. Consequently, when a test chart under white light is presented, the patient may accept the smallest blur circle of the first rays to impinge the retina, which under the fogging system would be those with the longest focal length, usually the red. At this stage, the letters of the line before the patient might be readable, although the habitual focus of the yellow light would still be before the retina.

(1) The average total range between the focus of the red and violet bundles is estimated to be 1.80 D. The range from red (of 5,790 to 8,000 A.U.) to yellow (of 5,460 to 5,790 A.U.) varies from a P.P. of –1.50 for the former to –0.25 for the

latter. From that yellow to green (of 4,458 A.U. to 5,790 A.U.), the variation is to a P.P. of the latter of + 1.50.

b. The range of the various chromatic foci introduces the possibility of physical or optical variations in accommodation which would greatly confuse the accepted principles of refraction. However, it appears that the average patient ordinarily selects one band, usually the yellow, as the criterion for normal or customary vision, and that variations in refraction are judged from the standpoint of the relative focus of that particular color.

(1) This assists in understanding the variations in amplitude of the presbyope and in acuity of the myope. The former may make his interpretation from the transference of the foci of one color to the next and appear to accommodate for different distances. The latter may be quite myopic for the yellow band, but still learn to select the red foci with a resulting increase in acuity. Subsequent changes in lens power may merely shift the various foci to his retina without activating accommodation or changing the acuity.

(2) However, the average patient who places the yellow focus upon his retina would find that the red or red-orange and the green or green-blue foci were almost equally out of focus. One would tend to focus as far back of the retina as the other would in front of it, or more accurately, each would cast blur circles of approximately equal size.

(3) While this principle could be used to determine the spherical refraction initially, it is ordinarily used in conjunction with the usual routines of refraction as a check upon the subjective response under white light and as a means of determining both the range of powers which provide approximately equal acuity and the lens which places the yellow focus upon the retina – this latter being assumed to be the precise refractive measurement of the eye.

c. The usual procedure employed is that of determining the most plus or least minus which enables the patient to read his best line under ordinary illumination. The chart is then illuminated so that identical letter charts side by side are presented, one seen or lit in green and the other in red light.

(1) The patient is requested to compare the two charts to determine whether the letters are clearer or blacker in one color than in the other.

(a) Usually, since the maximum fog for the line read is in effect, the red chart seems better, which indicates that the yellow focal plane is still in front of the retina.

(b) The plus power is consequently reduced until either the two charts appear equal or the next reduction of lens power makes the green chart better.

(c) If the fog has been reduced too greatly, the green chart will appear better. It is safer in such instances to add sufficient plus to make the red distinctly better and then reduce the plus until the point of equality is reached.

d. Davies (1957) tested a number of non-presbyopes and presbyopes for red/green preference, both on letters and symbols, uncorrected, and at various stages of the routine of correction.

(1) He found that one-half of the uncorrected hyperopes selected the red or equality, and 6% of the corrected hyperopes selected the green; 50% of corrected hyperopes selected the red, and the balance selected equality; 90% of the apparently corrected

hyperopes required a –0.25 D. lens to reach either equality or green preference. If the binocular balance had been conducted on black and white charts first, less alteration was needed in the bichrome test.

(2) Myopes showed an overwhelming red preference. Occasionally, some selected equality. Few selected the green. Monocularly, only 2.1% of corrected myopes, or 0.7% binocularly, preferred the green; 70.1% of the myopes monocularly, and 75.7% binocularly, were balanced by the addition of a ± 0.25 D. sphere, if they were not previously equal. Only one case needed as much as a –0.50 sphere and only 1.8% needed plus power. As with the hyperopes, if the balance had first been performed on black and white letters, fewer changes were required. Over-corrections of minus seldom exceeded 0.25 D., with a few reaching as much as 0.50 D.

(3) At near, usually the green or equality was found. The targets were seldom in the red. If the red was preferred, it indicated an over-correction of plus at near. Where the eyes differed, no correlation was found with either dominant eye or type of phoria.

(4) Davies drew the following conclusions:

(a) Monocularly, selection of the red or equality does not indicate the type of refractive state in the uncorrected eye. Green does indicate hyperopia.

(b) Binocularly, the color selected does not indicate the refractive state of the uncorrected eye.

(c) A hyperopic eye, preferring the green, is probably under-corrected. If it should prefer the red, it is not necessarily over-corrected.

(d) A myopic eye, preferring the green, is probably over-corrected, but if it prefers the red, it is not necessarily under-corrected.

(e) If a black and white equalization is performed to the best acuity, the red preference need not be significant.

(f) A preference for red at near is significant and indicates an over-correction of plus for near.

(5) He suggests the following places in the examination procedure to perform the red/green test:

(a) At the point of unaided vision. If it is better than 20/50, the green will indicate hyperopia.

(b) After equalization of the black and white targets. A preference for the red, if not equalized, should switch to the green with a –0.25 sphere.

(c) At the near point.

e. For proper effectivity, the brightness of the chart is required to be at a high test level and the surrounds at least moderately illuminated.

f. Causes of failure

(1) Mandell and Allen (1960) found that the intervals between the bichrome ranges of the major charts varied greatly. American Optical Co. charts presented an interval of 0.36 D., Bausch and Lomb charts, also 0.36 D., and the H. & L. charts, 0.50 D.

However, one AO chart differed in background from another with the green 1.58 times brighter than the red.

(2) Murrell (1955) found that the comparative brightness very often affected the results. He found the test much more accurate at 53 inches. Pascal notes that if the astigmatic interval is equal, less, or greater than the chromatic interval, the circle of least confusion is still placed at the middle of the yellow. An equivalent sphere which lies between the red and the green should be the desired objective.

3. *With Distant Cross Cylinder*

a. Schneller (1966) reports a technique for checking the validity of the sphere at distance with a cross cylinder. A dial of lines similar to a clock dial or a T chart is placed before the eye. The cross cylinder is placed with the axis 90 before the completed Rx.

(1) The patient is fogged, the plus is reduced, and the patient is requested to report whether *all* the lines appear clear at the same time or whether some lines appear clearer before others.

(2) If the vertical lines appear darker before the horizontal, the spherical plus power is reduced until the lines appear equal. If the horizontal lines appear darker, additional plus power is required.

(3) The technique assumes that astigmatism has been properly and completely corrected.

C. Other Factors Involving the Sphere

1. The final choice of the actual sphere depends upon the use the patient may desire to make of his correction, the exigencies of his work or habits, and the nature of his complaints. If the problem is entirely one of near work, fogging within the range of the check tests which still permits fairly good vision under white or normal intensity of light may be preferable. If he is required to have the keenest possible vision at far, it is best to leave him "in the green" or avoid the possibility of fogging.

2. Another factor involved in all the tests is that the usual test distance is rarely in excess of twenty feet and more commonly between ten and fifteen. At twenty feet, some 1/6 D. of accommodation may still be wanted. At fifteen feet almost 0.25 D. is required. Forcing the plus to the maximum may result in apparently perfect placement of the focus at the test distance due to the negative relative accommodation elicited for this small amount of required accommodation. When the patient restores his attention to objects at a greater distance, as he habitually does, he may become conscious of the slight blur which the extra plus, due to the NRA, provokes. Consequently, where it is desired to provide the maximum acuity at far, the best correction can advisably be reduced slightly, or if bichrome testing is used, the patient had best be left slightly "in the green" rather than balanced.

a. Since actual optical infinity is unattainable, the distance of 6 meters has been widely accepted as the ideal test distance, partly because such a distance is probably the maximum within the economic potentiality of test room construction, partly because its dioptric value is close to the minimal lens equivalent of 0.12 Diopter, and partly because Snellen and others deriving acuity charts utilized that distance as the numerator distance for the acuity fraction. Hofstetter had long pointed out that with the use of modern projectors which can present the test letters in reduced version of the standard test letter sized chart for whatever distance of projection is chosen, the use of 6 meters (or 20 feet) is irrational. Twenty feet is not actually synonymous with 6 meters, but even more 1/6 diopter value cannot be compensated for, – 1/8 diopter is insufficient, and 1/4 diopter too great. On the other hand, use of a test distance of 4 meters or 13 feet finds a much closer match for feet and meters, and also computes to an exact overcorrection of .25 diopters, which can be readily and automatically allowed in the final correction. The use of a four meter test distance makes more sense from both its precise optical value, therefore, and the exigencies of space utilization.

IX. CHECKING CYLINDER WITH CORRECT SPHERE

A. Acuity Method

1. With the correct sphere in place and the attention directed to the best lines, the cylinder may be rotated slightly to either side and an attempt made to determine the position of best acuity. This is fairly good in higher powered astigmatism but not very easily determined in low powers.

2. The power of the cylinder may be increased or decreased upon the same basis. Since such a change will vary the location of the circle of least confusion, the sphere should be altered to half the amount of the cylinder in the opposite manner so that the same spherical equivalent is maintained and the circle is kept on the retina. As the cylinder is increased by –0.50 D., for example, increasing the sphere by +0.25 D. will keep the circle at the same position. This permits judgment of the acuity based upon the actual size of the focal circle rather than upon marked change in both size and position.

3. Posner (1951) recommends a method of checking the axis of the cylinder based upon the fact that if the head is tilted, the corresponding torsion of the eye lags from 4 to 16° behind the tilt. Placing the correction with the cylinder in the trial frame, the patient is required to tilt the head some 30° to both sides. If acuity is better with the head tilted in one direction than the other, the axis of the cylinder is moved towards the better direction and the test repeated until equal vision results. The method is also indicative in cases of habitual head tilting, checking the finished correction, and determining a change in axis for near vision. Walton (1951) also comments that a cylinder off axis will affect vision more than torting the head ordinarily will; therefore, the Posner test may be considered quite indicative.

B. The Rotating Cylinder Method

1. Linksz (1942) describes a method of checking the cylinder for axis and amount by rotating the correcting cylinder. The method is based upon the principle that if two cylinders are placed so that their axes do not coincide, a set of resultants is produced which creates both new spherical and cylindrical powers and axes. If the powers of the two cylinders are not equal, the position of the axis of the new cylinder is correspondingly influenced.

2. The astigmatic state of the eye may be considered one cylinder and the correction cylinder of the eye the other, and the combinations of the two developed by geometric optics. The cylinder of the eye must be considered opposite in power to that of the correction.

a. When two equal cylinders of opposite sign are combined at oblique axes, the axis of the resultant cylinder lies not between them, but at a point 45° from the meridian between them.

3. By geometric optics, it is possible to determine the resultant sphero-cylinders of two equal or unequal cylinders with their axes placed at varying meridians from each other. The results of these calculations may be summarized as follows:

a. A combination of two cylinders with the axes not in coincidence results in a new astigmatic state consisting of a sphere of one sign and a cylinder of the opposite.

b. The larger the difference between the axis of the eye and the axis of the correcting cylinder, the larger the power of the resultant astigmatism.

(1) If the two cylinders are *equal* in power, a difference between their axes will produce a difference in power as follows:

(a) A difference of 30° will produce a resultant cylindrical equal to the originals.

(b) A difference of 15° will produce a resultant cylinder equal to one half the original.

(c) A difference of 5° will produce an error equal to 17% of the original astigmatism.

(2) If the correcting cylinder is too strong or too weak, it will still produce a new cylinder in proportion to the difference in axis but a smaller error of axis will be required.

c. The *smaller* the difference in axis, the *farther displaced* the axis of the induced resultant astigmatism from the axis of the eye's astigmatism.

(1) If the two cylinders are equal in power or if the correcting one is slightly stronger, as the correction cylinder is moved farther from the eye axis, the resultant cylinder moves closer to the eye axis but at only half the rate of progression.

(2) If the correcting cylinder is much stronger or weaker to any amount, the correcting cylinder must be moved a larger amount from the true position to induce a noticeable change in the resultant axis.

(3) The closer the power of the cylinder correcting the eye to the astigmatism of the eye, the more efficiently this procedure can be performed.

4. From the above it can be seen that if the correcting cylinder is placed slightly off axis, a resultant cylinder appears at approximately 45° from the midpoint of the ocular and correcting cylinders.

a. As the cylinder is rotated even farther from the ocular astigmatic axis, the resultant cylinder axis moves closer to the true astigmatic axis position.

5. *Checking the Axis*

a. The technique employs the Lancaster and Regan sunburst dial which has spokes spaced at 10° intervals. The patient is fogged approximately 0.25 D. to compensate for the minus power of the spherical-cylindrical combination which will result.

(1) Using a minus cylinder, the cylinder is rotated about the axis position. As the cylinder is placed before the eye, the patient is requested to report whether the lines are equal or whether some of them are blacker.

(2) If the cylinder is placed *precisely on axis,* the chart will appear as follows:

(a) If the cylinder power is correct, no black lines will appear outstanding.

(b) If the cylinder power is *stronger* than it should be, the lines on the chart which *parallel* the minus cylinder axis will be blacker.

(c) If the cylinder is too *weak,* the lines *perpendicular* to the axis of the minus correcting cylinder will appear blacker.

b. Linksz recommends that a power of cylinder be used either equal to or slightly stronger than the ocular astigmatism.

(1) If this cylinder is placed off-axis, a resultant cylinder with its axis on the opposite side of the ocular axis will be formed. The black lines will appear on the same side of the ocular axis as the displaced correcting cylinder.

(a) If a correcting cylinder is placed at 170 when the ocular cylinder is at 180, the resultant axis will be at 40, and the black lines at 130.

(2) If the cylinder is rotated farther away from the ocular axis, the resultant axis will move closer to the ocular axis, and the black lines will move in the same direction as the displacement of the correcting cylinder axis. If the cylinder is moved towards the ocular axis, the movements of the resultant axis and black lines will be opposite to that just described.

(a) If the correcting cylinder is now moved to 160, the resultant will have its axis at 35, and the black lines appear at 125.

(3) If the cylinder axis is moved *past the position of the true axis,* to the opposite side, the resultant axis will jump to the opposite side from its former position and the black lines will appear to also jump almost 90° away.

(a) If the cylinder axis in the above case is moved to meridian 10, the resultant axis will now be at 140, and the black lines at 50.

(4) Thus, the above illustration shows a swing of black lines from meridian 125, to 130, to 50, as the axis of the correcting cylinder is moved from 160 to 170 and past the true axis of 180 to 10.

(5) By repeating the procedure from both directions, the point at which the jump occurs can be narrowly delineated and the true axis determined.

c. When rotation of a cylinder does not produce this large jump of the black lines on the sunburst dial, the true axis has not been passed.

6. *Checking the Power*

a. The power is checked very simply once the axis has been located. The correcting cylinder is shifted 5° off the axis and the patient is asked to designate the position of the blackest lines.

(1) If the blackest lines appear close to the axis position of the cylinder, the cylinder is too strong.

(2) If the blackest lines appear closer to the perpendicular to the cylinder axis, the power is too weak.

(3) If the blackest lines appear about 45° from the cylinder axis position, the power is correct.

C. The Jackson Cross Cylinder

1. The Jackson (1932) Cross Cylinder technique is basically the same as that of the rotating cylinder insofar as the optical effects are concerned. Although recommended for the determination of astigmatism, it is also chiefly used as a check test for the astigmatic axis and power. Tour comments that the cross cylinder moves the focal lines in opposite directions in contrast to the fogging technique, which moves the entire interval of Sturm in the same direction, from ahead of the retina back to the retina.

2. The difference in principle is that the resultant cylinder due to two cylinders off axes, mentioned above, is further contrasted against a third sphero-cylindrical combination, the cross cylinders, which combinations produce another resultant which exaggerates the distortions even more.

a. If the cylinder is off the correct power and on the correct axis, the addition of the cross cylinders will produce a simple sphero-cylindrical combination which will combine with a spherical combination.

(1) If the eye is perfectly corrected, the addition of a +0.50 : –0.50 cross cylinder will merely make first one meridian hyperopic and the other myopic, and then will reverse the effects of the two. In either case, the circle of least confusion will be on the retina and the same size.

(2) If the patient is asked to read type, the type should look the same with the cross cylinders in any position.

b. If the correcting cylinder and ocular cylinder are the same power but are off axes, then a resultant sphero-cylindrical combination is set up at approximately 45° from the original axis.

(1) The new combination has a sphere of one sign and a cylinder of the opposite.

(a) Pascal (1950) notes that the power of the new meridian corresponding to the axis of a properly powered cylinder placed off axis is located at $\frac{90 + a}{2}$ degrees from the position of the cylinder axis, where a is the number of degrees from the true cylinder axis. That is, if a cylinder is placed 10° off the true axis, the resultant axis of like power is located $\frac{90 + 10}{2}$ or 50 ° from the misplaced cylinder axis on the opposite side of the true axis. If the true axis were at 80°, the cylinder would be at 70°, and the resultant at 120°. The opposite power is placed 90 – 50, or 40° from the misplaced axis, or at 30°.

(2) If the cross cylinder is placed obliquely to the axis of the assumed correcting cylinder, in one position the minus power of the cross cylinder will coincide with the minus power of the resultant combination of correcting lens and eye, while the plus power of the C.C. coincides with the plus power. This will produce even greater distortion of the blur circle. In another position, the plus of the C.C. will coincide with the minus of the resultant, while the minus of the C.C. coincides with the plus of the resultant, and a more uniform blur circle will result.

(a) If a patient has an astigmatism of 1.00 D. axis 90 and a correcting cylinder is placed at axis 75, a new resultant of +0.26 comb. –0.52 ax 37.5 is formed.

(b) If a –.50:+.50 cylinder is placed so that it is bisected by the assumed axis, one meridian will be at 30 and the other at 120.

(c) In one position, a new resultant of +0.75 comb. –1.50 axis 32.5 will be formed, while in the other a new resultant of +0.26 comb. –0.52 ax 112.5 will be formed. The latter will appear the better, and the axis of the correction cylinder will be moved towards the 120 meridian or from the erroneous position of 75 towards the correct one of 90.

3. *Technique for Axis*

a. In accordance with the above explanation, it can be seen that the comparison is one of distortion and blur, and consequently test letters are used. While various lines are recommended, a line slightly larger than the one the patient read at best is ordinarily recommended because of the potentially extreme resultants which might arise.

b. The C.C. is placed so that the two meridians of power are bisected by the axis of the correcting cylinder.

(1) In most apparatus, the handles are placed in this position, while the axis of the plus power is indicated by white dots, and that of the minus power by red dots.

c. The C.C. is rotated so that the meridian of plus power is now where the minus was and the minus where the plus was.

(1) If the correcting cylinder is at 90, the C.C. is first presented with the white dots at 45 and the red at 135; and then, the white at 135 and the red at 45.

d. The patient is asked to select the position of best acuity.

e. If one position is preferred, the axis of the minus correcting cylinder is then placed 5° closer to the meridian in which the red dots were in the preferable position. The C.C. is realigned so that the new axis position bisects it and the test repeated until a position of the correcting cylinder is found at which no preference is shown for either position of the C.C.

(1) If the above patient preferred the C.C. with the red dots at 135, the correcting cylinder would be moved to axis 95. The C.C. would be aligned so that one meridian was in the 140th and the other in the 50th. If repeating the test found the patient preferring the red dots at 140, the axis of the correcting cylinder would be moved to 100; if the patient preferred the red dots at 50, the axis would be moved half-way between its previous position at 90 and its present position at 95 to 92.5.

(a) If plus cylinders are used, the white dots of the C.C. serve as the guide.

4. *Technique for Power*

a. If the axis has been correctly located, the power can be checked very readily. The handle is shifted 45° so that the power of the C.C. now lies in the axis and perpendicular to the axis of the cylinder. The red dots will lie in the meridian of the axis, for example, and the white dots will lie at right angles.

b. The handle is rotated and the position of the dots is reversed. The patient is asked to determine, by viewing the test type, which position seems preferable.

c. If the preferable position is that in which the red dots coincided with the axis of the minus cylinder (or the white dots coincide with the axis of a plus cylinder), the power of the cylinder is increased and the test repeated. If the preferable position is the opposite, then the power is reduced.

5. It is obvious that the flipping of the cross cylinder merely lengthens or shortens the interval of Sturm. When the plus power of the C.C. coincides with the stronger plus meridian of the eye, and

the minus power of the C.C. with the weaker ocular meridian, the interval is lengthened; when the plus of the C.C. coincides with the weaker ocular meridian, while the minus coincides with the stronger, the interval is shortened.

a. If the cylindrical correction were –1.00 D. ax 90, then with a C.C. which was effectively –0.50 D. in one meridian and +0.50 D. in the other, the following resultants would obtain:

(1) When the minus power coincided with the ocular correction, the resultant would be +0.50 comb. –1.50 D.

(2) When the plus power coincided with the ocular cylinder, the resultant would be –0.50 sphere.

b. The comparison is then between either a circle, an oval, or two ovals, depending on the relative strengths of the astigmia and the C.C. In some instances, the comparison may be between two ovals with their axes at different angles, if the addition of the C.C. reverses the axis of astigmatism. When the cross cylinder test is performed under any amount of fog, both meridians of the eye are focused in front of the retina (although one may be on the retina and one in front in some cases), and the effect of the cross cylinder is likely to be that described. If, however, the cross cylinder test is performed when the circle of least confusion were on the retina, then the lengthening of the interval of Sturm would merely increase the size of the circle of least confusion while shortening it would decrease the size of that circle. Instead of a comparison of images composed of different types or sizes of ovals, the comparison would be of images composed of different sized blur circles (Pascal, 1940a and 1941). This position has been titled by Pascal (1950a) as the *position of meridional balance.* If additional cylindrical correction is either added or subtracted to the original correction during the C.C. test, the circle of least confusion is shifted from the retina, and the position of meridional balance is lost. Thus, in order to properly maintain this position during the test, it is necessary that a *spherical equivalent* be introduced for each change in power of the cylinder. This equivalent, established by Copeland, is merely the addition of a sphere of opposite sign and one-half the power of the cylinder added to the correction.

(1) Lindsay (1958) calculated the area of blur on the retina and found the range around the correct sphere beyond which conflicting answers will be given. The optimum sphere holds the circle of least confusion on the retina, but it is equally as dangerous to greatly under-correct as it is to over-correct during the technique.

(2) In a technique titled, *Meridional Balance Technique,* Pascal (1950a) utilized correcting cylinders in the form of cross cylinders. Thus, the proper position was maintained automatically. He recommended that the position of balance be established by the stronger plus sphere or weakest minus sphere which gave best acuity or by the spherical equivalent of the retinoscopy finding. The position may also be ascertained by the use of the duochrome test (Williamson-Noble, 1946). Coole (1952) also used a monochromatic background and Verhoeff circles to control the accommodation for the cross cylinder test. When the position of balance was found, the C.C. also was used to determine the *presence* of astigmatism where doubtful, as well as the power and position of a known astigmatism. The technique is described under Trial Case Accessories later in this chapter.

c. Williamson-Noble (1946) showed that the C.C. test performed *under fog* would result in images which emphasized the vertical or horizontal components of letters so that readability or interpretation was better possible even with greater distortions of the blur circles. Patients under fog viewing letters whose cognoscibility depended upon vertical strokes usually accepted a too great cylinder against-the-rule. His photographs indicated that the patient too much under-corrected in plus would likewise accept a too strong cylinder with-the-rule.

However, this latter ignored the dynamics of accommodation. The under-corrected patient was more likely to accommodate to place the circle of least confusion upon the retina, as was usually found in cases of moderate hyperopic astigmia. Hence, Copeland recommended that the C.C. test be performed with the patient "slightly in the minus," or just a step more than the criterion set by Pascal. Copeland's recommendation permitted the patient to choose the spherical equivalent of whatever sphero-cylindrical combination may have been determined before the C.C. test was applied. By either using the correction C.C. of Pascal or adding the appropriate sphere with each cylinder, the status was maintained during the test by the patient by utilization of his accommodation.

6. *C.C. and Line Chart (Reversal Test) (Pascal, 1952a)*

a. The astigmatic power may also be tested upon a line cross astigmatic dial, astigmatic T, or similar chart affording lines in the two principal meridians. The chart is presented so that one line of the cross or T is on the assumed axis. In contrast to the test with letters, the patient should be slightly fogged. The C.C. is placed as in the test for power with letters, and the relative blackness of each of the lines of the cross on the chart compared as the C.C. is flipped. If the power is correct, the line coinciding with the minus axis of the C.C. will appear blacker in each position. If the power is incorrect, the lines will appear approximately equal in one position, reversed from the above, or the extent of blackness will not be the same in both C.C. positions. Minus cylinder, with its axis coinciding with the minus axis of the C.C. when in the position where the coinciding line is not as black, is added to the correction.

(1) Whereas in testing with letters, Pascal recommended that the power of the C.C. should approximate that of the correction cylinder, in this test it was recommended that a weak C.C. should be used, not exceeding a ± 0.25 D. combination with a –0.12 sphere combined with a + 0.25 cylinder preferable.

b. The axis of the cylinder may also be checked by the C.C. and a line of a T chart *(Crisp-Stine Test).* A chart containing a cross with a marker at the intermediate position is aligned so that the marker coincides with the cylinder axis. The cross cylinder is placed as in the usual C.C. test for axis and rotated about this marker. The two lines composing the cross are compared for relative blackness. If the lines are not equal, the correction cylinder is moved towards the position of the cross cylinder axis which coincides with the nature of the power of the correction cylinder (a minus cylinder towards the minus axis of the cross cylinder or a plus cylinder towards the plus axis of the cross cylinder). For each move of the correction cylinder, the target chart is repositioned to the same degree. The Lebensohn arrow chart may also be used for this test. This is continued until both lines appear approximately alike.

(1) 0.04 D. of cylinder difference is manifested by a .25 D. cylinder placed 5° off axis, but patients are unable to tell the difference. The patient may call one of the lines "doubled" instead of blurred.

7. *Differences Between the Cross Cylinder Technique And Others*

a. In many instances, a variation is found between the cylinder determined by line chart or clock dial methods by rotating the cylinder and by the C.C. In the latter two, although the optics of both are concerned with combinations of oblique cylinders, it must be noted that one depends upon a sudden contrast of two blurs at approximately equal positions of arc, while the other depends upon a comparison of the best vision at one position with worsening vision, gradually introduced, up to a limit in either direction (Pascal, 1952). Some patients may be able to make a more accurate judgment in one procedure than the other, although the consensus seems to indicate that the sudden contrast (C.C.) is generally easier for determination. Likewise, the clock dial procedure depends upon the sensitivity and perceptiveness of the patient, particularly in small errors, and the degree of fog, while the C.C. depends upon relative interpretation by the patient while preferably under no fog (Pascal, 1940). Williamson-Noble (1946) believed that the C.C. test is the more reliable of the two when variation exists.

b. *Causes of error* (Borish, 1946 and 1960; Allen, 1959; Carter, 1966).

(1) Failure to fog to the circle of least confusion or achievement of the wrong spherical equivalent.

(2) Failure to keep the circle of least confusion on the retina by altering the sphere one-half of the power of the cylinder addition.

(3) Failure to explain to the patient that neither position is clear but to choose the clearer of two blurred positions.

(4) Speed of flipping may be wrong.

(5) Failure to allow time for accommodation to hold the circle of least confusion on the retina.

(6) Failure of communication.

(a) Identifying the wrong position, if flipped too fast, as first or second or this one or that one.

(b) Misinterpretation of "better as" as meaning squarer or blacker instead of clearer or more legible.

c. *Precautions are as follows:*

(1) Never work with the eye fogged.

(2) Be sure that the working cylinder (of the cross-cylinder) is not stronger than the correction cylinder.

(a) If close to correct, and the working cylinder is the same as the correction cylinder, a weaker cross cylinder should be used.

[1] This is also the best arrangement for conditions when the axis of the correcting cylinder is close to the true axis.

(b) If uncertain, and the working cylinder should be weaker than the correction cylinder, a stronger cross cylinder should be used.

[1] This is the better arrangement for conditions in which the axis of the correcting cylinder may be far from the true axis.

(c) If the working cylinder is weaker than the correction cylinder, alter the sphere to maintain the spherical equivalent as explained above.

[1] Reduce the minus spherical power or increase the plus spherical power by one-half the increase in minus cylindrical power.

(3) After finding the Rx, refine with the full working cylinder in place and with a low-powered cross cylinder.

(4) If a low cylinder is 90° off, the cross cylinder will verify the axis. Therefore check at 10° positions to each side to prove the axis.

(5) Errors may be caused by:

(a) Faults in the spherical equivalent before the eye.
(b) Excess of correction cylinder in relation to the working cylinder power.
(c) Extreme errors in position of the working cylinder axis.

d. Haynes (1957 and 1958) postulated that the scissors effect, observed in cross cylinder testing, was due to the fact that magnifications in one meridian of the cross cylinder varied from that of the other. The scissors effect, or the rotary deviation, varies as a function of the meridional angle of magnification. The differential rotary deviation, the differential meridional magnification, and the focal line effects decrease the sensitivity of the cross cylinder test. Hayes noted that two rotatable lenses were needed to avoid the presentation of one wrong face of the lens towards the patient when the cross cylinder is flipped.

8. *Methods To Help Avoid Error*

a. Besides the mentioned precautions concerning the mislocation of the circle of least confusion and the other potential errors, the chief problems seem to be in the choice of targets and misinterpretations by the patient and the examiner of "better" or "worse."

(1) Freeman (1955) used the Bichrome and the Landolt C just above the size of best acuity. He first unfogged on the red/green to the best acuity, added a –0.25 D. sphere for placing the circle of least confusion in proper position, and then employed the cross cylinders on the Landolt C's.

(a) The Landolt C will show a different appearance of the gap when the ellipse is either parallel to the axis or at right angles to the axis, but oblique positions may not show a clearly defined choice.

(2) Haynes (1958) recommended using a cross (similar to the Crisp-Stine test) as a target to eliminate the obvious magnification and related phenomena. Haynes (1957) also designed a *homokonic cross cylinder* which gave equal meridional magnification to further equalize the positions of the cross cylinder and the target's relation to it. This cross cylinder is not available for general use.

b. The author uses a technique similar to that previously used by Warman (1950) and Freeman (1954).

(1) Since one of the chief problems of the cross cylinder test is the fact that some aspect of memory is involved in the comparison, no matter how quickly the cross cylinder is flipped, a seen target is always compared to a recalled one. The use of letters of different acuity and the use of a legibility criterion instead of remembering if one letter, or line, or symbol looked better or not, helps eliminate some of the misjudgment resulting from this aspect. The author has used the following technique:

(a) First establish the best acuity with spheres only.

(b) Reduce the fog by –0.25 D. to be sure of the position of the circle of least confusion.

[1] If the patient is presbyopic, one should be careful not to err in the opposite direction by moving the circle of least confusion too far behind the retina.

(c) Direct the patient to exposed lines of the chart ranging in acuity from 20/50 to 20/15.

(d) Explain to the patient that he will see two blurred charts, but request him to indicate which is the better position by noting *which position of the C.C. allows him to read farther down the chart.*

[1] If in doubt, have the patient read the chart out loud in each position. The examiner may then judge which position is the best.

[2] Use *the actual legibility* of the various letters rather than blacker, clearer, or squarer, which may otherwise be the patient's criterion.

(e) If the results seem to vary irregularly from other cylinder indications, the circle of least confusion is probably not placed in the right relation to the retina. The starting sphere should then be varied by either adding slightly more minus or, if presbyopic, slightly more plus.

(f) For each position of the cross cylinder, wait for the best acuity to be revealed. If the patient is accommodating to put the circle of least confusion on the retina and accommodation slips, or the flip is too rapid, the circle may be off the retina in one position of the cross cylinder.

c. Simultaneous observation

(1) The obvious solution to the memory problem is the presentation of both aspects of the target at the same time. If the target, as seen through both cross cylinder positions, could be seen simultaneously, not only would memory be eliminated, but the nature of the target would no longer be so important. The following two modern developments have attempted this:

(2) *Matsuura Auto-cross* (available from Tobayo Optical Co. Ltd.).

(a) The device somewhat resembles a pair of opera glasses. Each cell contains power and axis refining controls.

[1] Behind these is a doubling device which creates monocular diplopia.

[2] A prong device engages the cylinder mechanism of the refractor, maintaining, automatically, a consistent relationship to the cylinder axis, so that the need to separately shift the device and working cylinder is eliminated.

(b) *Technique for axis*

[1] The dial is set to the axis indicator and the two side-by-side images are compared.

[a] If the right image is clearer, the cylinder and the device are rotated towards the position indicated on the right cell by an indicator. If the left is clearer, the rotation is toward the position on the left cell.

[b] When both images are equally distinct, the axis is correct.

(c) *Technique for power*

[1] The dials are set to the power indicator.

[a] If the right cell is clearer, minus cylinder is reduced. If the left cell is clearer, minus cylinder power is increased.

[b] When both cells or images are equal, the power is correct.

(d) The chief criticism of this device is that the prisms present the two targets at so great a separation that actually the eye moves from one to the other to fixate and compare rather than seeing them simultaneously.

(3) *The Simultans of Biessels* (available through Zeiss Distributors) (Figures XIX-7 and 8)

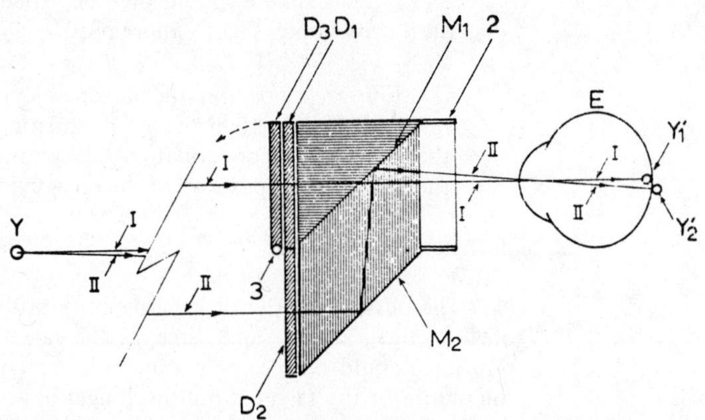

Figure XIX-7 – Simultans Optics (see text)

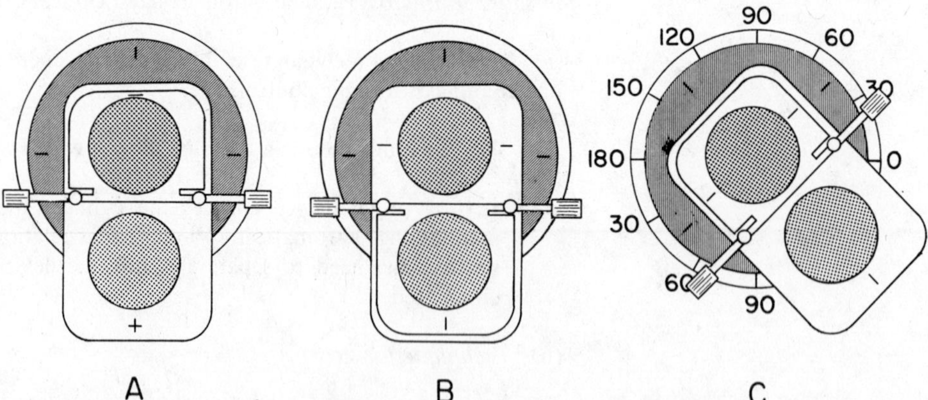

Figure XIX-8. A = Simultans with flip lens up to create a plus and minus sphere. B = Simultans with flip lens down to create two oppositely placed cross cylinders of equal power. C = Simultans oblique for test for axis for correcting cylinder at 90 or 180.

(a) As with the Matsuura Auto-Cross, this device attempts to eliminate the aspect of comparison by presenting the targets simultaneously. Also, since the last stages of visual acuity are non-linear, in comparison to linear changes of lenses before the eyes in 0.25 D. steps, simultaneous comparisons give a better criterion.

(b) Most systems using a biprism system still separate the images sufficiently so that the eye must move through a separating zone which requires memory for comparisons as if the images were successively fixed. Normally, the angle between these might be equivalent to 10 prism diopters. For true simultaneous comparison, it would be desirable to have the images contiguous.

(c) The Simultans test consists of a device in which reflecting prisms or mirrors are arranged so that two apertures present targets almost contiguously upon the retina. Seen from the front, the device again resembles a binocular, but as the illustration (Figure XIX-7) shows, the contruction attempts to avoid the separation usual in prismatic devices. Beam 1 passes through lenses D_1 and D_3, which, when combined, yield a +0.25 D. lens, and directly through a mirror M_1 to the pupil. Beam 2 passes through a lens, D_2, which has a dioptric power of –0.25 D., strikes a mirror M_2, is reflected from that mirror back to M_1 and is reflected at a slightly different angle from that which Beam 1 makes in passing through it. Both images, therefore, are in the same field of view without a dividing line. Sharpness of equal size blur circles can be compared if the eye is corrected to an emmetropic equivalent. If not, the images will be shifted towards positions in front of or behind the retina so that one image will be closer to retinal focus than the other. Figure XIX-7 illustrates these principles.

(d) Since both images strike the retina simultaneously and almost contiguously, the stimulus to accommodation is static. Actually, there is a prismatic difference of about 2/3 of a PD, and the fields slightly overlap; but since a target upon a common background is used, the backgrounds overlap and fuse, and only the targets are compared.

[1] To be compared simultaneously, the targets should fall on the central area within a 2/3 prism diopter angle or occupy an area on the retina which a 4 cm. object at 6 M. away, or a 2 mm. target at the reading distance would occupy. Such a placement of the images will scarcely require any movement of the visual axis for comparison.

(e) Biessels (1967) claimed that the spherical test alone has certain advantages in comparison to the bichrome test.

[1] Since the same color was used, any preference for red or accommodation for red was eliminated.

[2] The device can be built for any dioptric difference, even for low acuities.

[3] Accommodation is held more constant since double images appear as a combined single image. For example, two o's appear to form a figure 8. Since one portion of the 8 is in front of the retina, and the other behind it, accommodation tends to be held static.

(f) The complete device today employs a reflecting prism surface at the M_1 position instead of a mirror. In addition to the stationary lenses in the upper and lower apertures, a lens is provided so that it can be combined with either one of the stationary lenses by being flipped before one cell or the other. With the flip lens in the up position covering the top lens cell, a +0.25 D. sphere is formed leaving a –0.25 D. sphere in the lower lens cell. If the flip lens is combined with the lower lens cell, a cross cylinder with a minus axis at 180 degrees is created. In this position, the opposite lens cell exhibits a cross cylinder with a minus axis at 90 degrees. The actual power of the three lenses is as follows: D_1 is actually a +0.25 sphere combined with a –0.50 cylinder axis 90 degrees; D_2 is actually a –0.25 sphere; and D_3, which is flippable, consists of a +0.50 cylinder axis 90 degrees. When placed in front of D_1, it forms a +0.25 sphere. When placed in front of D_2, a cross cylinder of +0.25 –0.50 axis 180 is formed.

(g) The optical construction of the Simultans is such that the patient sees the lower image through the upper lens system and the upper one through the lower lens system. The markings on the instrument are so arranged as to compensate for this, so that the + and – signs before the apertures correspond to the position of the image seen by the patient and the lines indicating the minus axis positions of the cross cylinders are also marked according to whether the patient sees the upper or lower image, and not to the lens systems within that aperture.

(h) *Test for power* (Figure XIX-8 B)

[1] The Simultans device, with the cells exhibiting cylinder powers (flip lens down), is fixed in the aperture cell, and the axis mark of the upper aperture is aligned with the cylinder axis of the refractor. If the upper image is clearer, minus cylinder is added. If the lower is clearer, it is deducted.

(i) *Test for axis* (Figure XIX-8 C)

[1] The marker on the upper aperture is placed 45° from the axis of the cylinder axis as shown on the refractor cell (click position).

[2] If one image is clearer, the position of that image is noted. For example, upper-left, or lower-left, or however the device is placed.

[3] The aperture of the Simultans that corresponds to that position will, by its axis mark, indicate the position towards which the axis of the correcting cylinder is to be rotated. Since both the Simultans and the cylinder in the refractor will rotate together, all that needs be done is to rotate until the patient reports both images equally clear.

(j) *Test for spherical balance* (Figure XIX-8 A)

[1] If D_3 is now flipped into the up position, as previously described, a +0.25 D. and –0.25 D. power is the resultant in each of the cells. The targets can now be viewed as to which is brighter, and if the one seen through the +0.25 D. is brighter, a +0.25 D. is added to the correction. If the image seen through the cell containing the –0.25 D. seems to be the brighter, a –0.25 D. can be added to the correction. However, as in the bichrome test, the patient may accommodate 0.25 D. in order to balance the images. So after completion of the test, Biessels recommended that, without the Simultans, the patient be fogged and unfogged to the line of best acuity.

(k) *Test sequence*

[1] The test should be run in the following order: sphere, cylinder axis, and cylinder power.

X. EQUALIZING

A. After the subjective has been completed upon one eye, the procedure is repeated upon the other. At the conclusion of these monocular tests, it is well to attempt to equalize the clarity of vision.

1. This is due to the fact that a different state of relaxation of accommodation might have prevailed while one eye was under test than when the other was being tested.

   a. It should be emphasized that equalization actually applies to the status of the accommodation rather than to the visual acuity.

2. In most cases the acuity of each eye will be approximately the same. However, in frequent instances, the acuity of one eye will be markedly better than the maximum attainable for the other. Since this may be due to factors which are not strictly involved in the state of refraction, such as amblyopia ex anopsia, the relative comparison of the clarity of the two eyes cannot be be based upon the maximum acuity.

3. *Technique When Both Eyes Are Relatively Equal in Acuity*

a. The simplest but also least reliable method is that of occluding first one eye and then the other and asking the patient to select the better.

b. The two eyes may also be dissociated by vertical prism divided between the two eyes and presenting two images at the same time. It is well to take this test twice, with the prism placed opposite for each eye every time, so that distortions and preferences may not influence the reports.

c. Whether alternate occlusion or dissociation is used, the common technique is that of equalizing at a test line well above that of best vision. Usually the 20/40 line is chosen. Each eye is fogged 0.25 D. at a time until this line is blurred out for either. The fog is then reduced for each until the 20/40 line can be seen. The patient is then requested to compare the two. If amblyopia exists, equalization must be performed at a line easily read by the amblyopic eye at its best.

(1) When dissociation is used, as is preferable for better contrast, the prism may be reversed, as mentioned, without further change in the fogging lens.

(2) Additional plus in 0.25 D. steps is added to the better eye until the two are equally blurred.

d. If the pupils of the two eyes are of different size or if the refractive status is sufficiently different to introduce differences in image size, the test may not be effective.

e. If an additional 0.25 D. reverses rather than equalizes the preference, it is advisable to permit the dominant eye to retain the better vision.

f. After the vision is equalized at 20/40, both eyes are exposed to a single chart and the fog is reduced binocularly until the best acuity is attained.

g. It is well to repeat the bichrome or visibility check test binocularly at this point, although it will be found frequently that eyes which have been tested monocularly by those methods and which have reached equal lines of acuity are equalized without much further modification.

4. *Comparison of Monocular and Binocular Subjective*

a. Most frequently, the binocular test will result in slightly better acuity and slightly more plus acceptance than will the monocular.

(1) This may be due to an esophoria which is relaxed when the fusion faculty is brought into action and relaxes associated accommodative-convergence.

b. Occasionally, the binocular test will exhibit less plus than does the monocular.

(1) This is usually associated with an exophoria, which is relaxed under occlusion, but which requires convergence effort abetted by accommodation when both eyes are used.

5. *Indications of Unequalized Subjective Correction*

a. A plus lens may be added above the subjective to create a finite punctum remotum. The nearpoint test chart may be introduced and the farpoint for each eye measured. If these are unequal, the two eyes may not be equally corrected.

b. The same check may be made by either the dynamic retinoscope or by placing plus lenses before the eye until test type blurs at near. However, these tests may be influenced by unequal accommodation rather than by unequal refraction.

6. *Modification of the Equalization Technique*

a. The author utilizes a variation of the usual technique. Instead of exposing a 20/40 line of letters and blurring both eyes until that line is barely seen, he exposes an entire section of the chart from 20/50 to 20/15. This is the same target section used for the Jackson cross cylinder test, and as the equalization follows that test, the chart need not be changed.

(1) The chart is dissociated until two complete charts are seen. Prism must be equally divided before both eyes.

(2) The patient is requested to state whether both charts are equally clear.

(a) If one is clearer, +0.25 D. is added before that eye until the charts are equal or reversed. If reversal occurs, the dominant eye is left clearer.

(3) +0.25 D. spheres are added OU in successive steps, and the patient requested to state *at each step* if both eyes blur to an equal extent.

(a) If one eye blurs faster than the other, extra plus is added to the clearer eye to again equalize the charts.

(4) Sufficient plus is added to blur the top line.

(5) The eyes are then unfogged in –0.25 D. steps simultaneously and the patient requested to state if both charts clear to equal extents and each step.

(a) If one chart clears faster than the other, additions in +0.25 D. steps are added to the eye seeing the clearer chart to equalize them.

(b) Both eyes are thus unfogged to best acuity.

(6) It may be found that upon occasion a +0.25 D. is added to one eye at one stage and to the other eye at another stage.

(7) Where vision cannot be equalized, it is clearly evident to both examiner and patient so that future complaints of inequality are anticipated.

(a) The variations at different steps are not otherwise apparent at equalization at 20/40 only. The technique demonstrates frequently that equalization at 20/40 is often not equalization at 20/20.

(b) Since unequal accommodation is rare, the technique can scarcely induce accommodative spasm in one eye only, and as a step-by-step unfogging routine, often reveals added plus findings.

(8) The prism is removed at best visual acuity and the eyes fogged up binocularly and unfogged to best binocular VA.

(9) The same technique is also used with binocular polaroid systems instead of prism dissociation.

b. The cause of the changes from one stage to another is not clear. The author believes it may be due to variations of the hyperfocal curve and profiles of the caustics.

(1) Flom and Goodwin (1964) compared the stigma in the Badel optometers against the Clason projection. The comparison of the locus of the foci of the eyes against fog and the acuity of each eye indicated that equal conjugate foci and resolving powers for in-focus foveal images exhibit unequal resolutions for blurred imagery. They offered the following three possible factors as causes:

(a) Differences in pupil size, optical asymmetries, aberrations, and scattering of light result in unequal light distribution of the retinal image.

(b) Neural asymmetries, such as size differences of foveal receptor fields, mean that one eye may present a dominant signal.

(c) With blurred imagery, fixation is less accurate for one eye and acuity is impaired.

(d) Flom and Goodwin saw no assurance that accommodation was actually equalized under blurred conditions of perception by the addition of plus power to equalize acuity at the 20/40 line.

c. *The Goodwin Technique*

(1) Goodwin noted that Fry, Reese, and Flom found individual responses differ from plus lenses. Failure to obtain equality under fog with the same additions does not necessarily indicate an unequal accommodation.

(2) Goodwin preferred to present the patient to a line of fine acuity, to use the lowest possible prism, and to add a +0.25 D. to each eye for a relative decrease in clarity if both seemed equal.

(3) If one seemed better than the other:

(a) +0.25 D. was added to the better eye.
(b) If still unequal, –0.25 D. was added to the poorer eye.
(c) If still unequal, the –0.25 D. was allowed to remain before the poorer eye, and +0.25 D. was added to the better eye.
(d) If it is still unequal, the –0.25 D. is removed, and a +0.25 D. was added to the better eye. If this was still unequal, all the subjective findings were rechecked.

(4) Goodwin found that if the retinoscopy, the monocular occlusion, the prism dissociation, the bichrome, and the Turville were compared to an optometer, the Turville showed the highest agreement and the least variance and mean deviation.

(a) All of the techniques showed only a small variance except the bichrome. The bichrome seemed subject to color defects, to preference by myopes for the red, and to some green preference by presbyopes. The Turville and the polaroid techniques seemed to agree.

(5) In equalizing under conditions of amblyopia, he found that the eyes needed to be under a minimum fog with the respective smallest resolvable letters before each eye (not the same size due to the amblyopia). The critical interaction upon acuity may have a deleterious effect by reducing the acuity of the amblyopic eye. If binocular vision exists, a binocular technique is preferable, and fusion can be gained parafoveally.

(6) Gentsch and Goodwin (1966) compared several methods of equalizing vision.

These methods included static retinoscopy; monocular comparisons with +0.25 D. and +0.50 D. adds before the eyes; prism dissociation begun with an add of +0.75 D. and reduced to the best visual acuity; vertical dissociation blurred equally; bichrome under prism with a +0.75 D. sphere over the monocular subjective reduced to the smallest resolvable letters or equal red/green vision; the Turville Infinity Balance test of Morgan; and a comparison of the Haploscope with the Nagle optometer system for conjugate focus of each eye.

(a) Gentsch and Goodwin found that the Turville Infinity Balance test came within –0.25 D. of the Haploscope; actually, 0.22 D. ±0.09 D. The monocular and prism test showed 0.24 D. ±0.18 D. The prism dissociation showed 0.24 ±0.23 D. The retinoscope showed 0.29 ±0.26 D., and the red/green showed 0.32 D. ±0.44 D.

(b) Gross errors were possible by all methods, but the Turville Infinity Binocular test was the least likely to suffer them. The Turville Infinity Binocular test and the polaroid test agreed within 0.25 D. in the worst case.

XI. BINOCULAR TECHNIQUES

A. Septum and Similar Techniques (Bannon, 1965; Giles, 1965; Amigo, 1968)

1. Cyclodamia (D. Smith, 1930).

a. This technique was developed essentially to reveal accommodative spasticity (see techniques for adding plus to correction below) but is in a sense classified by Bannon as a binocular technique in which both eyes are exposed and are viewing targets.

b. The Jackson cross cylinder technique can be used with one eye at various levels of fog and unfog while the other eye is exposed under a +1.50 D. fogging lens.

2. Copeland (1940)

a. The eye not tested is fogged by a +2.00 D. lens instead of being occluded.

3. Sensitometry (1940)

a. The Luckiesh and Moss Sensitometer, (see Specialized Techniques), usually found 0.50 to 1.00 D. less plus than other techniques.

4. Sugar's method (1944)

a. Sugar used a Jackson Cross Cylinder on first one eye and then on the other with both eyes viewing binocularly.

5. Stigmatoscopy (1928)

a. One eye is tested while both fixate (again, see Specialized Techniques).

6. Humphriss or Immediate Contrast (1962)

a. Humphriss suspended foveal vision with a +0.75 D. lens for both the cross cylinder and duochrome test and a +1.50 D. lens for phoria tests. The test required a small four inch illuminated chart with a central letter or pair of letters for Duochrome testing.

b. He called it a *Psychological septum.* Peripheral fusion is held. The technique is used after the retinoscopy or monocular examination.

7. Mark (1962)

a. Mark used a technique similar to Copeland and Humphriss.

b. In cases in which the retinoscope showed a higher plus than the subjective, done with one eye occluded, he got better acuity and more plus if both eyes were open, even though one was fogged. He reversed the fog to test the other eye.

c. He assumed it was due to the overactive ciliary muscle, but it may be due to better fixation of the eye with the higher ametropia when both were employed binocularly.

8. Mallett (1966)

a. Mallett preferred to use a 1.00 D. cross cylinder to occlude the comparative vision of the eye not under test. He employed this while using his own test device, as described under Phorometry, for testing the cylinder axis and the power at nearpoint. He used a 0.25 D. cross cylinder before the eye under test.

9. Saul (1955)

a. Saul used three prism diopters base-down before one eye and three prism diopters base-up before the other, with a hand cross cylinder. Both eyes were corrected to the best visual acuity to check the axis and the power.

B. Turville Infinity Balance (TIB) (1946)

1. As obvious from the above, equalization of the two eyes, while of the utmost importance in influencing binocularity, has generally been a rather indeterminate and uncertain procedure. Since the action of accommodation must be controlled, some fog is required, but since the variations in aberrations between the eyes are uncertain, the degree of unfogging subsequently required for each eye is indefinite. Most clinicians have had the experience of carefully equalizing vision at the 20/40 level and then having the patient return with the prescription complaining of a slight blur in one eye. The ideal situation would be one in which the vision for each eye could be determined while both eyes functioned together. Not only equalization of vision but also the effects of torsion on the cylinder axis during binocular vision would be then readily apparent.

2. In 1936, Turville published a description of a technique which was further elaborated in 1946. While this technique has been widely heralded and accepted in the British Isles, its acceptance in the United States has been comparatively slow, and the method does not find widespread use as yet in this country. Part of the problem may lie in the fact that most American refractionists utilize test charts developed upon the principle of direct projection, whereas the British are more accustomed to test cabinets and mirrors. Morgan developed a test chart for the projector by which means the Turville technique can be used routinely.

3. The principle of the Turville system is that employed by the Remy separator or the Javal grid. In the original form, it consisted of a test chart with two fields of letters or test objects spaced 60 mm. apart, set at 6 M., and reflected to the patient from a mirror placed at a 3 M. distance. This mirror is bisected by a metal (now a ground glass) septum of 3 cm. width. The effect of the arrangement is demonstrated in Figure XIX-9.

a. As is obvious, one set of letters is seen by the right eye, while the other is seen by the left eye, the ground glass or septum occluding part of the chart from each eye. A black border about the chart as seen binocularly serves to invoke peripheral fusion, although central fusion is absent. The septum is, of course, also seen binocularly.

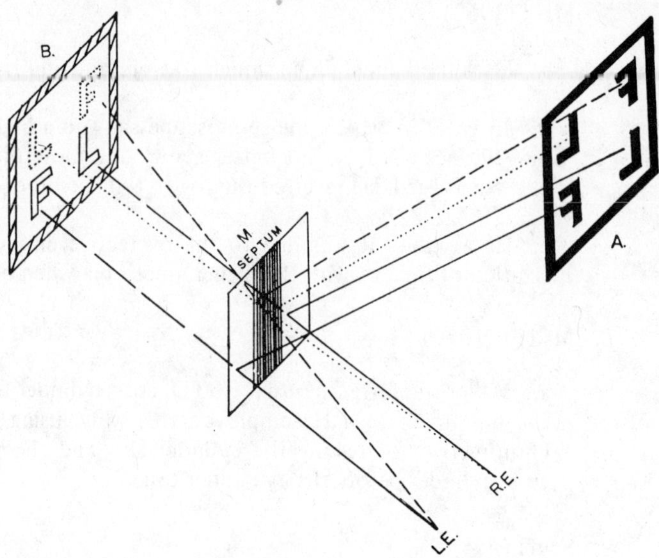

Figure XIX-9. Diagrammatic representation of Turville Infinity balance arrangement. A. Test chart, reversed. M. Mirror including septum. B. Projected representation of appearance of chart seen through mirror by patient. If septum is opaque, the lower letters of the test chart represent the projection to B, shown as open letters and indicated by solid and long dashed lines. The upper letters and short dashes and dots indicate how the opposite half of the chart is blocked for each eye. If septum is an inclined mirror, as in later Turville experiments, the short dashes and dotted lines indicate how a different part of the chart, (upper letters) is projected to position B giving the appearance indicated by all the letters on B.

4. A ready comparison of the acuities of the two eyes can be made. Small spheres can be added to either eye and the comparison noted. By using the C.C., the axis and power of the cylinder of either eye can be checked with the eyes functioning binocularly.

a. Since accommodation can only compensate at the nearpoint to 0.25 D. for a difference in the two eyes, the precise equalization may be extremely important. Morgan (1949) found by this method that the limit of variability statistically was, on the minus side, -0.20 ± 0.17 D. and on the plus side, $+0.15 \pm 0.09$ D. The test would seem exceedingly accurate for balancing to the extent of 0.25 D.

b. Comparing the results of his usual procedure with that found under Turville's device, Morgan found the following data:

(1) 20% of the cases showed a change of 0.25 D. in one eye.
(2) 2% of the cases revealed a change of 0.50 D. in one eye.
(3) 2% of the cases showed a change in axis of the cylinder of 10° or more.
(4) No case showed a change in cylinder power of as much as 0.25 D.
(5) 4% of the total cases showed a significantly different result by the Turville method.

5. Of great interest in the Turville method is the revelations of binocularity which the device

makes apparent. Thus, while peripheral fusion is maintained, the two test objects may draw together and even fuse in cases of exophoria, or draw far apart and even present two septums in cases of esophoria, or one line of letters may be slightly higher than the other in hyperphoria, or even one chart totally suppressed.

a. Using the 20/30 line as a guide, Morgan found that 98.6% of patients could detect a vertical difference of as little as 0.5 prism diopter of vertical displacement. Any vertical discrepancy may be assumed to be the evident hyperphoria and the correction prism prescribed.

(1) Morgan found only two such cases who could not tolerate the correction for other reasons.

b. Where the two targets move together or fuse, the amount of prism which restores them to their proper positions may be considered a measurement of insuperable exophoria, and prism base-in to that amount may be prescribed. Unfortunately, in esophoria, the patient is unable to clearly delineate the status due to the visibility of the septum.

6. *Technique*

a. *Position the chart (L and F) and the septum.*

(1) If these are seen separately and are level, no hyperphoria, exophoria, or suppression of the 20/60 letters exist.

(2) If the L and the F fuse, an apparent exophoria may exist.

(a) The chart with four letters and a peripheral lock should then be tried.

(b) If the charts can still not be kept separate, prisms may be needed to keep them separate.

(c) If prism is used, return to the L and F, using the peripheral lock.

[1] If the charts still cannot be kept separate, the smallest prism needed to keep them separate can usually be prescribed.

(3) If the L and the F are separated (esophoria), leave the amount of prism over 2 PD needed to fuse the letters.

(4) If the L and F are not vertically balanced one of the following may be present:

(a) Primary or true heterophoria may exist.

[1] The weakest vertical prism that aligns the two will probably be able to be worn.

[2] If over ½Δ, Lloyd suggested that the prism be used for correction. If less, it should be noted for later disposition.

(b) The disparity may be secondary and due to an inequality of visual acuity of the two eyes.

[1] A plus or minus 0.25 D. sphere may be added to one eye in an attempt to better equalize the vision. If this is the cause, the vertical disparity will disappear.

(5) If one side of the chart disappears, suppression exists, and the balance test cannot be performed.

(a) Larger letters may be tried, or, if added power restores the visual acuity with larger letters, an attempt may then later be made to restore it with the smaller ones.

(b) If fusion was restored with larger letters, the phoria should be aligned, and an attempt at altering the sphere should be made to see if misalignment then returns (Lloyd, 1950).

b. *The 20/20 letters are introduced, two for each eye,* bound by a binocularly seen peripheral band.

(1) If acuity is equal in both eyes, add +0.25 D. to each eye alternately as long as the letters remain clear until a final +0.25 D. addition blurs each eye.

(2) If acuity is better in one eye, add plus power to the poorer eye.

(a) If still not equalized, add plus to the better eye.

(3) If blurred but unequal, add –0.25 D. to the poorer eye.

(a) If not equalized, recheck the cylinder power with the cross cylinder.

(b) If still unequal, give the Rx approaching closest to equality or note the Rx accepted binocularly without the septum.

(c) If the patient is unable to equalize or select between the eyes with 20/20 letters, the 20/30 letters may be used.

(4) If one eye is amblyopic, equalization should be performed on a larger target.

(a) The power should then be reduced binocularly until the best eye gets best acuity.

c. *After equalization, recheck the vertical balance.*

(1) If there is no imbalance, any previously exhibited imbalance was not a primary deviation.

(2) If exophoria exists, use the mask for peripheral fusion to determine the primary phoria.

(3) If esophoria exists, remove the mask to measure the phoria.

(4) If a high vertical phoria exists, the Maddox rod may be needed to measure it accurately.

(5) If a cyclophoria exists, the letters will make an oblique line with each other.

(6) If the alignment is transitory, varying as the patient watches, note the amount of prism which aligns the two images at the first moment it is put before the eyes.

(a) Wait between prism changes until the eyes settle and retinal slip is not operating.

d. In a totally dark room the septum is visible. Also, very acute patients may note differences between the eyes of less than 0.25 D. or ½Δ.

e. Hyperphorias should be rechecked every few months since some portion may be latent.

f. *Where anisometropia exists,* the patient should note the vertical balance of the F and L with the chin turned both up and down.

(1) The stronger lens should be reduced until the letters appear level with the head in the habitual position.

g. *Finally, the septum is removed,* both eyes are fogged together, and then unfogged for best acuity.

7. By calling attention to appropriate charts, any testing method can be used, or each eye can be tested alternately with the accommodation better controlled.

a. A single lens can be used to check vertical disparity.

b. Similar targets, such as the Verhoeff circles, can be presented to each eye and used to test fixation disparity. Prism base-out is added before the eyes.

(1) If the peripheral fusion is strong, and the central image is far from the fovea of the non-fixing eye, base-out will elicit further fusional convergence, and the same balance will be restored as existed before the introduction of the prism.

(2) If the peripheral fusion is weak, and the central image is nearer the fovea of the non-fixing eye, the patient may fuse the two targets.

(3) A normal patient will overcome at least 2 PD of base-out.

(4) If no fusional movement is made, a small amount of base-in may be helpful.

(a) Morgan prescribed 1 PD for each 2 PD, that is, if the tests showed 3 PD or more of base-out accepted, no base-in was prescribed. If from 0 to 2 PD, 1 PD of base-in was prescribed, and if base-in was needed, the amount indicated was prescribed.

c. The tests do not always agree with the usual vergence tests.

(1) If the Turville test shows a low base-out acceptance, but the vergence tests show a high positive fusional reserve, prism will usually help more than orthoptics. But if both are low, either orthoptics or prism may be used.

d. Stereopsis can be tested by creating a slight disparity of both targets, and suppression can be noted.

e. Elom (1954) compared the results of the tests and retests within a period of 4 to 27 weeks of wear for prism prescribed according to the Turville techniques.

(1) If the history, the cover test, or the old Rx indicated a vertical prospect, Elom used the Turville septum and trial case prisms to level the charts.

(a) After the refraction, the phoria was tested by the Maddox rod cover test.

(b) The Turville technique was then used to level the targets, and the prisms that were indicated were fitted to level the fields.

(c) The Turville technique was also used for retest through the finished spectacles.

[1] If level, ½ PD was placed base-down before each eye to see if the target was displaced.

[2] If after the prism was introduced, the targets appeared releveled, additional prism was added until displacement was held.

[a] Elom considered this a legitimate increase in manifested phoria.

[b] Note, however, the resemblance to the compensatory reflex, described by Ogle (Chap. VI, XX).

(2) Three-fourths of the patients showed no increase in hyperphoria upon recheck, after wearing the Rx determined by the Turville technique. One-fourth of the patients needed ½ Δ of prism more to fully correct. Two patients required 1 Δ or more of prism to correct fully.

(a) Each of the latter had a lesser phoria at near than at far, but the prism found by the Turville method was incorporable in the distance Rx.

C. The Turville Dual Mirror

1. Turville later employed a dual mirror, the upper-half of which presented the TIB test and the lower-half of which presented a chart without a septum for monocular and binocular testing.

2. The monocular test was performed on the lower mirror for each eye, one at a time, and then the patient was referred to the upper mirror for the TIB test.

D. Morgan's Infinity Balance Technique (1949 and 1960)

1. Morgan first utilized Turville's technique on the Robinson-Cohen slide providing two columns of letters – one for each eye with a flat septum between them.

2. He later developed a special slide (AO No. 1217-21), usable without a mirror but with a bar septum between the patient and the chart. The septum was the same color as the chart and about 25 to 30 mm. wide, placed half-way between the patient and the chart. The septum was empirically set so that the right eye saw the right half and the left eye the left half of the chart.

a. The width of the septum can be accurately computed by Morgan's formula $S = \frac{cx}{d} + x = \frac{dp}{c+p}$ in which c = ½ of the width of each line on the test chart, d = the distance to the chart in cm, p = the interpupillary distance in cm., x = the distance of the septum from the patient, and s = the width of the septum.

(1) Since the occluded areas may overlap in midline without harm, a different septum is not actually needed for each interpupillary distance. An approximation is only required which can be determined by trial and error so that the large interpupillary distances will not have a binocular central field. This is easily done with split charts and a septum of the same color and illuminosity of the test chart.

3. DeLacey cautions that the Turville Infinity Balance test is actually under the control of the patient since the examiner cannot be sure of the separation of the targets for each eye, and the test

ordinarily uses 20/40 or 20/60 instead of 20/20 letters.

4. Brungardt (1958) found that using the Turville technique and with attention of the patient directed towards the chart seen by the better eye, an amblyopic eye would accept +0.75 D. more plus with an acuity of approximately 20/25 instead of 20/40 to 20/60. However, if the good eye was covered, the poorer eye visual acuity dropped back to 20/60.

E. **The Freeman Bichromatic Test** (1954, and 1955).

1. Freeman and Archer developed a chart which presented black Landolt C's and Verhoeff circles as well as letters; some placed on a red background, some on a green background, and some on a white background.

a. The chart could be used with a mirror or with a 35 mm. wide septum placed on the mirror.

2. *Monocular test*

a. The acuity is determined on the Landolt C's.

b. The patient is directed towards two panels of C's, one on a red and one on a green background presenting acuity letters from 6/24 to 6/6 in size.

(1) The preliminary sphere is determined by equalizing the panels.

c. The sphere is checked by what is known as the *sphere twirl* with C's on a red/green background as the target. The instrument used consists of a +0.25 and a –0.25 lens mounted on a wand. By twirling the wand, either of the powered lenses is presented before the eye in succession in a manner similar to the turning of a hand cross cylinder.

(1) If the +0.25 D. is before the eye, the red should appear better; if the –0.25 D., the green should appear better. If the targets and charts are not equalizable, the patient is left in the green.

d. Using the Verhoeff circles, a cross cylinder is introduced to determine the astigmatism. A +0.50:–1.00 cross cylinder is used when acuity is worse than 20/40, or for high astigmatism, while a +0.25:–0.50 cross cylinder is used for acuity better than 20/40 or for low astigmatism.

(1) The axes of the cross cylinder are presented in the vertical and the horizontal positions and the patient asked to make a choice. If there is no choice, they are then presented obliquely. If there is still no choice, no astigmatism exists.

(2) ,If a choice is found, a –0.25 D. cylinder is introduced with its axis in the position of the minus axis of the cross cylinder coinciding with the better position.

(3) The axis of this correcting cylinder is straddled with the cross cylinder in the usual way, and the axis position is refined.

(4) The cross cylinder is then aligned with its axis coinciding with the axis of the minus correcting cylinder, and the power is determined.

(5) Freeman cautions that one-half the power of the cylinder should be added to the

sphere of the opposite sign in order to maintain the midpoint of the caustic at the proper place on the retina. The patient must *not* be fogged.

e. After the astigmatism is corrected, the red/green sections are again used to rebalance the final sphere.

(1) A +0.25 D. is added, then a −0.25 D., to see if the color reverses with each. If it does, the final sphere has been reached. The +0.25 D. should be used first in order to hold accommodation constant.

3. *Binocular procedure*

a. The septum is now placed upon the mirror and the central part of the chart is used, as in the Turville technique. The outer parts of the chart are seen binocularly and act as a lock for fusion.

(1) The Verhoeff rings are fixated. The right two are seen by the right eye and the left two by the left eye.

(2) The cross cylinder test is now repeated for each eye.

b. The upper two rings now appear on a red background, while the lower two appear on a green.

(1) The right eye sees the right pair, one on red and one on green, while the left eye sees the left pair similarly placed.

(2) A +0.25 D. and −0.25 D. twirl is now performed before each eye, one at a time, for the final sphere.

(a) If not in the red, a +0.25 D. sphere is added to put the patient in the red.

(b) The patient is left slightly in the red.

(c) A reversal of the twirl should now make the green slightly better.

c. Accommodation is then checked on the black and white charts.

(1) The Landolt C's are used, and a +0.50 is added before both eyes.

(a) If this does not cause the C's to appear blurred, +0.25 is added to the Rx before both eyes.

(b) Again, the +0.50 is added, and if the charts do not appear blurred, the steps are repeated, a plus quarter being added each time until the addition of the +0.50 finally blurs the charts.

(2) With the Verhoeff circles on a red/green background, a final +0.50 is added before both eyes and left five seconds at a minimum.

(a) If upon removal the red is still better, accommodation has been relaxed as far as possible.

(b) However, if upon removal the green appears better, an added +0.25 D. is placed before the eyes, and the test is repeated until the red remains better.

F. **Banks** (1954)

1. Banks used a horizontal line of Landolt C's of decreasing size at the three meter distance as a target, with the head fixed in a headrest.

2. A 21-mm. wide septum was applied before the eyes.

3. He claimed that since the septum covered only one-half the foveal area, both foveas could see the rings.

a. This, he believed, enabled him to detect foveal suspension and to reveal disparity or slip.

G. **Binocular Diaphragm**

1. Fernandez, Edmund and Hunt (1955) used a diaphragm like a Bishop Harmon diaphragm incorporating Snellen's test types in the target. The results were similar to Turville's method.

2. The method enabled each eye to be tested while binocularly engaged.

3. Hyperphorias of 0.75Δ and up were revealed, and esophorias up to 3.0 to 3.5Δ were revealed.

4. The difference between the vision and the Rx found binocularly and that found with each eye separately was disclosed.

H. **The Hunt-Giles Far Point Test**

1. A monochromatic yellow/green filter was used.

a. Minus was added if the letters were blurred and plus if clear until the best letters on the chart were still just barely visible.

XII. POLARIZATION TECHNIQUES

A. **Dartmouth** used transparent filters and polarized astigmatic dials on an opaque background in 1939.

1. The filter was rotated so one eye saw the target while both eyes fused the background and the border.

B. **Leland Refractor** (1940) (Bannon, 1965)

1. Leland used polarized lights so that one eye saw objects but not a specific target seen by the other eye.

C. **Norman** (1950) (Bannon, 1965)

1. Norman used a projector which presented one eye with a vertical polarized target and the other eye with a horizontally polarized one. The charts were specially designed so that they were usable for various test procedures, from equalization to stereopsis. Both eyes fused the periphery of the charts, although only one saw the target under observation. He found a significant difference in binocular plus acceptance from that found monocularly (as Brungardt and others have reported).

D. **Schultz** (1950) (Bannon, 1965)

1. Schultz used a revolving drum which presented various charts. These were polarized into two halves – vertical and horizontal.

2. Filters were placed before the eyes which were smaller than the trial lens cells, so that peripheral binocular vision was observed. These filters also acted as a lock for fusion.

3. Increased illumination was necessary to make the test effective.

4. The usual routines were used for testing each eye, although both were constantly in use.

E. **Wilmut** (1951) (Grant, 1965)

1. The dimensions of the chart agree substantially with those of Turville's. Between two glass plates are two three-inch square polarizing sheets, set so that one polarizes vertically and the other horizontally. The non-polarized sections are blacked out, except for a rectangular strip and a narrow septum strip which acts as a lock for fusion.

2. This screen in placed three inches in front of the chart which is illuminated by two 60W strip bulbs located between the screen and the chart. The patient views the chart through two polarizing discs held before the trial frame.

a. Several different types of charts are utilized.

(1) One consists of an F and L, oppositely polarized. An exophore will see FL or E. If the polaroid filters are reversed before the eyes, the esophore will see LF, or E.

(2) Another contains four sections, the upper left and lower right being identically polarized, while the upper right and lower left are identically polarized, but opposite the other two sections. All four targets should be equally spaced from each other. If the patient has exophoria, the lower two come together while the upper two separate, while if esophoria is present, the upper two come together while the lower two separate. Wilmut believes that this will also discourage any voluntary convergence. Two vertical lines are also introduced to check cyclophoria.

(a) If the filters but not the targets are reversed, allowance for the type of phoria is made. Suppression may also thereby be revealed.

3. Wilmut has developed a similar apparatus using a trans-illuminated nearpoint chart for near testing. Here the spacing of the letters is such that their normal positions are assumed with a slight exophoria. He finds that reducing or increasing the add which still permits clear vision but which alters the phoria at this point, to be a valuable contribution of the technique.

4. Wilmut felt polaroid a better dissociator than the bichrome method because no variance of wave length influenced the acuity.

F. **Dowdeswell** (1952) (Grant, 1965)

1. Dowdeswell used two separate boxes – one polarized vertically and the other horizontally. One box exhibited the letter L and the other the letter F.

G. **Freeman** (1954)

1. For the far test, Freeman used a chart which contained panels of Landolt C's, with some on a red background, some on a green background, and some on a black and white background.

2. He used polaroid filters so each eye saw separate red and green targets peculiar to that eye.

3. Each eye could thereby be balanced separately, and both eyes could be equalized.

   a. He claimed that the accuracy could be checked to 0.12 D.

4. The technique is similar to that of the previous Freeman technique, but polaroid is used instead of a septum.

   a. As in the previous technique, black Verhoeff circles on a white background were used for the cross cylinder test.

H. **Cowen** (1955, 1959) (Grant, 1965)

1. Cowan objected to complete polarization of the targets, because by this approach and by placing of filters before the eyes, the over-all illumination was exceedingly reduced.

2. His charts were made with a linear polarizing film viewed through an analyzer and seen, when the polarizers were crossed, as black against a white background. One eye saw one chart and the other eye the other chart.

   a. The OD letters were polarized at 135°, while the OS letters were polarized at 45°. Some letters were seen binocularly to act as a foveal fusion lock.

   b. The analyzer may be rotated slightly either way without an unwanted image.

3. The method eliminated the need for a septum or a head support, and the phoria did not confuse the target. Otherwise, the conditions and standards for the Turville tests were optimally met.

4. The comparison of peripheral lock to foveal lock was found to indicate a need for greater prism when peripheral lock was used.

   a. The foveal lock held the eyes where the peripheral stimulus was insufficient.

5. Targets consisted of the following: an L and an F for the fusion test; Landolt C's, which could be seen without the red/green for the cross cylinder test or with the red/green for a spherical test, as in Freeman's technique; and a special chart of two dashes with a gap between, presentable vertically or horizontally for prism prescribing or phoria measurement (Figure XIX-10).

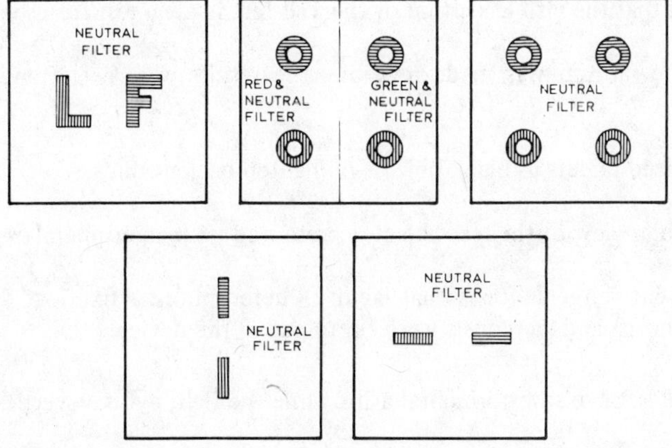

Figure XIX-10. Cowen's Polaroid Neutral Filter method.

I. Osterburg's Unit

1. This consisted of a projected chart, observed at the distance, with similar targets and techniques to Freeman's but polarized and in bichrome.

J. Stereo Background Refraction

1. *Frantz (1956)*

a. Frantz used targets polarized at axes 45 and 135 and additional color stereo 35 mm. slides. These slides were projected as a background for the polarized targets and were seen binocularly.

b. The polarized letters thereby consisted of targets, in symbols or letters, projected in the central area of a larger stereo picture.

c. Frantz claimed the vision was both more realistic and dynamic with better paramacular and peripheral fusion locks and was closer to the usual daily vision.

(1) Fixation disparity or suppression was more readily revealed.

d. The device can be used with any technique of binocular refraction.

2. *Phillips (1964)*

a. After the usual monocular refraction, the lines of the best acuity are projected onto a stereoscopic mountain scene or similar scene.

b. A polaroid filter occludes the lines from one eye.

c. A cross cylinder is used to check the cylindrical power and axis.

d. A vertical row of letters is then projected in which one half of the row is polarized for each eye.

e. Alignment of the vertical row for disparity or phoria, with or without the stereoscopic background scene, may be performed.

K. Polatest (Haase, 1961, 1962)

1. Haase claimed that the visible septum of the TIB test made a test for esophoria difficult.

a. When the septum was made invisible, the results were better and lower esophoria was found.

2. He used polarized targets as black objects on lighted backgrounds.

a. A uniocular view of the test object is presented with a peripheral fusion lock.

3. Twelve different targets for visual acuity, heterophoria, fixation disparity, aniseikonia, functional cyclophoria, and stereopsis were contained in the device.

4. In one test the left eye saw horizontal arms while the right eye saw vertical arms of a cross.

a. A deviation from the cross represented the heterophoria acceptably correctable with prism when normal correspondence existed.

b. Haase believed the difference of this test from the Maddox rod results was due to the "darkness rest position" of the Maddox compared to the "brightness rest position" of the Polatest.

c. He claimed that all prism Rx's determined by this method could be comfortably worn as a full correction.

d. Many procedures of the balance of the test were similar to the TIB procedures.

e. Cyclophoria tests, such as a pointer seen by one eye aligning with radial markings seen by the other, were also available.

L. The Vectograph (Grolman, 1965-66)

1. In discussing polarized slides, Grolman (1966) noted that polarizing techniques depended upon several different methods of manufacture. In one, polarized slides may be made by sheets placed over the slide and oriented at a different axis for each eye. The projector's aperture and the room provided the peripheral fusional stimuli.

a. This usually involves low visibility and low contrast since both the overlay and the analyzer cut out the light. Each eye also sees the counter lateral target as totally black, and finally, the test target design is limited to monocular fields, separately placed, which may be displaced laterally or vertically.

2. Another method of making polarized charts was by cutting the symbols themselves out of polarizing material. All polarized material was composed, Grolman noted, of a density filter film which absorbed light uniformly and of a polarizing film which exerted the polarizing property and absorbed light only in one meridian. Consequently, the density filter portion of the polaroid film, which tended to absorb the light uniformly, made the counter-lateral target visible against a non-polarized background, unless a neutural density background was provided. If such a background was provided, it provided an evenly illuminated background for the eye not seeing the target. However, the original target visibility was lowered for the eye that was seeing the target, and therefore only relatively gross symbols could be used.

3. The Vectograph symbols and characters were formed by a high resolution process and were deposited on a type of film of dicroic crystals as to present opaque images to one eye through the analyzer and a uniformly illuminated field to the other eye. They may be rotated out of alignment 20° before ghost images appear. If superimposed, each functions independently without optical interference of the other. The chart was constructed of vertical and horizontal lines placed at various areas, which were seen binocularly. Some of the letters or numbers were seen binocularly to help lock fusion centrally. The lines lock fusion peripherally (Figure XIX-11).

a. Letters, numbers, and lines were seen in such a manner that at one position of the chart, there were letters only for the right eye while the numbers and lines were seen binocularly. At another position on the chart there were letters only for the left eye while the numbers and lines were seen binocularly. Some charts presented some of the letters for the right eye and some of the letters for the left eye, and some charts present binocular dividers with identical charts side by side, one seen only by one eye and one by the other for equalization.

b. The first charts, in which one eye at a time saw the letters while both eyes saw the fusion symbols, can be used for ordinary monocular routines. The charts in which one eye saw one portion of the chart while the other eye saw an identical chart along side it, with the divider binocularly seen, could be used for equalization.

c. The chart in which some of the letters were seen by one eye and some by the other could be used for foveal suppression testing.

d. A non-polarized chart was also presented so that the binocular Rx could be determined with both eyes seeing together.

e. The clock dial, polarized so that one eye saw one portion and one another, was also contained on the chart.

f. A disparity test consisting of horizontal and vertical lines, forming a cross similar to that in the Polatest, was included. This was also presented with a circle and dot as a central lock for binocular fixation on another slide. Finally, a stereopsis test chart consisting of disparate circles was presented.

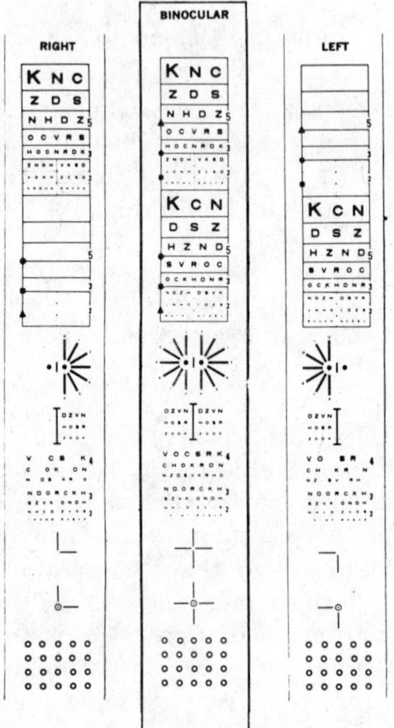

Figure XIX-11. Vectograph adult slide showing actual slide in center and adjacent portions seen by each eye.

4. The author uses this chart for a complete routine as described later. It can be used for any subjective routine, any fogging procedure with either both eyes active and fusion locked, or monocularly by eliminating the polaroid filter before the eye.

5. Grolman warned that the chart would appear dim unless care was taken that the angle between the projector, the screen, and the patient was such that the patient's head was within the angle of specular reflection. If the patient was placed so that he was outside of this angle, the contrast would be sharply diminished, and the chart would appear dark. Adjustment for vertical discrepancy must also be made. Therefore, if the projector was placed to one side, and the patient's chair was placed directly in front of the screen, the screen should be tilted slightly at one edge away from the wall so that this proper angle of reflection was attained.

6. Rosenberg and Sherman (1968) list the following advantages in the use of the vectographic binocular method:

a. Binocular problems may be revealed by differences in acuity taken binocularly as compared to that taken with one eye occluded; by binocular stability tests only available on the chart; and by disparity tests available.

(1) One-third of subjects tested showed a disparity different than the phoria finding of 1 to 5 Δ when no fusion lock was used. With a fusion lock, 35 of 47 subjects revealed 1 Δ or less difference than the phoria, while the other 12 showed more than 1 Δ. Tests of binocular balance are easier to perform with polaroid dividers than with dissociation. Stereopsis can also be tested.

b. No significant difference was revealed in the power of the cylinder but the axis did change in some subjects to some extent. (The difference in some instances in spherical power in cases of anisometropia has been noted earlier).

c. Disadvantages were mainly that tilt of the patient's head altered the placement of the targets, specifically causing the vertical separation to increase.

M. It is evident that many other procedures have been and yet remain to be developed upon the Turville premise. Morgan and Peters have made measurements of the amount of prism needed to cause the septum to double. This is not a duction or vergence test in the ordinary sense, and its significance remains to be investigated. The basis of prescription may be altered to coincide with changes increasing the stereopsis; prismatic corrections are apparently more reliably determined, and equalization seems definitely more exact. The modification of the reading correction, suggested by Wilmut, is a provocative usage of the technique.

1. Miles cautioned that binocular refraction might be misleading if strong dominance was present, or if one eye was markedly weaker, but otherwise, he found binocular refraction gave better binocular balance and that the axis of the cylinder was located while the eye was in the active muscle position.

XIII. RELIANCE UPON THE SUBJECTIVE

A. Where poor acuity, inability to cooperate, low intelligence, pathology or opacities, inattentiveness or any other interference with the proper reliance upon the patient's answers is found, the best procedure is to employ a correction determined by objective means.

B. A difference between the retinoscopy and binocular subjective may be due to the same causes which cause a difference between the monocular subjective and the binocular one, since the retinoscopy is basically monocular. Some rely exclusively upon the retinoscopy and others upon the subjective. While both schools have their adherents, the final criterion is the patient's satisfaction, and it appears reasonable that many factors of an optical nature may influence the retinoscopy so that its findings are not usable. The value of the patient's habitual interpretation and judgment of his own retinal stimulation must occupy too high a place in the function of vision to be totally ignored. Where a marked difference exists, and the subjective routine has been thorough and comprehensive, and the patient has been alert and responsive, the weight would seem to lie with the subjective.

1. Lienberger commented that fogging may increase lenticular astigmatism causing the finding to vary even further from retinoscopy and keratometry. Giles felt that if the subjective and objective did not agree, the retinoscopy had been performed off the visual axis.

2. Billson (1954) considered the retinoscopy more reliable and the subjective only a verification. However, Freeman and Hodd found that both retinoscopy and the subjective were usually equally reliable, but the subjective was preferable in markedly irregular cases.

C. It must be remembered that the image of the retinoscope is not only a finer image located at the choroidal plane, but also one dealing essentially with the central bundles of rays. In contrast, the image in the subjective is located at the retinal nerve layer and is the circle of least confusion of both central and peripheral rays. In addition, Pech (1933) showed that the reflected fundus rays of the retinoscope were practically monochromatic orange-red, whereas the average subjective was based upon the yellow rays of white light. There may exist a marked dioptric difference between the two.

1. The chromatic aberration of the eye may account for the difference in plus power of the retinoscope, since more plus is required to focus red than yellow. However, the posterior locus of the retinoscopy focus and the longer focal length of the central rays may tend to compensate for this. Discrepancies between the two, however, should be expected in either direction, since only chance would provide precise compensation of the elements involved in retinoscopy with those involved in subjective testing.

2. Some advocate the possibility of toxicity when the retinoscope shows less plus than the subjective. This deduction is based upon toxic action of the accommodation under the monocular retinoscopic test which is inhibited during the binocular subjective test. This would only be true if the monocular subjective showed a comparable accommodative action. Where the monocular subjective is not lower than the binocular while the retinoscopy is, the difference cannot be sought in accommodative action alone, or at least not in such action induced by monocularity. It is not unusual to find that the accommodation reveals a different status of relaxation during the retinoscopy than during the subjective and is usually on the order of an increased relaxation of the accommodation during the semi-somnambulant status of retinoscopy. The demand for subjective criteria may act to stimulate the accommodation, particularly since the patient is making a conscious effort to be critical and alert.

a. Where the retinoscopy shows less plus than the subjective, the only action of toxicity which might be effective, other than toxic accommodation, is in edematous effusion in the retinal-choroidal space. This might affect the relation of the focus of the subjective focus so that more plus was required to focus yellow light on the cones than red light on the pigmentary layer. This explanation is highly theoretical and it would seem more substantial to eliminate the consideration of toxicity from the explanation of the difference between retinoscopic and subjective findings in favor of the abundant supply of optical and interpretive factors.

XIV. SUMMARY OF THE STANDARD SUBJECTIVE TEST

A. Monocular

1. *Determine the Proper Amount of Fog*

a. Blur out dial or chart or use working distance over plus retinoscopy sphere.

b. Reduce to visibility of first dial lines or 20/40 test line.

2. *Determine Axis of Minus Cylinder*

a. Locate axis on clock or sunburst dial.

(1) Refine with movable V or comparison of adjacent lines.

b. Introduce movable T or cross chart.

(1) Refine axis by straddling principal meridians.

(2) Note broken square or step effect on dashed lines if used.

3. *Equalize Lines on T, Cross or Clock Dial*

a. Note reversal of lines, if any.

4. *Check Accuracy of Cylinder Correction Under Fog*

a. Fog and see if lines come out equally.

b. Use C.C. and see if opposite lines appear with reversal.

5. *Determine Proper Sphere by Unfogging*

6. *Check Sphere*

a. Intensity of illumination

b. Duochrome or bichrome

7. *Check Cylinder with Proper Sphere*

a. Rotating cylinder

b. Cross Cylinder

8. *Repeat on Other Eye*

B. Binocular

1. *Equalize*

a. Standard

(1) Fog to 20/50

(2) Reduce to 20/40

(3) Dissociate and add plus to equalize

(a) Add plus to better eye

(b) Leave dominant eye best if equalization is not possible

(4) Unfog binocularly to best acuity

b. Variation

(1) Dissociate by either vertical or lateral prism equally divided between the two eyes.

(2) Fog both eyes in +0.25 D. steps, up to acuity of 20/50.

(a) At each step, note if the blurred images are equally blurred.

(b) If one eye is less blurred than the other, add an additional +0.25 D. to that eye to see if it equalizes the blur.

[1] If it reverses the target, have the patient choose that position of lens powers which seems closer to equality.

(3) When 20/50 is reached, unfog both eyes in –0.25 D. steps again checking whether the acuity remains balanced at each step.

(a) If one eye clears faster than the other, add a +0.25 D. lens to that eye.

[1] If it reverses the clarity use the same criterion as in steps (2) (b) 1.

(4) Unfog until best V.A. is reached.

(a) Leave dominant eye with best acuity if equalization is unattainable.

2. *Check Binocular Correction*

a. Fog binocularity to 20/40 acuity.

b. Unfog to best acuity O. U. based on:

(1) Intensity of illumination

(2) Duochrome or bichrome

3. *Turville Infinity Balance Tests*

C. While several methods of performing each step are sometimes indicated, the practitioner may soon select those tests he finds most readily at hand or suitable to his equipment and facilities. He may also transpose the order of some tests, particularly the checks for cylinder and sphere. If he has more than one method at hand, however, he will find that he is better prepared because some patients will respond to one technique with more accuracy than to another. So long as he uses at least some means of performing each of the major steps, the technique may be considered adequate.

XV. COMBINED TECHNIQUE

A. A technique which the author (1946) has described provides a speedy combined routine which includes most of the steps outlined in the preceding sections in a continual procedure.

1. The author considers retinoscopy as part of the total routine and as the basis for beginning the subjective.

a. The sphere is built up with "with motion" until one meridian is neutralized.

b. The axis of the astigmatic meridian is determined with the retinoscope as accurately as possible. Since "with" motion is used, the axis of the minus cylinder lies at right angles.

c. Cylinders are not used but additional plus sphere is added until the second meridian is neutralized.

(1) This provides the plus spherical element of a combination of plus sphere and minus cylinder.

d. The difference between steps 1 and 3 provides a recording of the retinoscopic cylinder in minus, while the difference between step 3 and the working distance provides the sphere.

(1) These values are recorded as the retinoscopic finding.

2. Without removing the working distance the patient is directed to the dashed line cross of the Robinson-Cohen slide or the T chart of the Ferree-Rand projector slide.

a. The cross or T is aligned with the principal meridians of the eye as indicated by the retinoscope.

b. The working distance is reduced until one set of lines is distinct.

c. The axis of the cylinder is refined by straddling the principal meridians with the T or cross, and the arms are presented in the new principal meridians (see Rotary Charts for axis).

d. The two arms of the T or cross are equalized by addition of minus cylinder with the axis perpendicular to the darker arm. This provides a subjective astigmatic correction.

3. The Verhoeff circles are presented to the patient and the circles equalized in the red and green.

a. Usually this provides maximum acuity.

b. The test letter chart is presented and the acuity noted. If not normal or maximum, the fog is further reduced until the best lines are read.

c. This provides the spherical element of the correction.

4. The Jackson cross cylinder is introduced and the cylinder is refined again for axis and power on the test letters.

a. The spherical element, with non-presbyopes, is altered by adding –0.25 D. sphere.

b. The axis is always checked before the power and the spherical equivalent maintained.

(1) This provides a third reading for the axis and cylinder.

5. The patient is referred to the test chart, and the duochrome or intensity of illumination check is used to determine the best sphere.

6. It will be noted that each of the above steps moves into the next naturally and that there are provided three readings each – for the sphere, the cylinder power, and the cylinder axis.

a. Steps in the Above Which Provide a Spherical Estimate

(1) The maximum plus in retinoscopy less the working distance.

(2) The equalization of the Verhoeff circles.

(3) The duochrome applied to the line of best acuity.

b. Steps Which Indicate the Axis of the Cylinder

(1) The retinoscope

(2) The rotary cross or T chart

(3) The Jackson cross cylinder

c. Steps Which Indicate the Amount of Cylinder

(1) The difference between the two meridians in retinoscopy

(2) The equalization of the arms of the T or cross

(3) The Jackson cross cylinder

7. If a sunburst dial is available, the cylinder may be still further refined by the rotation described in Section X.

8. After this procedure has been performed for both eyes, the eyes are equalized, and binocularly brought to best vision; the duochrome test is repeated binocularly.

B. Concise Combined Technique

1. In recent years, the author has used a more concise combined technique which has served with great reliability. It has the advantage, particularly with older patients and children, of being completed before the patient becomes exhausted.

2. The retinoscopy is performed with spheres only. Plus is built up until the meridian of greatest plus is neutralized. In the course of doing so, the examiner notes the meridian of least plus as the spherical meridian and can readily mentally note the difference between this meridian and that of greatest plus as the indicated cylinder. If the eye is myopic, the stopping point is ultimately the meridian of least minus, although in the performance of the routine, the examiner may perform the retinoscopy, using spheres, through both meridians so that he may again record the indicated cylinder.

a. The meridian, therefore, of *greatest plus or least minus* is the starting point for the subjective routine.

b. The author does not remove the working distance lens or check the acuity with the retinoscopy. The merit of the retinoscopy is its indication to him of the refractive values, and he is not concerned with checking acuity at this time.

3. Starting at this point, the working distance is slowly reduced by a –0.25 D. at a time until the 1.50 D. for 26 inches or 2.00 D. for 20 inches has been totally removed. The patient, in the meantime, is directed towards the complete set of letters used for subjective testing (10/50 to 20/15).

4. Unless the astigmatism is above 1.50 D., acuity will usually come close to 20/20 or better without the cylinder, particularly in a young patient. If the patient is too old to compensate for the astigmatism, or if the astigmatism is greater than the 1.50 D., part of the cylinder indicated by the retinoscopy is placed at the axis indicated by the retinoscopy.

a. The patient is brought to the sharpest possible acuity by means of spheres only. Generally, to be sure that the bundle of rays is placed behind the retina, as necessary for the cross cylinder test which follows, an additional –0.25 D. sphere is added beyond the working distance value.

5. The patient is then directed to the group of letters comprising the test chart, and the cross cylinder is introduced with its axes vertical and horizontal. The cross cylinder is flipped and the patient asked to select the position of greatest legibility. If neither position is chosen, the cross cylinder axes are placed in the oblique meridians and again the patient is asked to choose. If again neither is chosen, astigmatism is not confirmed subjectively.

6. If one position is chosen, a –0.25 D. cylinder is placed with its axis coinciding with the minus axis position of the cross cylinder when the patient made his choice.

a. The cross cylinder is then presented before this –0.25 D. correcting cylinder and the patient requested to note whether or not a better position is still found. If both positions are equal, the –0.25 D. is assumed as the correct power at that moment. If the plus position of the C.C., when in coincidence with the minus correcting axis, is chosen, the cylinder is rejected. If the minus position is chosen, more cylinder is needed.

7. If the cylinder is accepted, the correction cylinder axis is then straddled with the cross cylinder axes, and the usual technique for determining the accurate axis of the cylinder is performed.

8. After the accurate axis has been found, the cross cylinder axes are again aligned with the correction cylinder, and the final power of the cylinder is determined.

9. When this stage is reached, plus sphere is then added to the eye until the chart is fogged to the upper line (20/50 or thereabouts) and then slowly unfogged again to best acuity. The red/green, or other method, is used to determine the spherical value giving the best acuity.

10. The same procedure is repeated upon the other eye.

11. With both eyes now having a spherical-cylinder value before them, the patient is directed towards the still fully exposed chart, which is now dissociated into two charts by prisms, and plus lenses are added before both eyes, as described earlier in the author's equalization technique, until the eyes are equalized line by line back up the chart and then equalized again line by line back down the chart to best acuity. If the Vectograph slide is used, the same technique is employed but prisms are, of course, not required.

12. Finally, with both eyes fusing binocularly, the patient is fogged back up to the upper line and then unfogged to best acuity and then again rechecked by either red/green or similar checking methods for the best acuity.

C. Allen used a similar technique to the author's, but placed the retinoscopy cylinder before the eye, as did Hebbard.

1. The sphere and the cylinder were left before the eye and reduced in power from the retinoscopy finding until the red/green was equal.

   a. In young people the spherical element was reduced by –0.50 or more.

   b. In presbyopes, the red was left equal to the green.

2. The cross cylinder was then used as described by the author.

3. If the cross cylinder was not responded to with reliability, Allen recommended the use of other subjective test procedures.

XVI. REFRACTION AT NEAR

A. The usual subjective routine does not concern itself with the differences which may be apparent in the correction when the accommodation and lines of sight are directed towards near vision. Many of the factors involved have been discussed in the chapter on Astigmatism. The near Rx is usually concerned essentially with determining an addition of power for presbyopia. Techniques for such additions are discussed in the chapter on Phorometry. However, since claims of variation of the amount of astigmatism particularly and even of the general Rx for near in non-presbyopes have been made, techniques have been developed for specific nearpoint testing and correction.

B. Since the limitations of lens production prevent modification of the correction for different distances, most practitioners do not see the object of attempting to determine the correction at near, as the differences in correction cannot be readily applied. However, in those instances in which the complaint is centered at the nearpoint, or in which a satisfactory prescription for distance provides little comfort at near without the incidence of accommodative difficulty, it may be necessary to determine the actual nearpoint correction and either use that or select an arbitrary compromise between the distant and nearpoint indications.

C. The simplest method for determining the astigmatic state at near is that of dynamic retinoscopy. However, this is subject to influence by the accommodative action, by the other somewhat moot factors which are involved in the procedure, and by the great possibility of error by the operator.

D. Pascal (1944) computed the variability of the astigmatic state and noted the following variations which were due to the optical properties of the eye and lens as ordinarily placed before the eye.

1. An astigmatic eye which was properly corrected for 20 feet developed a new error of astigmatism at all distances within that range.

a. The amount varied with the nature of the error, the extent of the error, the position of the correcting lens, the nearness of the object viewed, and with whether the amount of accommodation used was dependent upon the weaker or stronger principal meridian.

b. The axis varied with extortion of the eyes, cyclophoria, compensatory rotation if the head was tilted, and the plane of lens and direction of line of sight.

2. The change in power was usually low but may have reached as high as 0.50 D. The change in axis usually amounted to 5 to 10 degrees.

3. He suggested performance of the astigmatic test at an intermediate distance such as 50 cms. and also noted the axis during binocular fixation.

E. Hofstetter (1945) computed a formula which takes into account the distance of the correcting lens from the eye, the distance of the fixation object, and the power of the distance sphere in the principal meridians. From this formula a table was provided which facilitated easy computation of the astigmatic correction needed for near.

1. The calculations indicate that the significant changes applied to powers beyond the ordinary range of common prescriptions. Below are extracted those factors which would most commonly apply:

a. **TABLE XIX-3.**

Nearpoint or acc. stimulus	**Sphere**	**+5**			**0**			**−5**		
	Cylinder	**+5**	**0**	**−5**	**+5**	**0**	**−5**	**+5**	**0**	**−5**
	Distance of lens from eye									
16″ (2.50)	10 mm.	1.051	1.053	1.055	1.049	1.050	1.051	1.048	1.048	1.049
	15 mm.	1.079	1.083	1.086	1.074	1.076	1.079	1.069	1.071	1.083
	20 mm.	1.107	1.115	1.121	1.097	1.103	1.108	1.089	1.093	1.098
13″ (3.00)	10 mm.	1.062	1.064	1.066	1.059	1.061	1.062	1.057	1.058	1.059
	15 mm.	1.095	1.100	1.104	1.088	1.092	1.096	1.082	1.085	1.088
	20 mm.	1.129	1.139	1.146	1.117	1.124	1.130	1.107	1.112	1.118

b. The amount of cylinder for the given sphere was multiplied by the factor shown for the distance of the lenses from the eye and the working distance to determine the astigmatic correction at the near distance.

F. Fletcher (1954) pointed out also that near astigmatism may vary, owing to the spectacle astigmatism, independent of ocular astigmatism.

1. Spectacle astigmatism was slightly greater when the eye accommodates for a near object.

a. Young subjects may require as much as 0.50 D. more cylinder for near if the distance astigmatism is 4.00 D. or over.

2. Duke-Elder (1963) noted that due to the greater divergency of the near source, the cylinder may need to be stronger for the same effectivity at near. A + 5.00 D. cylinder at far needs to be +5.50 at near, and high astigmatic errors may need special near Rx's.

G. Bannon and Walsh (1945) have made measurements of the astigmatism at near by using a reduced reproduction of the Lancaster and Regan charts at the working distance. The status of accommodation has been maintained by the plus power indicated by the cross cylinder test at near. On the average, a +0.50 D. lens was added to the distant subjective to produce the necessary placement of the foci before the retina and the test conducted just as at the distance. The cross cylinders were also used upon both the chart and the letters at near.

1. As has been indicated by the computations of Hofstetter and Pascal, the astigmatism for near is generally greater than that for far.

2. The validity of the cross cylinder finding to establish the fog in view of the reports of Fry (1940) and others in regard to the status of accommodation during the cross cylinder tests is open to question. It appears that negative relative accommodation could disturb the position of the foci so that the results would be indefinite.

3. The results of Bannon's findings have been noted in the chapter on Astigmatism.

H. Techniques for Near Refraction

1. *Esdaile-Turville (1927)*

a. A reading card with separate lines of type parallel to each other, upon which a septum is mounted at 10 cm. from the card, is the basis of the test.

(1) The patient holds the card, and the septum permits each half to be seen by each eye separately, but simultaneously, with the peripheral field seen binocularly and serving as a fusional lock.

2. *The Turville Drum Unit (1951)*

a. This device is similar to Freeman's unit but used letters instead of Landolt C's.

3. *Lebensohn's check for near power (1949)*

a. Lebensohn used two parallel lines as a target, each 3 mm. long and 0.25 mm. wide, separated by a 1 mm. space.

b. He added a −1.00 D. sphere before the better or dominant eye if vision was equal.

c. A near reading add less +0.75 D. was placed before the eye.

(1) The patient should see three lines.

(2) Power in +0.25 D. steps was added one at a time until two distinct lines were seen.

d. The red/green rectangles, taken from a trial case, were used to perform a Duochrome test at near upon 4 pt. type.

e. If the Rx was correct for near, both a +0.25 D. or –0.25 D. lens should have been rejected as blurring the type.

4. *The Freeman Bichromatic Unit (1954) (Figure XIX-12)*

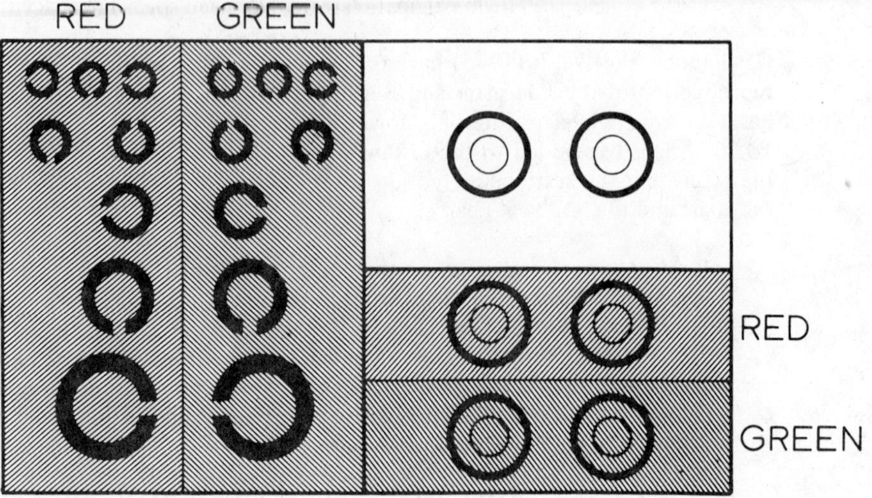

Figure XIX-12. The Freeman Bi-Chromatic Unit.

a. The unit follows the principles of the distance chart and includes targets which exhibit ordinary reading matter, Landolt rings, and duochrome and polaroid filters. The patient holds the unit in his hand at the usual nearpoint.

(1) To the right is a matched set of Landolt rings, one seen through a red and the other through a green filter.

(a) The presbyope should make the green chart out as better on the near test. Freeman makes the following assumptions:

[1] If accommodation lags behind convergence, the green will be clearer.

[2] If the accommodation overacts, the red is clearer since the presbyopes cannot adjust relative accommodation.

[3] If too much add is placed before the eye, the red is clearer and if too little, the green is clearer.

(b) Plus is added until a +0.25 D. makes the red better, and a –0.25 D. makes the green better.

(2) At the left of the chart is a panel of Landolt C's, in various sizes, for measurement of acuity at near.

(a) Polarization filters cover both halves of this chart, and using a polarizing visor, astigmia at near can be tested with the cross cylinders.

(3) At the lower right, the rings are paired and behind red and green filters. In addition, a polarizing screen can be introduced so each eye sees a separate pair of which one is red and one is green. The spheres can be equalized thereby monocularly and binocularly.

(4) An oblique tangent scale on the other side of the chart and a Maddox rod provide a means of judging vertical and lateral imbalance at the same time.

5. *The Freeman Drum Unit (1955) (Grant, 1965)*

a. This is a rotatable unit of which the first panel is identical with the first one of the bichromatic unit and is similarly used.

(1) The second panel consists of types of various sizes for checking the reading ability.

(2) The third side is an oblique tangent scale used with the Maddox rod.

(a) The position of the streak on the scale indicates both the horizontal and vertical phorias.

b. Side one can be used with polaroid for monocular checks and to balance accommodation for each eye.

c. The Worth four dot test with the polarizer is also included.

d. The Landolt C's can be used for acuity or for checking astigmatism at near with the cross cylinders.

6. *The Turville Near Balance Test (1950)*

a. The charts are reflected in an angled bisurface mirror held in a hand device at the usual nearpoint, which divides the field.

(1) The charts may be changed or placed at any distance. They consist of the usual Turville charts used at the distance but designed for nearpoint.

b. The mirror is dual and angled so that one part of the chart is reflected to one eye and the other to the other eye eliminating the need for a septum.

c. The angle of the mirror is equivalent to: $\frac{\frac{1}{2}\,\text{P.D.} \times 360^\circ}{\pi\ 2R}$

(1) The PD is the interpupillary distance, and 2R is twice the distance of the eye from the mirror.

d. The device is used to balance the spheres in presbyopia.

e. It may also be used for phoria and convergence tests.

7. *Wilmut's Near Polaroid Neutral Filter Balance Test (1951)*

a. Wilmut used a holder which carried slides and moved along a bar held by the patient by a handle before the eyes. The bar contained automatic stops at 40, 33, 25, and 20 cm.

b. Each nearpoint chart was made up of two panels with three lines on them of reduced Snellen, one panel set above the other. Either the upper or the lower panel might be seen by the patient or both might be seen simultaneously.

(1) Each chart consists of a mnemonic line for esophoria or exophoria testing, a

polarized line, O H P O, and also a third line of letters.

(2) On the upper chart, the right eye sees the PO, and the left eye sees the OH, and on the lower chart, the reverse.

(3) The unpolarized top and bottom lines act as a fusion lock.

c. If exophoria exists, one of the following occurs:

(1) The middle letters come together on the upper chart.

(2) The letters separate, with a line between them, on the lower chart.

d. If esophoria exists, one of the following occurs:

(1) The letters separate, with a line between, in the upper chart.

(2) The letters come together on the lower chart.

8. *Osterburg's Bino-Near Vision Test (Amigo, 1968)*

a. The unit is held in the hands for nearpoint positioning.

b. The device contains targets for stereopsis, the Worth test and the red/green test.

c. Polarization is used in the total technique in a similar manner as with Freeman's device.

9. *Goodlaw* (1961) developed a test at near utilizing polaroid filters and a card with a translucent polaroid target, which was illuminated from behind.

a. The targets consisted of the figures 2 and 3 under oblique polaroid, set at right angles to each other, with the 2 and the 3 placed one over the other in the center of a 10 X 10 cm. square. The borders of the squares also serve to lock fusion.

(1) As the illumination is reduced by the opaque card, the pupils dilate and reduce the depth of focus. This is revealed in a decreased range of the clear area from minus to plus blur point.

b. The device is used for revealing monocular tendencies as prism is added, as well as the usual nearpoint tests of monocularity and accommodation in a manner similar to those described for the preceding tests.

10. *Jaques*

a. Jaques employed a septum of 7 inches by 6 inches, made of white plastic, and fastened it parallel to the reading rod at the 7 inch mark, with two sets of reduced Snellen charts at 16 inches as targets.

b. He secured a monocular view of each group of letters but a binocular view of the peripheral areas.

c. He could check the astigmatism and equalize vision at near, as in the Turville or Freeman techniques.

A. Sensitometry

1. Luckiesh and Moss (1941, 1942, and 1949) developed a device for measuring the refraction subjectively which was based upon the relationship of the brightness-contrast threshold and the dioptric power of the eye. The apparatus consisted of a special target which was comprised of a uniform grey background containing a biconcave acuity target in the center. A diffuse vertical white streak of light served as a control for convergence without being a stimulus to accommodation. A gradient filter could have been introduced before either·eye. The size of the acuity target was constant but the contrast and brightness were varied by the gradient.

a. A +2.50 cylinder axis 180 is placed before the eye not tested. This obliterates the acuity target but permits the convergence control to assure fusion.

b. The gradients are reduced in density until the target is discerned.

c. Lenses in 0.50 D. steps from plus to minus 1.00 D. are introduced about the expected correction and the visibility is plotted.

d. The average visibilities when plotted should be symmetrical about an axis of maximum visibility with the apex indicating the correct dioptric power.

e. The test shows a very high reliability for repeats; the final Rx given is that permitting the highest visibility without accommodative action.

2. In a recent re-evaluation, Guth and McNelis (1969) reaffirmed the aptitude of the modified line target for sensitometric testing but noted that a disc as a target fell closer to the mean for the functional relationships of contrast and luminance applied to differently designed targets. It is necessary to distinguish between various criteria, such as detection of presence, which the disc and line meet, and discrimination of detail, which the usual test letters meet.

B. Stigmatoscopy

1. The stigmatoscopic method uses a point source of light as a target and is based upon the customary procedures of the optical bench. It is necessary to focus the point at a finite distance before the eye and hyperopes are artificially made myopic by the use of lenses. The conjugate point of the eye is determined by the smallest blur circle on the retina, represented by the finest focus of the point source. Astigmatism is measured by focusing each end of the interval of Sturm, at which positions the source appears as a fine slit or streak.

a. Bannon, et al. (1950), utilized an ophthalmo-eikonometer with half-silvered mirrors, upon whose arms slide housings containing the punctate targets. A target seen through the mirrors by both eyes is adjustable for varying fixation distances from 20 feet inward. Plus lenses are used to shorten the focal length of the eyes.

b. The targets in the sliding housings are varied for the condition of the eye.

(1) A monochromatic point is used for estimating the spherical error.

(2) Three such points in a row are used to determine the axis of the astigmatism.

(3) A single fine line is used to determine the power of the astigmatism.

(4) The dioptric power is determined by the reciprocal of the distance on the arm, the plus lens used, and other factors.

c. For a fixation distance of 20 feet, the emmetrope is found to require from –0.50 to 0.75

D. of correction. This is believed due to the spherical aberration of the eye.

d. The procedure shows a high reliability for retest and correlates highly with other methods. Although not readily adaptable to the usual clinical routine, it serves excellently for securing data concerning changes in refraction with variations of convergence; the refractive status at various fixation distances; the effect of different kinds of fixation targets; binocular as compared to monocular results; and similar laboratory accommodative-convergence experiments.

C. **Miller** (1961)

1. If a naive observer watches a single point source, as previously described under Stigmatoscopy, he can estimate the axis direction only if at least 2.75 D. of astigmatism exists. However, if the chart is rotatable, sensitivity is increased.

2. If two dots, equidistant from the center of rotation, are placed on a dial, they will form streaks. The streaks will remain parallel no matter how the dial is rotated, but as the dial is rotated, they will align with each other with great precision.

a. The best targets are monochromatic. Miller used one dot of yellow and one of green, both highly brilliant, with a low background illumination. The spots were 7 mm. in size and 38 mm. apart.

3. The tail of one colored streak should point to the tail of the other colored streak to determine the axis. If the correcting cylinder is placed 90° away, when the proper amount is reached, the dots become round. The test must be done under little or no fog so that the final sphere is not determined until the cylinder is equalized.

4. Miller actually used half a clock dial for the approximate axis, then placed his dial with the two holes in the approximate position and refined the axis with them. He used a dial which contained a V with a herringbone pattern in the V, the two spokes set 90° apart to determine the actual power. Both the V dial and the two-dot dial rotated together.

D. **Marquez** (1928)

1. Marquez used the principle of obliquely crossed cylinders and placed the retinoscopy sphere and the ophthalmometer cylinder before the eye while directing the patient to the clock dial. Cylinder was added according to the darkest line seen by the clock dial technqiue, but the resultant Rx was determined by combining the sphere and two obliquely crossed cylinders, rather than using just one. He claimed a greater sensitivity for the method.

E. **Velianoskopy** (Duke-Elder, 1963)

1. The target consists of a cross of very thin lines. A wire cross is centered before the eye and coincides in position with the target cross.

2. If there is no error, the target cross is seen slightly dimmed.

a. If a spherical error exists, the target cross arms appear doubled as if a dark shadow ran down the center of the lines.

b. With a 1.00 D. fogging lens, an interval will appear at the center of the cross.

(1) With no astigmatism before the eye, the interval appears equal in extent on both sets of lines.

(2) If astigmatism exists and the cross is placed at the correct axis, the intervals will be unequal, but the ends of the lines will be square.

(a) If the axis is incorrect, the ends have a slope.

[1] The direction of the slope will indicate the direction to rotate the crosses. The cross is rotated until both ends appear square again.

(3) Minus cylinder is added in a meridian parallel to the broadest shadow until the intervals are equal.

(4) Minus spheres are then added until the intervals or shadows disappear.

F. **Bachmaier's Technique** (1955) (Wiseman, 1955)

1. The test object consists of a wire cross emitting a red light with a bisecting line of green wire.

2. A Scheiner's disc with two apertures, one having a red filter and one a green one, is placed before the eye.

3. If emmetropia exists, the green wire bisects the red cross.

4. If ametropia exists, the green wire appears to one side of the center of the cross.

a. The wire is moved along a scale until it again bisects the cross, and the extent of movement indicates the error.

5. The apparatus can be rotated to test any meridian.

6. Advantages claimed are that the pinhole eliminates accommodation, the test distance is not critical, and no letter acuity is involved.

7. Samuel and McAlree tested the accuracy and found consistently less power than was revealed by other techniques, probably due to spherical aberration and the use of the periphery of the pupil. A correction factor of +0.37 ± 0.25 D. was needed. The variation in results at near and for distance showed that accommodation was not totally eliminated, since non-presbyopes showed +1.37 while presbyopes showed +0.216 difference in the test.

G. **Adams, Kadet, and White** (1966)

1. Four balls or diamonds, similar to a target used by Giles, made of lines which are vertical, horizontal, and oblique at 45° and 135° orientation, are used for locating the astigmatic axis and the power at far.

2. A Jackson cross cylinder test is also used on the 20/40 line.

3. The cross cylinder is finally used with the axes at 90 and 180 on an erect T chart.

4. All the results agreed closely enough to be accepted.

H. **Laser Refraction** (Knoll, 1966) (Goodwin & Thompson, 1967)

1. When coherent light from a laser hits a surface, it becomes scattered and produces real images of randomly changing interference patterns in front of the scattering surface and similar virtual images behind it.

a. The particular pattern seen is determined by the point in space conjugate to the observer's retina.

b. If the head is moved, the pattern moves with the head movement of the conjugate, if the conjugate is behind the surface, or opposite if the conjugate is in front of the surface.

c. Lenses can eliminate this movement and can neutralize the ametropia with respect to the scattering surface.

2. If the head is stationary, and the surface moves, the motion is more apparent. A slow-moving drum surface moves the pattern past the eye in the meridian of rotation of the drum.

a. In a test of 35 meridians, sensitivity for 29 was within ± 0.25 D. The test revealed more plus power in 15 of 25 meridians than did conventional methods.

3. The techniques, which can be observed by many at one time, consist of the observer viewing a small white drum with a 180° scale in back and a small opening in front. Behind the opening is a cylinder which may be turned in any axis. Its gold matte surface is illuminated by a beam of coherent light from a helium neon laser.

a. An oatmeal-like pattern of a red-light globe appears before the eyes.

(1) In myopia, the oatmeal pattern drifts towards the right and in hyperopia, towards the left.

b. One eye is occluded and the test lens added until the oatmeal pattern drifts in place.

(1) The cylinder can be rotated to different meridional positions to test for astigmatism.

c. Since the gold matte surface does not depolarize the light in reflecting it, polaroid filters and analyzers can be used to refract one eye while both eyes fuse commonly seen contours in the field of vision.

d. Baldwin and Stover (1968) found the laser as reliable and valid as ordinary subjective methods and comparable in results for adults. The technique was sensitive to changes of ± 0.25 D.

(1) It was not as utilizable as retinoscopy for a survey of children.

(2) Used at near, it seemed to reveal "with" motion, indicating that accommodation was not fully responding for the test point. It could perhaps indicate the extent of actual accommodative response.

I. **Jessen's Lighted Letters** (Jessen, 1969)

1. While not a radical departure from the usual test chart, Jessen has designed test charts for both near and far in which illuminated letters or symbols are portrayed against a black background. The charts reduce flare and are thereby reported superior for use in testing vision with contact lenses.

2. Polaroid, red-green, and the cross-cylinder are used with these in a fashion similar to techniques already described.

3. Charts for measuring lateral and vertical displacement are also available.

XVIII. DETERMINATION OF SPASTICITY

A. The criterion of a line improvement from 20/60 onward with each 0.25 D. change in the fog has been noted earlier. The patient may also report alternate blurring and clearing of the letters with the same lens. While this will not indicate the correct lens power, it is indicative of active accommodation and thus serves as a warning.

B. Specific Tests

1. *Comparison to Retinoscopy*

a. If the spherical element of the retinoscopy exceeds the subjective sphere in plus value beyond 0.50 D., there is a likelihood that the subjective does not represent the maximum correction of the eye.

2. *Punctum Remotum*

a. An artificially finite punctum remotum may be established with a plus lens. While relative accommodation may permit the target to be moved up to the focal length of this lens, if the target remains visible beyond that point, more accommodation for relaxation was available than the working distance provoked.

b. For example, if the eye were perfectly corrected and a plus 2.00 D. lens placed before it, the maximum relaxation would move the farpoint out to 20 inches. If the farpoint can be moved beyond that point, then the initial accommodation would exceed 2.00 D.

3. *Amplitude*

a. A similar test is that of measuring the amplitude of accommodation. If the amplitude is less than it should be, some of the accommodation may be in use at far.

(1) This test does not distinguish between deficiencies of the accommodative apparatus and accommodation used for the refractive state and at best would only be significant in large amounts of discrepancy.

4. *Effectivity of Lenses*

a. Since the power of a plus lens is increased as it is moved farther from the eye, the subjective correction may be moved away from the eye and the patient asked to note whether blurring of the chart occurs.

b. If the lenses can be moved away with no change in discrimination, spasticity may exist.

C. Techniques for Adding plus to the Correction

1. *Cyclodamia*

a. The technique of Dorland Smith which he called "cyclodamia" has previously been described (Bannon, 1947). It consisted essentially of correcting the eyes with the retinoscopic correction for both sphere and cylinder and then leaving the working distance before the eye while he prepared the subjective test.

b. The routine was first performed under excessive fog until the patient accepted the maximum plus which gave 20/200 vision. 2.50 D. was deducted from this amount and the balance recorded as the subjective.

c. The patient was then further unfogged until the acuity reached 20/40. 0.50 D. was deducted from this amount and the remainder was recorded as the subjective. If the resultants secured by both methods agreed, the true final Rx was assumed to have been determined.

d. The acuity was finally checked by reduction to best vision.

e. Smith classified the status of the refraction as follows:

(1) *Manifest or apparent* error was that revealed by a subjective with accommodation stable.

(2) The *full manifest* error was that revealed by the fogging method.

(3) The *static correction* was that revealed by cycloplegia.

(4) The *maximum apparent* error was that revealed by cyclodamia with better vision.

(5) The *approximate total or real* error was that revealed by cyclodamia with the poorer vision.

f. The fallacy in Smith's calculations lay in the assumption that a standard hyperfocal curve may be assumed for all eyes and extents of error and that a given amount of fog would reduce vision a standard amount. However, the technique may be considered the forerunner of many fogging and sudden blurring techniques since developed.

2. *Sudden Fog*

a. If during the routine, spastic action is suspected, a +2.00 D. lens is suddenly inserted before the lenses in front of the eye, the patient meanwhile observing a line of letters which could not be read at that moment.

b. After a few moments, the patient is directed to concentrate upon the line that he was attempting to read before the introduction of the high plus lens and the lens is suddenly removed.

c. Frequently it will be found that the line previously illegible is now read, although stubborn cases will report it visible at first and then blurring as they watch.

d. The amount may be disclosed by additions of 0.25 D. lenses to the plus and the repetition of the technique. The maximum addition through which removal of the sudden fog enables the line to be seen, even if only momentarily, represents the disclosed latency.

3. *Prism Base-In*

a. Where the binocular acuity appears poorer or requires reduction of plus to enable the patient to attain the same acuity as was attainable monocularly, it has been mentioned that exophoria inducing accommodative-convergence might be at fault. Such cases may accept more plus lens binocularly if the accommodative burden in assisting convergence is relieved by relaxing the convergence with the gradual addition of prism base in.

4. *The Dynamic or Delayed Subjective*

a. The simplest technique for disclosing the extra plus which the patient *will accept for steady wear* is the technique described by the author (1945) and also Baxter (1946), which consists of a simple combination of fogging and cyclodamia.

b. At the conclusion of the phorometry routine, the last test usually taken at near is the test of negative relative accommodation during which plus is added until nearpoint letters are blurred.

c. Leaving these lenses before the eyes, the nearpoint chart is removed and the patient's attention directed to the best line of letters seen during the subjective test, which are now badly blurred.

d. The plus lens before the eye is reduced until these letters are again visible.

(1) It is best to check this visibility point by the duochrome or other check methods used in determining the sphere during the subjective to be assured of the same degree of acuity.

e. Frequently, it will be found that the residue of this test exceeds the plus value found during the previous routine subjective.

XIX. TRIAL CASE ACCESSORIES

A. Among the other methods of determining the refractive status are special devices which are useful for specific purposes. While some of them are theoretically useful for defining the nature and extent of the refractive state, most of them are impractical but have merits which justify their employment upon occasion.

B. The Pinhole Disc (Lebensohn, 1950b)

1. The pinhole disc usually consists of an opaque disc with a 1 or 2 mm. pinhole in the center. The 2 mm. pinhole works well with bright light. A pinhole as small as 0.5 mm. will diffract enough to actually reduce acuity. Lebensohn (1950b) found a 1.32 mm. pinhole the best of a reasonably good range of sizes running from 0.94 to 1.75 mm. The standard trial case pinhole is usually 1 mm. in size.

2. The aperture of the pinhole influences the size of the blur circle formed on the retina. The finest pinhole would permit only the most central rays to enter, eliminating much of the caustic and providing a very small blur circle. Similar to the pinhole camera, which provides a fine image without actual focus of light by a lens system, the pinhole likewise tends to provide a good image without the necessity of a good focus by the ocular optical system. Consequently, it provides a good basis for determining the type of vision that a good focus should provide or whether an actual precise focus has been attained.

3. *Purposes of the disc*

a. To distinguish between causes of poor vision.
b. To check the final correction.
c. To estimate the nature and amount of refractive error.

4. *To Distinguish Between Causes of Poor Vision*

a. Whenever the entrance habitual or corrected vision is less than normal, the pinhole disc may be applied for information. Croyle (1950) used a 0.75 mm. pinhole for testing acuity better than 20/200 and a 1.0 mm. pinhole for acuity poorer than 20/200. In most cases, the pinhole is used for acuity poorer than 20/40, and the standard 1 mm. pinhole is usually employed.

b. The test is taken monocularly with the test chart exposed and the pinhole centered before the pupil of the eye. The patient may hold the pinhole himself or it may be aligned properly with his line of sight in the refractor. The illumination of the chart must be sharply increased when the pinhole is used.

(1) If the size of the patient's pupil is less than the size of the aperture of the disc or closely approximates it, the pinhole disc will not be indicative. The smaller the patient's pupil, the less value the pinhole test actually has. The better the acuity of the patient, the closer to 20/20, the less value the pinhole actually has. Presbyopes and hyperopic patients frequently present small pupils due to the accommodative effort, which not only enables their acuity to register far higher than the actual refractive status warrants, but also tends to invalidate the results of the pinhole test. The closer to the eye that the pinhole is held, the brighter the image will be and the less constricted the field of vision.

c. The conditions which may cause poor vision are the absence of a well focused image as in refractive states, amblyopia, opacities in the media, or fundus pathology.

(1) The pinhole disc will not improve vision where opacities in the media, edema of the retina, dystrophy, mature cataract, or vitreous haze exist. It likewise lowers the illumination and the resultant visual acuity in cases in which either an impaired light sense or macular lesions exist.

d. If the disc improves the vision markedly, the likelihood is that the poor vision is due to an uncorrected refractive state.

(1) Improvement alone may not rule out pathology since the poor vision may be due to a combination of pathology and refractive errors. Also, it may not indicate that lenses will likewise improve vision since the pinhole disc will give a greater improvement than lenses in cases where irregular astigmatism or conical cornea or discrete opacities exist.

e. If the disc does not improve vision, the cause of the poor vision is probably one of the conditions which will not respond to a lens.

(1) However, the cause may be amblyopia which may not respond to the pinhole but may to a lens. Also, if the initial acuity is fairly good, the introduction of the pinhole may actually reduce vision by reducing the intensity of the image. Should vision be reduced, a disc with a larger pinhole, provided it does not approach the pupil size, should be tried.

5. *To Check the Correction*

a. If the pinhole is placed before the final correction and the ametropia is properly or fully corrected, the pinhole should not improve the acuity further, but may actually reduce it due to reducing the intensity of illumination of the image.

(1) This assumes that the cause of poor vision is totally refractive.

b. If vision is further improved, the correction is not complete.

(2) If the pupil is widely dilated, the acuity may be improved even though the correction is adequate.

6. *To Estimate the Nature and Amount of the Refractive State*

a. *Holth's technique (kinescopy)*

(1) The patient is requested to hold the pinhole disc several inches in front of his eye and select a line on the chart for fixation.

(2) The pinhole is moved up and down slightly and the target observed through it for the direction of its motion.

(3) If the chart moves opposite to the movement of the disc, the error is hyperopia; if it moves with the disc, the error is myopia.

(a) The lens which causes the motion to cease corrects the ametropia.

(4) This requires a very acute observer and is useful only as a crude estimate.

(a) Emmetropes, due to spherical aberration, may also see a "with" motion.

b. The pinhole can also be used, if a cycloplegic is used in the eye, to estimate the refractive state within 0.25 D. by noting whether the size and distance of an optotype appears to be constant as the pinhole is moved away from the eye.

(1) If the size diminishes and the apparent distance increases, the condition is one of myopia.

(2) If the size increases, and the distance appears to decrease, the condition is one of hyperopia.

c. Nearpoint correction

(1) If the nearpoint target is withdrawn while the pinhole is moved before the eye until the point is reached at which the target movement apparently stops, the punctum proximum has been reached when the eye is presbyopic.

7. *Entoptic Phenomena*

a. If a bright surface is observed through a 1 mm. pinhole, an entoptic phenomenon may be revealed as the pinhole is moved about the pupillary area.

(1) Semi-transparent objects of indices greater than the media will appear as a bright object with dark outline.

(2) If the indices of the objects are less than that of the media, they will look like dark objects with bright outlines.

(3) If they are totally opaque, they will appear black.

C. The Stenopaic Slit (Croyle, 1950, and Hale, 1964)

1. The stenopaic slit consists of an aperture ranging from 0.50 cm. to 0.75 mm. in width and up to 15 mm. in length. The aperture limits the admission of light to approximately one meridian, being approximately the dimensions of a small pinhole in width.

2. It may be used practically to help determine the amount of the cylindrical state or to help determine the total refractive correction. Ordinarily it is used when the procedures of the accepted subjective tests are too confusing for the patient to interpret or when vision is so poor, due to high or mixed astigmatism, that the dials are not readily visible.

3. *Technique*

a. The patient is fogged and unfogged on the letter chart until the best possible acuity is attained.

b. The stenopaic slit is placed in front of the resultant lens and rotated until the position of best acuity is found. The meridian paralleled by the slit represents the axis of the correcting resultant minus cylinder.

(1) The slit is rotated to a position perpendicular to its best position. If astigmatism exists, this should provide poorer vision than it did in the previous position.

(2) The fog is reduced until the best possible acuity is attained. This represents a simple cylindrical correction for the meridian under test with the axis 90° from the position of the slit.

(3) The fog is restored and the slit rotated to the opposite meridian and the unfogging repeated until the same acuity is reached. The correction now represents a cylindrical correction for the second meridian.

c. By combining the two simple cylinders of d and e, a resultant sphero-cylindrical combination is produced which may be placed before the eye without the stenopaic slit.

d. The resultant can be fogged and unfogged to check that the maximum sphere has been attained. Also it is advisable to check the axis and power of the cylinder since the test introduced elements of the pinhole to the focus.

e. If irregular astigmatism exists, this device may permit the location of two oblique cylinders which can be combined to form the most useful sphero-cylindrical correction.

f. Heath (1959) recommended that the Landolt C or the letter O or a T chart be used as a target for this test, with the stem of the T chart kept parallel to the slit as it is rotated.

(1) He also suggested that the stenopaic slit can serve for retinoscopy.

g. The stenopaic slit is likewise useful for testing subnormal vision which is due to opacities, and in such cases may be attained in various widths, such as 1.5 mm., 3.0 mm. and 5.0 mm.

(1) Coulden (1950) reported a technique for irregular astigmatism, or opacities with the stenopaic slit, which was designed to differentiate pathological from physiological halos, if the latter were present.

(2) The stenopaic disc, with the slit in a vertical position, was passed before the eye.

(a) If the halo was physiological, it would split into sectors which recombine with a rotary movement as the slit passed before the pupil.

(b) If it was pathological, only a decrease in illumination would be reported.

h. The stenopaic slit could be used as a mechanical device with an inter-pupillary ruler to determine the vertex distance of the lens (Duke-Elder). The PD rule is passed through the slit, which is placed in the back cell of a trial frame, until it touches the lid. The thickness of the lid (approximately 1 mm.) needs to be added for the actual vertex distance.

D. Scheiner's Disc

1. This is a disc which contains two small pinholes spaced to fall within the average sized pupil.

2. It is used according to the geometric phenomenon observed by Scheiner, in which the entering rays are limited to small central beams so that they intersect at a plane other than their focal position, a single source provides two images.

3. Theoretically, a single source of light viewed through it will appear as a single source only if the rays are focused on the retina. If the rays are off the retina, the single light source will appear doubled, provided the light source is very small.

a. The lens which restores the source to its actual single appearance will then correct the ametropia.

b. In actual use, the device is not clinically effective.

4. Practically, this phenomenon may be employed to measure the punctum proximum of accommodation by having the patient view a small light source through the disc, while the light is brought closer to the eye. The point at which the light is seen double will indicate that the light is no longer focused on the retina and the linear distance of that point is converted into the dioptric value of the amplitude of accommodation.

a. As accommodation is stimulated, the pupil tends to constrict, and both apertures of the disc may not remain within the pupillary area. Also astigmatism may coincide with the position of the apertures producing confusing phenomena.

5. Croyle (1950) has suggested putting a colored filter before one hole of the disc and determining the refractive status by noting the position of the colored image.

a. If the colored hole is on the right of the disc, and the patient sees the same colored image on the right, which means that it is on the opposite side of the retina, myopia exists.

b. If the colored hole is seen on the opposite side to its position on the disc, which means that it is on the same side of the retina, hyperopia exists.

6. Allen (1966) devised a plastic, opaque rule (pupillometer) which contained pairs of transparent pinholes, separated vertically. Each pair was separated by an increasing increment of ½ mm. between the centers of the holes.

a. The patient viewed a bright surface with one eye with the stop held close to the cornea.

b. If the two holes appeared with a space between them, the rule containing the holes is moved towards a position where the holes were closer together. If the two holes appeared to the patient to be overlapping halos, the rule was moved until two holes were presented farther apart.

c. When a position was reached where the two holes appeared to barely touch so that the two halos made a crude figure eight, the distance which separated the centers of the two holes would measure the diameter of the pupil.

E. The Cobalt Disc

1. The disc is composed of cobalt glass which absorbs the central region of the spectrum and transmits the extremes. A white source of light will consequently be seen only by virtue of the transmitted red or blue wavelengths. These colors would form equal blur circles in the emmetropic eye when a light source located at 1.4 meters from the eye is viewed.

2. As previously noted with the duochrome test, an eye with a perfect focus would theoretically

have the yellow light focused on the retina, with the red and blue casting blur circles of approximately equal size. But if the eye is not in perfect focus, the yellow will be either in front of or behind the retina, assuming accommodation remains quiescent, and the blur circles of either the red or blue will be smaller than those of the other extreme. A white light viewed through a cobalt glass would reveal colored borders in accordance with the relative sizes of the blur circles of the two extreme wavelengths.

3. If a patient is asked to view a white light through a cobalt lens and accurately describe the appearance of the light, an interpretation of his refractive status can be made according to the following:

a. *In emmetropia* – a purple circle with light blue fringes.

b. *In hyperopia* – a blue circle with a light red border.

(1) *In simple hyperopic astigmatism* – a purple ellipse with red extremities.

(2) *In compound hyperopic astigmatism* – a blue ellipse with red extremities.

c. *In myopia* – a red circle with a light blue border.

(1) *In simple myopic astigmatism* – a purple ellipse with blue extremities.

(2) *In compound myopic astigmatism* – a red ellipse with blue extremities.

d. *In mixed astigmia* – a purple circle or ellipse with red extremities in one meridian and blue extremities in the other.

e. *In irregular astigmia* – an irregularly shaped oval of irregular coloring would appear.

4. Theoretically, the lens or lenses which restored the image to that described for emmetropia would correct the ametropia.

5. The cobalt lens may also be used as a check upon the reliability or accuracy of the final prescription to within + or –0.25 D. As described for estimating the refractive state, a small circle of white light is placed 1.4 or 1.5 mm. before the eye.

a. If too much plus has been placed in the correction, the patient will see a reddish dot with a purple fringe around it. If not enough plus or too much minus is in the correction, the patient will see a bluish central dot with a reddish border around it. If the correction appears to be accurate, he should see a purple area without the red dot in the center.

b. In cases of astigmatism, the image will appear as an ellipse, as previously noted.

6. Practically, the value of the chromatic dispersion revealed by the cobalt glass has been adapted to the standard bichrome and duochrome apparatus which has been previously described.

F. Red Lens

1. The red lens glass of the trial case may be used as a sudden interruption of fusion. It is introduced before one eye to see if diplopia is elicited.

a. Occasionally, it enables the examiner to determine if diplopia is at all possible where suppression is potential.

b. Likewise, where it does elicit diplopia, the rate of recovering single vision upon removal of the red glass may be significant.

2. It may also be used as a check for malingering where a duochrome test or a red/green chart is used. By placing the red glass before the eye seeing the green chart, visibility of the black letters can be determined for the eye suspected.

G. The Maddox Double Prism

1. The Maddox Double Prism consists of two prisms of five prism diopters power each, placed base to base so that the base line bisects the device. Images observed through it at a 6 mm. distance are separated by 60 cm.

2. It can be used to reveal a vertical deviation by noting that with both eyes exposed, three images are apparent.

a. If the central image is nearer to one of the double images seen by the eye with the Maddox Double Prism before it, a vertical deviation exists. If it bisects the double image seen by that eye, vertical orthophoria exists.

b. Similarly, if a lateral deviation is tested, the prism is placed so that the disparity is in the horizontal meridian.

c. A rotary prism can be used to attempt to align one of the units seen by the right eye to a position half way between the two images of the left eye. One of the problems that occurs with this technique is that there is a tendency to fuse one of the disparate images seen by the eye with the Maddox Double Prism before it, with the single image seen by the other eye.

XX. USE OF THE TRIAL FRAME

A. The danger of over-correction because of the limits of the testing distance has been mentioned. Also, the tendency of all techniques to force the maximum amount of plus before the eyes is obvious from the descriptions given. The student is again referred to the discussion of the habitual accommodative tendency of the average non-presbyopic hyperope under normal conditions and to note that while the full refractive correction must be determined for analytical and further purposes, the fact that a given amount of lens power may be accepted during testing or with a refractor does not insure that the same amount of power will succeed in automatically cancelling a habitual tendency to accommodate on the part of the patient through the finished spectacles.

B. In addition, the use of the refractor, while advantageous and expedient, may also place the lenses used during the test in a position which will vary from that of the lenses in spectacle form, despite efforts to adjust the instrument to a like position.

C. The author has consequently found it expedient to place in a trial frame the correction determined with the refractor, and check the patient's vision through this means on both the test letter chart and on objects seen through the window of his refracting room, located at vastly farther distances. This permits the patient to react to a more habitual set of circumstances insofar as his accommodative tendencies, the positions of the lenses on his face and the criteria of acuity are concerned. In many instances, a lens which seemed to give the sharpest vision through the refractor on the test chart must be unfogged an additional 0.25 D. before it seems to give the patient acuity at a block or so distance which is comparative to that with which the patient entered. The use of this procedure has been recommended to the writer, also, by many other practitioners.

D. In reverse, upon occasion, when the indications warrant the prescription of the maximum plus for nearpoint assistance, the procedure also surprisingly permits a lens which seems to blur slightly on the test chart to be accepted by the patient who is not too critical of long range vision.

E. The use of the trial frame in this way as the final criterion for the factors mentioned which might disturb the most careful technical examination is a procedure which assures, in the author's experience, not merely reasonable scientific accuracy, but also clinical success.

F. Fisher (1966) summarized some of the advantages of the trial frame for refining the Rx as follows:

1. A better vertex distance or one closer to that of the finished spectacles can be obtained.

2. A better Rx in situations in which torticollis may exist can be obtained.

3. Low phorias, particularly vertical ones, can be better measured with the trial frame than through the refractor.

a. The author has likewise found that where a vertical discrepancy is revealed in the rotary prisms of his refractor, it is safer, before prescribing or utilizing such a finding for prescription, to place the patient's spectacle Rx in the trial frame, direct the patient's attention to a small dot of light, and use a red glass and a Maddox rod and trial case prisms to remeasure the vertical discrepancy.

b. Usually, the amount of vertical discrepancy is less than that revealed by the rotary prisms of the refractor, and on some occasions, where a low vertical discrepancy has been revealed in the refractor, no vertical phoria is shown in the trial frame.

c. This may be due to the differences in distances between the prisms and the eye, the angle of the face of the refractor prisms, or to the fact that the trial lenses can be more accurately centered to the proper head position of the patient than in the refractor. Of course, the lenses must be centered for all patients in the trial frame, particularly when the strength of the lenses is marked.

4. Where a low visual acuity exists it is easier to demonstrate high additions and the close working range necessary for such additions.

5. It is easier to demonstrate the effects of changes in the prescription and/or orientation which may occur with them to the patient.

6. It is easier to orient cylinders, or demonstrate orientation, by either reducing the power or altering the axis position to eliminate tilts and other disturbances that sudden introductions of cylindrical powers may produce.

XXI. FACTORS AFFECTING RELIABILITY

A. Semantic Confusion

1. One of the chief causes producing error in the course of the subjective refraction is the lack of true communication between the patient and the examiner. It is common to use the terms, for example, "better" or "poorer" or "worse" as changes are made before the patient's eyes. To the patient, "better" or "poorer" or "worse" may refer to contrast, or to relative brightness, or to squareness of the chart, for example, in the cross cylinder test, rather than to the ability to see a line of smaller letters. Often, the patient watches one of the larger lines of letters and makes no attempt to read smaller letters as the lenses are changed, attempting to make his choice upon a criterion such as contrast or blackness of the letters. In the clock dial test, when the patient is asked for the blackest line, the patient may interpret blackest as synonymous with darkest, and darkest may become synonymous in his mind with dimmest or least bright. He may therefore choose that line which, rather than contrasting most greatly, has the highest amount of light reflection and contrasts poorly. It should be made clear to the patient that in tests in which the

legibility of the letters is to be the criterion, which is true when a letter or symbol dial or chart is used, the criterion is the legibility of the symbols or optotypes and not of contrast, squareness, blackness, or some other criterion the patient may choose to employ.

B. Psychological Blocks (Presberg, 1955)

1. The patient may be of the type who abhors revealing a mistake and may therefore subconsciously refuse to actually choose. Or, if he does choose, he may stick to the same choice persistently. For example, if asked continually to choose between position "one" and position "two," once having chosen position "one," he continues to stick to position "one" no matter how the changes in lenses vary the actual images.

a. In such cases, it may be better to refer in subsequent selections, to position "three" and "four," next to position "five" and "six," etc., instead of continually using the terminology "one" and "two." One of the possibilities, of course, is a semantic one. For example, in the cross cylinder, if the patient is asked to choose between the first and second positions of the cross cylinder, he may interpret the word "first" as meaning the original vision that he had before the cross cylinder was introduced, in which case, in his mind that always remains clearer than any of the subsequent choices which the cross cylinder presents to him.

2. The patient may be of the defensive type, relatively insecure, and may refuse to attempt to read past a given line in fear of making a mistake.

a. Many small children frequently exhibit this abrupt cutoff. The experienced practitioner is frequently faced with the child who has failed a school or other such similar survey test because of poor vision, but who, once his confidence is gained in the refracting room, exhibits perfectly adequate vision. The child has preferred not to attempt to answer rather than to make a mistake in front of the other children.

b. Some patients, given a choice between two blurred lines (as, for example, those which the cross cylinder presents), will refuse to choose because of the psychological transfer which makes them think that the blurred line that they have chosen represents the type of vision which their final Rx will provide them.

c. It is desirable that the patient be given to understand, in some manner, that he is perfectly able to choose wrongly without any loss of ego.

3. Part of the compensation for these factors can be provided by the techniques used in the examination. For example, rapid choices frequently cannot be demanded especially from aged patients, many children, and those who are defensive or afraid of error. The tests may have to be repeated or the opportunities for choice repeated several times. Other threshold techniques, such as reduced illumination for the measure of better acuity, or the red/green test, or other similar techniques described earlier may provide a means of avoiding necessity for psychological choice on the part of the patient. The patient should not be pressed to a point of perfection, and variations in the techniques used will allow the examiner, by himself, to perhaps make a choice from among the various answers that the patient gives him.

C. The Effect of Pathology

1. Where pathology exists, the refraction will usually vary from both the old refraction and from one refraction done at a different time from another.

a. The corneal integrity, the depth of the anterior chamber, and the iris plane for lenticular displacement or dislocation of the lens, should be checked.

(1) Concussion myopia (myopia following a blow to the eye or present sometimes in eyes of very low intra-ocular tension) may also show a change in the iris plane (see also Chapter III).

2. The refraction will often change suddenly and in a transient manner.

a. This is particularly noticeable in the presence of diabetes or of other diseases in which changes of either water or salt metabolism occur.

3. Suddenly appearing unexplained myopia should be checked specifically for either subcapsular lens opacities, the beginning of incipient cataract, or the beginning of keratoconus.

D. Some Factors to Consider in Formulating the Correction

1. The question of the necessity for the prescription of a very weak cylinder is one that is consistently pondered by the refractionist. Generally, it is considered safer to avoid the need or use of a weak cylinder unless a definite improvement in visual acuity results in its use. Even considering the sphere alone, it is generally considered safer to undercorrect rather than to overcorrect the ametropia. Where weak oblique cylinders are used, it must be remembered that even weak cylinders will produce an aniseikonic effect, and the resultant disorientation may produce more trouble than the correction is worth.

XXII. CONSIDERATIONS FOR SPECIAL CASES

A. Children (Hirsch-Wick, 1963; Herm, 1965)

1. It is noteworthy that preadolescent children seldom indicate asthenopia. Frequently, they appear in the refraction room because poor vision has been exhibited in some school or other survey, or the parents or teachers have noticed some difficulty with vision. Children whose acuity in the better eye exceeds 20/40 usually do not feel the need for prescription, and it is difficult, if one is prescribed, to make them wear the prescription. There is no need to be dogmatic in this aspect since if the ametropia is going to progress, it usually progresses identically with or without the wearing of the Rx. A child will wear the prescription as he himself feels the actual need.

a. Young children often do not attain 20/20 acuity even with a very low ametropia.

(1) High hyperopes (from 6 to 7 D.) often do not see well with or without the Rx.

(2) High astigmopes also see only to about 20/50, corrected.

(a) Such cases exhibit a condition known as *bilateral refractive amblyopia.* Sufferers from high degrees of astigmatism will often accept and wear the Rx, even though acuity is not apparently improved greatly.

(3) The anisometropes will often show no consistent pattern of acuity, except that where high monocular myopia exists, good acuity is seldom obtained in the myopic eye, even with the proper correction.

2. Wick (1963) noted that children responded with greater accuracy if tests were used which were specific as to "constant stimulus." For example, if a child was asked, "Is it blurred?" rather than "Is it blurring?" or "Is one dot above the streak?" rather than "Is it moving towards or away from the streak?"

a. The *Cover Maddox Rod technique* is a good technique for measuring phorias of children since at each exposure a fixed position of the dot and the streak is presented.

3. If the child is illiterate, it is simpler to present him with a chart using tumbled E's or Landolt C's and to place in his hands a plastic E or C and ask him to match the target rather than to name its position. Many children, as noted earlier, are chary of exhibiting ignorance or making a mistake, and rather than attempt to name an illiterate image, or picture of an object whose name or identity they are not sure of, they will prefer to pretend or act as if they cannot see it at all even though they actually do see it. With this technique, the procedure becomes a game, and even very young children of the age of three, are often able to quite assuredly match the positions on the chart, once it has been demonstrated to them with the plastic E or C.

4. For estimating the spherical changes, it is recommended that the changes be made in steps of +0.50 D. and that questions be asked in such a way that the answers can be a simple yes or no.

a. If a + 1.00 D. sphere is placed over the assumed final Rx, even the very young child should be able to observe that the targets have become blurred.

5. For the cylindrical correction, the total chart of tumbled letters, or E's or C's, should be exposed, and the child should be asked to read aloud to the best position for each position of the cross cylinder.

a. In very young children, an error of about 1.00 D. of astigmatism should exist before the ametropia is considered sufficiently significant for correction.

b. The acuity can be tested while the axis is rotated an equal number of degrees to each side of the assumed axis. If the acuity is not blurred equally upon the rotation to each side, the assumed axis is probably not correct.

c. The astigmatism should be checked both with the cross cylinder and without the cross cylinder. Acuity should be compared in both positions as follows:

(1) With the cross cylinder, the comparisons are performed as usual.

(2) Without the cross cylinder, a –0.75 D. cylinder can be placed at axis 90, or in the axis required by the error, and then rotated 90° away. The child should notice a difference in acuity with this test. If he does not, something is wrong about the assumed astigmatic correction.

6. A lack of "concordance" of the findings must be considered significant in determining the final correction.

B. The Aged (Hirsch-Wick, 1960)

1. Since the aged tend to fatigue very quickly, the examination should be done briefly and rapidly but without the impression of hurrying (Hirsch-Wick, 1960). The morning hours are generally better for elderly patients. If the findings do not seem clear, it is safer to retest again another day. During this retest procedure or during the examinaiton, individual tests should be reintroduced but the patient given sufficient time for a considered answer. Elderly patients have both good days and bad days. On some days, the patients are more tense or more worried about their vision than on others. This affects the results.

2. Generally, it is advisable to begin with the patient's old Rx and check by modifications, rather than to try to start a complete ıoutine from the beginning. Often, also, the trial frame is a better device to use than the refractor, since with it, the patient's working distance is more normal, the angle of the eyes to the lenses is an accustomed one; and the patient perhaps feels more at home and better understands what is desired.

a. As with children, it is frequently necessary to use steps of .50 D. for each change. This is usually true because the acuity itself has diminished sharply.

C. Poor Observers or Subnormal Vision (Tumblin, 1964; and Weber, 1965)

1. If astigmatic and similar dials are to be used, it is suggested that the examiner make drawings for the patient, making one line appear sharp and the others faint by blurring it with wet fingers so that the patient will know what he is expected to see.

2. The spherical component should be used following the retinoscope test, consisting of the retinoscopic spherical finding and a tentative cylinder. A cross cylinder, used on a T chart, is employed to refine the cylinder.

a. The patient can be unfogged until some of the lines of test letters can be seen at whatever distance is needed.

b. The 90 and the 180 position of the cross cylinders is preferable rather than some oblique positions.

c. The cross cylinders can be introduced and the unfogging continued until the lines reverse.

3. The patient can be referred to the letters larger than the best acuity and the correction again refined with a cross cylinder.

4. By tilting the head evidence of insurmountable phorias or diplopia can be revealed, and prisms can be prescribed as necessary for restoring single vision.

5. If the acuity is very poor, the refraction can be performed at near upon whatever charts will work, and then reduced by the working distance value.

a. The test may sometimes be repeated at different working distances.

b. The middle of the near range should be determined with the lens found and then the value of that nearpoint deducted in order to find the far Rx.

6. The cross cylinder can likewise be used for near tests.

a. The non-dominant or poorer eye should be occluded, and the tentative nearpoint Rx placed before the eye being refracted.

b. The patient should be referred to the 20/20 line on the nearpoint chart.

(1) If he cannot read it, the chart should be brought closer and the add increased by steps of +0.50 D. at a time until he can. If 20/20 is not attainable, the line of best acuity should be used for the final criterion.

(a) The additions should be reduced when this line is found, and the resultant power will constitute the near Rx for the size letter at that distance.

c. The actual add for near can be determined by taking a range of minus and plus add "blurout" and using the middle of the range for the add.

7. Another method of determining the refraction at near consists of unfogging to best acuity at

the nearpoint, introducing the T chart, and using the cross cylinder with it as has been described above for distant testing.

8. With all techniques, as with children and the aged patient, the patient should be given frequent rest periods and sufficient time to make an evaluated judgment.

REFERENCES

Abraham, S.V. (1951): Bell's Phenomenon and the Fallacy of the Occlusion Test. A.J. Oph. 14: 656.

Adams R.L.; Kadet, T.C.; and White, D.M. (1966): Comparative Study of Four Ball Cylinder Test, Jackson Cross Cylinder Test, and Near Cylinder Test. J.A.O.A., 37: 547.

Allen, M.J. (1950): Considerations of Criteria of Blur With Respect to Their Use In The Routine Examination. The O-Eye-O, 16 (2): 10.

**Allen, M.J. (1959): Cylinder Axis and Power Determination In Refraction, J.A.O.A., 30: 394.*

**Allen, M.J. (1960): Refractive Techniques At Distance And Near, New England, J. Opt., 11 (6): 137.*

Allen, M.J. (1966): Personal Communication (Pupil Measuring Device).

**Alpern, M.A. (1946): The After-Effect of Lateral Duction Testing on Subsequent Phoria Measurements. A.A.A.O., 23: 442.*

Amigo, E. (1968): Binocular Balancing Techniques, A.A.A.O., 45: 511.

Bachmaier, H. (1955): Cited by Wiseman, 1955.

Baldwin, W.R. & Stover, W.B. (1968): Observation Of Laser Standing Wave Pattern to Determine Refractive Status. A.A.A.O., 45: 143.

Banks, R.F. (1954): A Fovea Lock For Infinity Balance. Br. J. Phys. Opt., 38: 216.

**Bannon, R.E. (1946): A Study of Astigmatism at the Nearpoint With Special Reference to Astigmatic Accommodation, A.A.A.O., 26: 2.*

**Bannon, R.E. (1947): The Use of Cycloplegics in Refraction., A.A.A.O., 24: 513.*

Bannon, R.E. (1958): Recent Developments In Technique For Measuring Astigmatism, A.A.A.O., 35: 352.

Bannon, R.E. (1965): Binocular Refraction: A Survey of Various Techniques, Opt. Weekly: 56 (31): 5.

Bannon, R.E.; Cooley, F.H.; Fisher, H.M. & Textor, R.T. (1950): The Stigmatoscopy Method of Determining the Binocular Refractive Status. A.A.A.O., 27: 371.

Bannon, R.E. & Walsh, R. (1945): On Astigmatism, part III. A.A.A.O., 22: 210.

Baxter, N.M. (1946): A Suggested ''Dynamic'' Subjective Test. A.A.A.O., 23: 80.

Beach, S.J. (1948): Verified Refraction. J.A.M.A., Nov. 27.

**Berens, C. & Zuckerman, J. (1946): Diagnostic Examination Of The Eye. J.B. Lippincott Co., Phila.*

Biessels, W.J. (1967): The Cross Cylinder Simultans Test. J.A.O.A., 38: 473.

Billson, A.A. (1954): Subjective and Objective Refraction Compared. B.J. Phys. Opt., 24: 488, 619, 741.

Borish, I.M. (1945): Comments on A ''Delayed'' Subjective Test. A.A.A.O., 22: 433.

Borish, I.M. (1946): Subjective Testing. Indiana Opt. 18 (6): 5.

Borish, I.M. (1960): Comments About Subjective Refraction and the Importance of Communication. J.A.O.A., 31: 457.

Bothman, L. (1932): Homatropin and Atropin Cycloplegia: A Comparative Study. Arch. Oph. 7: 389.

Brecker, G.A.; Lewis, D. & Eastman, A.A.. (1959): Test Comparing a New With a Conventional Astigmatic Chart. A.J. Oph., 48: 118.

Brickley, P.M. and Ogle, K.N. (1953): Residual Assommocation. A.J. Oph., 36: 648.

Brungardt, T.F. (1958): Use of Turville's Subjective Technique: A Case of Anisometropia and Pseudo-Amblyopia. A.A.A.O., 35: 37.

Carter, J.H. (1966): Sensitivity Variations in The Jackson Crossed Cylinder Axis Test. Opt. Weekly, 575 (28): 29.

Carter, J.H. (1966-67): On The Significance Of Axis Error, Alumni Bull. Penn. Coll. Opt., 20 (3).

**Coole, W.A. (1952): Control of Accommodation In Subjective Routine Refraction. Br. J. Phys. Opt. 9: 161.*

Copeland, J.C. (1942): Locating the Astigmatic Axis Under Binocular Fixation. Ten Years of Optical Developments, Riggs Opt. Co.

Copeland, J.C. (1944): Personal Communication-Cross Cylinders.

Coulden, A.P. (1950): Useful Aids In Difficult Refractions. Opt., 120: 259.

**Cowen, L. (1954): Binocular Refraction. B.J. Phys. Opt. 16: 60.*

Cowen, L. (1955): Binocular Refraction – A New Application of Polaroid. Optician, Nov. 25.

Cowen, L. (1959): Binocular Refraction – A Simplified Clinical Routine. B.J. Phys. Opt. 16: 60.

**Crisp, W.H. & Stine, G.H. (1950): A Further Very Delicate Test For Astigmatic Axis Using The Cross Cylinder with an Astigmatic Dial and Without Use of a Letter Chart. Am. J. Ophth., 33: 1587.*

Croyle, F.V.N. (1950): The Pinhole or Stenopaic Opening. Opt., 119: 545.

Davies, P.H. O'C' (1957): A Critical Analysis of Bichromatic Tests Used In Clinical Refraction. B.J. Phys. Opt., 14: 170.

**Diamond, S. (1950): Pathology of The Refracting Media Which Influence the Refraction of the Eye, Australasian J. Opt., 33: 345.*

Duke-Elder, S.W. (1963): The Practice of Refraction, 7th ed., C.V. Mosby Co., St. Louis.

**Eastman, A.A. & Guth, S. (1958): A New Astigmatic Test Chart. A.A.A.O., 35: 461.*

**Elleman, H. (1950): A New Astigmatic Chart. Opt., 119: 551.*

Elom, F.T. (1954): The Results of Prescribing Prism From The Turville Test. Calif. Optom: p. 242.

**Emsley, H.H. (1944): Visual Optics. Hatton Press, Ltd., London.*

**Eskridge, J.B. (1958): The Raubitschek Astigmatism Test. A.A.A.O., 35: 238.*

Fernandez, R.H.P.; Edmunds, J.P. & Hunt, T.A. (1955): Binocular Diaphragm To Gain A Central Binocular Area. B.J. Phys. Opt., 39: 343.

Fisher, E.J. (1966): The Trial Case and Optometry. Opt. Weekly, 57: 33.

**Fletcher, R. (1954): Near Vision Astigmatism. Opt., 127: 341.*

Flom, M.C. (1966): New Concepts In Visual Acuity. Opt. Weekly, 57S

(28): 44.
Flom, M.C. & Goodwin, H.C. (1964): Fogging Lenses: Differential Acuity Responses In The Two Eyes. A.A.A.O., 41: 388.
Frantz, D.A. (1966): A Review of Three Dimensional Refraction. Opt. Weekly, 57 (1): 23.
*Freeman, H. (1954): Bichromatic Methods and Near Vision Refraction. O.J.R.O., 91 (16): 27.
Freeman, H. (1955): Working Method – Subjective Refraction. B.J. Phys. Opt., 12: 20.
Freeman, H. & Purdom, G. (1950): Analysis of the Cross-cylinder, Opt., 120: 375.
Fry, G.A. (1940): Significance of The Fused Cross Cylinder Test. Opt. Weekly, 31 (1): 16.
Garbus, J. (1949): Relative Merits of Cycloplegia and Manifest Refraction. Opt. Weekly, 40: 713.
Gentsch, L.W. & Goodwin, H.E. (1966): A Comparison of Methods For The Determination of Binocular Refractive Balance. A.A.A.O., 43: 658.
*Gettes, B.C. & Belmont, O. (1961): Tropicamide: Comparative Cycloplegic Effects. Arch. Oph. 66: 336.
Giles, G.H. (1965): The Principles and Practice of Refraction and Allied Subjects, 2nd ed., Chilton Co., Phila.
Goodlaw, E. (1961): A New Test For Binocular Refraction at The Near Point Working Distance. A.A.A.O., 38: 420.
Goodwin, H.E. (1966): Optometric Determination of Balanced Binocular Refractive Corrections. Opt. Weekly Suppl. 57: 47.
Goodwin, H.E. & Thompson, J. V. (1967): Theory of the Laser Optometer Opt. Weekly, 58 (52): 15.
Grant, J.E. (1965): A Survey of Some Methods of Refraction. Oph. Opt., 5: 387.
Grolman, B. (1966): Binocular Refraction: A new system. New Eng. J. Optom., 17 (5): 118.
Guth, S.K. & McNelis, J.F. (1969): Threshold Contrast As A Function of Target Complexity, A.A.A.O., 46: 491.
Haase, H.J. (1961): Complete Determination of Eyeglasses with Polatest. Werkzeitschrift 34: 8.
Haase, H.J. (1962): Binocular Testing and Distance Correction With the Berlin Polatest, (trans. by W. Baldwin in J.A.O.A., 34: 115.
Hale, J.R. (1954): Stereoscopic Vision. Opt. Weekly, 45: 1003.
*Haynes, P.R. (1955 & 1956): Use Of A Simultaneous Stimulus Situation With The Cross Cylinder For The Measurement of Astigmatism. Presented before the American Academy Of Optometry, North Carolina Section, Winston Salem, N.C., March, 1955; and before the Ohio Optometric Association, Cleveland, Ohio, 1956.
Haynes, P.R. (1957): A Homokonic Cross Cylinder For Refractive Procedures. A.A.A.O., 34: 478.
Haynes, P.R. (1958): Configuration and Orientation of Test Patterns Used With the Homokonic C.C. For Measurement of Astigmatism. A.A.A.O., 35: 637.
Heath, G.G. (1959): The Student Clinican. Indiana J. Opt., 29: 6.
Heath, G.G. (1964): Personal Communication.
Hebbard, F.W. (1967): Personal Lecture Notes, The Ohio State University.
Herm, R.J. (1965): Refraction of Children: I.O.C., 5.
Hirsch, M.J. & Wick, R.E. (1960): Vision of The Aging Patient, Chilton Books, Phila.
Hirsch, M.J. & Wick, R.E. (1963): Vision Of Children. Chilton Books, Phila.
Hofstetter, H.W. (1945): The Correction Of Astigmatism For Near Work. A.A.A.O., 22: 121.
Holth, Cited by Lebensohn, J.E., Editorial "The Pinhole Test," A.J. Oph., 33: 1612, 1950.
Hughes, W.L. (1941): Changes of Axis of Astigmatism in Accommodation. Arch. Oph. 26: 742.
Humphriss, D. (1963): The Refraction of Binocular Vision, Ophthalmic Optician, 3 (19) 987.
Humphriss, D. & Woodruff, E.W. (1962): Refraction By Immediate Contrast. B.J. Phys. Opt., 19: 15.
Jackson, E. (1930): How To Use The Cross Cylinder, A.J. Oph., 13: 321.
Jackson, E. (1932): The Astigmatic Lens (Crossed Cylinder) reprinted in Optical Developments, August.
Jaques, L. (1958): A True Macular Vision Test for Nearpoint. Instruction Booklet for Jaques Septum and Nearpoint Tests. Opt. Weekly, 48: 2297.
Jessen, G.N. (1969): Refraction With Lights Instead Of Shadows, A.A.A.O., 45: 667.
Knoll, H.A. (1966): Measuring Ametropia With A Gas Laser. A.A.A.O., 43: 415.
*Landolt, E. (1866): Refraction and Accommodation of the Eye. (Trans. E.M. Culver.)
*Laurance, L. (1926): Visual Optics and Sight Testing. 3rd Ed., School of Optics, Ltd., London.
*Lebensohn, J.E. (1936): Scientific and Practical Considerations Involved in the Near Vision Test with Presentation of a Practical and Informative Near Vision Chart. A.J. Oph., 19: 110.
Lebensohn, J.E. (1949a): Practical Problems Pertaining To Presbyopia. A.J. Oph., 32: 22.
*Lebensohn, J.E. (1949b): A Simplified Astigmometer. A.J. Oph. 32: 128.
Lebensohn, J.E. (1950a): A Simplified Astigmometer. Arch. Oph., 43: 905.
Lebensoh, J.E. (1950b): The Pinhole Test. A.J. Oph., 33: 1612.
Lebensohn, J.E. (1958a): Visual Acuity Tests for Near, Implication and Correlation. A.J. Oph. 45 (4, Pt. 2): 127.
Lienberger, E. (1949): Some Points on Correcting Astigmatism. Opt., 118: 515.
Lindsay, J. (1954): A Theoretical Investigation Into The Possibilities of Error In Measurement of Astigmatism By The Cross Cylinders. B.J. Phys. Opt., 11: 210.
Linksz, A. (1942): Determination of The Axis and Amount of Astigmatic Error by Rotation of The Trial Cylinder. Arch. Oph., 28: 632.
Lloyd, G.P. (1950): The Turville Infinity Balance Technique. S. African Opt. 17: 22.
Luckiesh, M. & Guth, S. (1949): A Sensitometric Method of Refraction – Theory and Method. A.A.A.O., 26: 367.
*Luckiesh, M. & Moss, F.K. (1940): New Methods of Subjective Refraction Involving Techniques in Static and in Dynamic Tests. Arch. Oph. 23: 941.
Luckiesh, M. & Moss, F.K. (1941a): A New Method of Subjective Refraction At The Nearpoint. A.A.A.O., 18: 249.
*Luckiesh, M. & Moss, F.K. (1941b): Characteristics of Sensitometric Refraction. Arch. Oph., 24: 423.
Luckiesh, M. & Moss, F.K. (1942): The Measurement of Visibility. J. Aeron. Sciences, January.
*Luckiesh, M. & Moss, F.K. (1943): Comparison of a New Sensitometric Method with Usual Techniques of Refraction. Arch. Oph., 30: 489.
*Mallett, R.F.J. (1966a): Fixation Disparity Test For Distant Use. Opt. 152: 1.
*Mallett, R.F.J. (1966b): The Investigation of Oculo-motor Imbalance. Oph. Opt., pt. 1: 6 (12): 586; pt. 2: 6 (13): 654.
Mandell, R.B. & Allen, M.J. (1960): The Causes of Bichrome Test Failure. J.A.O.A., 31: 531.
Marano, J.A. (1958): Color Mixing: A New Method For Testing Astigmatism. Opt. Weekly, 49: 1400.
Marano, J.A. (1959): Color Vision In Astigmatism. Opt. Weekly, 50: 1457.
Marano, J.A. (1962): Subjective Astig-

matism Determined In Minutes. Opt. Weekly, 53: 635.

Mark, H.H. (1962): On Accuracy of Accommodation. B.J. Oph., 46: 742.

Marquez, M. (1928): Lecciones de Opttalmolgia Clinic Julio Casano, Madrid. (Cited by Raubitschek, 1952.)

Matsuura, T.T. (1961): The Matsuura Auto Cross. Opt. Weekly, 52: 2153.

Miller, R.G. (1961): A New Test For Astigmatism: A Preliminary Report. A.A.A.O., 38: 681.

Morgan, M.W. (1949): The Turville Infinity Binocular Balance Test. A.A.A.O., 26: 231.

Morgan, M.W. (1960): The Turville Infinity Binocular Balance Test. J.A.O.A., 31: 447.

*Morgan, M.W. (1968): Accommodation And Convergence – 4th Prentice Lecture Am. Acad. of Optom. 45: 417.

Morgan, M.W. & Peters, H. – personal communication anent Turville technique.

Morris, G.G. (1950): Cycloplegia and Refraction. Australasian J. Optom., Jan. 30, 1249.

Murrell, S.C. (1955): An Evaluation of The Bichrome Test. N. Carol. Optom., July-August.

Norman, S.L. (1950): Binocular Subjective Refraction With The Polaroid Occluder. Opt. Weekly, 41: 1657.

O'Brien, J.W. & Bannon, R.E. (1948): Fogging Method – Comparative Analysis. A.J. Oph., 31: 1453.

Pascal, J.I. (1940): Fundamental Differences Between Crossed Cylinders and Line Chart Astigmatic Test Arch. Oph., 24: 722.

Pascal, J.I. (1941): The Jackson Crossed Cylinder. Arch. Oph., 25: 355.

Pascal, J.I. (1944): Intrinsic Variability of Astigmatic Errors. Arch. Oph., 32: 123.

Pascal, J.I., (1950): The Cross Cylinder Versus The Rotating Cylinder. Opt. World, 42 (7): 26.

Pascal, J.I. (1950): Cross Cylinder Tests – Meridional Balance Technique. O.J.R.O., 87 (18): 31.

Pascal, J.I. (1952a): The V Test For Astigmatism. O.J.R.O., 89 (4): 35.

*Pascal, J.I, (1952b): Studies In Visual Optics. C.V. Mosby Co., St. Louis.

*Pascal, J.I. (1953): The Pascal-Raubitschek Test For Astigmatism. J.A.O.A., 25: 491.

*Pascal, J.I. (1954a): The Preliminary Sphere In The Meridional Balance Technique. Opt. World, 42 (7): 26.

*Pascal, J.I. (1954b): Basis Of Objective and Subjective Cross Cylinder Tests. Opt. World, 42 (4): 18.

Pease, P.L. & Allen, M.J. (1967): New Contrast Visual Acuity and The Effect Of Ambient Illumination, Filters and Scatter. A.A.A.O., 44: 226.

Pech, J.L. (1933): Physiologic and Clinical Values of Chromatic Aberrations of The Eye, (trans. in Studies of Duochrome Refraction, B & L Opt. Co.).

Phillips, R.C. (1964): Stereo-Refraction. Penn. Optom., July-August, p. 9.

Posner, A. (1951): The Head Tilt For Astigmatism. A.J. Oph., 34: 1169.

Presberg, M.H. (1955): Psychologic Factors In Refraction. A.J. Oph., 39: 566.

*Raubitschek, E. (1952): The Raubitschek Arrow Test For Astigmatism. A.J. Oph., 35: 1334.

Rengstorff, R.H. (1966): Observed Effects of Cycloplegia On Refractive Findings. J.A.O.A., 37: 360.

Rosenberg, R. and Sherman, A. (1968): Vectographic Projecto Chart Slides, J.A.O.A., 39: 11.

Samuel, C.H. and McAtree, L.G. (1957): Investigation of a New Method of Subjective Refraction. Opt. Weekly.

Saul, R.J. (1955): Binocular Techniques. Opt. J. & Review, 192 (2): 88.

Schneller, S.A. (1966): The Colorless Bichrome – A Distance Cross Cylinder Test. Opt. Weekly, 57 (7): 38.

Schuman, M.N. (1964): Thesis on Marano Chart – Personal Communication.

*Sheard, C. (1923): A Dozen Worthwhile Points in Ocular Refraction. A.J. Phys. Opt., 4: 443.

Shlaifer, A. (1949): Cycloplegia – A Review of Its Use and Status In Refractive Practice. Penn. Coll. Optom. Alumni Bull., April.

Smith, Dorland (1930): The Estimation of the Total Refractive Error Without a Cycloplegic. Trans. Am. Acad. Oph. & Otol. 101: 127.

Sugar, S.H. (1944): Binocular Refraction with Cross Cylinder Technique. Arch. Oph. 31: 34.

Tait, E.F. & Sinn, F.W. (1936): The Effect On Ciliary Tonus Of Homatropine. A.A.A.O., 13: 140.

*Thorington, J. (1939): Refraction of the Human Eye and Methods of Estimating Refraction. P. Blakiston Co., Inc., Phila.

Tour, R.L. (1965): Astigmatism in Refraction, I.O.C., 5 (2).

Tumblin, J. (1964): Radical Refraction – presented to Tenn. Acad. Optom.

Turville, A.E. (1946): Outline of Infinity Balance. Raphael's Limited, Hatton Garden, London.

*Turville, A.E. (1950): Modern Developments In Subjective Refraction Technique. Optics, 90: 1.

*Turville, A.E. (1951): Some Recent Experiments On Infinity Balance. Trans. Int. Opt. Congress, London.

*Van Noorden, G.K. & Lipsius, R.M.C. (1964): Experiences With Pleoptics in 58 Patients With Strabismic Amblyopia. A.J. Oph., 58: 41.

Walton, W.G. (1951): Compensating Cyclo-torsion and Visual Acuity. A.A.A.O., 28: 84.

Warman, J.R. (1950): The Correction of Low Astigmatism. Opt., 119: 429.

Weber, J.M. (1965): How To Elicit Reliable Responses in The Subjective Examination of Poor Observers. A.A.A.O., 42: 732.

Wick, R.E. (1960): The Management of the Aging Patient in Optometric Practice, Hirsch and Wick, Vision of the Aged, Chilton Books, Phila.

Wick, R.E. (1963): Hirsch and Wick, Vision of Children, Chilton Books, Phila.

Williamson-Nobel, F.A. (1946): A Possible Fallacy In The Use Of The Cross Cylinder. Reprinted in Optical Developments, January.

Wilmut, E.B. (1951): The Use of Polarizing Filters For Infinity Balance Examination and Near Correction. Trans. Int. Opt. Congress, London.

Wiseman, K. (1955): A New Subjective Method Entirely Independent of Patient's Visual Acuity. O.J.R.O., Dec. 1, p. 34.

*Worfold, L. (1950): Binocular Refraction. Australian J. Opt., 33: 201.

Phorometry 20

I. INTRODUCTION

A. Those tests which deal with the determination of the power of accommodation and convergence, and particularly with the action of the two in relation to each other, may be loosely grouped under the common heading of phorometric tests. While specific devices other than the phorometer or refractor have been developed and can be applied to the determination of specific findings, and even trial case prisms can be used for some of them, the most efficient, smooth-flowing and commonly employed techniques involve the use of the rotary prisms which constitute the chief feature of the modern phorometer.

B. Mirror phorometers and stereoscopic devices are also employed, and usually with greater exactitude for laboratory and research investigations, but the prism phorometer remains the device of customary clinical usage with results reasonably accurate for most purposes and with a technique more readily understood by the untrained observer comprising the average patient.

C. Because the phorometer is employed for most tests which deal with the accommodative-convergence relationship, even such accessory tests as do not require the rotary prism, or could be performed as accurately and easily with other devices, are grouped and discussed in this same chapter.

D. Certain tests which properly are of concern in the consideration of accommodation and convergence, such as the nearpoint of convergence and the rotations and versions, have been considered previously because of their better placement in the routine.

II. TESTS

A. The customary phorometric tests include tests primarily activating convergence and tests primarily directed towards altering the stimuli to accommodation. In the chapter discussing the relationship between the two, it has been pointed out that some tests which apparently influence one, actually involve the other because of the association between them. However, for the sake of ready distinction, the tests may be segregated not by the function actually involved, but by the function towards which the change in stimulus is directed, although the student must keep in mind that the obvious response to the stimulus may not necessarily be the correctly interpreted one. By this criterion, the tests may be divided into several categories, as follows: (numerical symbols, used to identify the different tests in the widely used Optometric Extension Program are listed in parenthesis after certain applicable tests.)

B. Tests involving an alteration of the stimulus to convergence

1. *Phoria Tests at Near and Far*

   a. *Lateral phoria at far* (No. 3, No. 8)
   b. *Vertical phoria at far* (No. 12)
   c. *Lateral phoria at near* (No. 13A, 13B, 15A, 15B)
      (1) Known as Fusional Supplementary Convergence (F.S.C.)
   d. *Vertical phoria at near* (No. 18)

2. *Duction (Vergence) Tests at Near and Far*

   a. *True adduction or advergence (at far)* (No. 9)
   b. *Convergence (at far)* (No. 10)
   c. *Abduction or abvergence (at far)* (No. 11)
   d. *Positive Relative Convergence (at near)* (No. 16A)
      (1) P. R. C.
   e. *Positive Fusional Reserve (at near)* (No. 16B)
      (1) P. F. R.
   f. *Negative Relative Convergence (at near)* (No. 17A)
      (1) N. R. C.
   g. *Negative Fusional Reserve (at near)* (No. 17B)
      (1) N. F. R.
   h. *Vertical Ductions or Vergences (at far and near)* (No. 12, 18)

C. Tests involving a change of stimulus to accommodation

1. *Tests of Indefinite Response*

   a. *Dissociated or monocular cross cylinder* (No. 14A)
   b. *Binocular cross cylinder* (No. 14B)

2. *Tests of Definite Response*

   a. *Amplitude of Accommodation* (No. 19)
   b. *Positive Relative Accommodation* (No. 20)
      (1) P. R. A.
   c. *Negative Relative Accommodation* (No. 21)
      (1) N.R.A.

D. Other Tests

1. Gradient Test
2. Fusional Recovery Test
3. Cyclophoria Tests
4. Stereopsis

III. PHORIA TESTING

A. The phoria test is designed primarily to indicate the position of rest of the eyes when fusional convergence is relaxed. To accomplish that purpose, the so-called fusion impulse must be suspended. This can only be accomplished by the presentation of targets so designed that no similarity exists between the images received by each eye, or by placing the targets in such a manner that both cannot fall within the fusion fields of the two eyes at the same time. Under such circumstances, provided accommodation is not in use, only the tonic convergence remains active, hence phoria tests are also frequently termed tonicity tests.

1. If fusion is completely dissociated, as is done in the usual clinical phoria tests, the phoria disclosed is known as the "dissociated phoria." It is this phoria which is commonly referred to simply as the "phoria" in most phorometric procedures. If some form of fusional stimulus is maintained, as is employed in the derivation of the phoria by means of disparity tests, the phoria is then known as the "associated phoria."

a. As shown in studies by Ogle, Martens and Dyer (1967), these two need not agree and may actually be contradictory in individual cases.

B. Dissociated Phoria Techniques

1. Various techniques, based upon varying methods of interrupting fusion, are used. The most common ones are described below. In some instances, the variation in technique involves not so much a different means of dissociation as a different method of measuring the result.

2. Scobee (1952) summarizes the ideal conditions of the ideal test for heterophoria.

a. The patient should be rendered emmetropic and must have been in that state long enough to possess a normal accommodative-convergence ratio. Scobee estimates that for the perfect result, the correction should have been worn a month before the test.

b. He should be in a normal state of physical fitness and unaffected by fatigue, illness, etc.

c. The test should not involve apparatus which precludes relaxation or be so dull as to decrease attentiveness.

d. Head and body should be in the primary position and should not be subject to postural strain.

e. Fixation of the dissociated eye should not be stimulated, the background should be free of marks or figures which would either confuse the patient or incite a fusional impulse.

f. The conditions of the test must be reproducible by other observers or the same observer on different occasions.

3. It is obvious that the ideal test conditions are seldom met in the ordinary routine. However, Hofstetter (1952) points out that two primary conditions must be met in the choice of a phoria test procedure. One, the test must have repeatability – the results must be comparable if taken at different occasions or by different examiners; two, the test must have validity – a variation of conditions should produce a consistent variation of the response, and the order of response should be compatible with the indications of other tests. Hirsch (1948) also adds that the test should be easy to administer, and if taken at the nearpoint, should require accommodation to a consistent extent equal to the reciprocal of the test distance.

a. Morgan (1960) found that tests for the distance phoria showed a high reliability even when the time interval between tests was many years.

(1) *Reliability* would indicate that the test measured the same thing each time, while *validity* would indicate whether it measured what it was supposed to measure.

b. Morgan (1955) divides the sources of error in the test procedures for all tests as:

(1) *Systemic* – due to errors built into the device itself or inherent in the device used.

(2) *Personal*

(a) Poor judgment on the part of the patient
(b) Poor timing of the test (too quick or slow)
(c) Pre-judgment by the examiner to conform to a theory or to the calibration system of the device.

(3) *Mistakes*

(4) *Random errors* – the sum of a number of small variations due to uncontrollable variables.

c. The errors in measurement of distant heterophorias were found to be approximately 1.5 prism diopters. The standard deviation varied from ± 1.1 PD to ± 2.8 PD with the mean S.D. ± 1.5 PD and a variance of about 2.3 PD.

4. In the endeavor to meet the conditions of the ideal test, a great number of diverse modifications have been developed, varying from simple or little equipment to devices specially contrived for the sole purpose of making a measurement. These devices fall into four groupings:

a. Tests which exclude the field of view of one eye from the other eye, as the cover test, the Maddox Wing test, the amblyscope, polaroid, and rod septums, etc.

b. Tests which dissociate by distorting one image, as the Maddox rod test.

c. Tests which dissociate by displacing the images, as the Von Graefe test.

d. Tests which utilize after images, as the Bielschowsky tangent test.

5. Various investigators have checked the common phoria tests for repeatability, reliability, and for comparisons of test to test. Scobee and Green (1951) considering the cover test as the ideal test, despite the finding of Ludvigh (1948) and others, that the test does not appear reliably measurable within 1 or 2 Δ, statistically compared various standard phoria tests to the cover test. They disclosed the following correlation coefficients:

a. TABLE XX-1

At twenty feet:		At 13 inches:	
Von Graefe test	*+.82*	*Von Graefe test*	*+.72*
Maddox screen test	*+.81*	*Maddox screen*	*+.48*
Maddox rod test	*+.81*	*Maddox wing*	*+.68*
		Thorington	*+.77*

b. For phorias at 20 ft. with the Maddox rod test, a reliability coefficient of +.95 for lateral and +.92 for vertical was found. This seems to indicate that if the test conditions are controlled, the phoria finding is exceedingly reliable and unvarying from one time to the next. However, the screen Maddox rod test appeared unreliable at nearpoint. Intermittant screening uncovered less phoria than no screening.

(1) Hirsch (1948) and Hirsch and Bing (1948) in a further study likewise found a

high reliability for the phoria at nearpoint taken by the Von Graefe method (with a large E and with fine type) and a Thorington test modified as described later. The cover test, screen Maddox rod, and Maddox wing did not meet the necessary criteria for nearpoint tests. Hirsch found the modified Thorington even more reliable than the von Graefe with better control of accommodation and greater repeatability. The modified Thorington gave the highest repeatability finding, although it also produced a lower actual value. This might be due to either the fact that readings from prisms are greater than the actual prismatic effect of the prism, or partly due to the fact that the Thorington test made a greater demand upon accommodation. Illumination did not appear important.

(2) Goodlaw (1961) likewise found the modified Thorington more reliable than the screen Maddox rod test or the red-green test.

(3) Weymouth (1963) also compared the results of the von Graefe, the Maddox rod, and parallax tests and found little difference in the results if accurately done.

(4) Soderberg (1968) reported a coeffficient of correlation between the Von Graefe test and the Maddox rod, upon 100 subjects, of .9375 for the far tests, and .913 for the near tests.

(a) He used the rod and prism upon opposite eyes with the Maddox rod test, and the cover-uncover technique for both the Von Graefe and Maddox rod at near.

c. Other investigations have been made of the effects which minor variations in technique produce upon the results. Thus Green and Scobee (1951) investigated the Maddox rod test in regard to the effect which the rod and prism before the same eye produced as compared to the rod before one eye and the prism before the other. The differences for lateral phorias were very slight but for vertical phorias they recommend that the technique used be specified with the finding. Bedrossian, (1952) checking the effects of utilizing a red glass, notes that red and white images most successfully interrupt fusion, while red and blue ones tend to fuse. Scobee and Green (1951) also investigated the use of a red as compared to a white Maddox rod and noted that a red Maddox rod reveals more esophoria or less exophoria than does a white one, possibly because of the fact that the eye is hyperopic for red, and accommodates when it is used. Also, the size of the streak of the Maddox rod test at near does not appear to influence the test, although Hirsch (1948) found that with the von Graefe test at near, a difference due to accommodative demand existed in performing the test when the target was a large E as compared to a fine fixation target.

(1) The effect of accommodation on the phoria was tested by Daugherty and Geraci by varying the prism in fixation from one eye to the other in both anisometropes and isometropes. A significant difference was revealed only when the anisometropia exceeded 2 sigmas. Sloan and Rowland (1951) also found that the optical stimulation of the testing distance was not a significant source of error.

(a) However the Gradient Test reveals a definite response in most cases to accommodation at least at the near test point.

(2) Weymouth (1963) comments that a totally dark room or unfigured wall is desirable. Sloan and Rowland emphasized that test targets should be seen against a uniform, dark background.

(a) Maddox recommended that 4 foot candles be used for the Maddox rod test. Soderberg (1968) comments that if the room is totally dark, the apparent streak appears to be close to the eye and stimulates psychic convergence.

(3) Morgan (1955) suggests that the test be performed by occluding one eye to further disrupt fusion; then expose and note the position of the targets; occlude and add prism; expose and note if a closer alignment exists; occlude and add prism; repeat the steps until the targets are aligned upon exposure.

IV. LATERAL AND VERTICAL PHORIAS

A. The patient is correctly seated behind the refractor at the conclusion of the subjective technique. The distant test chart is presented.

B. Von Graefe Technique (Figure XX-1).

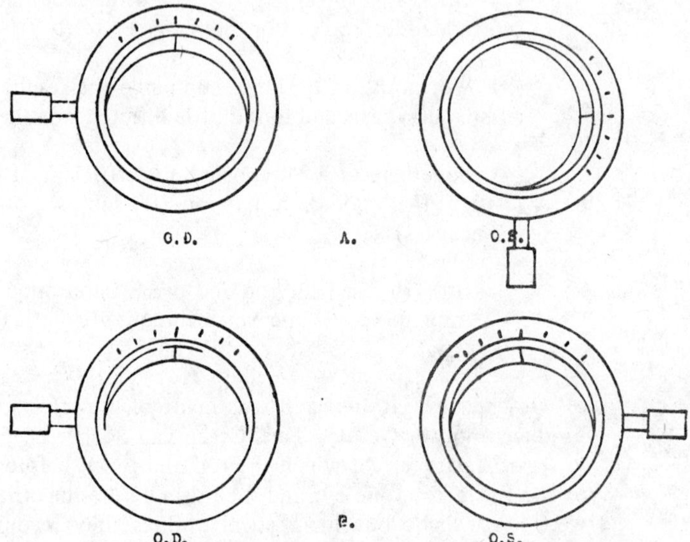

Figure XX-1 – Rotary prisms in position for phoria and duction tests (seen from in front). (A) Prisms in position for phoria tests; prism before right eye measures lateral phoria, while O.S. prism dissociates; O.D. prism dissociates for vertical phoria, while O.S. prism measures. (B) Prisms in position for lateral ductions, either base-out or base-in.

1. *Lateral Phoria*

a. The most commonly used technique and one which is suitable for both near and farpoint testing is that which employs a dissociating prism over one eye and a measuring prism over the other.

b. The rotary prisms are placed before the eyes so that the prism before the right eye can be turned either base-out or base-in, while that before the left eye can be turned either base-up or base-down.

c. A single line of test type of best acuity is presented on the distant test chart. This line may be used for both the lateral and vertical phoria.

(1) Some clinicians prefer to employ an isolated letter or a horizontal row for the vertical tests and a vertical row for the horizontal tests. The results do not differ too greatly since, in most cases, it is impossible to obscure the margins of the chart itself, which act as peripheral incentives to fusion. Consequently, a totally dissociated state is not actually achieved under ordinary clinical conditions, but the practical results are sufficiently useful despite that flaw if proper technique is employed.

d. The prism over the left eye is turned to an extent of 5 or 6 prism diopters base-up. This places the image on the retina of that eye above the upper limits of the useful fusion field and projects the line of letters below that seen by the right eye, producing dissociation.

(1) If a vertical phoria exists coincident with the direction of the dissociating prism, the amount may be insufficient to produce diplopia. If the patient does not report diplopia, the prism should be increased in amount until he does. A patient who suppresses vision in one eye may not report diplopia even with large amounts of prism. Such patients must be handled in a different manner.

e. As the eyes assume the phoric position, the two images will drift apart in a lateral direction. The measuring prism before the right eye is now turned to its full extent base-in (towards the nose), displacing the image of the right eye towards the patient's right.

(1) Should there be a very large exophoria, the amount of power of the rotary prism may be insufficient to move the target to the right of the lower one. In such cases additional prism base-in will be required, either from the trial case or the fixed prism powers of the refractor battery.

f. The patient can now be informed that two images exist, the upper of which is to the right of the lower. He is requested to notify the examiner when he observes the upper target precisely above the lower one.

g. The prism base-in before the right eye is slowly reduced until the patient has aligned them.

(1) If the residual prism before the right eye is 0, the condition is orthophoria; if the prism base is in, the condition is exophoria to the amount indicated on the prism scale; if the prism base is out, the condition is esophoria to the amount indicated.

h. Since the chart acts upon the peripheral fusional impulses, it is advisable to repeat the test, but this time the measuring prism is turned base-out, moving the upper target to the left of the lower one. The same procedure is followed, the prism being reduced until the two targets are aligned one above the other. An average of the two readings is taken for the final phoria.

(1) Since unusual conditions may give rise to extraordinary results in some patients, it is recommended that where a large contradiction of the two findings is found, the tests be repeated several times to eliminate the findings which are distinctly haphazard.

i. Some recommend that the finding always be taken from "within" the phoria. This involves a more cumbersome procedure without insuring any more accurate results.

(1) After the dissociation and the report of diplopia, the patient is requested to state the position of the upper target in relation to the lower one before any prism is introduced before the right eye. If the upper target is to the right, esophoria exists and prism base-out is slowly increased until the two targets align. If it is to the left, exophoria exists and prism base-in is slowly added until the targets align.

(a) This technique can be simply applied by remembering that a prism displaces the target towards its apex. Consequently, if the image appears to the right and it is desired to move it to the left to place it above the other, prism apex-in (base-out) is needed, if it is to the left and must be moved towards the right, prism apex-out (base-in) is needed.

(b) A similar over-simplification may be applied to the end result after the targets have been aligned. The apex of the prism at that point indicates the direction of original deviation. For example, if the targets appear aligned with 2 Δ base-in before the eyes, the apex points out and the condition is exophoria (out-turning). If the prism were to read 1 Δ base-out at the moment of alignment, then the apex pointing in would indicate a condition of esophoria (inward).

j. Upon occasion it will be found that the subject reports the approach of the upper target close to a position directly above the lower target, and then, before the examiner can accurately decide upon the amount, reports the upper target has either crossed to the other side or lapsed back again in its original direction of displacement. Two possible causes can be offered for the phenomenon.

(1) The patient has been fixating upon the lower target and as the upper one approaches alignment, he shifts his fixation to the upper one. Since the action of the various extra-ocular muscles varies slightly depending upon the position of the eye away from the primary position, a shift from the eye with a vertical prism before it, and thus declined, to an eye not declined but with prism base-in before it, and thus abducted, may present two entirely different balances of the binocular innervations. This would be particularly apparent where, as is likely, the subject shifts up and back from one target to the other in an attempt to determine the precise point of alignment.

(a) It is recommended that the subject be instructed to keep his attention solely upon the lower target (for lateral measurement) and merely report when the upper target appears, as seen peripherally (out of the corner of his eye), to be above the one at which he is looking.

(b) For vertical measurements, the laterally displaced target is fixed and the one noted peripherally is vertically displaced.

(2) Another possible cause is that the patient's attention wanders and he varies his accommodation while the test proceeds. This might take the form of an increase in accommodation at distance (myopia of empty space) or of either an increase or decrease at near.

(a) As the test is taken, it is well to emphasize to the subject that the print or configuration of the target being used for fixation be kept as clear as possible at all times. The writer has found that if difficulty is exhibited, the patient can be asked to read the print aloud while the prism measuring alignment is being turned, and repeatability will be markedly improved.

(3) A potential third cause is associated with problems attached to the lack of fusion and is better dealt with under strabismus.

2. *Vertical Phoria*

a. The prism before the right eye is now turned base-in to its maximum, separating the two targets again with the upper to the right.

b. The patient is now instructed to inform the examiner when the two targets are at exactly the same height.

c. The prism before the left eye, set at 5 or 6 Δ base-up, is slowly reduced in strength until the patient reports that the two targets occupy the same relative heights.

(1) If the residual prism is zero, the vertical phoria is orthophoria; if the base is up (and the apex points down), the condition is recorded as right hyperphoria (or left hypophoria); if the prism is turned until the base is down (and the apex up), the condition is left hyperphoria (or right hypophoria).

3. It will be noticed that both the lateral and vertical phorias are measured with a single setting of the prisms, the one before the right eye placed to exert lateral prismatic effect and the one before the left eye placed to exert vertical prismatic effect.

a. The left prism dissociates vertically and the right prism measures for lateral phorias.

b. The right prism dissociates horizontally and the left prism measures for vertical phorias.

4. The same setting of the prisms is used for all phoria tests at near by this method. Instead of the row of letters or line or box at far, a nearpoint card is used at the sixteen inch working distance. This card may present a reduced Snellen chart as the target, a round black spot, a diamond shaped group of letters, or a small row of letters. The attention of the patient at the nearpoint should be sufficient to demand the most exacting vision. Consequently, a device presenting a target which demands that accommodation be active and maintained is preferable as a nearpoint target. The reduced Snellen chart, the other letter devices, or a series of fine lines which the patient must count provide such a target.

a. Unless accommodation is held fixed, the nearpoint phoria as noted above, may vary and fluctuate as the uncontrolled accommodation increases or decreases the accommodative-convergence. If the acuity is insufficient to assure fixation of accommodation upon the target used, a target of sufficient sized letters or markings to insure the maximum use of accommodation should be provided.

C. Maddox Rod Technique

1. Another common method of measuring a phoria at the distance is by means of the Maddox rod. The original Maddox rod was a simple cylindrical rod evolved from the Maddox double prism. The eye cannot focus the excessive divergent bundle due to the short focal length of the glass rod (Figure XX-2; Eggers, 1959). Linksz (1950) offers another explanation of the optical effects of the Maddox rod which is easier to accept (See Fig. XX-3).

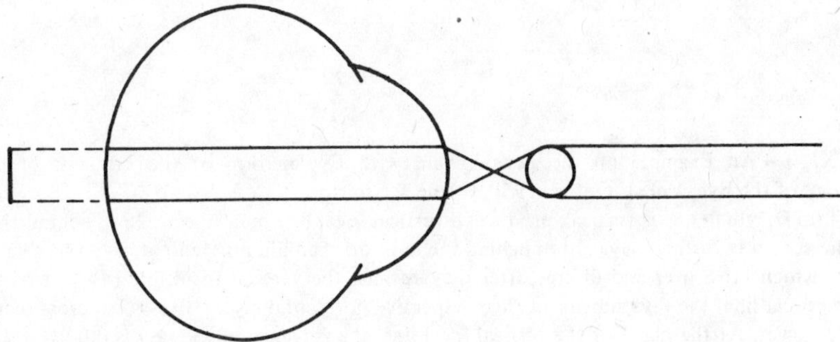

Figure XX-2 – Principle of Maddox Rod

a. The modern Maddox rod consists of a parallel series of adjacent simple cylinders of such power as to provide the appearance of a single streak when a small source of light is viewed through it. The streak is formed at right angles to the axis of the cylinder and is of the width of the original source. By placing the rod over one eye only, dissociation is accomplished by providing two images of such different form, one to each eye, that fusion is impossible.

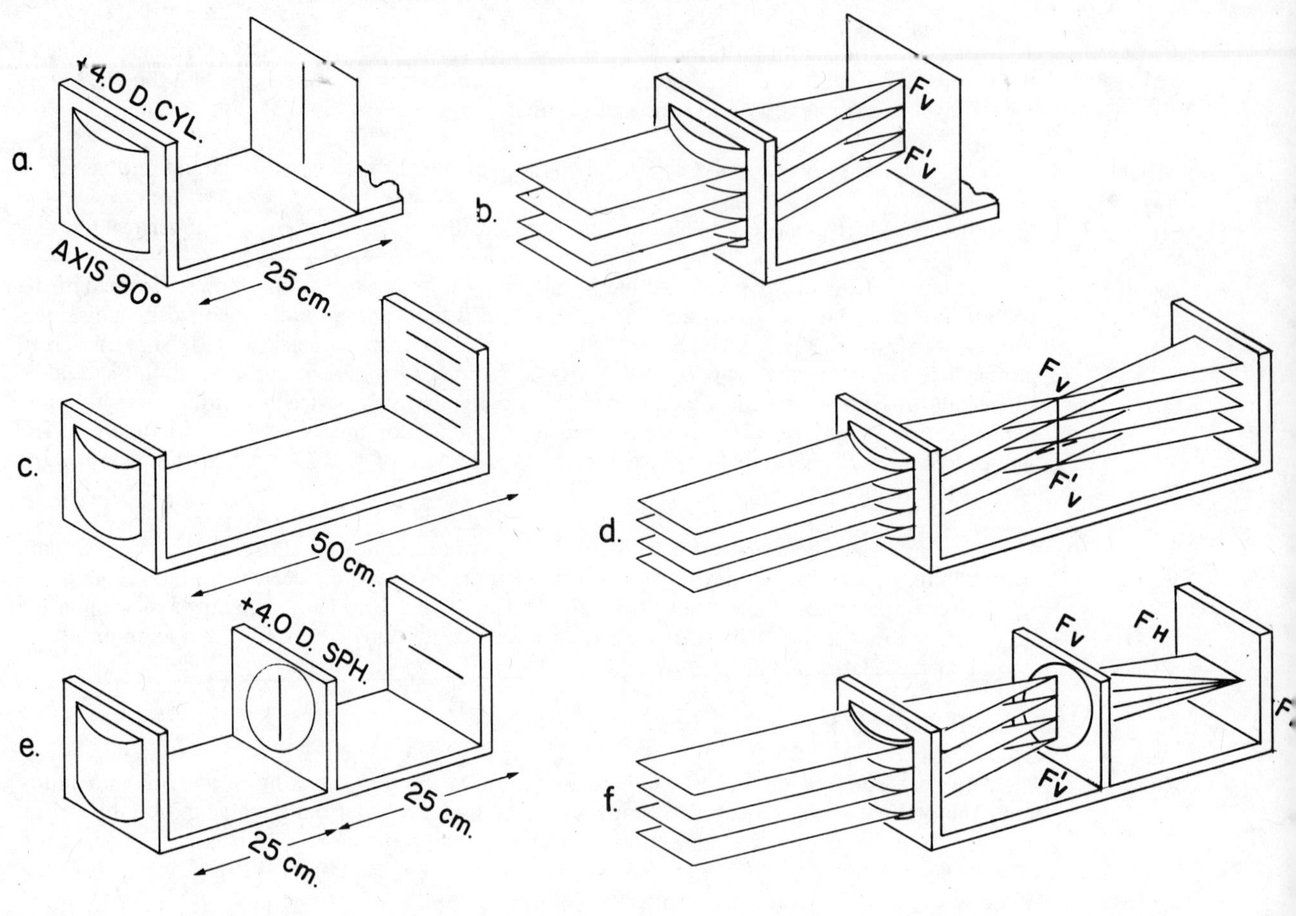

Figure XX-3 – An Example on the Lens Bench, with Explanation of the Principle of the Maddox Cylinder (from A. Linksz, Physiology of the Eye, Vol. 1, Optics, 1950, Grune & Stratton, N. Y.)

A +4.00 *D* cylinder, axis vertical, produces a vertical focal line on a screen .25 m behind the lens (*a* and *b*).

If the screen is further, say, .50 m behind the lens, only an illuminated patch can be seen (*c*). This illuminated patch is caused by the rays which cross over and diverge after they formed the vertical focal line (*d*). Converging toward the focal line and diverging from the focal line, the rays remain in their respective horizontal layers. In vertical cross sections the cylindric bundle of rays has no vergence power. At the plane of the vertical focal line, the vergence of the rays is 0.00 *D* in the vertical, ∞ in the horizontal. A +4.00 *D* spherical lens placed into the plane of the vertical focal line cannot have any effect upon the rays contained in the individual horizontal layers. They cross over and diverge as if no lens were present to interfere with them. On the other hand, the vergence of the horizontal sheets to each other is zero. They are parallel. The plus power of the lens makes these parallel sheets converge towards its own second principal focus without being able to interfere with the divergence of the rays within the individual sheets. The sheets become inclined toward each other and meet in a horizontal line on a screen placed at the *second* principal focus of the *second* lens (*e* and *f*).

If it is assumed that the first lens represents the Maddox cylinder, axis vertical and that the second lens of diagrams *e* and *f* represents the refracting system of the eye while the screen of the same diagrams represents the retina, the above represents the simplest explanation of how the Maddox cylinder, axis vertical, produces a horizontal line image on the retina.

Dissociation is further abetted by using either a red glass Maddox rod or a white Maddox rod before one eye and placing a red glass before the other eye.

(1) If a red Maddox rod is used, less exo or more eso may be found because accommodation is increased for the red light.

(2) Also, since the line may seem nearer, proximal convergence is induced.

2. *Lateral Phoria*

a. The Maddox rod is placed with the axis horizontal before the left eye. A red glass is placed before the right eye. The patient is directed to view a small spot of light at the distance. He should see a red spot and a vertical white line.

b. A rotary prism is placed before the right eye and turned base-in sufficiently to move the spot to the right of the streak.

c. It is reduced in power until the streak appears to pass through the center of the dot.

(1) The resultant position of the prism is interpreted exactly as in the Von Graefe technique.

d. Since a stimulus to fusion does exist because of the equal spatial borders of the streak and the spot in their horizontal dimension, the test may be repeated, as in the Von Graefe technique, by placing the spot to the left of the streak with prism base-out and realigning the two, using an average of the findings for the recorded result.

e. Also the resultant may be determined from "within" the phoria by placing the prism at 0 and noting on which side of the streak the spot appears. If the spot is to the right, prism base-out is needed; if to the left, prism base-in is required to align the two.

3. *Vertical Phoria*

a. The Maddox rod is rotated until the axis is vertical, producing a horizontal line. The prism before the right eye is rotated to provide either base-up or down.

b. The prism is turned to 5 Δ base-down and the patient should report a horizontal line with a red spot above it.

c. The power of the prism is then reduced until the streak again passes through the spot and the final interpretation is made from the resultant position of the prism at that point.

d. As with all phoria tests, it is well to repeat the test with the displacement in the opposite direction and accept an average of the findings for the actual recording.

4. The Maddox rod technique provides a ready method for the farpoint phoria, securing its dissociation by means of varying images rather then displacement and consequently employing only one prism for measuring.

5. The *Screen Maddox test* is recommended as a more reliable way of performing the Maddox rod test.

a. The Maddox rod and a red glass are placed as for the usual test.

b. One eye is occluded, and prism placed before it according to the deviation previously noted.

c. The position of the dot and the streak are noted when the eye is exposed.

d. Each time the prism is altered, the eye is occluded so that no motion of the target is observed in contrast to the rotary prism technique.

e. When the proper prism is before the eye, removal of the card will expose the dot bisected by the streak.

6. Green and Scobee made some comparisons of various alterations of technique (1951):

a. The Maddox rod and prism were both placed before the same eye in one technique and before separate eyes in another.

(1) The prism or rod were both placed before the right and then the left eye.

(2) The prism and rod were reversed also at different times.

b. For the lateral phorias at far, it is safer to designate the technique used if findings are being compared.

c. For vertical phorias at far and near, it is necessary to indicate the technique used.

d. For lateral phoria at near, all techniques are comparable, and one can be substituted for the other.

e. Lebensohn (1955) recommends that the prism be placed over the Maddox rod and the red glass over the other eye to insure constant fixation of that eye.

7. The Maddox rod is not commonly used at the nearpoint because of the difficulty of providing a light source as target and because the question exists as to whether a dot of light does or does not provide sufficient stimulus to accommodation to hold the test to validity.

a. Vodnoy describes a hand-held Maddox rod which can be employed for testing the reading distances at eccentric angles and at all points of the motor field in combination with trial case prisms or a prism bar (1964).

b. Bannon suggests that a spotlight or a penlight be used as a target for near tests (1943).

D. Thorington Method

1. The Thorington (or Prentice) method, in contrast to the Maddox rod technique, is more suitable for nearpoint testing and also requires only one prism. But this prism is a displacing prism and not a measuring one. This is due to the nature of the target, which is on the order of a stereoscope phoria target.

a. The target consists of a series of numerals and letters arranged in a horizontal row so that the distances between the individual markings are equivalent to the displacement of 1 prism diopter at the sixteen inch test distance. The markings are arranged so that the central position is occupied by a vertical arrow with the letters on one side and the numerals on the other (Figure XX-4).

b. A prism is introduced before the left eye with sufficient base-up effect to double the target.

c. The patient then reports two rows of figures, one above the other. As his lateral phoria becomes evident these rows will drift apart laterally.

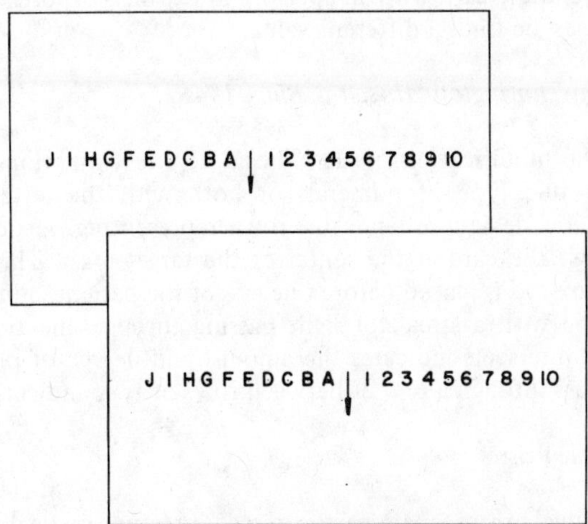

Figure XX-4 – Prentice phoria test. Upper chart seen by right eye. Displacement to left indicating eye turns to right, or exophoria exists. Each symbol represents 1 prism diopter, indicating 6½ exophoria.

d. When the rows stabilize in position, the patient is asked to note to which letter or number in the lower row the arrow of the upper row points.

(1) If the arrow of the upper row points to the arrow of the lower row, the condition is orthophoria.

(2) Since the displacement is in the opposite direction of the deviation of the eye and the upper target is seen by the right eye, if the upper arrow moves to the left, pointing to the letters, the eye has moved to the right and exophoria exists. If the upper arrow points to a number, esophoria exists. The amount is indicated by the distance of the figure under the arrow from the center.

2. The *vertical phoria* is taken upon a companion target which has the figures arranged in a vertical row. Dissociation is accomplished by the use of sufficient prism base-in to provide diplopia. If the left arrow points to letters above the center, right hyperphoria or left hypophoria exists. If it points to numerals below the center, right hypophoria or left hyperphoria exists.

a. Since prism base-in is used over the left eye, the target on the left will be seen by the left eye, while that on the right will be seen by the right eye. The arrow of the left target will point to figures on the right target. Consequently, if the arrow points to letters above the center, the right target has moved down, meaning the right eye has moved up; if it points to numerals below the center, the right target has moved up, meaning the right eye has moved down.

3. While the Thorington method is not so subject to peripheral fusion because of the targets themselves, it is subject to the patient's awareness of the close identity of the two targets and the realization that the two should center precisely. Consequently, more psychic convergence is manifested with this test than with the others. The results seem to indicate less of either esophoria or exophoria than is shown in the same cases by the other methods, indicating a tendency towards consciously centering the two arrows and the respective figures by volitional effort.

4. Mills (1950) considers the numerals in this test too large to properly stimulate accommodation. He also feels that the edges of the card act as a stimuli to fusion. By using a screen between

the patient and the card with an aperture in it which exposes the arrow and numerals, but conceals the card edges, he finds a different value.

5. *Modified Thorington (Hirsch & Bing, 1948)*

a. The modification of the Thorington test mentioned earlier consists of using a card of either fine type of numerals or both with the letters on the card representing various prismatic deviations and the rows representing vertical deviations. A fine hole is drilled through the card at the center of the target mass. This hole is illuminated from behind. A Maddox rod is placed before one eye of the patient, and the resultant view is that of the card of type with a streak of light passing through the type. The letter or numeral which the streak intersects indicates the amount and degree of phoria. If the rod is rotated, the streak will pass through a row or between rows of type indicating the vertical phoria finding.

E. Maddox Double Prism

1. The double prism separates the target into two vertically separated images. In principle, the other eye should see a third image of the target half way between the two, if no vertical phoria exists.

a. If orthophoria is present, the three targets are aligned.

b. If eso or exophoria exists, the central target will be displaced to right or left of the other two accordingly.

c. If a vertical phoria exists, the center target will appear closer to the upper or lower target of the pair and in extreme cases, may fuse with one of them.

d. In cyclophoria, the two images will not form a vertical line but an oblique one, or will not form a parallel plane including the single image of the other eye.

F. Duane Cover Test

1. A test frequently used for estimating the existence of phorias quite quickly is the cover test or parallax test. The test may be performed by either objective or subjective observations, although the former requires practice and close observation, while the latter requires a patient of sensitive discrimination and comprehensive awareness of the results desired.

2. Because of the fusional factors of the other methods of testing, such as the limiting borders of the chart upon which the targets are displayed or the similarity in form and construction of the targets themselves, complete dissociation is seldom achieved. The obviously most certain disruption of fusion is attained by occlusion of one eye, for this eliminates any factor of binocular vision due to fusion desires or reflexes.

a. Advantages of the cover test are that it is objective; fusional innovation is completely controlled; it can be used in all directions of gaze; it is not affected by apparatus, and it can be measured despite suppression. The chief disadvantage is that its accuracy depends upon the observer's ability to judge the amount of deviation.

3. The technique is simple in that the patient is requested to observe a distant source of light, preferably as small as can be readily provided, and the operator merely places a card or other occluder before one eye. The operator must, however, assume a position which enables him to see the movement of the occluded eye, both behind the occluding card and after it is removed.

4. The technique consists of merely occluding and exposing one eye and then the other or the two alternately for several repetitions while the eye undergoing the occlusion is observed.

a. If no motion of the occluded eye is noted at either the moment of occlusion or the instant of exposure, no phoria is considered to exist.

b. If the occluded eye turns out at the moment of occlusion, exophoria exists. Likewise, if the eye is observed to make a slight movement nasalward when re-exposed, exophoria exists. If the eye turns inward under occlusion and outwards when re-exposed, esophoria exists. If it turns upwards under occlusion and downward when exposed, hyperphoria is evident, whereas opposite movements would exhibit hypophoria.

(1) As the eye is occluded, fusion is interrupted and the eye assumes the position of tonic rest. Since the other eye is fixed upon the target, the entire phoria is assumed by the occluded eye. The first motion, under occlusion, is the movement of the eye to the position of rest, when fusional innervation is relinquished.

(2) When the eye is re-exposed, fusional innervation is provided to restore the macula to the position of stimulation by the target. The eye consequently moves in an opposite direction to return the line of sight to the fixating position from its tonic position.

c. *The Duane Parallax Test*

(1) Some patients may be aware of the instant diplopia and may notice a movement or jump of the target as the eye returns to the fixing position. The movement of the target will, by the laws of projection, be in an opposite direction to the movement of the eye. This movement, or *phi phenomenon,* is measured by adding prism until it is eliminated.

5. The cover test is limited in that discrepancies of less than 2 pd require almost expert attention for discovery and even then are not frequently detectable. Also distinction must be made between movements which indicate phorias and those which indicate intermittent or constant strabismus of varying types. This distinction will be treated in the chapter on Strabismus.

6. The amount of phoria may be measured, if movement is noticed, by placing a prism before the eye being occluded, with the base opposite to the movement under occlusion (or in the direction of the recovery movement under re-exposure). If the movement continues, the amount of prism is increased until an amount of prism equal to the imbalance is reached. At that point no fusional innervation is required when both eyes are exposed since the prism permits fusion with the eyes in the tonic state. Occlusion and re-exposure will elicit no movement. However, it is advised that sufficient prism be placed before the eye to reverse the movements. That is, if occlusion elicited a movement outwards, and exposure a recovery inwards, the prism should eventually arouse a movement inwards under occlusion and a recovery outwards.

a. Sloan (1954) notes that the prism measurement is only accurate in low powers, since to be accurate, the displacement should be performed at the center of rotation of the eye.

(1) Both centrads and prism diopters are based upon the assumption that all bending is done at only one surface of the prism.

(2) To avoid problems, the prism should be held as close to the eye as possible.

b. Sloan recommends that 1 Δ be deducted if motion is reversed under 5 Δ and 2 Δ be deducted if it is over 5 Δ.

c. If both a vertical and lateral deviation is exhibited, both should be neutralized simultaneously.

d. Both eyes should be covered and exposed to reveal anisophoria.

7. Possible errors in the test are due to accommodation being active, to latent deviations, to improper prism positions, to fatigue, and to failure to maintain central fixation.

8. Small degrees of error or anomalous correspondence may confuse this test. Flom (1958) suggests some unusual situations observed with it.

a. In the unilateral test, in which one eye is covered and the other observed,

(1) if there is less than 6 prism diopters of movement (flick) when the preferred eye is covered and no movement of the preferred eye when the other eye is covered, a unilateral strabismus of under 6 Δ is likely;

(2) if the occluder is alternated back and forth before the eyes after the correcting prism is placed before the eye, movement of the eye just exposed will be revealed, indicating a motion greater than the "flick" previously exhibited in the unilateral test.

b. If the unilateral test is repeated with the correcting prism added before the non-preferred eye, and no "flick" is noticed, it is an apparent strabismus case. If a "flick" is noticed (opposite in direction), it is a fusion case and non-strabismic.

(1) In strabismus, the preferred eye will fixate, and the non-preferred assume or hold a strabismic position.

(2) In fusion, both the preferred and non-preferred eye will move in response to the introduction or removal of the occluder and prism, first to assume a phoric position when fusion is disrupted and second, to restore fusion when occlusion is removed.

c. The original "flick" may be due to:

(1) a large fixation disparity associated with large heterophorias, but otherwise normal vision;

(2) a constant strabismus wherein the fusion free deviation is reduced, but not completely eliminated by motor fusional movements related to a non-harmonious anomalous correspondence with a small angle of anomaly (see chapters on Strabismus).

9. Another use of the cover test is an estimate of fusional reserve for young or elderly patients who either cannot respond to the tests later described or who would be fatigued by them (Morgan, 1960). The cover test as described above will reveal if fusion exists at far by virtue of the return movement for fusion when the occluder is removed (assuming a movement away occurred when it was introduced).

a. At nearpoint, the same test can be applied with 8 prism base-in to allow for the near phoria.

b. The fusional reserve can be estimated by placing 10 prism base-out at the nearpoint and again noting if fusion is regained upon exposure of the occluded eye.

G. The Anisophorometer

1. A portable device for use with the Maddox rod at near has been introduced by Oberman

(1967) which he calls the Anisophorometer. This consists of a calibrated scale extending to each side of a fixation light. The scale is calibrated to read directly in prism diopters. Turning it 90° either laterally or vertically enables lateral or vertical phorias to be tested. A streak seen by one eye intersects a figure on the scale, representing the phoria. Oberman claims that this device can accurately be used for nearpoint phoria testing, although some drifting of the streak was reported due to variations in accommodation.

2. The device may also be used to measure phorias in the various cardinal directions of gaze, and thereby reveal anisophoria, if present. The extent of displacement from the primary position recommended by Friedenwald (1936) is 20°, the usual limit of ocular rotations before head movement is added.

H. General Considerations Concerning Dissociated Phorias

1. Since the various techniques differ in the type of target, the method of measuring, and other features, *exact* repetition of findings from one technique to the other is seldom found. However, the repetition of successive tests even by the same methods is also not *exact* since many other factors besides the technique may be involved. For standardization, the usual technique employed most widely is that of Von Graefe, principally because it enables the operator to measure the phorias at either far or near without altering the uniformity of his procedure. The other techniques should be in the examiner's grasp, since different subjects may not respond with equal success to the same techniques.

2. *Influence of Kinesthesis*

a. Morris (1960) and Stern (1953) both experimented with the influence of a target held or touched by the hand of the subject as the test was taken.

(1) Morris found 2 PD less exo with the screen Maddox rod technique for untrained observers but little effect upon trained observers.

(2) The reliability for repeat findings for prism diplopia tests, screen Maddox rod and modified Thorington was increased.

(3) Stern found both esophoria and exophoria decreased with kinesthetic apprehension.

b. Stern reports a greater than chance increase in convergence but is not sure if the increase is due to proximal convergence or increased accommodative-convergence.

3. The phorias at far and near are consequently all taken by the same methods with the exception of the distance of the target and of the lenses before the eyes.

a. Habitual lateral phorias at far and near are taken with either no lenses or with the original entering corrections of the patients.

b. The same tests are taken with the new correction found in the refraction.

c. The near lateral phoria is also taken with the total lenses found under the dissociated cross cylinder test and with the total lenses found under the binocular cross cylinder test.

d. The vertical phorias, at far and near, are usually taken with the newly determined correction.

4. *General Rules For Phoria Testing*

a. The target always appears displaced opposite to the direction in which the eye turns, or the eye has deviated in the direction opposite to the apparent shift of its target.

b. The base of the prism is always placed in the direction of the apparent displacement, or the apex in the direction of the deviation of the eye to measure the phoria.

c. The corollary to b: The apex of the prism always indicates the direction of deviation of the eye when the position of phoric balance is attained, as when the targets are aligned.

5. *Special Considerations*

a. If acuity is too poor for the nearpoint phorias without additional help, the nearpoint phorias should be taken through a reading add. Frequently the binocular cross cylinder finding is sufficient for the purpose.

b. If suppression prevents one technique from being employed, a different technique may be successful. Devices to discourage suppression, such as a red glass before one eye, an increase in the amount of the dissociating prism, alternate occlusion of the two eyes or, if necessary, alignment of the gross outlines of a peripheral target may be used.

(1) Alternate occlusion is used by first occluding one eye and then the other and attempting to determine the error by the parallax displacement similar to the Duane cover test. Prism is introduced as described in that test.

c. Giles (1965) recommends that the lines of sight be depressed for near phoria tests. This would include potential effects of the lenses and of the other muscles in the net result (see Sections V, D. and VI, E).

d. Since the phorias are often tested in the phorometer or refractor through the rotary prisms, and with the lenses in the cells of the refractor, the prismatic effect of the lenses, particularly if the instrument is not decentered for the nearpoint interpupillary distance, and the lens power is high, should actually be included in the value of any prism test performed. However, this is seldom done although especially recommended when the values are applied to diagnostic systems such as graphical analysis.

I. Associated Phorias

1. The associated phoria is determined by techniques utilized to measure and describe the phenomenon known as fixation disparity (Ogle, 1950; Ogle & Prangen, 1951; Martens & Ogle, 1959; Carter, 1957-1964; Hebbard, 1961-1962; Ogle, Martens & Dyer, 1967).

a. The target for one technique is illustrated in Figure XX-5 (Martens & Ogle, 1959).

b. The right eye observes the lower vertical line, known as a Nonius Line, through a polarizing filter corresponding to the direction of polarization of the line. The left eye observes the upper Nonius line through a filter which is polarized to correspond to the lines' polarization. The upper line is invisible to the right eye, and the lower one is invisible to the left eye. The horizontal axis bisecting the plane between the lines is visible to both eyes.

c. The lower line is exposed, by means of a shutter, for short intervals of about 0.25 second, and the subject is asked to judge whether the lower line appears directly beneath, or to the left or right of the upper line.

(1) The position of the lower line is adjusted at each exposure until an average position, within limits, is obtained whereby the two images are judged to be aligned.

d. The actual displacement of the lines, measured in an angle subtended at the eyes of the subject, in minutes of arc, represents the fixation disparity.

2. If prism is increased base-out and base-in, in known amounts, the extent of disparity normally changes as the amount of prism is increased. A representational curve of the relationship may be graphed as shown in Figure XX-6.

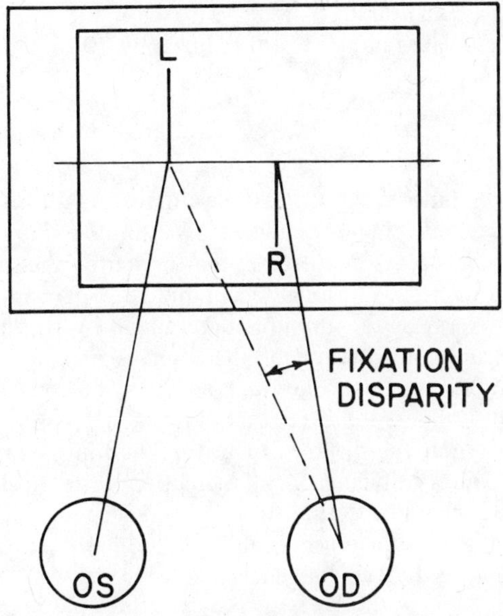

Figure XX-5 – Test Method For Fixation Disparity (From Martens, T.E. & Ogle, K.N.: A.J.Oph., 47[1], 1959, 455-463)

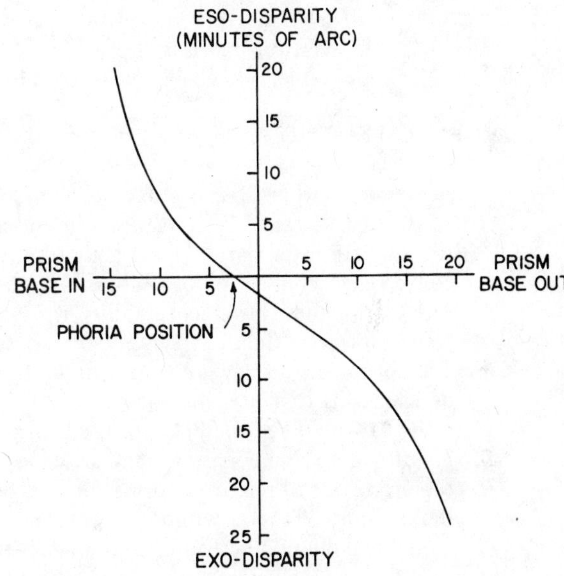

Figure XX-6 – Curve Showing Disparity In Minutes Of Arc For Various Prism Values.

a. The disparity usually agrees, (although not always) with the direction of the dissociated phoria.

b. If prism base-out is increased, the fixation lags behind or the disparity indicates less convergence than the prism calls for (exo-disparity) while if prism base-in is increased, the fixation lags behind and the disparity indicates less divergence than called for (eso-disparity).

c. The position of zero disparity will indicate that prism value which actually represents the position of balance, or the phoria position.

(1) In Figure XX-6, this is found at 2 Δ base-in, representing 2 Δ exophoria.

3. While the curve shown is most frequently observed, it is not the only one possible (Ogle,

Martens, Dyer, 1967). The test can be performed with fixation at a near point, and with the lines so organized as to measure a vertical discrepancy as well, by addition of prism base-up and base-down.

4. As mentioned above, the "associated" and "disassociated" phorias are often in agreement in direction, if not in amount, but do upon some occasions actually contradict each other. In such circumstances, Ogle believes that the true state of convergence is more truly noted by the disparity method.

5. Although polaroid devices such as the vectograph slides, and techniques such as Turville's do indicate fixation disparity, most test methods commonly in use do not. The techniques available likewise do not provide accurate means of measuring the extent of disparity. Prisms, generally the only readily available means, do not provide sufficient refinement for accurate notations of small disparity changes, and since the prisms must be used to provide increases in the stimulus conditions themselves, the measurement is absorbed in the procedure. It seems apparent that a needed development in phorometry is a precise and ready means of establishing the amount and direction of the "associated" phoria in the routine examination process.

a. Tubis (1954) however, in comparing a polaroid test of disparity with the dissociated vertical phoria test, concludes that the dissociated phoria test if reduced by 20 to 25% of its value, is a reliable measure of imbalance.

V. VERGENCES (DUCTIONS)

A. Tests of the vergences by means of prisms are commonly known as the ductions. Adduction is considered a test of convergence and abduction a test of divergence. However, the limits exhibited by the adduction tests are not the acutal limits of convergence. As discussed in the chapter on the subject, convergence consists of the sum of various innervations, tonic, fusional, accommodative, and psychic. The total actual convergence ability is usually far in excess of the amounts determined by the duction tests. However, ductions serve the purpose of indicating the nature of the reserves of convergence available at the distance of testing under the fixed conditions of the other factors. Thus, if a convergence deficiency is exhibited by means of a duction test, it might indicate that convergence is subject to ready fatigue when the eyes are used for attentive vision at the distance of testing, within the range of fatigue of accommodation at that same distance. The significance of the duction tests is chiefly, therefore, one of relative information, providing some concept of the status of convergence in relation to the accommodation, without always indicating the total convergence ability. Ordinarily, however, ineffectual duction performance is associated with a poorer total convergence ability.

B. The duction tests provide an easily accessible means of measuring and approximating the actual convergence function by the use of prisms. As the images of the target are moved from the foveas, the fusion reflex moves the foveas to the position assumed by the incident stimulation. In adduction the movement of the eyes is inward just as in the ordinary change of fixation from a distant to a near target; in abduction, the movement is outward. The target is always presented in the median plane of the lines of sight.

C. While trial case prisms might be used, their presentation involves many other factors which become obvious as the duction tests are comprehended. The best devices for the measure of ductions are the rotary prisms which increase the convergence or divergence in gradually varying amounts within the range of the fusion field without allowing the fusion to be consciously interrupted. However, due to their construction, and to the position of the rotary prisms in relation to the lenses before the eyes and their distance from the eyes, also to the distance of the target from the prism, the eyes do not actually usually turn as much as the prism reading indicates. This is further complicated by the fact that the graduations of distance on the instrument reading-rods of different makes are not calculated upon the same basis. Another factor (Hirsch, 1949) is that some rotary prisms are calibrated up to 30 Δ and some to 15 Δ. On both types, the examiner exhibits a tendency to read the calibrations to the nearest even figure, although the tendency is more marked on instruments calibrated to 30 Δ. For practical purposes, the prism reading on the scales is accepted as a measure of the actual turning of the lines of sight but such values will not agree with more critical laboratory methods of measurement. It would seem to be essential to have both the construction and calibrations of different refractors made uniform in these details and for the refractionist to learn to apply corrective calculations to these inherent discrepancies.

1. Duction findings may be influenced, according to Morgan (1960), in a number of ways.

a. The findings can be influenced by the effort expended, which may be incited beyond normal by the examiner.

b. The speed with which the rotary prism power is increased will influence the finding recorded.

(1) The amplitude of fusional convergence first rises abruptly and then descends as the angular velocity of the stimulus increases (Ludvigh & McKinnon, 1968). Large versional movements can move at the rate of 500°/sec.,. while small versional movements achieve 100° to 200°/sec. In contrast fusional movements achieve a rate of only 6°/sec., probably due to the different kinds of muscle fibers activated.

(a) Within 0.2 seconds, at the rate of 6°/sec., the stimulus is 1.2° off the fovea.

(b) Upon five different subjects, utilizing a speed varying from 1/8 to 6°/sec., the maximum vergence for all subjects was attained when the stimulus was moved at a rate just under 1°/sec.

c. The tests preceding will influence the findings, particularly if the tests are taken quickly one after each other.

d. The aperture of the lens in the refractor may appear to occlude as prism is introduced, and more so if the instrument is thicker. The interpupillary distance may need to be altered as prism is increased.

e. A qualitative value as well as a quantitative one may be significant.

2. Since, in most cases, lenses are placed before the eyes and behind the prisms before the duction tests are performed, centering of the eyes in the instrument apertures is necessary to avoid modification of the prismatic reading by induced prismatic power of the lenses, although some modification is unavoidable. This is particularly true in the nearpoint tests, and generally, a reduction of 4 mm. is required for the average P.D. to center the lines of sight through the back lens for nearpoint testing.

a. As the patient attempts to maintain fixation on the target while the prism power is increased, it is obvious that the lines of sight move closer to the apex of the prism. In so doing, they pass through a portion of the correction lenses in the refractor which is farther and farther from the optical centers of the lenses. The induced prism power of this shift alters the actual true reading of the vergence under test. Fry (Haines, 1952) has worked out the formula for the following graph which applies a correction factor to the values actually read from the scales of the measuring prisms. The power used on the scale is the average power of the two lens combinations before the eyes, as applied to the 180th meridian (Figure XX-7).

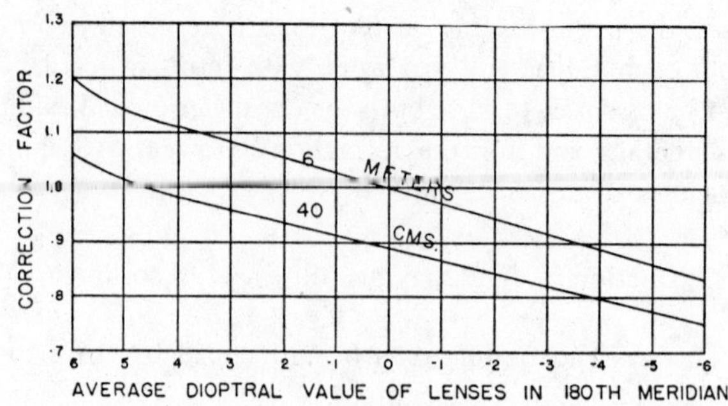

Figure XX-7 – Fry's Correction Factor For Prism-Lens Combination Readings.

b. Pascal (1952) points out that the value of the prism at near is not the same as at far. Lessened rotation of the eye is required behind a prism when fixing at near. This can be computed by:

(1) The percentage of loss of effectivity is equal to $\frac{100\ Xd}{L}$ where d is the distance of the prism from the eye in mms. and L is the distance of the object from the eye in cms.

(a) For example, if the object is at 40 cms. and the prism is 25 mms. in front of the eye, the loss is $\frac{25}{400}$, = 6.25% of loss.

(b) If the value found were 10 Δ, the true value would be 9.35 Δ.

c. While few reports of unanticipated prismatic effect of lenses in the modern refractors have been made, a large number of examiners utilize phorometers or trial frames in which trial case lenses are used. Schillinger (1951) analyzed a large number of trial case lenses for determination of unwanted prismatic effects due to misplacement of the optical centers of the lenses. He found the following results:

(1) Of 568 non-precision spheres, 244 or 42.9% exhibited a decentration error of 0.5 Δ or over. Of 580 precision spheres, 75 or 12.9% exhibited a decentration error of 0.5 Δ or over. Of 54 non-precision cataract trial case lenses, 25 or 46.2% exhibited an error of 1 Δ or over, whereas 4 of 62 precision cataract trial case lenses (0.5%), exhibited the same error. While most such errors are found in lenses of higher powers, the number of induced apparent vertical imbalances seems materially affected. Also, since the trial case lenses are round, and placed in varying positions from time to time, the element of error introduced by their use is incalculable.

(a) Chin and LaRich (1966) could find no significant effect on the duction findings of oblique cylinder corrections and implied oblique aniseikonia.

(b) Giles suggests that the influence of anisometropia can be noted by comparing the phorias with and without the Rx before the eyes.

D. Procedure for Lateral Ductions (Vergences) (Figure XX-8).

1. The patient is correctly positioned at the conclusion of the phoria tests. Both prisms are placed before the eyes so that the power can be directed either base-out or base-in.

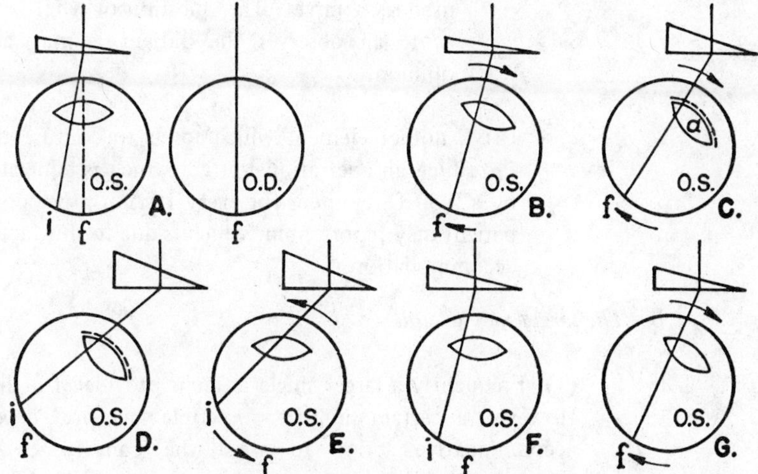

Figure XX-8 – Diagrammatic representation of movements of eye during duction tests. (A) Both eyes in primary position, illustrating displacement of image by prism before O.S. (B) Movement of fovea of O.S. to image point, maintaining single vision. (C) Continued movement of fovea with increased prism; action of accommodation, *a*, to assist convergence, producing blur point. (D) Break point, showing placement of image by prism beyond range of accommodative assistance to convergence. (E) Eye assuming rest position, fovea moving away from image point of prism producing break, causing images to separate more widely; accommodative-convergence relaxes and image clears. (F) Reduction of prism during recovery, showing image placed at limit of fusion area with eye in rest position. (G) Recovery movement of eye, fovea moving to position of image impinging fusion area in (F), producing single vision again. Arrows represent movement of fovea and front of eye.

2. The patient is directed to print of the just readable size at far and to a similar target or reduced Snellen chart at near. He is instructed to inform the examiner when any one of the following events occurs:

a. *The print may blur.*

(1) This would be due to a change in the status of accommodation. As previously discussed, this is assumed by some to indicate the appearance of convergence–accommodation, that is, accommodation forced into action by the action of convergence. It seems to definitely indicate the exhaustion at that point of the fusional convergence which has operated independently of accommodation. The blur point, if found, is noted as the limit of fusional convergence.

(a) As Allen (1950) has pointed out, the use of the term "blur" is one which does not afford a certain criterion to many untrained observers. As seen later, most nearpoint test-type targets are too far removed from the minimal stimulus stage to be critical, and the patient must determine for himself just what is meant by "blur." A range of focus equivalent to + or –.50 D. has been found as the average over which a blur may not be reported. Allen recommends that targets of fine lines, used also by Morgan, Neumueller and others, in which the lines would fade to a uniform gray field, be used for tests involving a 'blur' criterion.

[1] Giles (1965) reports that Adamson, however, found that the blur point apparently began at the same point, no matter what size type was

used as a target. The question of what is understood as "blur" and how acute an observer the patient is may account for the differences of opinion.

(b) Another element which tends to confuse the "blur" point is that prisms introduce an aberrational effect which is equivalent to the distortion produced by a 0.50 D. cylinder for every 10 Δ of prism power for a 3 mm. pupil size. The patient may report a blur which is due to this factor rather than to any change in accommodation.

b. *The target may double.*

(1) Frequently a larger single letter is provided for this purpose if a blur is reported. However, a certain number of people have not developed the faculty of inciting accommodative action to assist the convergence and do not report a blur. Consequently, it is best to provide a target which serves for both the blur or the break (diplopia point) at the same time. A single fine letter may be provided or a row of letters and a vertical line or any combination which provides both an adequate and fine enough target for noting the blur and a non-confusion target for noting the break.

(2) If no blur is reported, the break point rather than the blur point represents the limits of fusional convergence. However, if a blur has been reported, the break point represents the limits of both fusional and accommodative-convergence for that test, the accommodative-convergence being the difference between the blur and the break points.

c. *The target may neither blur nor double but may simply move to either side.*

(1) In the event of suppression, the image in one eye will be ignored. The other eye will perform a simple refixation of the light deviated by the prism so that both eyes will be making versional movements rather than performing a vergence movement. Since the target will appear to be deviated towards the apex of the increased prism power, the patient will merely observe an apparent displacement of the target. The suppressing eye can be determined by noting the fact that the target is moving in the same direction as the apex of the prism before the seeing eye.

3. When diplopia is elicited, the patient is then requested to report when single vision is regained. *This point is known as the recovery.*

a. When fusion is disrupted, the eyes tend to return to either the tonic state at far or to the fusion-free state at near, reaching a position determined by tonic, psychic and accommodative-convergence innervation. At this point the image of one eye may be on the fovea, but that of the other eye is peripherally located. Reduction of the prism now brings the displaced target closer to the fovea in the latter eye. (Actually, since the prism before both eyes is reduced, the effect is gained by both reduction of the prism and corresponding versional movements of both eyes.) At a given point, the displaced image is placed within the fusion field of the non-fixing eye and fusional innervation is stimulated to provide a necessary movement to restore the target to the fovea. Thus, the actual value of the recovery point is to measure the limit of the fusion field in that direction, and the true dimension of the fusion field would be the recovery value, with allowance for the position the eye assumed under dissociation (the phoria).

4. The procedure consists then of increasing the prism power slowly before both eyes, as equally as possible, until the blur and the break points are reached, or the latter alone if no blur is manifested, and then reducing the power until the recovery points are reached.

a. The amount of prism at which the blur was determined is recorded as a separate value. The break and recovery are recorded as a fraction in which the break is the numerator and the blur the denominator, as 20/13.

b. When base-out prism is applied, the blur at far is known as the True Adduction; at near as the Positive Relative Convergence (PRC).

c. With base-in applied, no blur is expected at far, since a relaxation of accommodation, which should not be in employ at far, would be required. At near, since accommodation is being employed, the blur point results from a relaxation of the accommodation and is recorded as the Negative Relative Convergence (NRC).

d. The break/recovery fraction is recorded at far, for base-out as the Convergence or Adduction test; for base-in, as the Abduction test. At near, for base-out, as the Positive Fusional Reserve (PFR); for base-in as the Negative Fusional Reserve (NFR).

5. *To summarize,* the lateral ductions are taken:

a. *At far*

(1) Base-out to blur.
(2) Base-out to break and reduced to recovery.
(3) Base-in to break and reduced to recovery.

b. *At near*

(1) Base-out to blur.
(2) Base-out to break and reduced to recovery.
(3) Base-in to blur.
(4) Base-in to break and reduced to recovery.

c. The tests are taken as a continuous process. That is, once the distance target is in place and the prisms in position before the eyes, the patient is instructed to report either the blur, the break or the movement. Prism base-out is increased, and when the blur is noted, the increase is smoothly continued until the break is found. The patient is then instructed to report the recovery and the prism is decreased. When the recovery point is reached, the patient is told to report the same phenomena, the prism is quickly reduced to 0, and base-in is increased until the results are secured. The same continuity is repeated at the nearpoint upon an appropriate target, such as a reduced Snellen chart, or a vertical row of letters, or box of letters.

6. If suppression occurs, the suppressing eye is noted. Sometimes a further increase in prism power may elicit diplopia by removing one image from the suppression field. In such cases a recovery point may be determined, although that point may measure the limit of the suppression field rather than the fusion field.

7. It is advisable to halt briefly at the break point to allow the eyes to return to the position of

rest. Otherwise an immediate reduction may overtake the eyes as they are in process of returning to that position and the recovery finding will not only be much higher than it should be, but will vary with the rate of operation of the examiner so as to be totally inconsistent from one time to the next.

E. Procedure for Vertical Ductions

1. The testing for vertical ductions involves factors not as dominant in affecting the results of the lateral ductions. As has been mentioned, the vertical functions are fusional reflexes of a limited degree and because their total span is small and the average rotary prisms calibrated in units which are correspondingly very large, various effects of the stimulation to the respective muscles and the balance of the eyes are reflected in disproportionate amounts. The sustained or continuing contraction of the muscles last stimulated has been mentioned previously. This produces the effect of a reduction in the value of the antagonistic duction which follows the original duction tested. Some estimate that a period of up to 20 or more minutes is required before the tonus is restored to normal so as to provide an accurate finding for the second duction. However, Walsh (1946) states that repetition of the second test several successive times will aid in establishing the true finding which is supported by consistency of the results.

2. Another point of debate is whether it is necessary to test the vertical ductions for each eye separately in both directions or whether the findings taken upon one eye in both directions or upon both eyes in the same direction are sufficient. Bielschowsky (1939) believed that because of the latent residual contraction, the findings taken upon separate eyes would differ from the comparative finding taken upon one eye. Others compromise by dividing the prism between both eyes, but this neither eliminates the question of residual contraction, actually involving both eyes in accordance with Bielchowsky's premise, nor facilitates the reading of the comparatively gross calibrations of small amounts in dividing them between two prisms.

   a. The most common clinical technique employs one prism only over one eye. Right supraduction and left infraduction are comparable, and right infraduction and left supraduction should likewise be equivalent.

   b. Some recommend that only the break point be recorded. However, most clinicians recommend that both a break and recovery point be noted. The author has found some instances in which a disparity between the recoveries seemed more significant than that revealed by the break points.

3. The technique is relatively simple. Since accommodation is not usually involved in the vertical movements, no blur point is manifested. Attention is directed to either a single fixation target or a horizontal line of letters at either near or far, depending upon the status of the routine, and the prism is increased before one eye.

   a. If base-down before the right eye is increased, the right supraduction is being measured. The patient reports diplopia and the prism power is reduced until the recovery of single vision. The same fractional notation is used as for lateral breaks and recoveries.

   b. The prism is then increased with the base-up to measure the right infraduction and the same notations are made.

   c. If desired, the examiner may then repeat the procedure with a prism before the left eye.

d. For continuity, the vertical ductions at far are taken immediately after the lateral ductions at far by rotating the prisms from the lateral base effect to a vertical base effect. If a row of letters has served as the target, this need not be changed. The vertical ductions at near are also taken after the lateral ductions at near by the same adjustment of the rotary prism positions. The reduced Snellen chart can be used as the target. If a vertical line has been used for the lateral duction target, it should be replaced by a horizontal line for the vertical duction test.

VI. RELATION OF PHORIA TO DUCTION FINDINGS

A. It will be recalled from Chapter VII that both the lateral phorias and ductions are concerned with disclosing the various types of convergence stimulation. The phoria exhibits, by virtue of its discrepancy from the orthophoric position, the amount of fusional convergence, either positive or negative, which the patient must use to attain binocular fixation of the target. The duction, up to the blur point, measures the reserve of fusional convergence still available after fixation has been attained. Consequently, it would be expected that a patient exhibiting a high degree of exophoria, and requiring that amount of positive fusional convergence to achieve binocular fixation, would reveal a lesser positive reserve of fusional convergence than if the condition had been orthophoric. The same patient, if he had exhibited esophoria, might reveal a higher reserve than if orthophoric. The total positive fusional convergence would actually consist of the value of the base-out blur point plus the exophoria or minus the esophoria, while the total negative fusional convergence value would equal the base-in blur point plus the esophoria or minus the exophoria.

1. The phoria might then be stated to indicate the "demand" for ordinary use of the fusional convergence, while the duction opposite to it would indicate the "reserve." The amount of the reserve will vary to some extent with the "demand." Consequently, it is frequently noted that cases of high exophoria will exhibit base-in duction findings which are quite high in value, while the base- out duction findings are relatively low.

2. Where a wide discrepancy is observed in the duction findings in the two directions and the phoria is comparatively negative, the possibility of a latent imbalance should be considered.

B. This is particularly true when the vertical phorias are compared to the vertical ductions (Walsh, 1946). The lateral ductions are subject to voluntary influences and the action of both accommodation and psychic influences, but the vertical ductions ordinarily are of a fairly stable amount and usually equal in both directions. If a right hyperphoria exists, it would be expected that the right supraduction would exceed the right infraduction. Usually the disparity is in an amount which agrees reasonably well with the extent of vertical deviation. Consequently, if no vertical phoria is exhibited, but a discrepancy is found between the opposing vertical ductions, it is frequently assumed that a latent vertical phoria exists.

1. A large number of factors seem to affect the vertical phorias and ductions. Much emphasis has been placed upon these because of their dominant role in visual discomfort and the difficulty of appropriate correction. Whereas lateral deviations can be often ignored when the contrasting vergences are sufficient in amount, or corrected by lenses or training, most vertical discrepancies are neither fully revealed upon first test, nor respond to the same procedures employed for the lateral deviations.

2. The relationship between the phoria and duction is considered more exact in the vertical direction. Also, the influence of the duction, where it precedes the phoria, is much more evident. In reverse, a habitual vertical phoria also seems to affect the range of the vertical ductions. Thus,

Fry and Ellerbrock (Allen, 1950) found that the middle of the range of the ductions varied with the phoria. Tubis (1954) also regarded the balance of the duction break points as a good subsidiary indication supporting the implication of the vertical phoria test, although he recommended that the prism power found be reduced by one-third of its value. He found the recovery value to be of little significance. Ogle and Prangen (1953) also found that up to a vertical discrepancy of 6 Δ, most subjects will compensate and reveal ductions which balance or which, if the discrepancy is induced, equal those previously exhibited. This compensating ability enables an adjustment in the oblique gaze similar to that made by patients wearing anisometropic corrections. Where no such compensation is evident, an actual retinal image distortion or permanent mechanical anomaly may be present.

a. In contrast to the opinion that the vertical duction test may influence the vertical phoria test when taken in that immediate sequence, the influence of vertical ductions and phorias upon lateral phoria tests taken immediately following appears to be slight or non-existent (Booth, Lofgren and Thome, 1965). As seen later, this permits great flexibility in the placement of these tests in the routine examination procedure.

b. Ellerbrock (1949, 1950) has pursued the different factors entering into the vertical divergencies. He finds that the amplitude of the test is dependent upon displacement of parallel horizontal borders, that peripheral diplopia will influence the extent, and that increasing the peripheral diplopia by increasing the targets, will exhibit a summating effect to a point. A single foveal stimulus produces the least effect. If stimuli are applied peripherally for an opposite fusional demand, the extent of the duction is diminished, in proportion to the closeness of the peripheral stimulus to the fovea. Also, the form of the stimulus varies the amplitude, and unequal magnification reduces it. Other factors which influence the amplitude of vertical divergence include the rate at which the disparity is introduced, the faster rate producing a lower range; the intensity of the stimulus, which affects the after-discharge rate more than the extent of the contraction; and the length of time the divergence is maintained, which up to a point, influences the rate at which the targets disappear. The size of the total pattern also influences the amplitude within limits by reinforcing the central image.

C. Marlow (Bielschowsky, 1939) originated a procedure known as prolonged occlusion based on the premise that latent deviations could not be revealed by temporary and momentary methods of interfering with fusion. This technique is used in all cases in which neither a refractive or convergence disorder is discovered which accounts for the patient's subjective complaints. First one eye is totally occluded for a period of one week and then the other eye is occluded for an equal period. Since this is the absolute interruption of fusion, latent imbalances due to spastic muscular action should be relaxed. The repetition of the phoria tests after this period has been found to reveal imbalances of much higher amounts than were originally revealed, or discrepancies of fixation when previous testing revealed none. The procedure is particularly significant if the symptoms of discomfort present when both eyes were used disappear under or during the occlusion.

1. Chavasse maintains that the total heterophoria never changes in a given individual, but that fatigue, stress, etc., results in the conversion of latent heterophoria to manifest heterophoria and that the latter is what is measured by usual tests. The occlusion procedure is designed, evidently, to reveal the total heterophoria. However, much controversy surrounds the test, and opinions vary from those of Abraham (Scobee, 1952), who considers the test merely a subjective test for Bell's phenomenon and not a test for latent heterophoria, to Cushman and Culver (1953), who state that in no case did occlusion bring out any imbalance in a patient who did not actually have an imbalance. Bannon (1943) has suggested that while the occlusion test may alleviate the symptoms,

other causes than imbalance may be the source of the difficulty, and where no subsequent imbalance is found upon retest, aniseikonia should be suspected.

a. Tonicity for fusion did not disappear immediately following occlusion in 74% of the cases (Ellerbrock and Loran, 1961). Residual tonicity thereby affects the measurement of hyperphoria, and the eye under cover does not invariably turn upwards.

D. Another procedure often recommended is that the actual heterophoria be ignored and the range of the ductions be averaged to establish the actual balance point (Ellerbrock & Fry, 1941). Duke-Elder (1949) and Abraham (Scobee, 1952) recommend this procedure, but Scobee (1952) quotes the work of Haessler to indicate that, in regard to lateral balance, the degree of heterophoria is not determinable by such a method. Kratz (1951), however, did find a relation between the lateral phoria and the abduction at far which revealed that the abduction differs from 8 to 11 Δ from the phoria, with a mean of 9.4 Δ. In regard to vertical heterophoria, the procedure is more acceptable, but the effects of the ductions upon the phoria, and inversely the adaptation of the duction range to the phoria, as discussed above and in other chapters, makes an interpretation on this premise also suspect. Almost all recommendations call for the compensating duction to be taken first where a vertical heterophoria is disclosed.

1. Commonly, if the vertical phorias are orthophoric in amount, the vertical ductions are not taken. That this procedure may ignore the significance of latent hyperphorias is obvious. However, the residual contraction of the vertical muscles following the first duction, previously noted, may result in unequal ductions more frequently than should be evidenced unless the cautionary retesting advocated earlier is performed. On the other hand, the work of Ellerbrock and Fry (1942) demonstrated that a compensatory mechanism for the induced vertical deviations of anisometropic lenses may exist and that vertical imbalances may correct themselves.

2. Ogle and Prangen (1951) by means of "associated" vertical measurements, determined the existence of an ability, on the part of most persons, to adapt to or compensate for relatively large vertical discrepancies, similar to the discovery of Ellerbrock and Fry (1942), and Ellerbrock (1950).

a. The wearing of a correcting vertical prism, did not, after a given time, displace the position of the disparity curve from its pre-prism position, as might have been expected. It was possible to increase prism in steps not exceeding 2 Δ at any one time, up to a total of at least 6. Even at that stage, not only did the disparity curve occupy the very same position which it had previously, but the dissociated phoria, as measured by the Maddox rod test, was also the same as it had been prior to the application of prisms. Likewise, the same symmetric and normal range of vertical prism vergences were revealed.

(1) The data show that a large hyperphoric imbalance is induced when vertical prism is added which, as the fusion is maintained, decreases until the stress returns to its formal level. At this point the muscle balance between the eyes is no longer affected by the prism.

(a) The time required for compensation of 2 Δ steps for seven subjects ranged from three to ten minutes.

(2) If the 6 Δ of prism is removed, diplopia will exist for a period of from 2 to 16 minutes, then become a phoria in the original direction of stress, and finally return to the original state.

(a) The rate of recovery for the seven subjects was from two to three times longer than the time required for the original compensating process.

(3) Those patients who reveal hyperphorias, and have this slow compensating ability will reveal the same phoria as before wearing a correcting prism for some time.

(a) Such cases have been earlier explained (see above) in various ways, usually as "latent" hyperphorias whose full error was slowly revealed by the wearing of the partial correction. Upon each subsequent examination, within limits, the prism was increased, only to have the next examination again reveal the hyperphoria.

(4) Some patients exhibit only a partial compensatory ability or no compensatory action at all, and will thereby accept the vertical prism prescribed and reveal either no subsequent vertical phoria or an altered one, utilizing the prism to gain relief from symptoms due to the hyperphoria.

b. It is evident that the eyes, when reading a newspaper or book, look towards oblique points to each side at which vertical divergence must take place. The amount of such divergence at near may reach 3 Δ at some laterally and vertically displaced points, varying in the type of divergence from one to the other, as from up and left to up and right.

(1) Maddox rod tests reveal an immediate reflex compensation for these variations, which is not the normal vertical fusional amplitude, since tests of this at these positions of fixation reveal the usual and normal ratio of supra and infra vergences. This compensation may also apply to the varying vertical divergences produced by anisometropic lenses before the eyes during different directions of gaze.

c. The "rapid' reflex is probably exhibited during clinical tests of vertical divergences (ductions). As the prism is introduced at a fairly rapid rate, the eyes lag behind the extent of fixation disparity, and also reach a definite endpoint.

d. In contrast, the "slow" compensating reflexes are separate from the other, reach a greater range, and serve as a new base line from which all further vertical eye movements are executed. The normal amplitudes, measured clinically, represent only the maximums within which this slow stabilizing compensatory mechanism can begin to operate.

3. Carter (1963, 1964 and 1968) also describes a similar compensating mechanism for lateral phorias, indicating that if prism is prescribed for a lateral discrepancy revealed by the disparity method and if after 15 minutes, the same disparity is now shown with the prism as was exhibited without it, the compensating mechanism indicates that prism in the prescription will serve little purpose.

E. Nadell (1964) analyzed the relationship of lateral and oblique muscle action to vertical imbalances. The reinforced lateral action of the obliques in extortion and of the vertical recti in intortion accrues in vertical deviations resulting from the recti at 23° outward gaze and only from the obliques at 51° inward gaze.

1. The measured phoria would depend upon the fixation distance and interpupillary distance.

2. The use of a lateral prism to dissociate would cause the fixing eye to deviate and the associated eye to follow concomitantly. The amount of prism used to dissociate and its direction could influence the vertical phoria.

a. A moderate amount of base-in will test the obliques of the other eye, while a large amount will test the vertical recti.

b. A moderate amount of base-out will test the vertical recti of the other eye, while a large amount will test the obliques.

3. The more prism used to dissociate, the more likely a vertical discrepancy will be found because one set of muscles becomes less efficient.

4. As the vertical muscles also help in lateral movement, correction of vertical discrepancies may help the lateral ductions.

VII. OTHER PROCEDURES

A. Special Instruments.

1. The phorias are frequently taken upon various types of survey instruments developed chiefly for quick routine in school or industrial placement. Many opinions are available, but Sloan and Rowland (1951) maintain that where the tests are properly designed to exclude peripheral visibility, which clues the distance and provides fusional stimuli, the findings on these instruments correlate about as well with clinical tests as the different clinical tests do with each other, insofar as the far lateral phoria tests are concerned. The near lateral phoria tests are more variable, while the vertical tests do not agree nearly as well. All devices and tests were uncertain for mild vertical phorias and Sloan and Rowland recommended re-testing of the vertical phorias. The technique of each instrument is specific for the instrument and does not require explanation here.

2. In a previous chapter, a variety of special nearpoint test devices employing a binocular principle have been described. These are used to test both phorias and vergences as well as the nearpoint correction and other aspects of fusion, accommodation and binocularity. The oldest method, of whose principles most of the others employ variations, is the Esdaile Turville Equilibrium test (Turville, 1934).

a. *The Esdaile Turville Equilibrium Test*

(1) Turville describes a special apparatus which resembles in principle a Remy separator, consisting of a card of print, dotted lines and other symbols with a bar parallel to the card to act as a septum. This septum is adjustable for different interpupillary distances and also for either 40 or 33 cm. fixation.

(a) The spherical power and cylindrical power of the correction can be checked in a manner similar to that employed in the Infinity Balance technique (see previous chapter).

(b) The dotted line indicates the vertical balance, being continuous in orthophoria. Vertical discrepancies are first checked by altering the sphere before one eye, indicating an aniseikonic cause rather than a muscular one. In a similar manner the cyclophoria may be noted by tilting of one of the sections of the dotted lines. Alteration of the amount and axis of the cylinder is attempted to correct such an indication.

b. *Polarized Turville Balance Technique (Wilmut, 1951)*

(1) In the previous chapter a description of the Wilmut modification of the Turville test has been given. Wilmut has developed several methods of determining not so much a measure of the imbalance as a method of correcting or alleviating imbalances. These will be considered in the chapter on Analysis and Prescription.

3. *The Eskridge Flip-Prism Test (1961)*

a. Eskridge employs a 3.00 prism diopter prism mounted in a cell with a long handle like the hand-flip cross cylinder.

b. A spot of light or a 20/40 letter is used as a target.

c. A trial frame is placed on the patient and his head is maintained erectly and with avoidance of head-tilt.

d. The prism is first presented before one eye base-down and then with the base reversed to the base-up position.

e. If diplopia occurs either way:

(1) The prism is presented base-down for 2 seconds and base-up for 2 seconds.

(a) As it is repeated, the patient is asked to compare the extent of diplopia.

(b) If a difference in the extent of diplopia in one direction of the prism than in the other is revealed, vertical phoria exists.

(2) The apex position represents the phoria.

(a) A greater discrepancy with the apex up reveals hyperphoria; with the apex down, hypophoria.

(3) Loose hand prisms are added until the vertical separation is balanced in both directions.

(a) The prism required to do so measures the extent of phoria.

f. The test correlates 0.97 to the Turville results, whereas the Von Graefe test usually exceeds the Turville finding by ½ prism diopter.

(1) Peripheral fusion usually lessens the vertical phoria, and Eskridge summarizes that the rule of thumb habit of reducing the prism found for the correction may be due to the fact that a higher value is usually found in the unfused state.

g. Where the test showed "gliding," wavering or movement of the targets while disparate, occlusion revealed a higher phoria. "Gliding" may therefore indicate a latent vertical phoria.

4. *Bishop Harmon Test (Giles, 1965)*

a. The test consists of a card of letters printed along a horizontal line which is viewed by the patient through an aperture that is variable in width.

(1) The scale is set for the interpupillary distance at 40 cms.

(2) The aperture is narrowed until binocular vision is lost and the letters begin to double.

5. *The Mitchell (1953) Test* is simpler and consists of a rule, a rectangular septum and some nearpoint cards. The aperture is moved along the rule, occluding varying areas of the card, until binocular vision is lost.

a. The card, at the reading distance, consists of eight letters in two groups of four each with an oblique line crossing between the groups. The upper portion of the line has two red circles on it. The lower has two green ones (Figure XX-9).

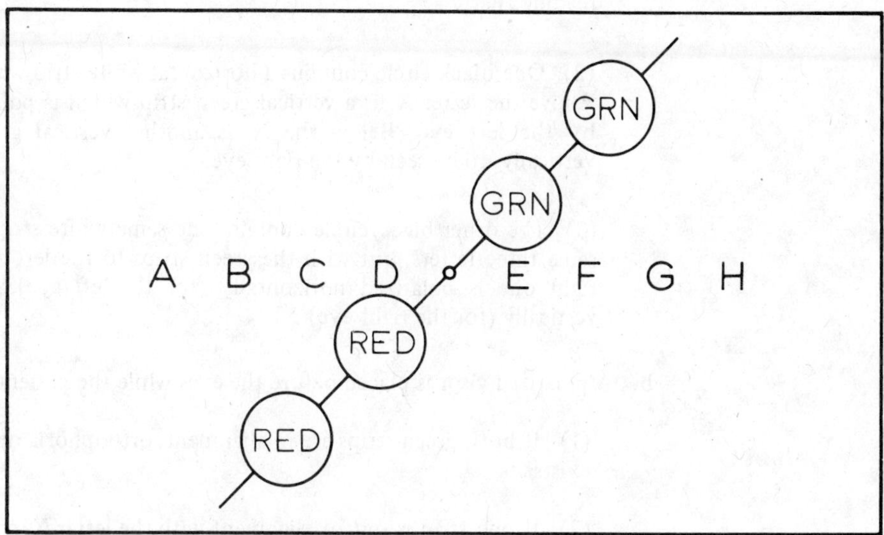

Figure XX-9 – Mitchell Card for Fusional Stability

b. A 30 mm. septum is moved away until only a small area is seen binocularly as a macular fusion area. If the card is moved too far, part of the nearpoint card is obscured.

(1) The patient should hold fusion at a distance comparable to his interpupillary distance.

(a) If fixation is at 40 cms. with a 30 mm. aperture card, the card should reach a point away from the eyes proportional to the interpupillary distance. For example, $\frac{30}{60}$ X 40 equals the distance the septum should reach from the test object, which would be 20 cms.

(2) If moved beyond that, the test card will break into two parts which will overlap or separate according to the phoria.

(a) The aperture card is moved away from the test card until fusion returns.

(b) The further the septum from the calculated maximum position on the rod according to the interpupillary distance, the weaker the fusion stability.

c. Mitchell maintains that foveal vision is maintained until interrupted, whereas in the Turville infinity balance, peripheral vision holds binocularity while both foveas are occluded.

6. *The Maddox Wing Test (Giles, 1965)*

a. A Remy separator-like instrument presents a white finger pointing vertically upwards and a red arrow pointing to the left, to one eye. The other eye sees a horizontal row of figures in white and a vertical row in red. The figures are calibrated to read in degrees of deviation, and the positions of the arrow and finger indicate the phorias.

7. *The Mallett Fixation Disparity Test*

a. The unit consists of a box similar to the Freeman or Turville-Eskridge units, in that it is held at the accustomed nearpoint distance by the patient.

(1) Two reading charts contain two black circles, one placed in the center of each reading chart.

(2) One black circle contains a horizontal white strip which contains the letters OXO. Above the letter X, is a vertical green strip which is polarized horizontally to be seen by the left eye. Below the X, is another vertical green strip which is polarized vertically, to be seen by the right eye.

(3) The other black circle contains the same white strip, running vertically, with the same three letters, but with the green strips to the left and right of the letter X. The right one is polarized horizontally (for the left eye) and the left one is polarized vertically (for the right eye).

b. A polarized visor is placed before the eyes while the patient views the left circle.

(1) If both green strips are in alignment, orthophoria or "compensated" heterophoria exists.

(2) If one strip is out of alignment with the letter X, according to laws of projection, the direction of displacement indicates the lateral uncompensated heterophoria and retinal slip.

(a) Both green strips may slip from the X indicating a binocular slip.

(3) A tilt of one or both green strips will exhibit cyclophoria, according to the laws of projection.

(4) The other circle is used to measure the presence of vertical heterophoria.

c. The minimum prism or sphere which eliminates the slip is the correction.

(1) For exophoria, the weakest base-in prism or minus lens which aligns the strips is added to the Rx.

(2) For esophoria, the minimum base-out prism or plus lens is used, except that plus lens in excess of the working distance value is not used.

(3) Cyclophoria at near may be due to the infra-vergence position of the eyes.

(a) It may induce a change in the desired astigmatic axis position for near.

d. Suppression may be revealed by the total absence of one of the green strips. It is further tested by the introduction of a chart which contains several three letter lines of decreasing angular size, the middle letter of which is visible to both eyes. Some peripheral circles are also visible to both eyes. The remaining letters are visible to each eye according to their polarization.

e. Other Uses

(1) Mallett measures the ACA by noting the amount of prism which corrects the slip present, and comparing it to the lens power which does likewise. If slip is not present, he compares the least prism and lens power which induces it.

(2) The dominant eye is usually revealed by the fact that it is not the one which exhibits the slip.

(3) The Freeman ± 0.25 D. spherical twirl can be used to check the power of one eye by using a 1.00 D. cross cylinder to inhibit vision in the other. Mallett prefers this to a fogging lens or polaroid for testing one eye in binocular position.

(4) By pushing up the device, using fine type and a vertical line, the nearpoints of both accommodation and convergence can be measured.

f. Bichromatic Balance Test

(1) A special chart, illustrated in Figure XX-10, can be used for a bichromatic test.

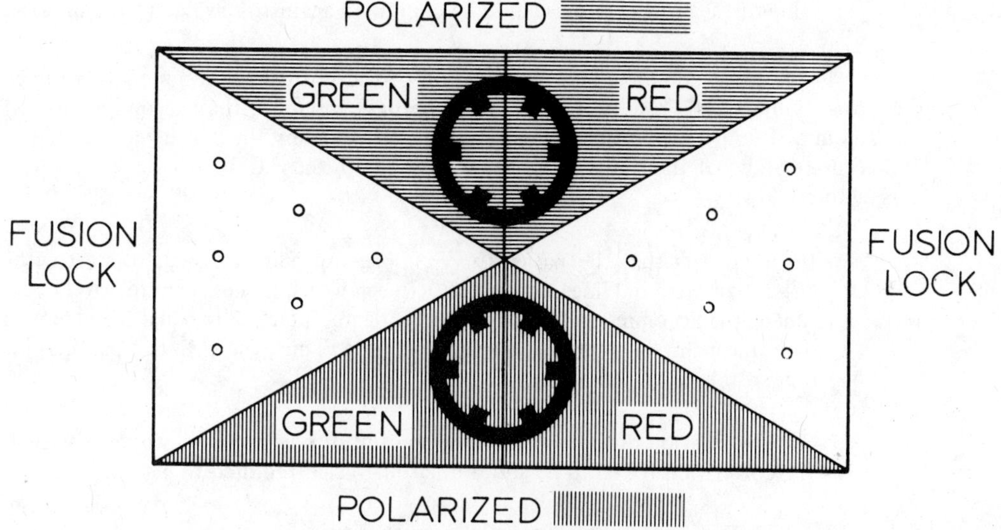

Figure XX-10 – Mallett Bichromatic Chart.

(a) Using the polaroid visor, each eye can be tested for equal clarity of the cog in both the red and green backgrounds.

(2) The device also enables accommodation to be equalized insofar as effort at near is concerned.

g. A stereopsis test chart consisting of white symbols on a black background, one column polarized for one eye, and the other for the other eye, is revealed under dim illumination with prism base-out of 3 prism diopters used to fuse the columns.

(1) By reversing the visor, the displacement can be reversed, enabling the examiner to check the response.

8. See also Turville, Wilmut, Freeman, and related devices in Chapter XIX (Subjective Testing).

VIII. ACCOMMODATION TESTS – CROSSED CYLINDERS

A. The cross cylinder test is a test of indefinite response in that the accommodation may be inhibited, stimulated or apparently not respond at all. The theory of the test is somewhat analogous to that of the phoria test in that the accommodation should be suspended with the retina in the interval of Sturm created by the C.C., and a perfect focus should be impossible, just as the convergence is suspended by dissociation. The theory then assumes that since no true focus can be placed on the retina, the accommodation will relax an amount free of convergence, or an amount equal to the excess strain, if any, of accommodation. The relaxation would place both foci behind the retina, and the addition of plus lenses would then restore the circle of least confusion to the retina, marking the critical measuring point.

1. The accommodation not relaxed would be held fixed by the convergence in the fused C.C. test and would be the difference between the original value of the working distance and the amount of plus added with the C.C. in place.

2. This "relative accommodation" would leave an amount of convergent-accommodation in play, which by an assumption of reciprocal action of the two functions should be equal to the accommodative-convergence still maintained under a phoria test at the same distance. Hence, the value of the cross cylinder would be computed against the value of the phorias.

B. Fry (1940a) conducted an investigation of the status of accommodation under the influence of the cross cylinder. His results indicate that the basic premise, that accommodation is controlled by the amount of convergence-accommodation which is fixed by the convergence at the time of the test, is not accurate and that the status of accommodation with the C.C. before the eyes depends upon a number of factors.

1. It appears that the patient may choose any point of focus to start with, that is, the vertical lines, the horizontal lines, or a point between which makes them relatively equal. As plus lenses are added, the accommodation changes to a degree practically equal to the power added, maintaining the same point of reference originally chosen. Thus, the C.C. test parallels in a modified form the tests of relative accommodation.

2. The relation of the phoria to the amount of plus accepted was also statistically determined and the correlation found to be about one-fourth that required to be significant.

3. The cross cylinder test is influenced then by:

a. A desire for clear vision manifested by a preference for either set of lines or equal clarity.

b. A tendency to compensate for the phoria by increasing or relaxing accommodation to induce a change in accommodative-convergence.

c. The psychological awareness of the nearness of the target.

C. The fused cross cylinder finding is also used to help determine a near add. The calculations are again based upon a certain relationship of accommodation and convergence as expressed by a comparison of the phoria with the C.C. finding. Fry (1940b) in a study of the use of the C.C. for this purpose and by these means, analyzed 100 cases in which the subjective prescription alone had been prescribed satisfactorily. The grand average indicated that the method of determining the add by means of the phoria seemed to verify the procedure. But when individual cases are studied, it is found that adds ranging from −1.50 to +1.25 could have been determined. The solely accurate value of the C.C. for determining the nearpoint prescription seems to be in cases of absolute presbyopia, in which cases the gross C.C. finding serves as the add. In partial presbyopia, the C.C. finding, *without modification,* may approximate the add, and it is used in that manner.

D. Westheimer (1958) also points out that the clarity of one or the other set of lines is not a determinant of accommodative activity, since accommodation is usually either excessive or insufficient for the distance.

1. In presbyopia, the technique as usually used is adequate.

2. For non-presbyopes, Westheimer suggests removal of the cross cylinders between each lens

change and reintroducing them at the lens change, until the lines appear alike. This might avoid a possible accommodative action based upon clarification of one set of lines only.

3. It is doubtful, however, if this is a significant factor in the average case.

E. Dissociated Cross Cylinder Technique

1. The T chart is presented to the patient at the working or nearpoint test distance.

2. The cross cylinders are placed before both eyes with the minus axes at 90°.

3. Prism base-down is placed before one eye and prism base-up before the other, and the amount increased equally until the patient reports two T charts.

4. The patient is requested to note the upper chart and relate whether the lines running up and down (vertically) or those running across (horizontally) are blacker, or if the two are equal.

5. If the horizontal lines are darker, a plus .25 D. sphere is added before the eye and the patient requested to repeat his observation.

6. The patient is then referred to the lower chart and the same request and procedure is employed.

7. The attention is alternated from one chart to the other with each step of additional .25 D. The additional power is added until the two sets of lines appear equal.

   a. Some clinicians recommend that sufficient plus be added to force a reversal and make the vertical lines blacker. The power is then reduced until equality is again produced.

8. If one eye equalizes before the other, the eye not equalized is presented with additional power until it is.

   a. The acceptance of unequal power may be due to unequal accommodation but is usually due to either unequal balancing of the subjective correction or to improper cylindrical correction of one of the eyes.

9. If the vertical lines are originally darker, most clinicians do not add minus since the accommodation can readily compensate for it. However, some men do add and record a minus value.

10. The gross addition remaining before the eyes is used for associated phoria test.

F. Binocular Cross Cylinder Technique

1. Since the binocular technique usually follows the dissociated one, the dissociating prisms are removed and the patient should see a single T chart through the dissociated C.C. findings.

2. The C.C. are replaced if they have been removed for the phoria with their minus axes again at 90°.

   a. Some do not remove the C.C. for the phoria but leave them in position for this test. Whether the presence or absence of the C.C. influences the result is debatable, although it would appear that a phoria taken upon a target requiring sharp vision, with the C.C. in place, would be inaccurate. Such clinicians frequently avoid this contretemps and use the T chart as the phoria target. The indefinite accommodation required plus the strong fusional stimuli such a chart presents would theoretically tend to discredit their results.

3. Since the dissociated findings are already before the eyes, it will be frequently found that the vertical lines appear blacker and that the plus must be reduced to regain equality. The power is reduced before both eyes at the same time. If the lines are equal or the horizontal lines are darker, plus is added binocularly until reversal is attained and then reduced to equality.

4. Some men prefer to build up plus and either remove the dissociated findings before beginning the binocular or take the binocular findings, which usually reveal less plus than the other, prior to taking the dissociated test.

5. The total findings determined by the binocular test are used for the associated phoria, following the test.

G. Other Considerations

1. Since the lines constitute rather gross targets, a finer sense of discrimination is frequently evinced if the illumination is reduced fairly close to the threshold.

2. The immediate reaction to the C.C. may be one of accommodative effort in an attempt to equalize the lines. It is advisable to wait a moment before questioning the patient to permit the accommodation to stabilize.

3. Total presbyopes or nearly total presbyopes will frequently find both sets of lines so badly blurred that the choice may be made upon the basis of psychological preference, usually for the vertical lines. If plus is added and the images brought closer to the retina, the actually blacker horizontal lines will be selected, and additional plus is required to equalize the two sets.

4. The gross binocular C.C. findings may be used as a preliminary tentative add for presbyopia.

5. If no lens equalizes the two sets of lines, the lens which barely leaves the vertical blacker is used as the finding for the test.

6. While it is common practice to ask the patient to indicate which lines are "blacker", the author has found that some patients will always choose the horizontal lines because the vertical lines, even if clearer than the horizontal ones, often are described by the patient as appearing "brown" or "reddish" colored. In such cases, even when the horizontal lines appear more blurred than the vertical, the patient will indicate that they are nonetheless, the "blacker".

a. To avoid this, the author has taken to using the phrasing: "Which of the two sets of lines, the one running sideways or the ones running up and down, appear to stand out better or to contrast better?" The question of relative color is thereby unimportant.

IX. RELATIVE ACCOMMODATION

A. Although the existence of accommodation which does not arouse convergence innervation is not universally accepted, the appearance of such accommodation is presented by the tests thereby erroneously named tests of relative accommodation.

B. Positive Relative Accommodation (P.R.A.)

1. The patient is directed to the nearpoint chart utilizing the finest visible type.

2. He is requested to report when the type appears to be blurred. Since a gap between the first appearance of the blur and sufficient blur to make the print incomprehensible usually is found, the clinician may use either as the stopping point for both the positive and negative tests, but should use the same one for both tests. The first blur, although more valuable for analytical purposes, is

rather difficult to define and most clinicians find the blur-out point more readily determinable.

3. Minus lenses are added in .25 D. steps before both eyes until the blur is reached.

a. Since, as the limits are approached, the effort of accommodation may be sluggish, the examiner should wait a moment before deciding that a given power measures the limit of the test.

4. The amount of minus added above the lenses previously before the eyes is recorded as the finding.

C. Negative Relative Accommodation (N.R.A.)

1. The procedure is identical with that for P.R.A. except plus lenses are added.

D. The fact that convergence remains fixed while accommodation varies with the addition of plus and minus lenses has been interpreted to indicate the exhibition of accommodation free of convergence. However, what may actually take place is that as accommodation is increased with the addition of minus lenses, accommodative-convergence is increased also. The fixation is maintained by the utilization of the negative fusional convergence to secure binocular fixation at the nearpoint test distance. As additional minus is added, and additional accommodation-convergence is induced, the total negative fusional convergence is ultimately activated. At that point, the further response of accommodation to more minus would induce sufficient accommodative-convergence to produce over-convergence and diplopia. Since the patient desires to maintain single vision, he does not accommodate further and the next addition of minus creates a blur. In the same way, the addition of plus lenses relaxes the accommodation and reduces the accommodative-convergence. This is compensated by an increase in the positive fusional convergence. At the critical point, the reserve of positive fusional convergence is exhausted, and further relaxation of accommodation would produce an under-convergence or diplopia. The patient, therefore, does not usually relinquish additional accommodation, and permits the next plus addition to blur him.

1. Occasionally a patient is found who continues to respond to the changes in lens power even beyond the critical points and reports diplopia without blurring rather than a blurred single target. This report is as good a criterion for the test as the other.

2. The lens which creates the blur or diplopia is recorded for each finding.

E. The subjective determination of relative accommodation seldom agrees with the objective findings. The discrepancy is ascribed to the ability of the patient to interpret the blurred images even after the focus has been removed from the retina. Consequently, the P.R.A. and N.R.A. findings are almost always excessive by this discrepancy for comparison and correlation with other tests involving the accommodative-convergence.

X. AMPLITUDE OF ACCOMMODATION

A. The simplest method of measuring the amplitude is that of Donders, and Duane, in which a target of the best acuity is moved towards the eye until it is blurred, and the distance of the target at that point from the eye is converted into diopters. When taken binocularly, the target is presented on the median line; when taken monocularly, it is presented directly before each eye.

1. The test is always taken monocularly for each eye and also binocularly.

2. Several discrepancies of this method have been noted in Chapter VI, but the chief deficiency by ordinary procedures is the fact that the target size is fixed, and as it is brought closer to the eye, the letters subtend at a successively larger angle. The findings taken by this means may therefore be somewhat higher than otherwise.

B. Another method of taking the amplitude is Sheard's method of adding the value of the nearpoint distance to the result of the P.R.A. finding. When done binocularly, this is scarely reliable, since the P.R.A. finding is affected by the extent of the relative convergence rather than the limits of the accommodation. If done monocularly, however, convergence is eliminated, and the technique produces fairly consistent results (see Chapter VI).

1. The Optometric Extension Program recommends that since the addition of minus power tends to reduce the size of the target, the target should be moved closer to the eye, to 13 inches rather than the usual 16-inch working distance. However, the addition to the minus power found is still interpreted as that of the 16-inch distance so that the finding is noted as –2.50 D. combined with the actual total of minus lens power required to blur.

C. In taking either the amplitude or the P.R.A. and N.R.A., advanced presbyopes may not be able to see the target equivalent to their distant acuity, which should be the size used at near, without plus lens assistance. A plus lens of sufficient power to enable them to see the letters may be introduced. However, the value of this lens must be subtracted from the amplitude and the positive relative accommodation test, and added to the negative relative accommodation test to record their true values.

1. Since in the relative accommodation tests, the ideal add would be one which required the use of one-half the accommodation, the end results of the two tests would equal each other in such presbyopic cases if the correct add were before the eyes at the time of testing. Consequently, in presbyopes, the add used to assist the patient is frequently not subtracted or added to these findings, but the actual findings found with the add are recorded and a notation made beside them indicating that the add was in place. If they are equal, it is a clue towards the determination of the proper add. The assisting lens is always, however, deducted from the amplitude value found with it.

D. One of the chief inconsistencies of all nearpoint tests depending upon maintenance of precise accommodation is the discrepancy between the actual accommodation interpreted as the reciprocal of the test distance and that which the patient may actually be using, due to blur interpretation, etc., as previously discussed. Another discrepancy is due to the nature of the test types used (Berens & Fonda, 1950) (see also Chapter X).

1. A commonly used nearpoint card is one developed upon the test-types arranged by Jaeger. J1, the smallest, subtends a 5′ angle at 45 cms. (17-18 inches), and when moved closer is far from a precise stimulus to accommodation. At 9 inches, J1 actually represents visual acuity of 20/40, and at 4½ inches, 20/80. Thus, an amplitude of 8 to 10 D. might be easily recorded. The Jaeger types consist of twenty different sizes, graded by number, and principally determined by the sizes of type available. Different editions are not consistent, the character of typeface varies, and the letters are not square, and of unequal diameter and vary in dimensions and definition even in parts of the same letter. A printed reduced Snellen chart, also in common use, also employs a 20/20 line which subtends a 5′ angle at 45 cms. and utilizes variations limited by the print face available. (See Chapter X).

2. The ideal test chart would be one which is photostatically a reduction of a proper series of letters varying in accurate size and form to letters which subtend the required angles for distances far inside the common nearpoint test distance. Thus, a card with 20/20 letters for 5 inches, factored back to type for 30 inches or so, would enable the examiner to require fixation upon the appropriate type size as the card was moved closer for the amplitude test. Berens and Fonda (1950) and Lebensohn (1936) have developed a card which more closely meets the desired ideal. Others have employed cards using line gratings and similar small separations of targets drawn finer than most available nearpoint test cards.

E. A final notation concerning the results attainable in tests of accommodation must deal with the position of the lines of sight during such tests. The association between added convergence ability and directing the vision down may also affect the accommodative performance. Ripple (1952) notes that accommodative ability is greater when the eyes are directed inward, still greater when they are directed downward, and greatest when both directions are combined.

XI. OTHER TESTS

A. Fusion Check Test

1. The Fusion Check Test is a quick routine test to assist in determining whether the complaint originates from excessive difficulty in maintaining binocular fixation.

2. The procedure of the test consists of creation of a condition of dissociation and then observation of the ease and rapidity with which the fusion is regained when the causes of dissociation are removed. The interpretation of the results are purported to reveal the facility and fusional "desire" of the patient.

3. Dissociation is gained by placing a vertical prism of 6 pd base down before one eye and a red glass before the other while the patient has both eyes shut. A small circular light serves as a target for the farpoint test and a dot on a card serves as the target at the nearpoint.

4. When the patient is requested to open his eyes, two targets are seen, one red and one white. The prism is suddenly removed when one of several results may be noted:

   a. The two dots may combine almost instantaneously into a single spot, being pinkish in color at far or on a pinkish background at near.

   b. The dot may appear as a single white or red dot at far or on a white or reddish background at near.

   c. The two dots may slowly come together or may remain apart.

5. If a single dot is seen on a pink background (or of a pink color if at far), it is assumed that fusion is good, since the recovery was rapid and instantaneous.

   a. Since the red and white may blend in such a way as to seem almost white, it is necessary to proceed farther in such cases in order to determine whether fusion or suppression has taken place. The red glass is suddenly removed and the dot or background should appear slightly greenish due to the after image if the red dot has been part of the original image. If the red dot has been suppressed, the color of the dot will not alter. However, at near, where the background of the card supplies the color clues, the periphery may not be suppressed even when the dot has been and the color will usually change in either type of vision.

6. If the dot is red, the white dot has been suppressed.

7. If the dots slowly drift together, fusion is only fair, while if they remain apart, fusion is poor.

8. The rotary prisms may be used if desired to restore single vision in those cases in which no single target is seen, one prism introducing vertical and the other horizontal power, according to the patient's description of the position of the two targets. The prism is slowly increased until fusion is restored and the amount required may serve as a guide to the inclusion of prism in the correction.

9. Bedrossian (1952) found that the introduction of a red lens without vertical prism before one eye would usually break fusion in almost 50% of the normal cases. Further, he declared that the ease with which the diplopia was manifested bore little relationship to the amplitude of lateral ductions. The diplopia, although agreeing in order with heterophoria in 92% of the cases, revealed

a disparity which was the same in amount in any direction of gaze. The test has achieved great popularity as a quick check test for fusional ability, but if Bedrossian's findings are accepted, should still be viewed with scepticism.

a. Red and blue could be fused easily, blue and white less easily, and red and white least easily.

b. Suchman (1968) recommends it as an easily employable test for young children, but cautions that errors in "color naming" may confuse its interpretation.

B. Cyclophoria

1. The presence or absence of cyclophoria should be determined prior to measuring the vertical phorias if the dissociation technique by means of lateral prism is used for the latter. This is due to the fact that ordinarily a single letter or block of letters such as a Snellen chart is used as a target for the phoria. The actual alignment of the targets is consequently based upon equal heights of the uppermost margin of the targets and the vertical position of one of the images is partially dependent upon the cyclophoria. The error induced is demonstrated by the accompanying illustration (Figure XX-11). If cyclophoria does exist, it is better to measure the vertical phorias by the Maddox rod technique, which is not influenced by the torsion.

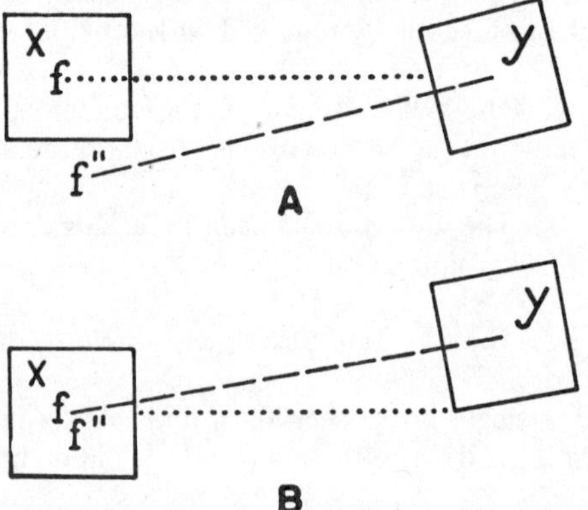

Figure XX-11 – Cyclophoria including error in measurement of vertical phoria by dissociation method. (A) Usual report of equality of height of targets; position of horizontal axes and foveal points indicate actual error induced by form of measurement. (B) Actual alignment of foveal points of projection at equal heights, showing apparent appearance of inequality of height of targets. Dotted line represents plane of horizontal meridian of fixing eye; dashed line indicates plane of horizontal meridian of non-fixing eye. x is image seen by fixing eye; f representing projection of fovea; y image seen peripherally by non-fixing eye; f'' representing foveal projection.

2. A double or bi-prism may be used to determine the cyclophoria. This prism is placed before one eye with its base line horizontal. The patient is requested to fixate a horizontal line or row of letters, which is seen by the eye with the bi-prism before it as two lines or rows vertically separated. When the other eye is exposed to the target, a third line or row appears between the other two. If no cyclophoria exists, this line should be parallel to the others. If the central line is not parallel to the lines between which it lies, cyclophoria exists and can be determined by noting that the torsion of the lines is opposite to that of the eye.

3. A simpler method and one more commonly used is that of placing a Maddox rod before each eye and comparing the two streaks for parallelism or perpendicularity.

a. If the axis of one Maddox rod is placed horizontally and that of the other is placed vertically, a cross should be seen. The arms of the cross should appear at right angles to each other.

b. If both rods are placed with their axes in the same meridians, a vertical prism is required to dissociate them. Two lines will then be seen which should lie parallel.

c. If cyclophoria is demonstrated, one of the Maddox rods can be rotated until the lines are either perpendicular or parallel as the method used requires, and the calibrations of the extent and kind of cyclophoria can be read from the Maddox rod indicators.

d. The line always appears perpendicular to the axes of the cylinders comprising the rod so that the rod is readily rotated once the position of the line is known.

4. If a vertical phoria exists or a lateral phoria is exhibited, the lines will be displaced in accordance with the phoria. In using the double prism, the single line of one eye may be fused with either of the double ones of the other eye if sufficient vertical phoria is present. In using the Maddox rod for the cross images, either phoria may move one arm very close to the end of the other so that the image scarcely resembles a cross. However, the perpendicularity of the angle at which they meet should still be discernible. If the Maddox rod is used with a dissociating prism and a large lateral phoria seems to place the two lines so far apart that judgment of parallelism is difficult, the rods may be reversed in position so that vertical lines are produced which can be dissociated with prism base-in or base-out.

C. Stereopsis

1. Various tests of stereopsis are employed. Many require specialized equipment.

a. *The Howard-Dolman test* is basically a test whereby two vertical rods are viewed from a distance and aligned from in front at what appears to be an equal distance from the observer. The linear distance from the observer of the movable rod from the fixed rod serves to grade the stereoptic acuity.

b. *Stereoptic cards* with test patterns at various separations may be used in a stereoscope. A refractor or trial frame with prisms added may be made into a stereoscope. Usually the distance separating the targets exceeds the pupillary distance and prism base-out is needed. Prism is added until the three images are seen, the center one of which is stereoptic. Plus spheres equivalent to the distance of the chart from the eyes are added.

c. *The Verhoeff stereopter* consists of three rods of different widths: 2, 2.5, and 3 mms. One rod is either nearer or farther than the other two by 2.50 mms. The varying sizes allow a large choice of angular subtenses. The different sizes also give clues opposite to those offered by accommodation and retinal disparity.

(1) Verhoeff (1963) has also introduced a kinetic test consisting of a chart of two holes of 37 mms. diameter placed 61 mms. apart. Figures viewed through these change position and move ahead with a change in disparity apparently through elimination of part of the surround.

2. Results of various test devices for stereopsis are frequently not comparable, indicating that certain clues may be present in one and absent in another, or that different things may be tested or enter into the testing. Sloan and Altman (1954) compared the Howard-Dolman, the Verhoeff and various stereoscopic devices and tests to each other and reported the following:

a. *Auxiliary Monocular Clues*

(1) The monocular threshold of the Howard-Dolman test was 5 times that of the binocular. Size and accommodation were influenced, but the disparity of the targets was the chief influence. Monocular clues of vergence of light and angular subtense agreed with the disparity.

(2) Stereopters and vision testers also depended essentially on disparity, but the lack of differences in size of targets might create false monocular clues and give poor findings.

(a) Bleything (1957) reported, however, that the size of the targets did not alter the stereoscopic localization.

(3) The Verhoeff test might offer a conflict between clues from disparity when the targets were such that more distant targets were wider than near ones and the clues from the visual angles of the targets. Different subjects showed varying results.

b. *Distance of Test Targets*

(1) In all angular units, the distance from the unit may affect the results. The stereopter gave a false indication of good stereopsis because of the short test distance.

c. *Effect of Aniseikonic Errors*

(1) A constant error, if aniseikonia exists, appears in the rod test. In the Verhoeff test, it is not so influential, as the face of the instrument and rods provide a plane of reference. The plane of the steropsis tests may be rotated, but judgment is not affected.

d. *Other Differences*

(1) Luminance of background, lateral separation of targets, luminescence of targets, fixed steps in the stereopter, may all affect the results.

(a) The printed *Fixed settings* of disparities in stereoptic cards predetermine the scoring basis.

e. *Summarization*

(1) Various tests agreed in from 79 to 92% of the cases in selecting good or poor depth perception.

(2) Poor performance on all tests is usually due to low visual acuity, suppression, tropias, possible heterophorias, or lack of skill or effort of motor adjustments (as in the Howard-Dolman test).

(a) The Howard-Dolman test does not reveal intermittent loss of binocularity as a cause of poor judgment.

(3) Bleything also reports that adding minus or base-out shifts the localization to increased distance. The stereoscopic size increases with the localization distance at a slightly greater rate than predicted by the visual angles subtended for each distance measured.

3. *A device designed by Hofstetter,* known as the Stereotest, consists of a translucent plate mounted on a flashlight which contains three 10 mm in diameter opaque dots, which appear equally spaced in a triangle form when the disc face is viewed. One dot was actually on a rod which was 9 mm long, and the other on a rod which was 18 mm long, while the third dot was on the face of the disc. Since most patients referred essentially to one of the dots only, Hofstetter later altered their placement so that one dot remained at the 9 mm extension but both the others were at the surface of the plate.

a. The device is held facing the subject at a distance of ± 5 feet, at eye level and aimed at the point between both eyes. The examiner occludes the face of the instrument with a large blank card and rotates the flashlight to position the dots randomly. He then exposes the face for one or two seconds, records the face immediately so the subject cannot study the dots, and asks the subject to locate the protruding dot.

(1) The test is repeated for six random positions as described above, and a subject with stereopsis should correctly locate the protruding dot every time.

(2) A subject who fails three or more times does not exhibit stereopsis.

(3) A subject who fails one or two of the six exposures may be given as many as two additional series of six exposures each. If he does not pass all six in one of the series, he does not exhibit stereopsis.

b. The ultimate threshold of stereopsis can be attained by varying the distance of presentation. A chart giving both careful instructions for the above test and a chart of seconds of arc per distance of test accompanies the instrument, although the seconds of arc can be determined by the formula, $\frac{P \times R}{d^2} \times 206{,}265$ where P = the interpupillary distance of the subject, R = the dot displacement from the disc; and d = the test distance.

c. Koetting and Mueller (1962) made a version of the instrument in which several transparent discs took the place of the pegs and the dots were painted or attached to the surfaces of the discs. The flashlight illumination tended to reflect back from the anterior discs to the dots on the discs behind, changing the brightness of the dots and cluing the subject that the darkest dot lay farthest frontwards. Some minor variations in the above were specified in technique and in separation of the dots but the basic test principle of Hofsetter's was employed.

4. Sloan and Altman (1954) found that the monocular clues to the differences in distance may indicate that these monocular clues contribute substantially to binocular depth perception, although the sensitivity to uniocular clues alone is much poorer than to binocular clues of retinal disparity.

5. Emmes (1961), using the Wirt polaroid stereopsis test, noted that pre-presbyopes scored one step higher than presbyopes.

D. Gradient

1. The gradient test is basically a test of the accommodative-convergence relationship. Since the relationship of the two is generally constant for the individual, so that for a given total convergence, a given proportion of accommodative-convergence is involved with a given accommodation, a change in the stimulation to accommodation at a fixed distance would result in a change in the amount of accommodative-convergence. This change would be revealed by a compensating alteration in the amount of fusional convergence supplied. The amount of fusional convergence in use can be measured by the phoria, in which fusion is interrupted, and the eyes return to the status determined by tonic, accommodative and psychic innervation.

2. If a pair of eyes using a given amount of accommodation is dissociated and the phoria measured, and if the accommodation is then altered a known amount and the phoria is remeasured, the change in the phoria would be due to the change in fusional convergence, which would in turn be exactly equal to the change of the accommodative-convergence which had been associated with the alteration of the accommodation. Hence, the change in the phoria would indicate the amount of accommodative-convergence associated with the accommodation. As this is assumed to be a constant, it would apply equally for all amounts of accommodation and one measurement would suffice to indicate the nature of the relationship.

3. This relationship is expressed as a ratio, Accommodation/Accommodative-Convergence, and this ratio is known as the ACA ratio. Thus, if a change of 1.00 D. of accommodation altered the phoria by 2 pd, the ratio would be expressed as 1.00/2; if 1.00 D. altered it 4 pd, as 1.00/4, etc.

4. *The gradient test* consists then of a phoria taken with a known amount of lens before the eye to alter the accommodation.

a. The conclusion of the lateral phoria test at near, when the images are aligned and the lateral phoria is indicated on the measuring prism, 1.00 D. lenses are added to the subjective before both eyes.

(1) Morgan recommends adding minus lenses rather than plus lenses for more consistent results.

b. The patient is asked whether the targets are still one above the other. If they are not, the prism is altered in accordance with the new position of the upper target (seen by the eye behind the measuring prism) until they are again aligned.

c. The difference between the original phoria and this new amount of phoria is recorded in relation to the 1.00 D. lens as the gradient.

d. Since, if 1.00 D. altered the phoria 3 pd, 2.00 D. would alter it 6 pd, and so on up to the limits of accommodative-convergence used at that distance, a standard lens value may be used for all cases. The author prefers to use 1.00 D. and usually records merely the change of the phoria as 2 pd, since the relationship of 2 pd for each diopter is obvious. If more than 1.00 D. is used, the fraction should be reduced to one diopter so that the relationship can be expressed as "so much accommodative-convergence for each diopter of accommodation." If 2.00 D. were used in all cases and a change of 8 pd. were found, it should still be expressed as 1.00/4; that is, a 4 pd ACA for each diopter of accommodation.

5 While the ACA ratio is reasonably constant in and for the individual, it is not constant for all individuals, and the ratio must be determined for each specific patient (see Chapter VII).

E. The Lancaster (1939) Test

1. The phoria may also be differentiated from paretic involvement by taking the phoria at various fixation positions in the field. The vertical findings should be checked with both erect and tilted head positions where vertical imbalances are suspected, since a typical head tilt usually compensates for vertical paresis. Usually, a nine field examination employing the tangent screen, with and without head tilt, is used and is further described in the chapters on strabismus. However, a simple procedure can be utilized as described by Lancaster.

2. The patient views a white screen while wearing spectacles containing one green and one red lens. With a green and red spot projected on the screen, the patient will see only one fused spot, but the difference between the two on the screen measures the phoria.

a. Brock (1963) places 17 red dots in various areas of a ruled red screen and uses a red flashlight to locate any designated area. The patient sees the screen through a green lens. Disparity can be measured in various loci of the field.

b. A nearpoint adaptation fits on the reading rod for measurements with the head held naturally and the eyes cast down.

3. If two streaks are used, both vertical, the angular positions of the streaks, if they are not fused, assist in determining the paretic muscle involved.

a. Morgan (1960) suggests using a hand-held Maddox rod and light and noting the disparity of the vertical streak as the light is moved laterally, then of a lateral streak as the light is moved vertically.

(1) This is particularly recommended when elderly patients are tested.

(2) Chart of Disparities and Related Affected Muscles in various parts of field (see also Chapters VII & XXXI).

(a) TABLE XX-2

Vertical Separation Torsion	*L.S.R.* *R.I.O.* *L.I.O.*	*R.S.R.* *L.I.O.* *R.I.O.*	Vertical Separation Torsion
Left Separation	*L.L.R.* *R.M.R.*	*R.L.R.* *L.M.R.*	Right Separation
Vertical Separation Torsion	*L.I.R.* *R.S.O.* *L.S.O.*	*R.I.R.* *L.S.O.* *R.S.O.*	Vertical Separation Torsion

4. Fields (1963) also describes a slide for the Lancaster test which consists of two 1 to 2 mm. holes separated by 6 to 8 mms., one containing a red filter and the other a green one and projected on a screen. A red and green filter is placed before each eye, respectively.

XII. SUMMARY

A. A facile phorometric routine is that which permits the tests to slide readily into each other with the least changing of targets, alterations of equipment, or positioning of the refractor, and yet does not involve tests in such an order that one may influence the results in the next, as, for example, what vertical ductions might do to the vertical phorias. The author has found the following order one which serves well:

1. *Tests at far*

a. The target usually recommended has been either one line of type of best acuity, or a small square or circle of light with one or more letters of the line of best acuity within it. The author, has in recent years, used the entire section of the projected chart, ranging from the approximate 20/50 to the 20/15 lines of letters. This eliminates the need to change the chart from that used for subjective testing to that used for phorometry, and back again for the "delayed subjective." While the larger chart does involve a greater peripheral area, and does require a slightly larger dissociating prism, the results have not seemed sufficiently different to require the more time consuming changes the previous forms of targets would require.

b. *Phorias at far*

(1) The prisms are placed before the eyes so that the vertical rotary prism is before the left eye, and the horizontal one before the right eye.

(2) Vertical phoria at far

(a) The right prism dissociates and the left measures as previously described.

(3) Lateral prism at far

(a) The left prism dissociates and the right measures. No change in prism placement, target, etc. is required.

c. *Ductions*

(1) Since the distant ductions are often reflected in the near ones, and since the

duction findings may influence the subsequent nearpoint phoria values, the ductions at distance are not taken at this time.

2. *Tests at Near*

a. The refractor is adapted for the nearpoint tests by narrowing the space between the cells so as to reduce the interpupillary distance by approximately 4 mm. The nearpoint rod is brought into place presenting the nearpoint target at 16 inch working distance. This target may be a small line of letters, a group of letters of the same size, a set of small lines, or a reduced Snellen chart. The author uses a card which contains a reduced Snellen chart on one side, and a T chart on the other. However, similar cards are available containing targets of ruled lines, groups of letters, etc. The main objective is to have available a target which will insure accommodative action is maintained during the tests, and which will permit easy transfer of targets for the desired tests.

(1) The patient is directed to the letters or target of best acuity. If presbyopia exists, and the letters comparable to the acuity at far cannot be deciphered, a size which can be read is used for the early phoria tests until the add needed for better acuity is known.

b. *Phorias At Near*

(1) The prisms are in position (following the distant phorias) without further change for the nearpoint phoria tests, as soon as the nearpoint target is presented.

(a) The vertical phoria at near is first taken, just as for distance.

(b) The lateral phoria is then taken.

(c) The Gradient

[1] When the lateral phoria at near is found, the prism over the right eye is left at its measuring point which aligns the upper target over the lower.

[2] Minus 1.00 D. lenses are added before both eyes and the patient reports whether the upper target remains directly above the lower or is displaced, and if so, in which direction. The −1.00 D. lenses must be removed after the test.

[3] The measuring prism need merely be adjusted to realign the targets.

[4] If the patient is presbyopic, the gradient is not taken, but a phoria is taken with the cross-cylinder values before the eye, later, when these have been determined.

(d) Phorias With Cross Cylinder Findings

[1] See below. Not taken at this time.

c. *Cross-Cylinder Test*

(1) Binocular Cross-Cylinder

(a) The prisms are rotated to the zero value, but left in position. The nearpoint card is rotated to present the T Chart. The C.C. are introduced before the eyes.

(2) Dissociated Cross-Cylinders

(a) The prisms before the eyes are used to dissociate. The right prism must be rotated so that its action becomes vertical, and the prism amount divided equally before both eyes.

d. *Phorias with Cross Cylinder Findings*

(1) In effect, these are another version of the gradient test.

(2) All reports of correlation indicate that these phorias have very little value or implication within the recommended procedure of some to use them to determine the nearpoint addition. The author does not take them at all although they can be taken with very little additional adjustment after each of the above tests, since the prisms are already before the eyes.

(3) In presbyopes, where the gradient has not been taken immediately following the lateral phoria, the add based upon amplitude and the above cross cylinder *gross* values is before the eye for the successive tests. If the C.C. findings do not approximate the add which is indicated by the amplitude, the plus addition is modified until it does. Usually, the C.C. value is reasonably close to the required amount so that the plus added in presbyopic cases during those tests can be used for the remainder of the tests. If the amplitude has revealed the patient to be non-presbyopic, the plus of the C.C. is removed.

(4) The phoria at near is repeated with the add for presbyopic patients. If a gradient was taken earlier, as in non-presbyopes, this phoria is omitted at this time. The accommodative-convergence relationship of the presbyope can be approximately determined from this version of the tests by comparison to the original phoria at near prior to the add.

(a) If the phoria is taken with the binocular cross-cylinder findings alone, and the dissociated cross cylinder findings are not usually taken (a policy the author generally follows except where lack of equalization is suspected), the prism positions are those of the preceding phoria tests and are automatically in place for the phoria with the cross-cylinder findings.

(b) If the dissociated C.C. findings are taken, the prisms will have been altered so that equal vertical prism is before each eye. If phorias are then desired, the right prism will have to be rotated back to its position for phoria testing (from vertical action to horizontal action).

e. *Amplitude of Accommodation*

(1) The prisms are reduced to zero power, but not removed. The push-up method is used, whereby the reduced Snellen Chart (or other target of best acuity) is moved towards the eye. Since this follows the C.C. test, care must be taken not to forget to remove the cross-cylinder.

(a) The binocular test is first taken.

(b) When the binocular nearpoint is found, the card is removed a slight distance away and the monocular test is taken, by occluding first one eye, and moving the card in, then removing the card slightly again, and occluding the opposite eye (exposing the first) and moving it in.

(c) The patient's attention must be directed at all times to the print or lines of best acuity.

f. *Ductions At Near*

(1) Lateral Ductions

(a) The C.C. being removed, the T chart is replaced with the original nearpoint letters. (In presbyopia the add is in place and the letters should be equivalent to the distant acuity.) The prisms are arranged for horizontal power. No other adjustment is needed.

(b) Since the Negative Fusional Reserve affects the Positive Fusional Reserve less, if taken in that order, than if taken in reverse, the author takes the N.F.R. test before the P.F.R. test.

(2) Vertical Ductions

(a) The prism need merely be rotated for vertical power.

g. *Relative Accommodation*

(1) Positive (P.R.A.)

(a) The prisms are now removed. The other arrangements are in place for this test.

(2) Negative (N.R.A.)

(a) No other adjustment is required.

3. *Delayed Subjective*

a. When the blurpoint of the Negative Relative Accommodative Test has been found, the nearpoint chart is lifted, and the patient's attention directed to the distant test chart, and to the letters of best acuity previously established. The lenses are unfogged to best acuity.

4. *Cyclophoria*

a. Although not always taken, this test can be readily taken just after the Delayed Subjective.

(1) If the prisms are in position of vertical action, following the nearpoint vertical ductions, the Maddox rods need merely be introduced before both eyes, and prism power divided equally to dissociate the eyes.

(2) The Maddox rods are removed and the prism restored to zero for the vertical ductions which follow.

5. *Ductions at Far*

a. Since the prisms have been left before the eyes in the position of the last prism test (vertical ductions), the duction tests can be taken upon the distant target.

(1) Vertical Ductions At Far

(a) The prisms are in place for this, and the test need merely be performed.

(2) Lateral Ductions At Far

(a) If the vertical ductions were taken, the prisms need be rotated so that their action is now lateral.

(b) As at the nearpoint, the Abduction is taken before the Adduction.

(c) If the vertical ductions were not taken at either near or far, and many examiners do not take them unless a hyperphoria is disclosed, the prisms will be found, following the Delayed Subjective, in the positions of the nearpoint lateral ductions and will not be required to be altered for the distant ductions.

b. The author seldom takes the ductions at far since, as noted earlier, their indications are often included in the nearpoint ductions. However, where an analytical system is to be used, or if a predominant imbalance is revealed in the phorias, the ductions are taken to confirm the indications.

6. *Stereopsis*

a. If a chart for stereopsis at distance requires lateral prism to create a fused stereoptic pattern, the prisms are already in position after the distant lateral ductions and can be easily introduced to create the pattern.

b. If it is to be taken at nearpoint, it can be taken at any point after the prisms are in horizontal power position, since it interrupts the routine because it requires a special target. Similarly other special tests can be taken at appropriate places in the routine, preferably where they least interrupt the flow of procedure from one test to the other.

B. Some considerations which influence the tests should be kept in mind. Not every patient will understand what the examiner wishes, and variation in technique will be required. Also, the vertical tests may be influenced by the judgment of the patient, who may have his own concept of what constitutes a "level" position. This may be particularly true if a cylinder is introduced in the subjective to a patient who has not had his astigmatism properly corrected before, and where other types of meridional or over-all aniseikonia are induced.

C. The diagnostic system which the practitioner prefers may also indicate the order and totality of his routine, as will be seen in the later chapters.

D. Finally, the routine will vary with the experience and personal likes of the examiner and with the type of equipment which he employs. So long as the necessary tests are included, and the total routine does not become overwhelmingly fatiguing and burdensome to the patient, the results will be fairly satisfactory. In the author's opinion, a minimum clinical routine subsequent to the refraction should contain the following:

1. Vertical Phoria at Far
2. Lateral Phoria at Far
3. Vertical Phoria at Near
4. Lateral Phoria at Near
5. Gradient (in non-presbyopes)
6. Cross-cylinder (binocular)
7. Cross-cylinder (dissociated) (optional)
8. Lateral phoria at near with add (usually binocular C.C.) (in presbyopes)
9. Amplitude of Accommodation

10. Negative Relative Convergence
11. Negative Fusional Reserve
12. Positive Relative Convergence
13. Positive Fusional Reserve
14. Vertical Ductions
15. Positive Relative Accommodation
16. Negative Relative Accommodation
17. Delayed Subjective
18. Cyclophoria at Far
19. Vertical Ductions at Far
20. Abduction
21. Adduction
22. Convergence
23. Stereopsis at Far

a. Either the Gradient or Phoria with add is taken, depending upon state of presbyopia.

b. The Vertical Ductions are optional, depending on the vertical phoria or other indications.

c. The cyclophoria test may be omitted upon occasion, depending on symptoms, etc.

d. If the optional tests are omitted, the prisms still remain in position for continuity of performance without unnecessary alteration of position.

REFERENCES

Allen, M.J. (1950): Consideration of Criteria Of Blur With Respect To Their Use In The Routine Examination. The O-Eye-O, 16 (2): 10.

Bannon, R.E. (1943): Diagnostic And Therapeutic Use Of Monocular Occlusion. A.A.A.O., 20: 345.

Bedrossian, E.H. (1952): Significance Of Red Lens Diplopia. A.J. Oph., 35: 1356.

Berens, C. & Fonda, G. (1950): A Spanish-English Accommodation And Near Test Card Using Photoreduce Type. A.J. Oph., 33: 1788.

Bielschowsky, A. (1938): Disturbances of the Vertical Motor Muscles of the Eye. Arch. Oph., 20: 175.

Bleything, W.B. (1960): Factors Influencing Stereoscopic Localization. A.A.A.O., 37: 327.

Booth, S.M., Lofgren, J.R., & Thome, C.D. (1965): The Effect Of Vertical Ductions On The Near Lateral Phorias, Thesis, College of Optometry, Pacific U., June, 1965.

Brock, F.W. (1963): New Method For Testing Binocular Control. J.A.O.A., 34: 443.

Carter, D.B. (1957): Studies of Fixation Disparity. I. Historical Review, A.A.A.O., 34: 320; II. Apparatus Procedure and the Problems of Constant Error, A.A.A.O., 35: 590; III. The Apparent Uniocular Components of Fixation Disparity, A.A.A.O., 37: 408.

Carter, D.B. (1960): Fixation Disparity With and Without Foveal Fusion Contours, A.A.A.O., 41: 265.

Carter, D.B. (1963): Effect of Prolonged Wearing of Prisms. A.A.A.O., 40: 265.

Carter, D.B. (1964): Fixation Disparity and Heterophoria Following Prolonged Wearing of Prisms, A.A.A.O., 42: 265.

Carter, D.B. (1968): Notes On Fixation Disparity, J.A.O.A., 38: 1103.

**Charnwood, Lord: Fusion in Binocular Vision. B.J. Phys. Opt. 11: 65.*

Chin, L. & LaRich, L. (1966): A Study of Effects of Oblique Meridional Magnification upon Ductions. Opt. Weekly, 57: 61.

Cushman, B. & Culver, J. (1953): Prolonged Occlusion. A.J. Oph., 36: 76.

**Dayton, G.O. Jr., Jones, M.H. (1964a): Analysis Of Characteristics of Fixation Reflex In Infants By Use of Direct Current Electro-oculography, Neurology. 14: 1152.*

Dayton, G.O., Jr., Jansen, G. & Jones, M.H. (1962): Abstract, Invest., Oph. 1: 414.

**Dayton, G.O., Jr.; Jones, M.H.; Aiu, P.; Rawson, R.A.; Steele, B. & Rose, M. (1964b): Developmental Study Of Coordinated Eye Movements In The Human Infant, I & II, Arch Oph., 71: 865, 871.*

**Doherty, B.A. & Geraci, M.J. (1964): Comparative Phoria Measurements. Opt. Weekly, 45: 1479.*

Duke-Elder, S.W. (1949): Textbook Of Ophthalmology, Vol. 4, C.V. Mosby Co., St. Louis

**Duke-Elder, S.W. (1963): The Practice Of Refraction, 7th ed., C.V. Mosby Co., St. Louis.*

Eggers, H. (1959): The Maddox Rod Phenomenon. Arch. Oph., 61: 346.

Ellerbrock, V.J. (1949): Experimental Investigation Of Vertical Fusional Movements. A.A.A.O., 26: 327, 388.

Ellerbrock, V.J. (1950): Tonicity Induced By Fusional Movements. A.A.A.O., 27: 8.

**Ellerbrock, V.J. (1952): The Effect of Aniseikonia on Vertical Divergence. A.A.A.O., 29: 403.*

Ellerbrock, V.J. & Fry, G.A. (1941): The After Effect Induced By Vertical Divergence. A.A.A.O., 18: 450.

Ellerbrock, V.J. & Fry, G.A. (1942): Effects Induced By Anisometropic Corrections. A.A.A.O., 19: 444.

Ellerbrock, V.J. & Loran, D.F.C. (1961): Limited Occulsion And Hyperphoria. A.A.A.O., 38: 359.

Emmes, A.B. (1961): A Statistical Study Of Clinical Scores Obtained In The Wirt Stereopsis Test. A.A.A.O., 38: 398.

Eskridge, J.B. (1961): Flip Prism Test For Vertical Phoria. A.A.A.O., 38: 415.

Field, K.K. (1963): A Simplified Homemade Lancaster Test. J.A.O.A., 34: 461.

Flom, M.C. (1958): Some Interesting Eye Movements Obtained During The Cover Test. A.A.A.O., 35: 69.

Friedenwald, J. (1936): Diagnosis and Treatment of Anisophoria. Arch. Oph. 15: 283.

Fry, G.A. (1940a): Significance Of Fused Cross Cylinder Test. Opt. Weekly, 31 (1): 16.

Fry, G.A. (1940b): Nearpoint Corrections From 14B Findings. Opt. Weekly, 31 (2): 48.

**Fry, G.A. (1941): An Analysis of the Relationship Between Phoria, Blur, Break, and Recovery Findings at the Nearpoint. A.A.A.O., 18: 393.*

Giles, G.H. (1965): The Principles And Practice Of Refraction. 2nd ed. Chilton Books, Phila.

Goodlaw, E. (1961): A New Test For Binocular Refraction At The Nearpoint Working Distance. A.A.A.O., 38: 420.

Green, E.L. & Scobee, R.G. (1951): Position Of Risley Prisms In Maddox Rod Test. A.J. Oph., 34: 2, pt. 1: 211.

Haines, H.M. (1941): Optometric Research, J.A.O.A., 10: 151, etc.

**Harker, G.S. (1960): Two Stereoscopic Measures Of Cyclorotation Of The Eyes. A.A.A.O., 37: 461.*

Hirsch, M.J. (1948): Clinical Investigation Of A Method Of Taking Phorias At Forty Centimeter. A.A.A.O., 25: 492.

Hirsch, M.J. (1949): Clinical Notes On Accuracy Of Reading Rotary Prisms. A.A.A.O., 26: 27.

Hirsch, M.J. & Bing, L.B. (1948): The Effect Of Testing Method On Values Obtained for Phorias at Forty Centimeters. A.A.A.O., 25: 407.

**Hirsch, M.J. & Wick, R.E. (1960): Vision Of The Aging Patient. Chilton Books, Phila.*

Hofstetter, H.W. (1952): Comments On Phoria Measurements. The O-Eye-O, 18 (2).

**Jaffee, I.W. (1960): The Action And Use Of The Maddox Rod. J.A.O.A., 31: 451.*

**Jaques, L. (1957): Hyperphoria Testing – A Constant Inconsistency. Opt. Weekly, Jan. 3, 11.*

Koetting, R.A. & Mueller, R.C. (1962): Evaluation of A Rapid Stereopsis Test. A.A.A.O., 39: 299.

Kratz, J.D. (1951): Clinical Significance Of The Abduction Findings. A.A.A.O., 28: 11.

**Kratz, J.D. (1960): The Cover Test In Optometric Practice. J.A.O.A., 31: 453.*

Lebensohn, J.E. (1955): Nature Of Innervational Hyperphoria. A.J. Oph., 39: 854.

Linksz, A. (1950): Physiology Of The Eye, Vol. 1, Optics, Lea & Febiger, New York.

**Ludvigh, E. (1949): The Amount of Eye Movement Objectively Perceptible to the Unaided Eye. A.J. Oph. 32: 649.*

Ludvigh, E. and McKinnon, P. (1966): Relative Effectivity of Foveal and Parafoveal Stimuli in Eliciting Fusional Movements of Small Amplitude. Arch. Oph., 76: 443.

**Maddox, E.E. (1893): The Clinical Use of Prisms, 2nd Ed., John Wright & Co., Bristol.*

**Maddox, E.E. (1907): Tests and Studies of the Ocular Muscles, Keystone Publ. Co., Phila.*

Mallett, R.F.J. (1966a): A Fixation Disparity Test for Distance Use. Opt., 152: 1.

Mallett, R.F.J. (1966b): The Investigation of Oculomotor Balance. Oph. Opt., pt. 1, 6 (12): 586, pt. 2 6 (12): 654.

Mallett, R.F.J.: The Mallett Fixation Disparity Test. Mark 2. Archer-Elliott, Ltd. London.

**Mark, M.J. (1954): A Fixation Target For The Cover Test. O.J.R.O., 91 (2): 40.*

Mills, G. (1950): Designing A New Near Muscle Balance Test. Opt., 119: 115.

Mitchell, D.W.A. (1953): Investigating Binocular Difficulties. B.J. Phys. Opt., 10: 1.

Morgan, M.W. (1955): The Reliability Of Clinical Measurement With Special Refrence To Distant Heterophoria. A.A.A.O., 32: 169.

Morgan, M.W. (1960): Anomalies of the Visual Neuromuscular System of the Aging Patient and Their Correction. Chap. 7 in Vision of the Aging Patient, ed., Hirsch & Wick, Chilton Books, Phila.

Morris, F.M. (1960): The Influence Of Kinesthesia Upon Near Heterophoria Measurements. A.A.A.O., 37: 327.

Nadell, M. (1961): The Measurement Of Vertical Phoria. Opt. World, 49 (5): 28.

Oberman, T. (1967): In Anisophoria, "Don't Spare the Rod." 58 (47): 21.

**Ogle, K.N. & Martens, T.G. (1957): On the Accommodative Convergence and the Proximal Convergence, Arch. Oph., 57: 702.*

**Ogle, K.N. & Prangen, A. de H. (1951): Further Considerations of Fixational Disparity and The Binocular Fusional Processes, A.J. Oph., 34, pt. 2.: 57.*

**Ogle, K.N. & Prangen, A. de H. (1953): Observations On Vertical Divergence And Hyperphorias. Arch. Oph., 49: 313.*

Ogle, K.N., Martens, T.G., & Dyer, J.N. (1967): Oculomotor Imbalance In Binocular Vision and Fixation Disparity, Lea & Febiger, Phila.

**Osterberg, H. (1964): Binocular Refraction and Measurement of Phorias for Distance and Near Vision. Optica Int'l 20.*

**Pardon, H.R. (1962): A New Testing Device For Stereopsis. J.A.O.A., 33: 510.*

**Parks, M.M. (1963): Diagnostic Procedures In Pediatric Ophthalmology: Ocular Diagnosis Motility. I.O.C., 3: 4.*

Pascal, J.I. (1952): Selected Studies In Visual Optics. C.V. Mosby Co., St. Louis.

Ripple, P.H. (1952): Variations Of Accommodation In Vertical Directions Of Gaze. A.J. Oph., 35: 1630.

Schillinger, R.J. (1951): Hyperphorias Induced By Trial Lenses. A.J. Oph., 34: 1150.

Scobee, R.G. (1952): The Oculorotary Muscles. C.V. Mosby Co., St. Louis.

Scobee, R.G. and Green, E.H. (1946): A Center For Ocular Divergence; Does It Exist? A.J. Oph., 29: 422.

Scobee, R.G. and Green, E.H. (1947): Tests for Heterophoria; Reliability of Tests; Comparison between tests; and Effects of Changing Test Conditions. A.J. Oph. 30: 436.

Scobee & Green (1951): See Chapter 21.

**Sills, R.A. (1960): Correspondence in A.J. Oph., 49: 1063.*

Sloan, L.L. & Rowland, W.M. (1951): Comparison Of Orthorater and Sight Screener Tests Of Heterophoria With Standard Clinical Tests. A.J. Oph., 34: 1363.

Sloan, L.L. & Altman, A. (1954): Factors Involved In Several Tests of Binocular Depth Perception. Arch. Oph., 52: 524.

Sloan, P.G. (1954): The Cover Test In Clinical Practice. A.A.A.O., 31: 3.

**Snydacker, D. (1962): The Maddox Rod Test – A 10 Year Followup. Trans. Am. Ophth. Soc., 63: 595.*

Soderberg, D.S. (1968): An Evaluation In The Use Of The Maddox Rod, J.A.O.A., 39: 473.

Stern, A. (1953): The Effect Of Target Variation And Kinesthesia Upon Near Heterophoria Measurements. A.A.A.O., 30: 351.

Suchman, R.G. (1968): Visual Testing Of Preverbal and Nonverbal Young Children, A.A.A.O., 45: 642.

Tubis, R.A. (1954): An Evaluation Of Vertical Divergence Tests On The Basis Of Fixation Disparity. A.A.A.O., 31: 644.

Turville, A.E. (1934): The Esdaile-Turville Equilibrium Test. Ellis Opt. Co., Croyden.

Verhoeff, F.H. (1963): A New Kinetic Test For Binocular Stereopsis. Arch. Oph., 69: 436.

Vodnoy, B.E. (1964): Utilization Of The Hand Held Maddox Rod, A.A.A.O., 35: 681.

Walsh, R. (1946): The Measurement And Correction Of Hyperphorias In Refractive Cases. A.A.A.O., 23: 373.

Westheimer, G. (1958): Accommodation Levels During Crossed Cylinder Tests. A.A.A.O., 35: 599.

Weymouth, F.W. (1963): An Experimental Comparison Of Three Common Methods Of Measuring Heterophoria. A.A.A.O., 40: 497.

Wilmut, E.B. (1951): The Use Of Polarizing Filters For Infinity Balance Examination And Near Correction. Trans. Int. Opt. Song., London.

SECTION IV
ANALYSIS AND PRESCRIPTION

21 Analysis and Prescription

I. SOURCES OF DISCOMFORT

A. The refractionist faces two different corrective instances, the first of which is obvious to the patient and the second of which is dependent upon the patient's trust and faith in the refractionist (Hirsch, 1963).

1. On the one hand, he can improve the visual acuity, eliminate the asthenopia or headaches, or improve visual performance.

2. On the other hand, he can correct errors which could become worse and which might cause another anomaly to develop.

a. Correction can be made with a device which improves only while it is worn, as a minus lens, or with a device which is not needed later (as prism training).

b. Hirsch suggested calling application of the first form *neutralization,* as it did not really correct, and of the second type, *corrections.*

(1) However, the term *correction* has become so widespread as an application of a lens Rx (lens correction or spectacle correction) that it is here suggested that applications of the first order be continued to be called *corrections* while those of the second category be titled *cures.*

B. The basic conditions, obvious to the patient, which the refractionist must correct are either insufficient vision for far or near, discomfort when using the eyes, or a combination of both. Ordinarily, poor vision, with the exclusion of pathological defects, is due to either myopia, absolute hyperopia, astigmatism, anisometropia, or presbyopia. The correction of these can be based upon a reasonably reliable criterion insofar as improvement of vision is concerned, since both the patient and the examiner can be fairly positive of an improvement of acuity alone.

1. Usually, if the refraction has been done with reasonable accuracy and skill, the subjective finding, or in some circumstances the retinoscopy finding, will represent the correction providing the best acuity at far. Unless other involvements such as presbyopia or accommodative insufficiency are evident, this same correction will also provide maximum acuity at near. If presbyopia is manifest, the procedure for determining the assistance for the nearpoint which provides satisfactory vision has been discussed.

C. However, the refractive correction alone cannot be predicated, without other analysis, to also provide comfortable vision or to relieve symptoms of discomfort when the original vision was satisfactory. Even assuming an accurate refraction insofar as can be determined at the time of testing and based upon the acuity, the following causes of discomfort may still be uncorrected and unrevealed until further analysis of the entire examination is made:

1. *In myopia,* simple full strength corrections serve for lower or medium ametropias, in the writer's experience (as well as in that of Hirsch, Duke-Elder, Morgan and many others). Few other symptoms are apparent and all concepts agree that the lens "corrects" or "neutralizes" the ametropia. Disagreement lies in the area of prevention and "cure."

a. As previously discussed, various attempts, methods, and trials for effecting "cure" have been advocated. As Hirsch stated, "The best cure for myopic progression seems to be in growing older."

b. Uncorrected myopia may call for action of the lids and orbicularis muscles, producing fatigue about the orbit and brow.

c. Corrected or over-corrected myopia may induce over-accommodation because of the changed value of the accommodative unit.

d. Correction of high myopia may reduce the retinal image size and affect acuity.

2. *The lower or moderate hyperope* reveals no visual symptoms but may reveal headaches or other asthenopic symptoms, particularly if attempting to see at near. As Giles (1965) pointed out, small errors could cause difficulty for some patients. There is little evidence to show that much difference (except for symptoms, if present) is made by wearing or not wearing a correction. A "cure" might be predicated for full-time wear, insofar as it might help to maintain a normal accommodation-convergence relationship and fusion.

a. Flom (1963) emphasized that while fogging lenses in a correction have been advocated in attempts to neutralize accommodative spasm, the blurred distant vision often merely interfered with binocularity and may have caused an increase in esophoria. There was no proof that over-correction would make latent hyperopia manifest.

3. *Astigmatism* may produce blurred vision, asthenopia, discomfort, and headaches. The astigmatic correction not only relieves these, but may act as a cure in both assisting binocular vision and in preventing a type of low grade amblyopia in which uncorrected visual acuity may be less in later years than if it had not been corrected.

a. Changes in the axis of strong astigmatism may produce prismatic effects different than those that the patient has grown accustomed to. Knoll (1960) found that a change in a minus 3.50 D. cylinder from 20° to 15° in both eyes induced a prismatic effect of ½ prism diopter vertically (see Chapters dealing with lenses for formula).

4. *Anisometropia*

a. The Rx may be "curative" in that it definitely provides better binocular vision since both eyes would be difficult to coordinate otherwise. Discomfort may also result from low ametropias and the resulting prismatic effects and aniseikonia.

(1) If not previously corrected, loss of orientation and fusional problems may result.

5. *Presbyopia or accommodative insufficiency*

a. Accommodative causes of asthenopia may result from either one, even though the distance correction is reasonably adequate. In such cases, the fatigue or complaint will be manifested and associated with near use of the eyes.

(1) One potential problem not discernible in tests at 16 inches is the difficulty the actual working distance may cause. This is not only to be considered with adults and presbyopes, where the application is obvious, but with children. Hurst (1964) studied the eye at the book or desk distance of a number of school children of different age levels. The mean eye to desk distance of primary children was 5.7 inches, increasing with age to the senior grade where it was 10.5 inches.

6. *Lateral or vertical imbalances*

7. *Fusional deficiency*

8. *Photophobia*

D. The causes of discomfort such as astigmatism and hyperopia and failure to equalize vision have been discussed in the chapters on the subject and in the chapters dealing with the specific refraction procedures. Ordinarily, the average competent examiner arrives at a prescription which compensates for these possibilities. The induced effects of anisometropia insofar as imbalances are concerned have also been noted, and will be further considered under imbalances. Also, presbyopia is ordinarily readily corrected unless complicated by convergence insufficiency. Photophobia will be treated under tinted lenses.

1. Accommodative difficulty in the young non-presbyope, the various types of imbalances and convergence deficiency, as well as fusional problems, require the employment of the techniques discussed under phorometry and the addition to or modification of the correction indicated by the refractive procedures alone. The consideration of these problems constitutes the major portion of the analytical routines or methods now prevalent.

E. Basic Differentiation of Causes

1. Of the probable causes of discomfort noted, it can be readily realized that some would be present if only one of the eyes were in use while others depend entirely upon the use of both eyes together. Because the refractive procedures deal mainly with the eyes from the standpoint of each eye separately, even though equalization and anisometropia are considered, and since the procedures dealing with the determination of the refraction are among the best developed of those employed, it is not surprising that Snell (1953) found that, in a statistical analysis of the prevalence of headaches among strabismic and monocular patients as compared to binocular patients, the great percentage of cases having discomfort rested with the binocular ones. Since, in many instances, doubt may exist as to whether the cause of discomfort lies with the refraction or with the problems involved in binocularity, a simple diagnostic technique can be employed to assist in the determination of the proper cause.

2. *Occlusion*

a. Marlow (1932) first proposed occlusion to help determine the true imbalance, as has been noted in previous chapters. However, he also found that the complaints which were attributable to such imbalances disappeared during the occlusion procedure. Bannon (1943) suggested, along with others, that occlusion could serve as a diagnostic aid to suggest the presence of aniseikonia. If the complaint disappeared under occlusion and no deficiency of convergence or imbalance was disclosed to account for the difficulty, aniseikonia may have been evident. Morgan (1960) warned that vertical imbalances disclosed after occlusion, however, may sometimes merely be a manifestation of Bell's phenomenon and incorrect.

(1) In any event, whenever occlusion relieves the complaint, the cause may be sought in the existence of some handicap to easy binocular vision. If the occlusion does not relieve the complaint, the cause may be considered to be either an error in refraction, photophobia, or accommodative in origin.

(a) Since the error in refraction may exist in either eye, occlusion should be employed, as has been recommended, first upon one eye and then upon the other for an equal period.

(2) Flom (1963) noted that minus may cause headaches when first applied to myopes, more because of convergence and fusion problems than of accommodative ones. Occluding one eye will often relieve the headaches.

b. Conditions which occlusion would not relieve and which must be analyzed from the standpoint of the refraction or near correction are as follows:

(1) Uncorrected hyperopia or myopia

(2) Over-corrected myopia or hyperopia

(3) Under- or over-corrected astigmatism

(4) Presbyopia

(5) Accommodative insufficiency

(6) Photophobia

c. Conditions which occlusion would relieve are as follows:

(1) Lateral imbalance

(2) Vertical imbalance

(3) Convergence insufficiency

(4) Poor fusional ability

(5) Aniseikonia

(6) Anisometropia, induced by the correction

(a) As previously noted, Fry and Kehoe (1940) have demonstrated that most patients learned to compensate for such imbalances so that in most instances no discrepancy was revealed. However, upon the occasion of first correction and during the learning period, some difficulty may be encountered.

II. THE DISTANT CORRECTION

A. The initial correction from which the final correction is determined, is that which would constitute an adequate correction if the eyes were used only for distant vision. This is usually the subjective correction, although it may be modified by further considerations.

1. Basically, this correction consists of the most plus or least minus which gives the maximum acuity at far.

a. Spasticity, pseudo-myopia, and other forms of hypertonic action of the accommodation at far have been considered earlier. As previously remarked, unless a previous correction of equivalent strength has been worn without relief of the symptoms, an increase in plus power, even if not corrective of the total hyperopia, will often prove satisfactory for distant wear.

(1) If the discomfort can be attributed to *esophoria at far* due to accommodative excess, additional plus might be required even if acuity is at first reduced.

b. Accommodative action due to astigmatism should be relieved by the subjective correction which usually represents the best astigmatic correction. However, indications of under-corrected astigmatism, revealed at the nearpoint or by discrepancies of large amounts between the ophthalmometer, retinoscopy, and subjective corrections may require modifications of the cylinder indicated in the subjective test.

(1) Similarly, wide discrepancies between the subjective corrections indicated by different techniques such as the cross cylinder and the clock dial, or the indication of a high cylinder in a patient who has never previously worn one, must be treated with caution. Generally, the weaker the cylinder which does not reduce the acuity too markedly, the safer the prescription.

(2) If a very strong correction not previously worn improves vision, the spherical element above will not usually bother too greatly, even though the change in image size will disturb distance judgment for a while and should be explained before the lenses are prescribed.

(a) The cylinder, if very strong, will, as previously noted, create a much greater disturbance of orientation, and Humphriss (1950) recommended that only one-third the power of a strong cylinder be initially applied and that power be increased gradually in subsequent prescriptions.

(b) The spherical equivalent with a proportion of cylinder giving about the same acuity or giving the most *relative* improvement in vision may be used (Humphriss, 1950).

[1] The sphere and different increasing fractions of the cylinder may be tried (as a 4th, a 3rd, a half, etc.) by noting the increase in acuity with each fraction. The portion giving only a slight increase in acuity need not be prescribed.

(c) The axis may also be rotated in slight amounts and the change in acuity noted. The closer it can be brought to 90 or 180° without loss of visual acuity, the less oblique distortion. The patient can walk about with the Rx in the trial frame and observe if distortion is bothersome.

c. If the problem lies at the nearpoint, a fuller spherical Rx may be given than for distance. However, small minus cylinders, contrary to initial expectations, often improve nearpoint acuity.

d. If the patient has worn an Rx previously and the change is marked, the same concepts may be applied to the differences between the two Rx's.

2. The chapters dealing with the refractive procedures have considered many of the possible discrepancies which might nullify the distant prescription's value. However, the careful examiner will usually arrive at a basic prescription which will be adequate for the distant vision. In most instances, the examiner will find that the patient has either not worn a correction previously or will find sufficient difference between the old correction and the new one to assure him that he is either providing better distance vision or the same vision with less accommodative effort required. Under such circumstances, the examiner may concentrate upon the prospect of the status of the convergence to assure himself of having recognized any other possible causes of ocular discomfort.

B. The other major factor to consider at the distance is that of lateral or vertical imbalance. Except in very high discrepancies, lateral imbalance is not frequently a cause of discomfort insofar as distant vision is concerned, and where it is, its indications are fairly predominant. Vertical imbalance is, however, a larger contributor to visual difficulty than is frequently conceded.

III. VERTICAL IMBALANCE

A. Since a vertical imbalance is ordinarily manifested at both the far and near test distances, it may be considered, as a whole, independent of the distance for which the correction is designed.

1. Upon occasion, however, a variation is found at different distances in the amount of the vertical phoria. This may be due to paresis of one or more of the particular muscles involved in assisting convergence or the effects of accommodation and the ACA ratio. Also, Morgan (1960) pointed out that both lateral and vertical prismatic effects varied as the eye looked through different parts of the prism, which convergence at near required them to do. If the test was made through lenses and spectacles or a trial frame, the lines of sight may be at least 8 mms. below the optical center of the lenses.

2.. Morgan (1954) challenged the matter of the reality of the vertical discrepancy by several questions.

a. *Was there a complaint that reflected a possible vertical imbalance?*

(1) If there was a history of previous unsatisfactory Rx's not too different from that now found, or if the old Rx contained prism power, or if diplopia was present, a discrepancy should be expected (Eskridge, 1963). Likewise, intermittant blurring of print, loss of the proper line in reading as the eyes moved from one line to the next, and head tilting or torting were further clues. A "pulling" sensation was often connected with muscular anomalies. Wrinkling of the forehead, elevation of the eyebrows, and facial muscle tension were also evidence of the condition.

b. *Was the finding an artifact of the test method or a true malfunction?*

c. *Was the measurement valid?*

(1) A vertical phoria revealed with a refractor should be checked with the trial frame using a Maddox rod, red glass, and trial case prisms. Often the phoria was of a different amount or totally refuted. A subjective cover test through which ¼ PD was noted could also be applied. The Turville method of validating vertical needs appeared best.

(2) One of the problems pertaining to the use of prisms clinically was that of actually determining the true visual direction rather than the prism diopters marked on the refractor or placed in the trial frame, since these varied in their effect upon the true visual direction with their distance from the center of rotation, position of the object,

and plane of the surface. Pratt (1962) noted two applicable clinical methods as follows:

(a) Ogle's – in which the prism value was corrected by the formula (1 -hp), in which h was the distance of the prism from the center of rotation and p, the distance of the object from the same center (all in meters).

(b) Alpern's – in which the formula was $\frac{t}{[(1 - .027D)(t + s) + .027]}$ in which t was the distance of the object from the spectacle plane, s was the distance of the prism from the spectacle plane, D was the dioptric power of the spectacle lens, and .027 was the assumed distance of the center of rotation from the spectacle plane. All distances were given in meters.

d. *Was the deviation constant or non-concomitant?*

(1) If a deviation is found, it is often well to test in the other eight directions of the nine field examination. The test should be repeated with each eye fixing separately, since non-comitancy will reveal a different refractive state if the affected eye fixes.

(2) Even in comitant deviations, the head was tilted down for esophoria, up for exophoria, and to lower the perceived image on the side towards which the head is tilted (Eskridge). In esophoria or orthophoria, the head tilts towards the hypophoric eye, and in exophoria, towards the hyperphoric eye.

(3) In paresis, the head usually tilted if the obliques were involved. It turned towards the field of action of the paretic muscle, while the eyes turned in the direction opposite that of the main action of the affected muscle.

3. Parks (1958) presented the following routine technique for determination of isolated cyclovertical muscle palsy:

a. The primary deviation is noted, leading to a choice among four muscles in each eye.

b. The muscle involved is determined by noting if the diplopia increases in the field of vertical action of the affected muscle.

(1) A choice of two muscles is presented at this stage, one in each eye.

(a) The suspected muscles are: the inferior rectus in one eye and the inferior oblique in the other, or the superior rectus of one eye and the superior oblique of the other.

(b) If the ametropia is long standing, and especially if in the fixing eye, contractures and hypertrophies may lead to misjudgments in this primary test.

c. Bielschowsky's head tilt is used to determine the exact eye and muscle. (See also Chapter XXXI).

(1) *If the head is tilted to the right,* the right intorters, the superior rectus and the superior oblique contract, while the left extorters, the inferior rectus and the inferior oblique contract.

(2) *If the head is tilted to the left,* the right extorters, the inferior rectus and the inferior oblique contract, while the left intorters, the superior rectus and the superior oblique contract.

(3) *If tilted to the right:*

(a) O.D. turns up

[1] O.D. intorter cannot pull down

[a] Superior oblique weak

(b) O.S. turns up

[1] O.S. extorter cannot pull down

[a] Inferior rectus weak

(c) O.D. turns down

[1] O.D. intorter cannot pull up

[a] Superior rectus weak

(d) O.S. turns down

[1] O.S. extorter cannot pull up

[a] Inferior oblique weak

(4) *If tilted to the left:*

(a) O.D. turns up

[1] O.D. extorter cannot pull down

[a] Inferior rectus weak

(b) O.S. turns up

[1] O.S. intorter cannot pull down

[a] Superior oblique weak

(c) O.D. turns down

[1] O.D. extorter cannot pull up

[a] Inferior oblique weak

(d) O.S. turns down

[1] O.S. intorter cannot pull up

[a] Superior rectus weak

d. Looking in and down, as in reading, causes an extorsion due to action of the internal rectus, but this does not cause trouble or discomfort. Small degrees of cyclotorsion may not cause discomfort (Duke-Elder, 1963).

B. The normal expected reactions for the vertical vergences and phorias are that orthophoria should be revealed vertically at both near and far and that the supraductions and infraductions should be from 3 to 4 pd for the break with about half that amount for the recovery. Also, the supraduction should balance the infraduction.

1. Where the phoria is unaffected by accommodative-convergence, the actual phoria finding may be assumed to represent the vertical deviation.

2. Where the phoria varies from far to near and a near lateral phoria is prevalent, the phoria finding may not equal the mid-point of the duction finding and will actually represent the vertical balance when the eyes are in the lateral phoria position and not directed towards the point of fixation.

a. Scobee (1952) described a differentiation of vertical heterophoria at far and near by performing the distance test with the lines of sight in the primary position and the near test with the lines of sight depressed and converged. A vertical imbalance at distance depended principally on the balance of the vertical recti, while the one at near depended principally on the vertical obliques. Heterophoria, due to paresis or other malfunction of the specific muscles, could thus be more accurately ascribed. However, the problem of the determination of *anisophoria,* described by Friedenwald (1952) as a varied phoria finding in different directions of gaze, was actually more closely associated with true strabismus, considered in later chapters, than with heterophoria as here regarded. Some differentiation was made between pathological anisophoria, in which paresis or spasticity of a muscle or muscles was the cause of the difference in heterophoria, and that anisophoria due to the different prismatic effects of anisometropic corrections. Friedenwald maintained that an aniseikonic patient was given anisophoria by the iseikonic correction. Non-pathological anisophoria was partially correctible by prism segs in bifocals, slab-off prisms, different corrections for far and near, iseikonic corrections (when not the original source of the anisophoria), and by the patient moving the reading matter towards the position of least heterophoria.

(1) Pascal (1949) commented that eventual contracture of the antagonist would make a pathological hyperphoria resemble a comitant one, if the tests were made in the primary position. He suggested that a simple check could be made by noting a change in the amount of heterophoria when the patient observed the target and the head was tilted backwards.

b. Posner (1951) recommended that *alternating hyperphoria,* in which the non-fixing eye deviated to a different extent upon alternating the fixation, be measured by using a Maddox rod alternately before both eyes and averaging the two results for a final prescription. Thus, if with the right eye fixing, the finding were 3 Δ of the left hyperphoria, and with the left eye fixing, the finding were 1 Δ of the left hyperphoria, the resultant would be 2 Δ of the left hyperphoria.

3. Ordinarily, the *phoria* will represent a discrepancy *equivalent* to the discrepancy of the *vertical ductions.*

a. If 1 pd of right hyperphoria is found, it will usually be disclosed that the right supraduction is, for example, 5 pd, while the right infraduction is only 3 pd, the supraduction having gained 1 pd while the infraduction has lost 1 pd from the balancing point.

b. Where the convergence influences the vertical phoria, however, this may not be the case and the ductions may reveal a different extent of vertical alignment than does the phoria, as noted above.

C. As has been noted in the chapters dealing with vergences and phorometry, the true vertical imbalance may not be revealed by the temporary suspension of the test during the routine, and the full correction may not be manifested until several prism prescriptions have been worn over a period of years. Occlusion will frequently reveal the full extent of the phoria, but when occlusion is not employed, the fact that the correction, in the form of vertical prism, may have to be increased from one examination to another may not indicate anything more than that the full extent of the deviation, hitherto concealed is becoming manifested. Many practitioners have become mistakenly alarmed by the fact that the vertical phoria seems to increase with the wearing of vertical prisms. Walsh (1946) stated that the partial correction seemed to permit eventual exhibition of the full error, and that the wearing of vertical prism did not tend to increase the amount of error beyond the extent which would have been revealed had the full error been discovered originally.

1. However, Ogle and Prangen (1953) and Carter (1963) found that patients exhibited the same phoria and fixation disparity after wearing prisms as they revealed before, regardless of the amount and direction (within limits) of the prism worn.

2. If the associated vertical phoria test is determined by the disparity method (similar to the technique employed for the lateral associated phoria – see Chap. XX), and if a vertical prism, not exceeding 2Δ is placed before the eye, and a sufficient time allowed, the disparity curve with the prism beforythe eyes will be found to equal that found before the introduction of the prism in a number of individuals.

a. If the prism is again increased by an amount not exceeding 2Δ, this additional prism will also be compensated for. Another 2Δ (totalling 6Δ) can be added to some subjects, and still again be compensated for.

(1) This compensation can occur if the subject had little or no vertical imbalance initially as well as if he had one.

(2) The rate at which the compensation takes place varies from 3 to 10 minutes after the prism is introduced.

(3) The vertical vergence tests taken with the prism before the eyes reveal values equal to those originally disclosed before the introduction of the prism, an effect noted with dissociated phorias by Ellerbrock and Fry (1941) and Ellerbrock (1949, 1950).

b. If the total prism is then removed, diplopia is immediately manifested, lasting from 2 to 16 minutes in different subjects, and resulting in a large hyperphoric stress in the previous direction of forced divergence, when fusion is first regained. However the eyes ultimately return to the original vertical state which existed before any introduction of prism.

(1) The rate of recovery is from two to three times as long as that required in the original compensating process.

c. If while the prism is before the eyes, the dissociated vertical phorias (such as the Maddox rod test) are measured it will be found that an almost complete compensation is also revealed by this test. However, recovery after prism removal, in the absence of fusion stimuli, may not be completed within 2½ hours.

3. In some subjects, only a partial compensation may take place, so that the disparity curve measured after the prism is worn falls between the original pre-prism position and that which would be equivalent to the prismatic displacement.

4. If an individual fixates a page of print, rotating his eyes up and to the left, across the page to up and to the right, and ultimately from down and to the left to down and to the right, as is done in reading the page from top to bottom, the amount of vertical divergence between the lines of sight of the two eyes when looking at these oblique and elevated or depressed positions can be calculated and in some positions may reach as much as 3 of vertical hyperphoria.

a. Tests of disparity at these points indicate no such hyperphoria, and vertical divergence tests at those points reveal equal amplitudes of divergence in both directions. Similar results are found when measured in different directions of gaze through anisometropic corrections before the eyes.

5. Ogle, Martens & Dyer (1967) postulate that two types of vertical compensating mechanism exist, a rapid one used to compensate for oblique elevations and depressions or for anisometropic corrections, and a slow one enabling some people to compensate for existing hyperphorias or for imbalances introduced by vertical prismatic effects.

a. The usual clinical tests of vertical divergences are performed too rapidly to exhibit the latter, and their endpoint is an expression of the former.

(1) The hyperphorias and vertical vergences are the same after introduction of prism as they were before.

b. For those subjects who do not possess this slow compensatory mechanism, or reflex for vertical prisms, hyperphorias will be reduced and corrected in strict proportion to the prismatic power introduced.

c. The physiologic mechanism may be associated with a variation of the structure of the retinal lattice of one eye – elements closer together, for example, in the superior region than in the inferior one – and thus result in the exhibition of a vertical phoria despite the presence of the compensatory reflex.

6. Clinically it would appear that the utility of a prism prescription would depend upon whether the slow compensatory reflex could be demonstrated. If demonstrated, prism would prove useless and unnecessary.

a. Since a time element has been established, the presence of the reflex could be tested by placing the refractive correction in a properly centered trial frame, measuring the vertical deviation, introducing the correcting prism, allowing the trial frame to be worn for an hour or so, and then remeasuring the phoria and the vertical ductions with the correction before the eyes.

(1) If the original phoria was again revealed, and the ductions were balanced, the compensatory mechanism existed, and prescription of correcting prism was unnecessary.

(2) If the prism appeared to eliminate the phoria, no compensating mechanism would be revealed, and the prescription of the prism would be indicated.

7. The accepted conclusions concerning the value of occlusion and of the revelation of the "full" error after partial correction by repeated examinations (vis. Walsh above) may need reexamination in view of the concept expressed in the slow compensating reflex.

D. Not all authorities agree on the amount of correction initially required for vertical phorias. Giles (1965) suggested 2/3 the amount for distance and 3/4 the amount found at near. Morgan (1954 and 1960) recommended correcting the full amount, particularly for the aged if suppression or deviation were utilized. He permitted a partial amount on occasion, but warned that care should be taken not to interfere with the head tilt, usually due to a torsion and not a vertical imbalance. When tested in the trial frame, the amount should be nearly equal to the vertical deviation. Posner (1951) suggested correction of all or nearly all the phoria. Some authorities felt that minor vertical discrepancies may be ignored, while Walsh, Bielschowsky, and Lancaster, among others (as previously noted) felt that the measuring devices employed for vertical discrepancies were too gross and that even variations of ¼ of a prism diopter were significant. Morgan stated that small errors often created trouble when full correction was not attempted.

E. Determining the prism

1. Several methods of determining the prismatic correction for vertical discrepancies are prevalent.

a. Where the deviation is constant at both far and near and the phoria discrepancy agrees with the ductions, the actual amount of prism which will relieve the phoria may be used.

(1) Eskridge (1963) recommended the Flip Prism value be used for prescribing the amount of correction.

b. Where the imbalance indicated by the phoria and that indicated by the ductions disagree, most authorities recommend that the correction be based upon the prism which equalizes the vertical ductions.

(1) Since the phoria may not be expressive of the total imbalance, the ductions may be the preferable indication of the actual discrepancy. However, the patient usually makes an effort to compensate for the phoria and this effort may develop sufficient residual vertical duction balancing the phoria to also conceal part of the error. Usually the balance of the vertical ductions is the goal desired until subsequent tests reveal the concealed error, if any.

(2) The prism necessary may be simply determined by the following formula:

$$\frac{\text{Base-down to break} - \text{Base-up to break}}{2} = \text{Correcting prism.}$$

(a) The prism is Base-down if the resultant is plus and base-up if it is minus.

(3) Tubis (1954) found that balancing the vertical duction break points served as a good subsidiary to the indications of the vertical phoria, although he recommended that the prism power be reduced by one-third its indicated value.

c. Since the residual contraction often conceals inequality of the ductions, the author has also noted the discrepancy of the two recovery points. Usually these will agree with the break points to the extent of half the breaks. Upon occasion, findings which indicate fairly equal breaks will reveal unequal recoveries.

(1) As the recovery points represent the limits of the fusion field, and it is assumed that the eyes drift to the phoric position after dissociation, it is obvious that the recovery points, which should be anatomically equidistant from the fovea, will vary in accordance with the phoria. For this reason many authorities ignore their implications as mere confirmations of the phorias. However, upon occasions, the recovery points do not agree with the phorias but either contradict or exceed the phoria indications. This might be indicative of the insufficient relaxation of the musculature to permit resumption of the phoria position, or an induced phoria following the severe excitation of the duction tests, or perhaps a fuller revelation of the true imbalance due to opposite stimulation of one duction as opposed to the habitual compensating contraction of the other. Until the role of the recoveries is more fully defined, they

cannot be totally ignored, and in the author's experience, where the recoveries agree most closely to the indication of the phoria, the prism is most readily accepted subjectively.

(a) Tubis (1954), on the other hand, did not find the recovery points of value as compared to the break points.

2. A simple technique for the determination of the vertical correcting prism which is reported by almost all users as highly reliable and indicating a correction almost wholly wearable is that previously described in the chapter on Subjective Techniques under the *Turville Infinity Balance Technique.* In this method, as both eyes observe the companion charts and the acuity is equalized by changes in the correction, such discrepancies in vertical balance as might be due to aniseikonic effects are readily determinable and sometimes alleviatable by changes in the spherical element of one eye. Where a definite vertical misalignment of the charts is evident, that prism which balances the two charts is reported as the correction prism.

a. Elvin (1954) evaluated changes in the prismatic corrections determined by the Turville Technique in 40 patients at median intervals of 6.3 weeks. He found that 29 required less than ½ prism diopters of alteration, that 9 required as much as a half prism diopter, 1 required 1 prism diopter and one required 2 prism diopters. Of these, ¾ required no actual change in the corrections, one-fourth required a half a prism diopter of change and only 2 patients needed their correction actually changed as much as one-half prism diopter. Both of these latter patients had a deviation fully corrected at distance, which decreased at the reading level.

b. Carter (1968) emphasizes that if the patient shows a lateral phoria of over 4 it is difficult to assess the true vertical phoria by any dissociated technique accurately, due to the variation of muscle action when the eye is directed to different directions of regard. An indicated vertical discrepancy may be solely due to false vertical inequality based upon the secondary actions associated with lateral rotations.

3. The author has employed *a subjective method,* also utilized by Morgan, for determining the acceptance of prism. This consists briefly, of presenting a correcting prism in the trial frame while the patient observes, binocularly, the best type for distance and or near. as the case may require, and of requesting the patient to report his reaction. As Sheard (1923) mentioned, any case in which the binocular visual acuity was less than the monocular, or where a clear binocular definition was not obtained, or the vision binocularly was not as comfortable or as easy as it was monocularly, should be investigated for imbalances, particularly vertical.

a. The correcting prism is presented with the base-in varying positions before both eyes so that the psychological influence of an addition to the correction may not predetermine the patient's reaction, since some will respond affirmatively under any situation.

b. If the patient reports improvement in acuity, better fixity of wavering margins of the chart, or subjective relief when the prism is placed with its base in agreement with the phorometry tests and definitely denies the prism when it is placed with its base at variance to those indications, the author has considered the responses as definitive in regard to the inclusion of the prism in the correction.

c. Where the error varies between that indicated by the phoria test and that indicated by the ductions, the prism is tried in varying strengths and the power most efficacious used.

d The same subjective method is also used to check the inclusion of lateral prism, which will be discussed later in this chapter.

e. In variance to the above, Carter (1968) maintains that, while the reduction of disparity by prism usually results in a slight increase in acuity, it is usually inconclusive in cases of exophoria or hyperphoria.

4. Sheard recommended that the prism be placed before the non-dominant eye, but Fry (1945) suggested that dividing the amount equally before both eyes, with the bases necessarily opposite, had less tendency to distort and disturb the orientation of space perception.

a. If the prism exceeded six diopters, according to Walsh, the prismatic lenses were too cumbersome and distorted too much for inclusion in the correction. In cases exceeding that amount, surgery may have been necessary.

(1) However, occasional reports of large amounts of prism being worn with apparent success appear. Emmes, (1968) describes a case of a patient fitted over a period of five years with vertical prism, increased from 5 to 20, for the distant wear, and fitted with 27 vertically with 4 base in for near, with all indications of fusion.

b. Lebensohn (1955) stated that a hypophoria at near required correction more than did one at far.

5. Since rotary prisms are calibrated in 1 or ½ pd markings, and these are placed so close together as to be difficult to read accurately in relation to the patient's time of response, some of the more precise determinations may not be readily practical. It would seem that improvement in the devices for measuring vertical discrepancies should be forthcoming if the small irregularities previously noted are às significant as claimed.

6. The correction of the calculated vertical prismatic imbalance in cases of anisometropia often proved to be unsuccessful (Bannon, 1955). Anisometropic lenses have unequal prismatic effects at the distance of 10 mms. below the optical center, which is the nearpoint intersect. It is incorrect to assume that the eyes will make the same angular depression or that the visual axes are depressed by the same amount. A precalculated correction may add to, rather than subtract from, the problem It is important to measure the vertical phoria and the fusional amplitudes while the patient is actually looking through the reading intersect, preferably with the old Rx, as a trial frame or phoropter introduces other problems. A penlight and Maddox rod can be used.

a. As noted earlier, anisometropic patients exhibited a capacity for compensating for vertical prismatic inequalities at the straight forward and reading positions (Bannon, 1955; Ogle and Prangen, 1954). This compensation was used to maintain single binocular vision in vertical imbalance and in peripheral portions of the lens. Anisophoria may often be revealed if the lenses are removed. The phoria may balance the prismatic effects of the lenses, revealing no apparent phoria through them.

(1) Ogle (1956) also noted that if the inherent vertical anisophoria was opposite, but approximately equal to, the prismatic effects introduced by lenses, no significant hyperphoria would be measured through the lenses. Lebensohn (1955) found no prism as often as some prism was required for the correction of anisometropic anisophoria and thereby concluded that it was unwise to correct to the computed vertical prism difference in anisometropic lenses. On occasion, the residual heterophoria persisted through the lenses.

IV. LATERAL IMBALANCES

A. Lateral imbalances include discrepancies of the order of esophoria and exophoria at either far, near, or both. A lateral imbalance of itself is not necessarily significant as is true of vertical imbalances, unless it is of marked degree or supplemented by deficient duction findings.

1. In considering the effects of lateral imbalances, the major indications are frequently provided

by the phorias, and the supplementary information is garnered from the ductions.

B. Intimately related to the simple appearance of lateral imbalances, is the question of convergence insufficiency and the problem of inequality between the accommodative and convergence burdens. Much of the present day analysis is based not upon the specific indications of the phoria and/or duction tests but upon the comparison of the status of the accommodative and convergence functions. This latter involves analysis of the various tests of each function in a joint determination of the particular one under stress. In such an analysis, esophoria and exophoria are considered not as conditions which require correction in their own right, but as symptoms, along with the other tests, of which of the two functions, accommodation or convergence, requires assistance.

C. The probable comprehensive analysis combines the proven considerations of both approaches, i.e., considering the specific imbalances in their own right, considering whether such imbalances are found or not, and considering the probability of over-all functional deficiency.

1. While it is likely that the phoria and duction will both indicate true deficiencies, it may be possible to find an imbalance indicated by the phoria with sufficient duction to compensate, and in reverse, to find little phoria with a deficient duction for close work.

D. The attempt to determine from the tests, other than the refractive ones, some indication of either accommodative or convergence deficiency has evolved along the lines of a graphical consideration of the ranges and limits of the two functions. Such graphic interpretations have been used in the attempt to determine the thoroughness of the refraction, analyze the relationship of the accommodative-convergence, and establish the limits of the *zone of comfort* or *zone of clear binocular vision.* Another approach has been that of establishing a series of *norms or expecteds* for each test and attempting to determine discrepancies, by deviations, from these norms. This latter has developed into analytical *"types"* or *"syndromes"* concerned mainly with establishing the need for additional accommodative or convergence aids. Before the question of either lateral imbalances or functional deficiencies can be considered, it is advisable to note the significance and development of the analytical graphs and the imports derived from them.

V. ZONES OF COMFORT

A. The zone of comfort has been described by a large number of investigators beginning with Donders in 1864 and including Pereles in 1889, Nagel in 1880, Landolt in 1886, Percival in 1892, Howe in 1907, Sheard in 1928, Fry in 1937 and 1939, Hofstetter in 1945, and Fincham and Walton in 1957. Not all of these are considered here, but the following considerations may serve to indicate the trends and emphasis these have taken.

1. It must be remembered that all tests upon which the zones and norms are based are stimulus values and not response values. This creates artifacts which are obvious in the following discussions.

B. Donders (1864) (Figure XXI-1)

1. Donders is credited with being the first to graph the limits of accommodation for given amounts of convergence. He tested the positive and negative relative accommodation at varying distances and also the nearpoint of accommodation. This latter he took by two methods, the maximum nearpoint at which single binocular vision could be maintained and the monocular nearpoint, disregarding binocular vision. He used only tests of the relative accommodation. The diagonal representing equal points for accommodation and convergence is called *Donders' line.*

a. From this diagram Donders postulated that the accommodation could be maintained only for a distance at which the PRA is relatively great in comparison to the NRA.

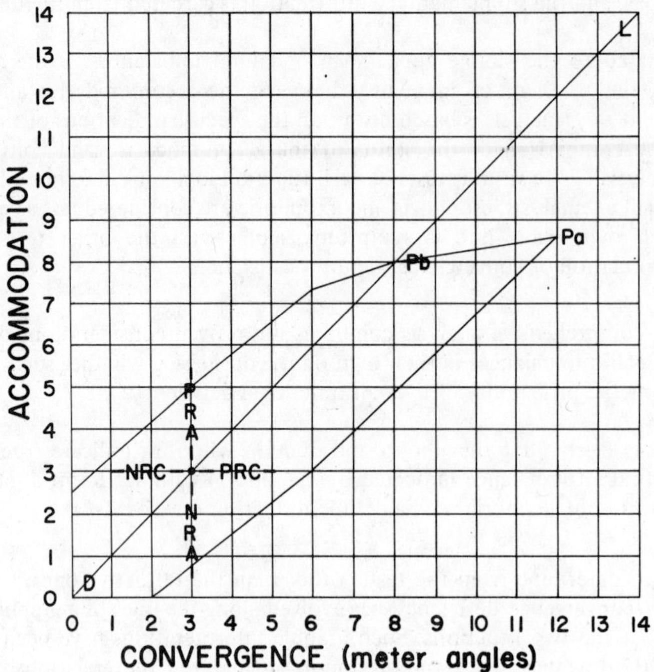

Figure XXI-1 – Donders' diagram of zone of single clear vision (after Neumueller). *DL* Donders' line of equal accommodation and convergence; *Pb* binocular punctum proximum of accommodation; *Pa* monocular punctum proximum of accommodation. *Pa* represents maximum amplitude of accommodation and punctum proximum of convergence.

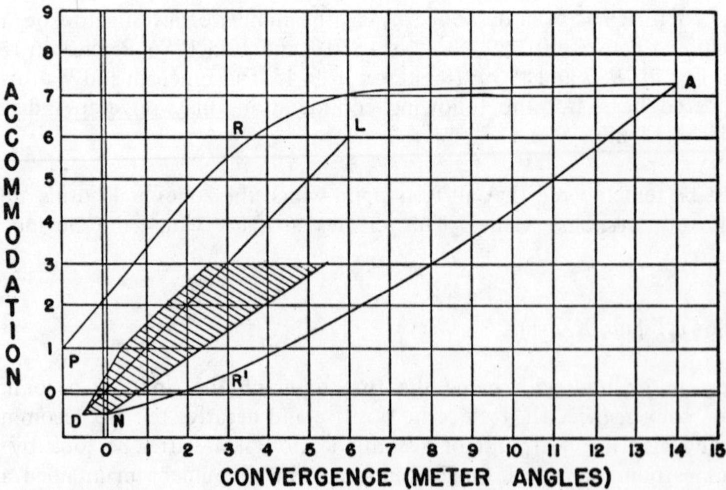

Figure XXI-2 – Percival's zone of comfort (after Sheard). *DL* line of equal accommodation and convergence; *PRA* relative positive amplitudes of accommodation; *NR'A* relative negative amplitudes of accommodation; *A* nearpoints of accommodation and convergence; shaded area, zone of comfort.

(1) While this criterion is useful in aiding the determination of presbyopic additions, it is subject to fallacy since most younger people have a PRA which far exceeds the possible maximum NRA. Even an uncorrected hyperope with symptoms of accommodative stress will reveal, if not near presbyopia, a PRA in excess of the NRA.

2. Alpern (1962) commented that Donders' line was curved because the data for accommodation were specified at the spectacle plane, while those for convergence were specified at the center of rotation. Plus lenses shifted the curve further to the right and minus further to the left.

C. Landolt (Hofstetter, 1945) later added to this diagram tests of the positive relative convergence and the negative relative convergence.

1. A number of other investigators also charted the area of single clear vision. From all of this there developed a companion postulate that the convergence could only be maintained for a distance at which the PRC was relatively great compared to the NRC.

D. Percival (1928) (Figure XXI-2)

1. Percival developed a graph of the accommodation and convergence from which he attempted to make direct clinical applications.

a. Landolt had predicted that not more than one-third of the absolute range of convergence could be exercised continually without fatigue.

(1) The amplitude of convergence in meter angles needs to be three or four times greater than the convergence demand in meter angles to meet Landolt's criterion.

b. Percival applied the concept of the relative range of convergence rather than the absolute range. He created the term *area of comfort,* which he defined as follows:

(1) The area of comfort occupies the middle third of the total relative range between the limits of 0 and 3 meter angles of convergence. Above 3 meter angles this definition does not hold.

(a) According to Percival's postulate, the Donders' line should fall in the middle third of the total range of positive relative convergence plus negative relative convergence.

(b) If the base-out blur point were 14 pd, the base-in blur point were 10 pd, and the fixation were at 16 inches, the fixation point would fall in the middle third as shown:

Base-out (PRC) Base-in (NRC)

14 13 12 11 10 9 8 7 | 6 5 4 3 2 1 0 1 2 | 3 4 5 6 7 8 9 10

No. 16A — Fixation — No. 17A

E. Sheard (1928) (Figure XXI-3)

1. Sheard plotted the zone of comfort using the relative convergence and accommodation at both far and near but including also the phorias, as indicative of the fusional convergence required to secure fixation at the desired point. This concept is the first to conceive of the *point of demand* as other than the Donders' line and to recognize the relationship of the physiologic indications of the phorias and ductions.

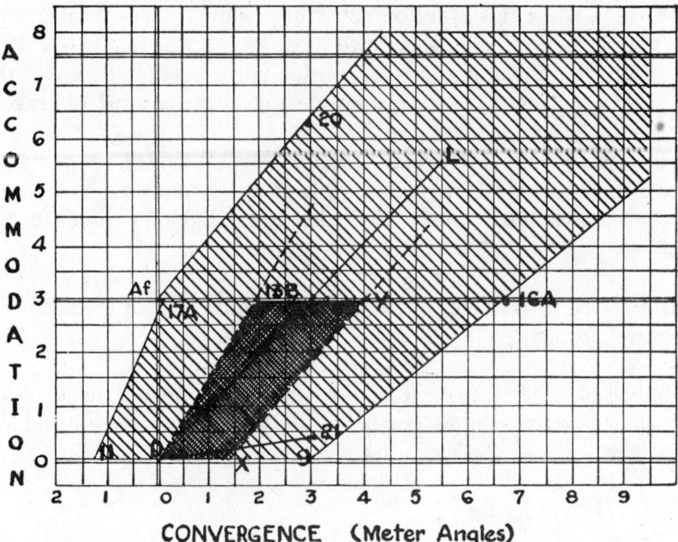

Figure XXI-3 – Sheard's chart of relative ranges of accommodation and convergence for 6 M and 33 cms. *D* center of coordinates, negative relative accommodation at far; *Af* positive relative accommodation at far; *11* negative relative convergence at far; *9* positive relative convergence at far; *16A* positive relative convergence at near; *17A* negative relative convergence at near; *20* positive relative accommodation at near; *21* negative relative accommodation at near; *D,13B,Y,X,* Percival's area of comfort; *13B* nearpoint exophoria; *DL* line of equal accommodation and convergence.

a. In exophoria, fusional convergence has to bring the eyes from the tonic status to the fixing point at far and assists in arriving at the fixing point at near. The base-out to blur finding gives an indication of the fusional convergence held in reserve and the base-out finding plus the exophoria indicates the total positive fusional convergence.

b. In esophoria, fusional divergence must be used to bring the eye to the fixing point, and the base-in to blur test measures the fusional divergence in reserve. The sum of the esophoria and the base-in blur finding equals the total fusional divergence or negative fusional convergence.

2. Sheard postulated that in order to maintain comfort, the fusional reserve must be twice as great as the fusional use or demand. This criterion may be stated as follows:

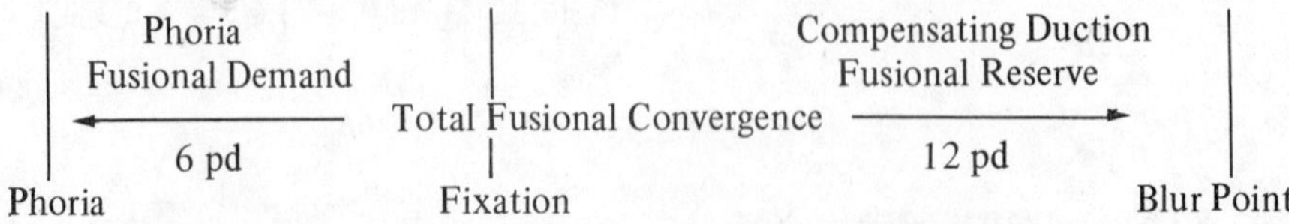

a. The total fusional convergence must be at least three times the phoria.

b. The fusional reserve must be at least twice the fusional demand.

c. The compensating duction must be at least twice the phoria.

(1) For exophoria, the compensating duction is base-out; for esophoria, base-in.

3. Comparison of Sheard's and Percival's criteria indicate that both state the same thing whenever the phoria position falls in the middle of the blur point range, and that a discrepancy arises only when the phoria position varies from the exact middle of the range.

a.

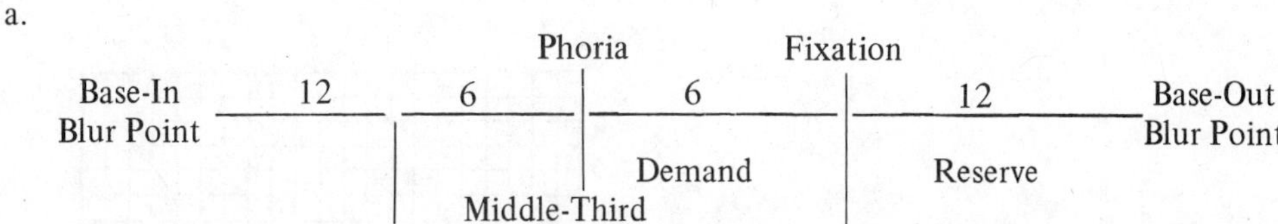

4. The work of Haines (1938) showed that the positive and negative fusional blur points varied with the phoria, the positive fusional convergence increased with exophoria, and the negative increased with esophoria. This may be due to the fact that the patients have developed the compensating function to balance the discrepancy. However, since the two vary with the phoria, the indication was definite that the middle point of the total fusional range could not be taken as an accurate indication of comfort. In a similar manner, Hofstetter (1945), in developing a graphic representation of the zone of clear binocular vision, found that whenever the patient's findings agreed with both Percival's and Sheard's criteria, comfort was found, but in two cases in which the findings differed between the indications of the two criteria, Sheard's criteria were more reliable.

5. The fact that comfort is had by patients with extreme cases of imbalance which do not appear compensated by the contrary ductions may indicate one of the following:

a. Comfort can be had with less than two-thirds the fusional convergence held in reserve.

b. The blur points are not adequate expressions of the limits of fusional convergence.

c. The role of accommodative-convergence may not be fully appreciated.

F. Neumueller (1946) (Figure XXI-4)

1. Neumueller objected to the use of Donders' criteria and Percival's criteria on the grounds that each established a relationship between supply and demand upon the basis of an independent comparison of each function. Based upon the preliminary work of Tait (See Chapter XX), Neumueller conducted further investigations of his own upon the relationship and indications of the four blur point tests, P.R.C., N.R.C., P.R.A., and N.R.A. He used a target consisting of test objects which used the ability to discriminate between two fine lines as the criterion of blur instead of letters, thus eliminating the matter of familiarity with the letter organization of words which may affect subjective tests of this order.

2. Using these tests, he developed a relationship of the four findings based upon a reciprocal action of the accommodation and convergence which closely paralleled that found by Tait.

a. According to these data, he described the parts of convergence as the reflex accommodative-convergence and the supplementary convergence or fusional convergence which would correspond to Tait's physiologic exophoria. This latter, Neumueller believes, is also expressed by the negative relative convergence test. In a similar manner, the accommodation is comprised of convergent-accommodation and of supplementary accommodation, which would be expressed as the negative relative accommodation test.

3. Since the accommodative-convergence and convergent-accommodation would be reciprocal, the supplementary accommodation and fusional convergence would exhibit a relationship for normal total uses of equal accommodation and convergence.

a. This might be expressed as follows:

Total accommodation=convergent-accommodation + supplementary accommodation. TA=CA+SA.
Total convergence=accommodative-convergence + fusional convergence. TC=AC+FC.

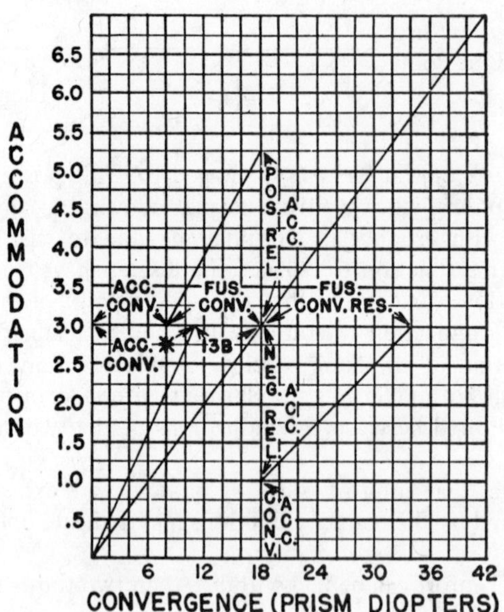

Figure XXI-4 – Neumueller's chart of accommodative and convergence functions. *Acc-Conv.*, accommodative-convergence in use at near, as shown by total convergence less 17A value; *Acc-Conv.;** accommodative-convergence in use at near, as shown by total convergence less physiologic exophoria; *Fus-Conv.*, fusional convergence in use at near as shown by *17A; 13B,* fusional convergence in use at near as shown by physiologic exophoria; *Fus. Conv. Res.*, reserve of positive fusional convergence as shown by *16A; Pos. Rel. Acc.*, reserve of focus or supplementary accommodation at near as shown by *20; Neg. Rel. Acc.*, focus or supplementary use at near as shown by *21; Conv. Acc.*, convergent-accommodation in use at near as shown by total accommodation, less *21* value.

(1) If convergent-accommodation was assumed to equal accommodative-convergence, it would be obvious that if the total accommodation and total convergence were equal, the supplementary accommodation would also equal the fusional convergence.

(a) That is, if TA=TC and CA=AC, then SA must equal FC.

b. While the CA and AC are not assumed to be equal, according to Tait, (See Chapter XX), a definite reciprocal relationship does exist between them. If such a relationship exists, then a correlative relationship should exist between the supplementary accommodation or negative relative accommodation and the fusional convergence or negative relative convergence.

(1) For example, if the CA were twice the proportion of the TA that the AC was of the TC, then the SA would be half the proportion of the TA that the FC was of the TC, with TA = TC.

4. The table given shows the correlation between the tests of the negative relative accommodation and negative relative convergence which Neumueller found. From that correlation he derived the following relationship (for 13 inches):

TABLE XXI-1

Acc.-conv.	Conv.-acc.	Neg. rel. conv.	Neg. rel. acc.
16	*2.50*	*2*	*0.50*
14	*2.00*	*4*	*1.00*
12	*1.50*	*6*	*1.50*
10	*1.25*	*8*	*1.75*
8	*1.00*	*10*	*2.00*
6	*0.75*	*12*	*2.25*
4	*0.50*	*14*	*2.50*
2	*0.25*	*16*	*2.75*
-	*00*	*18*	*3.00*

5. From the above premises it is obvious that if the accommodation were being employed to an amount greater than the convergence was, the TA would be greater than the TC, and the parts comprising the TA, such as the CA and SA, would be greater in actual amount than the parts comprising the TC, such as the AC and FC. Consequently, the NRA would show a higher finding than the NRC would show related to it by the above table.

a. Thus, if the NRC were to show 8 pd and the NRA were to show 2.50 D. instead of the 1.75 which the above table indicates related to the NRC, an excess of 0.75 D. would be revealed. Such an excess would be explained only by an assumption of a greater total accommodation in employ or an undercorrection of the hyperopia.

b. Since with each increase of the lens power a corresponding change is made in the relationship of the NRA and NRC, only one-half the discrepancy or 0.37 D. would be indicated as needed to balance the two or correct the full error.

c. Neumueller notes that the total relative convergence should actually include the distant phoria as is done by Tait in determining the physiologic exophoria. But since most distant phorias fall between 2 of esophoria and 2 of exophoria, the discrepancy would rarely be more than 0.25 D., which he states is too narrow a tolerance anyway. The indications of the relationship which he employs are mainly those of revealing whether the case is fully corrected or if over-use of accommodation still exists. The amount determinable cannot be established within 0.25 D. in any case.

6. The following main groups are found:

a. *Those in which an undercorrection of the subjective correction is indicated.*

(1) While Neumueller does not state any specific handling of such indications, such findings might point to over-stimulation of convergence.

b. *Those in which the findings indicate an increase in plus power.*

(1) The inclusion of such power in the distant Rx depends upon the acuity affected, the temperament of the patient, the constancy of wearing of the correction, the demands of the patient's occupation, and also the Positive Relative Accommodation.

(a) Where the PRA is lower than 2.00 D. for people up to age thirty or 1.50 D for pre-presbyopes above thirty, the additional plus is advised in the form of a bifocal, as also is the case when the symptoms at near are severe and the full correction at far intolerable.

7. Insofar as the indications of the PRC are concerned, Neumueller believed that it should exceed the NRC or the phoria, whichever is higher.

8. Finally, Neumueller attaches little value to the matter of the actual extent of the accommodative-convergence association. Since the analysis depends upon the relationship of the two relative findings of the functions, which are not associated, and since both, in the properly corrected case, will vary in their established reciprocal relation, the matter of whether the hook-up is tight or loose is not a factor.

G. Fry (1937, 1938, and 1943) and Hofstetter (1945)

1. The work of Fry and of Hofstetter has resulted in a delineation of the zone of clear single binocular vision which avoids the discrepancies found by earlier investigators. The previous charts were based mainly upon typical clinical methods of determining the blur points. These methods did not allow for the depth of focus or the ability to recognize letters despite their blurred focus and so did not precisely designate the points at which accommodation actually varied. By using the haploscope and special targets, a finer discrimination is possible, and Hofstetter indicates that recognition of blur does not occur until the accommodation has altered the focus to an extent equal to one-half the depth of focus of the eye. This amount can be averaged as approximately one diopter, and if this allowance is made for each limit of accommodation, a reasonably definite figure for the zone of single binocular vision can be determined.

2. *Plotting the Graph* (Figure XXI-5) (Abel, 1951)

a. The graph consists of a calibrated chart in which the x axis or abscissa represents the demands upon convergence and the y axis or ordinate represents the demand upon accommodation. The superior horizontal axis represents a prism scale for 40 cms., while the inferior axis represents a prism scale for distance testing or 6 meters. The left vertical scale represents the actual stimulus to accommodation. The right vertical scale (not shown) can be calibrated to show the difference between accommodation through the subjective finding, usually represented as zero, and any other test distance or lens power used for testing.

(1) First blur points are represented by circles, blur out points (not generally used), by solid circles, phoria findings by x's, break points of ductions by squares, and recovery points, when used, by triangles.

(2) In the various illustrations and samples, the symbols used for the tests are those utilized by the Optometric Extension Program, and used here because of their brevity. The numerals indicate the tests as follows: No. 8, Lateral Phoria at far; No. 9, True Adduction; No. 10, Convergence at far; No. 11, Divergence at far; No. 13B, Fusional Supplementary Convergence (phoria at near); No. 14A and 14B, Dissociated and Binocular Cross Cylinder; No. 16A,Positive Relative Convergence; No. 16B, Positive Fusional Reserve at near; No. 17A, Negative Relative Convergence; No. 17B, Negative Fusional Reserve at near; No. 19, Amplitude of Accommodation; No. 20, Positive Relative Accommodation; No. 21, Negative Relative Accommodation.

b. *The Demand Line*

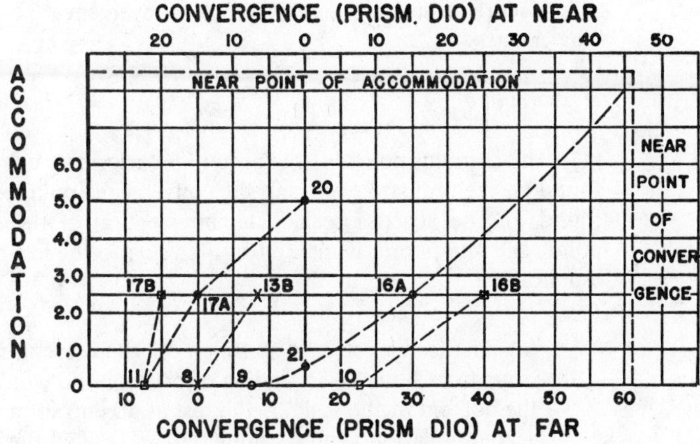

Figure XXI-5 – Graphical plot of findings (after Fry). Prism notations to left of O indicate base-in or exophoria; prism notations to right of O indicate prism base-out or esophoria; findings on O accommodation level refer to lower horizontal scale; findings at 2.5 level of accommodation refer to upper horizontal scale; *9,21,16A* positive limit of zone; *11,17A,20* negative limit of zone; *8,13B* slope indicating ACA ratio.

(1) Donders' line is plotted by computing the stimulus to accommodation and convergence.

(a) For accommodation

[1] The subjective is used as zero stimulus and the reciprocal in diopters of the distance of test used to determine the other points of the line.

(b) For convergence

[1] The convergence may be determined by the accommodative demand X 6.

[2] It may also be determined by the following formula:

$$\frac{\text{Pupillary Distance in mm. x 10}}{\text{distance in cms. + 2.7 (distance in cm. from spectacle plane to center of rotation)}}$$

(2) Since the demand line is relatively constant and has been demonstrated in previous graphs, it is not illustrated in Figure XXI-5 and subsequent figures.

c. *The borders of the area of accommodation and convergence*

(1) The left margin of the chart and the bottom margin of the chart represent two of the borders of the area of accommodation and convergence.

(2) The upper border is determined by projecting a horizontal line from the ordinate point representing the stimulus to accommodation at the maximum amplitude of accommodation.

(3) The right border is determined by projecting a vertical line from the abscissa

point representing the stimulus to convergence at the maximum amplitude of convergence.

d. *The phoria line*

(1) The stimulus point for the accommodation through which the phoria was taken is found on the ordinate scale, and the convergence point representing the test distance is found on the abscissa scale. The intersection of these two represents the demand point, and the phoria is marked by its value to the left if exophoria and to the right if esophoria.

(a) If the subjective is considered as zero accommodative demand, and the test is made at 6 meters, a finding of orthophoria would be marked at the 0 point on the bottom of the scale. If the test at 40 cms. is made through the subjective, the accommodation is now stimulated 2.5 D., and the phoria value would be marked on the horizontal line corresponding to that stimulation. It would be marked to the left, if exophoria, and the right, if esophoria, of the 0 on the upper horizontal scale representing 40 cms.

(b) If an add of +1.00 were used, the upper horizontal scale would still be employed if the test distance were still 40 cms., but the horizontal line used would be that corresponding to accommodative stimulation of only +1.50, the 2.50 value of the distance less the add, while if a phoria were taken through a −1.00 add to the subjective, the line chosen would correspond to an accommodative stimulation of 3.50, the 2.50 values of 40 cms. plus the extra minus, and so forth for various lens values.

(c) If a test were taken with the subjective at 33 cms., then the line corresponding to an accommodative stimulation of 3.00 D. would be used and the zero point of the convergence scale would correspond to the 18 Δ mark on the bottom horizontal scale. The zero point for a test at forty inches would correspond to the 6 Δ point on the bottom scale, for twenty-six inches it would be the 9 Δ point on the bottom scale, and so forth. These points are indicated by the Donders' line, when it is drawn into the graph. Esophoria would always be so many Δ to the right of that point, and exophoria so many Δ to the left, according to the finding.

(d) If two different refractions are used and the findings through both graphed on the same chart, then one of the refractions is assumed to be the zero position and the other is graphed as a change in accommodative stimulus. The amount of change in stimuli is determined by reducing both refractions to their spherical equivalents and noting the difference of the average values of the two eyes.

(e) The phoria line is represented on the graph as a fine line, with a sometimes shaded border to include all valid phoria findings.

e. *The vergence lines*

(1) Base-out findings, stimulatory to convergence, are plotted to the right of the demand point at the distance tested. Base-in findings, inhibitory to convergence, are plotted to the left of the demand point. (As seen above, this point is zero on the bottom scale for 6 meters, zero on the top scale for 40 cms., and located as described for the phorias for other distances.)

(2) Corresponding blur points are connected by a segmented line, as are correspond-

ing recovery and break points. If no blur point is evident in a given test, its break point is used as a blur point value.

(3) The breaks and recoveries can be connected, even if blurs are presented, to check the slope of the phoria and blur line (Heath, 1959). Hofstetter (1954) stated that the transitions of the zone tend to make the blur test at distance unreliable and limited in usefulness. The "breaks" are the lower limits of the left-hand curve and the upper limits of the right-hand curve. Low recoveries or absence of the blur points may be interpreted to indicate a low quality of fusion.

f. *Accommodative blur points*

(1) The minus lens add to blur is plotted, as an additional stimulus to accommodation, above the test distance point at the zero value of the test distance. Thus, if taken at 40 cms, it is plotted *above* the line representing 2.50 D. of accommodative stimulus – under the zero value on the upper convergence scale. Since minus lens to accommodation is equivalent to prism base-in to convergence, the segmented line representing the base-in blur points is extended to include this finding.

(2) The plus lens add is calculated from the same point as the minus but its own value is *below* that point, since it reduces the accommodative stimulus. As a plus lens acts equivalent to prism base-out, the line connecting the prism base-out blur points is extended to include this finding.

(3) The line including the minus lens and base-in prism blur points may be called the Relative Convergence Inhibitory line, while the one comprised of the plus lens and base-out prism blur points may be called the Relative Convergence Stimulatory line.

3. *The Zone of Clear Single Binocular Vision*

a. The zone of clear, single binocular vision may now be noted as lying in the area delineated by the zero line to accommodation as the bottom boundary, the amplitude of accommodation as the upper boundary, the relative convergence inhibition (RCI) line as the left boundary, and the relative convergence stimulus (RCS) line as the right boundary.

b. Flom (1954) also spoke of the Zone of Single Binocular Vision, in which the left boundary is represented by the Negative Fusional Reserve and the right one by the Positive Fusional Reserve, that is, by the break points of the vergence tests rather than the blur points. These limits are not usually used for the zone under discussion.

(1) The left or negative side of the zone is limited by the limits of negative relative convergence and positive relative accommodation; the right or positive side of the zone is limited by positive relative convergence and negative relative accommodation.

c. The general form of the zone is somewhat like a parallelogram. If the various tests are taken with various lens powers before the eyes at varying distances, and the total zone is plotted, it will be found that the upper limit of the zone is determined by the amplitude of accommodation, while the extreme right-hand limit depends upon the amplitude of convergence. The area represented by the RCI and RCS lines represents the width of the zone.

(1) The RCI line shows a straight section, with a somewhat curved section at its top, and a short vertical extension at the bottom, while the RCS line shows a straight section with a somewhat curved section at the bottom and a short vertical extension at the top. The deviations of each line from the direction of the bulk of the line is due to the depth of focus of the eye, as indicated in Figure XXI-6.

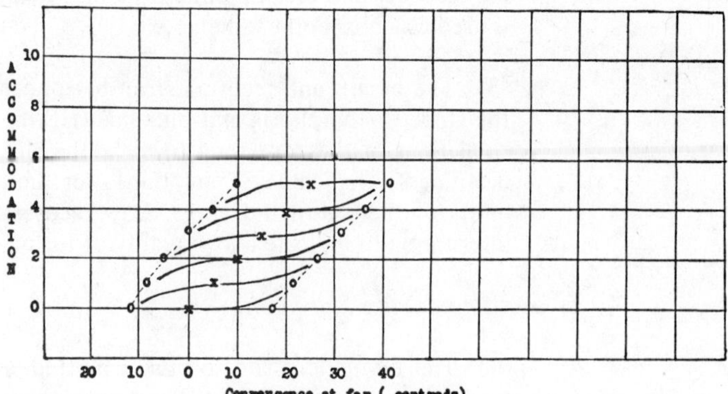

Figure XXI-6 – Width of zone at different levels of accommodation (after Hofstetter). *O* respective base-in and base-out blur points; *x* phoria positions; lines, indicate range of clear vision; dotted line, indicates lapse in findings due to depth of focus.

(a) Clinical emmetropia, representing the bottom of the zone, should be plotted at a point of accommodative activity of 0.50 D. or 0.75 D.

(2) The phoria line representing the ACA ratio is approximately a straight line and will parallel either or both the RCI or RCS lines. The right hand or RCS line may also be affected by, and its slope determined in part by, the convergence-accommodation rather than the accommodative-convergence, although in general the accommodative-convergence is of greater importance. If the phoria line paralleled only one, it would therfore usually parallel the RCI line (Morgan, 1968).

d. While the theoretical zone was represented as a parallelogram in the main, with the positive and negative slopes parallel to each other and the phoria line, the actual clinical zone was described more accurately as shown in Figure XXI-7 (Manas, 1955).

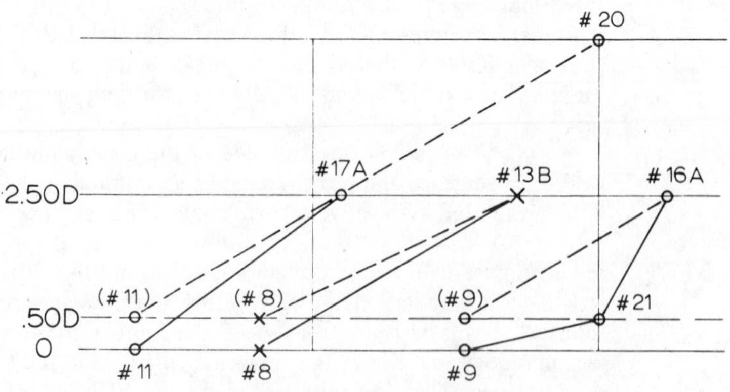

Figure XXI-7 – See text.

(1) If O.E.P. tests No. 11, No. 8 and No. 9 were plotted at 0.50 D. of active accommodation, as indicated in the drawing, it would be observed that the zone assumed a shape much closer to the predicted form with relatively parallel borders and phoria lines (Morgan, 1968).

(2) The ACA may be determined from either of the following formulas:

(a) $\frac{15 - \text{No. } 11}{2.50 - \text{No. } 20}$ or

(b) $\frac{15 - \text{No. } 8 + \text{No. } 13\text{b}}{2.50}$

e. *Certain conclusions about the zone may be drawn:*

(1) *Position*

(a) The lateral position of the zone is established by the phoria line, particularly by the distant phoria. In a few instances, the entire zone appears to change position, but such changes seem associated with periodic strabismus, often when the subject is unaware of the condition and suffers no symptoms from it.

(2) *The Height of the Zone*

(a) The height of the zone, affected by the amplitude, may decrease with age. Since the convergence-accommodation ratio changes with age and this affects the ceiling and the positive side of the zone, both will also vary with age.

(b) If the true amplitude of accommodation is greater than the manifest amplitude, the accommodative line, representing the height of the zone, will extend to the right beyond the right limiting border of the zone.

[1] Alpern (1950) explains this projection as not fusional convergence, as it might appear to be, but as accommodative-convergence. While the response to accommodation is absent, the stimulus and association continue and remain co-linear with the phoria lines, even though neither are straight lines any longer.

(3) *The Width*

(a) The width of the zone represents the range of relative convergence. The width may be varied by training, particularly on the positive end (base-out).

(b) Where changes in the width are brought about at one level of accommodation, it is equalled at all other levels of accommodation. A patient given training with accommodation at zero shows as much increase in the range at other levels as at the zero level of accommodation.

(c) Variations in range are not followed by variations in position of the phoria.

(4) *The Slope*

(a) The slope is linear throughout a middle range but varies from it at the extremes.

(b) The slope bears no relationship to ametropia.

(c) The slope indicates the accommodative-convergence relationship for the individual.

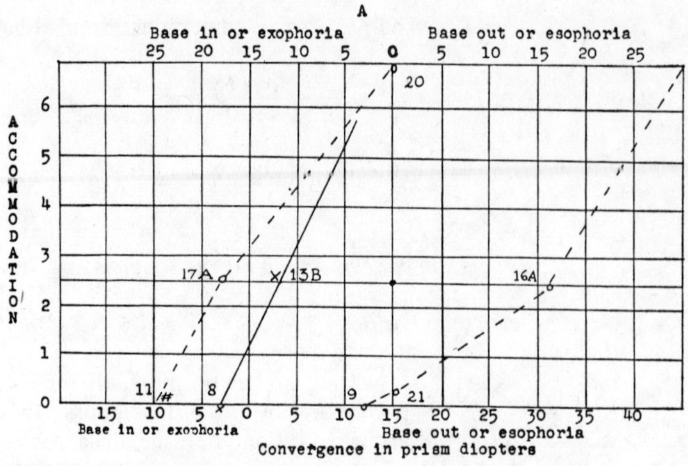

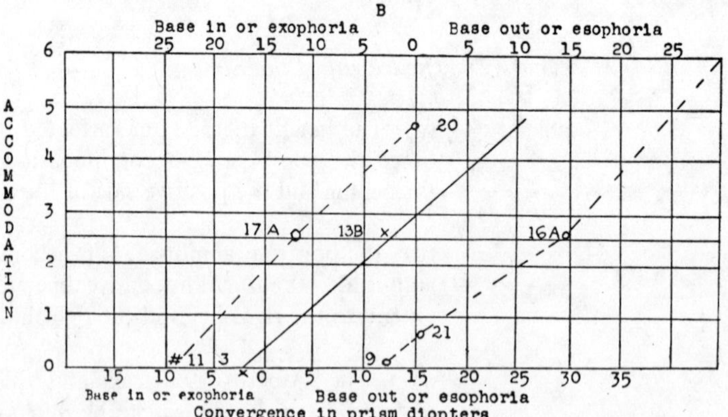

Figure XXI-8 – (A) Graph showing slope of case with low accommodative convergence ratio. Note high phoria at near and width of relative ranges. (B) Graph showing slope of case with high ACA ratio. Note low near phoria and limited relative ranges.

[1] It can be seen that the slope is the graphical representation of the gradient, that is, the determination of the ACA by the use of phorias at different levels of accommodation (Figure XXI-8).

(d) The ACA ratio or gradient may be determined either arithmetically or graphically. The former has been described, but the latter requires the use of the graph.

[1] The point on the stimulation to accommodation line intersected by the phoria slope line is used as the start of a perpendicular to the stimulus to accommodation line.

[2] This perpendicular is dropped to the zero stimulus line.

[3] The number of Δ from the phoria position on the zero line to the place on the zero line struck by the perpendicular is noted.

[4] This amount divided by 2.5 gives the gradient per diopter of accommodation.

4. Morgan (1968) considered that the *zone was, in principle, generated as follows:*

a. The actual accommodation will appear to be reciprocal to the working or testing distance, but the response is really some 0.50 D. less.

b. If base-out prism is added, the increasing convergence tends to stimulate accommodation, but the stimulus for clear vision prevents an increase until the limits of positive relative convergence are nearly reached. As this limit is approached, the functions of accommodation and convergence are at or near a relationship which would have been achieved by action of the convergence-accommodation. If clear vision is now lost, convergence and accommodation will change with respect to the convergence-accommodation relationship and not with respect to the accommodative-convergence relationship.

c. If base-in is added, a decrease in convergence occurs which tends to inhibit accommodation. The stimulus for clear vision prevents this from acting until near the limits of negative relative convergence. If convergence is to be decreased more, accommodation will change and the rate of increased loss of convergence will be determined by the accommodative-convergence. Convergence-accommodation could not be a factor as the amount of accommodation in play would always be greater than the amount stimulated by the convergence in play.

d. As minus lenses are added in the determination of positive relative accommodation, accommodation is stimulated as is accommodative-convergence. Bifixation is now maintained by the utilization of negative relative convergence at or near the limit of accommodation. The total available negative relative convergence has been used up. Addition of more minus lens power will not result in a further significant increase in accommodation and the fixated target will become blurred.

e. As plus lenses are added, accommodation decreases as does accommodative-convergence. This loss of accommodative-convergence is made up by the utilization of positive relative accommodation. This will continue until either all available accommodation is inhibited or until all available relative convergence is utilized. The limiting factor may be accommodation, rather than relative convergence.

f. If accommodative-convergence and convergence-accommodation are similar, the sequence of events becomes difficult to interpret. The details of the stimulus-response pattern may vary with the individual.

5. Hofstetter's Proposed Revision Of The Analytical Graph (Figure XXI-9)

a. In a recent paper (1968), Hofstetter has proposed a revision of the format of the analytical graph upon which the zone is charted. These modifications include:

(1) Reversal of the ordinates

(a) Accommodation would be presented along the x axis or abscissa and convergence along the y axis, or ordinate, in opposite positions to that of the accustomed graph.

(b) This would permit the ACA slope to more properly approach the conventional mathematical slope formula where a high ACA is nearer the vertical while a low one is nearer the horizontal.

(c) The representation of convergence on the y ordinate allows the various types of convergence to be plotted against the more apparently single function of accommodation, as is conventional in graphic methods.

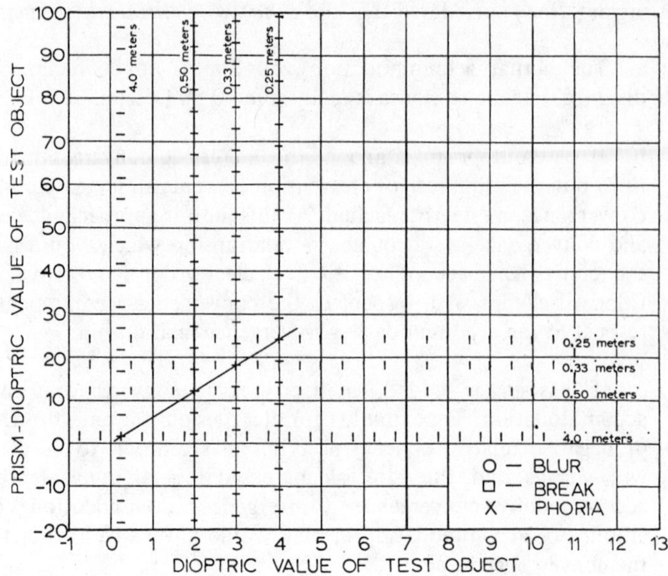

Figure XXI-9 – Hofstetter's Revision of Graph for Plotting Zone of Comforts (see text).

(2) Scale values for the tests at 0.25, 0.33, 0.50 and 4.0 meters.

(a) The close distances represent distances favorably used for many test procedures or of importance in modern industry, while the 4.0 meter distance represents a true work distance with a dioptric value expressible in commonly used units. (See Chapter XIX, Subjective Test Methods.)

(b) The omission of a 0.4 meter scale does not interfere with the plotting of data taken at that distance, since the position is easily determined on the graph.

(3) Titling of the abscissa as "Dioptric Value Of Accommodation Stimulus."

(a) This more truly expresses the actual test conditions than does the previous title, "Stimulus To Accommodation."

(4) Titling of the ordinate as "Prism-diopter Scale of Convergence Stimulus."

(a) This expresses a truer specification, in terms of parallelism of the lines of sight, for the scale at all test distances.

(5) A demand or Donders' line is included, as before.

(a) Plus lenses are represented by displacements to the left of the line.

(b) Minus lenses are represented by displacement to the left of the line.

(c) Prism base-in is indicated by displacement below the line.

(d) Prism base-out is represented by displacement above the line.

(e) Each scale is graduated in terms of diopters and prism diopters from their intersection with the demand line.

VI. VALIDITY OF THE DATA

A. Proximal Convergence

1. The graph can be shown to demonstrate the amount and influence of proximal convergence by the simple expedient of testing at infinity and using minus and plus lenses to achieve the changes in accommodative stimulus and then re-testing with the same procedures at a near point. The shift in the zone from one position of tests to the other will be equal to the influence of proximal convergence. The major shift will be noted in the slope line and the RCS line, which will be displaced but remain parallel under both test distances.

a. Burman (1956) attempted to utilize a simplified version of the graphical method by adding a +1.00 and a −1.00 lens to the subjective findings and recording four different phorias. He used these to determine the lateral position and slope of the zone. He considered the distance findings more reliable and equivalent to the near if allowance for convergence is made and derived the width of the zone from them. He then measured the positive versions at near, added plus lenses to secure negative relative accommodation, and with the nearpoint of convergence determined the right slope of the zone. The amplitude of accommodation provided the height. As he ignored the entire matter of proximal convergence, the validity of the graph he derived may be questioned.

B. Reliability of Patient Response

1. As Hebbard (1952), Heath (1959) and Hofstetter have emphasized, whatever system of analysis used, it was subject to the potentiality that the data upon which the analysis was being made were totally unreliable due to the fact that the patient was not a trained observer, the examiner made errors in calculating or recording, or the circumstances of the examination may have been misleading. Consistency of the findings depended upon repeatable measurements and evidence of the existence of established relationships between the findings. Inconsistent findings should be readily apparent so that remeasurement could be made upon the occasion. Either some type of norm for reference or the graphical summary of the tests lended itself best for this purpose.

a. Morgan (1968) commented that from a clinical point of view, the methods based on the original Maddox concepts, if not exactly precise as seen in this discussion, were still acceptable, especially in the ranges of accommodation and convergence used for normal vision.

2. The graph should meet the previously indicated standards in regards to its approximate shape, the form of the various lines, and the parallelism between them. If it does not do so, different tests or distances of test should be employed to attempt to secure more reliable results. Also, the reliability of the findings may be checked in another way. With only two findings for phorias or blur points, in the ordinary routine, one cannot be used as an indication of the reliability of the other. But if extra findings are taken, such as the gradient phoria or phorias with the P.R.A. and N.R.A. findings in place, and the relative blur points are also taken with those powers, the findings which fail to conform to a straight line indicate unreliability of the data. This may be due to the operator's technique or to the patient. Close checks should be kept on the criteria which may induce these deviations. The after effects of duction tests or orthoptics are evident, and tests taken after their application may need to be repeated. Likewise, the influence of fusion may require the repetition of the phoria test from both the base-out and base-in sides and an average established. Usually repetition of a test will indicate the extent of reliability. Despite such discrepancies, a general agreement of the findings even if a slight variance from a true line is shown is sufficient for the purpose.

3. Successive tests upon patients who reappear for periodic examinations can be graphed to indicate the actual reliability of any of the data. If the subjective correction is altered from one

time to the next, the difference between the two is indicated in the graph by noting a change in accommodation. Likewise, a test taken with the habitual or no correction before the eyes and the same test taken with the subjective before the eyes must be graphed accordingly.

a. Flom (1954) reported a narrower zone after the first correction of anisometropia, which later widened. He suggested that the latter was the truer measurement and the earlier data were invalid.

b. If a patient entered with no Rx and a phoria, No. 3, indicated 2 eso, while a subjective of +1.00 was found, which revealed a No. 8 finding of 1 exo, the graph would show the stimulus to accommodation 0 with the +1.00 finding (No. 8), but a stimulus to accommodation of 1.00 D. for the No. 3 finding.

(1) For example, the following set of phoria findings would graph (Figure XXI-10) as follows:

Entrance Rx, 0; subjective, +1.00; 14A, +1.50; 14B, +1.75; No. 3, 3 eso; No. 8, 1 exo; No. 13A, 6 exo; No. 13B, 6 exo; No. 15A, 7 exo; No. 15B, 8 exo.

c. If the same patient entered a year later and now showed these findings, they would be entered (Figure XXI-10) as follows:

Entrance Rx, +1.00 new Rx, +2.00; No. 14A, +2.75; No. 14B, +2.25; No. 3, 0; No. 8, 2 exo; No. 13A, 6 exo; No. 13B, 8 exo; No. 15A, 12 exo; No. 15B, 10 exo.

d. As can be seen from Figure XXI-10, the ACA slope is not varied even though the findings scanned casually seem to show a difference in the phoria position upon successive examinations. Also it can be seen that at least one of the findings is not reliable because it is too far from the phoria line.

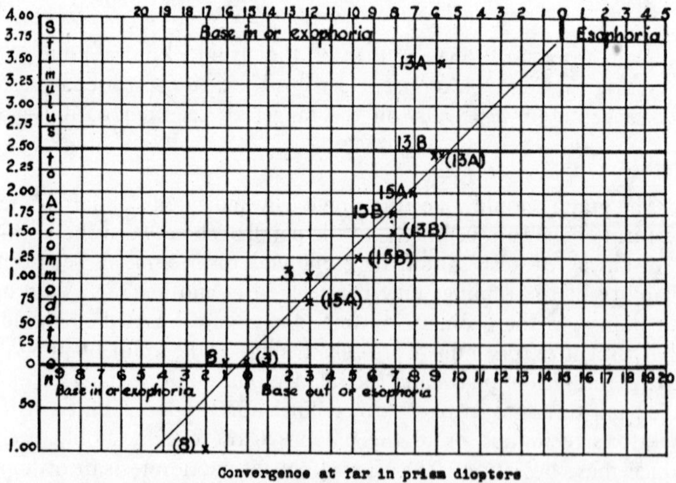

Figure XXI-10 – Graph of phoria findings of two separate examinations of same patient showing basic ACA slope and reliability of findings. "X" indicates graphic position of finding. Basic Rx. +1.00; *3, 8, et al.* findings of first examination; *(3), (8), et al.* findings of second examination. All phorias placed on accommodative equivalent of lens power in comparison to basic Rx of +1.00 for far; for near, same, plus stimulation of working distance (2.50 D.). Finding *13A* of first examination definitely unreliable; finding *(8)* of second, doubtful.

e. In another example, a zone in which the slope was so great that the demand line crossed the inhibitory line at the left, indicating a need for base-in prism, the position could have been due to an invalid finding due to reluctance to accommodate accurately for the near phoria test, rather than to a convergence problem. If accommodation were exercised, the zone would swing over (Heath, 1959).

C. Problems of accommodation and convergence

1. The specific problems involved in convergence are treated in the next section. The graphical method lends itself to the application of the following conditions because the width of the zone is readily apparent in relation to the phoria positions, the ACA ratio is obvious, and, upon occasion, drastic situations are emphasized by intersections of the slope and relative convergence lines. Based on the known characteristics of the zone, inferential diagnosis was applicable in terms of qualitative deficiencies in fusion or accommodation (Heath, 1959).

a. In general, where the slope indicates a high ACA relationship, it is likely that either plus lens power or prism base-out or both may be required above the subjective, while where the slope indicates a low ACA relationship, minus lens power or prism base-in may be required. However, other factors should first be considered before applying this rule sweepingly.

2. Hofstetter illustrated diagnostic use of the zone with a case in which a complaint of eyestrain at near revealed the following data. These data are plotted on an accommodation-convergence graph in Figure XXI-11.

a. Position a on the graph represents the condition with no Rx worn at distance.

(1) 3.50 esophoria at far; 3 pd base-in; 19 pd base-out.

b. Position b on the graph represents the situation with no Rx worn for near.

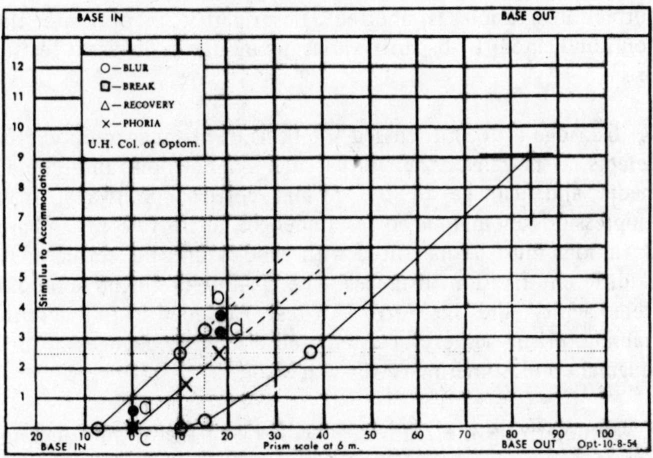

Figure XXI-11 – A Plot of Accommodation and Convergence Findings. The circles represent limits of clear single binocular vision. The X's represent phorias. The heavy dots labeled *a, b, c,* and *d* represent demand points referred to in the discussion. The heavy vertical line and heavy horizontal line in the upper right hand corner represent the maximum convergence and accommodation respectively.

(1) 10 esophoria at near; base-in is 0; base-out is 27 pd.

c. Position c represents the old Rx at far.

(1) Orthophoria; base-in is 8 pd; base-out is 10 pd.

d. Position d represents the old Rx at near:

(1) 5 esophoria; 5 pd base-in; 22 pd base-out.

e. a and b definitely do not meet either Sheard's or Percival's criteria and d fails to meet it slightly. Only c qualifies. If an add of +0.50 at near is supplied, a position between Sheard's and Percival's requirements would be met.

VII. SPECIFIC REGARD OF LATERAL IMBALANCES

A. While considerable success is enjoyed with the prescription of vertical prism, it is almost axiomatic that prescription of lateral prism is fraught with risk. Base-in prism enjoys some degree of success, but base-out prism is seldom worn with satisfaction. Consequently, many maxims regarding the prescription of lateral prism have arisen, and as will be seen, many systems for determining an acceptable amount have been developed.

1. Giles (1965) recommended that prism be prescribed only when it would reduce discomfort or diplopia, not otherwise alleviated, or aid orthoptics. He preferred its use particularly for mature patients, where altering the spherical power of the correction would not abet the condition. Base-out prisms were recommended only as a last resort, and never over one-half the distant phoria for distant wear only.

2. Flom (1963) commented that base-in prism relaxed convergence and induced vertical discrepancies due to the unbalanced action of the superior and inferior rectus when the eyes were diverged.

3. Morgan (1960) and Carter (1968) reported that prism is better accepted if the deviation agrees in direction with the fixation disparity and that if the disparity is overcome by prism or lens correction, fusion is abetted. If disparity is opposite the phoria, in direction, prism is contraindicated. If disparity varies in amount in different tests, Carter suggests training rather than prism.

4. Eskridge (1963) discussed the basis of prism correction criteria at length. Problems arose from defects in the sensory apparatus; such as ametropia, amblyopia, eccentric fixation, opacities of the media and damage to the retinal cortical pathways; from integrative anomalies, such as suppression, anomalous correspondence, horror fusionis and aniseikonia; or from motor processes. Deviations must be measured with validity and the status of fusion amplitudes likewise measured at different fixation distances. The quality of fusion should also be noted, e.g., recovery point, stereo-acuity, and the Worth Dot test. All aided in this determination. The choice between visual training, prism, surgery or attempted effects of changes of the lens correction became a matter of judgment and, sometimes, trial and error.

5. Summarizing the reasons, Textor (1949) gave the following provisions for prescribing lateral prism:

a. When the history indicates other therapies have been unsuccessful.

b. Where the symptoms include occasional diplopia, vertigo, gastrointestinal symptoms, panoramic headaches (in moving vehicles or watching motion) and are persistent and consistent.

c. Where the phoria is anatomical in origin and does not vary as do the innervational types or indicate pathological origins.

(1) These are constant in different directions of gaze, consistent upon re-test, and exhibit a physiological exophoria and not an esophoria.

d. Where the positive fusional amplitude is exceedingly poor.

B. The various forms of lateral imbalance which may create discomfort may be segregated into the following categories:

1. Orthophoria at Far, with Imbalance at Near

a. *Exophoria at near*

b. *Esophoria at near*

(1) Associated with a low amplitude of accommodation

(2) Normal amplitude of accommodation

2. Esophoria at Far, with Imbalance at Near

a. *Esophoria at near or low exophoria*

(1) Hypertonic accommodation

(2) Toxic esophoria

b. *High exophoria at near*

3. Exophoria at Far, with Imbalance at Near

a. *Exophoria at near*

(1) Fatigue or weakness of convergence

(2) Accommodative-convergence

(a) Normal

(b) Low

(3) Undeveloped accommodation

(4) Presbyopia

C. Orthophoria at Far

1. *With Exophoria at Near*

a. The manifestation of exophoria at near is, as has been explained earlier, merely an indication of the portion of the total convergence which is fusional in nature. Since this depends essentially upon the accommodative-convergence relationship, such an exophoria may be altered chiefly by changes in accommodation. Such exophorias are not a source of trouble, if the fusional reserve qualifies according to the previously noted criteria of reserve in relation to demand. Where the fusional convergence reserve is deficient, it can readily be built up by orthoptics or, on occasion, prism base-in may lessen the demand itself.

(1) Giles recommended that the amount of correction be determined by either:

(a) The physiological exophoria less the phoria

(b) The gradient test less the norm

(c) Sheard's criteria

(d) One-fourth of the near exo

(e) Of the above, Sheard's criteria are usually accepted as the method with greatest validity.

2. *With Esophoria at Near and a Low Amplitude of Accommodation*

a. If the accommodative mechanism is impaired so that a given innervation to accommodation does not produce the dioptric change which it should, it is evident that increased accommodative innervation will be required. Such innervation will also increase the attending accommodative-convergence so that the convergence will tend to overfix the mark. Single vision may be attained by the use of negative fusional convergence, which may balance or compensate for the excess accommodative-convergence, but dissociation will neutralize the fusional convergence and permit the eyes to assume the esophoric position.

(1) Such impairment may be due to age (presbyopia), paralysis, ciliary involvements, or toxic effects. If due to lack of training in the use of accommodation, such as is found in high errors of refraction, the amplitude may be built up and will reduce the esophoria which is based upon the accommodative-convergence ratio; but if due to an actual impairment of the mechanism, the only method of reduction of the nearpoint esophoria is by means of a bifocal which reduces the total accommodative innervation.

(2) Near-point esophoria in myopic children, due to fuller minus correction, was usually reduced or eliminated with constant wear of the minus (Flom and Takahashi, 1962).

3. *With Esophoria at Near and a Normal Amplitude of Accommodation*

a. While no ready explanation other than a possible abnormal ACA ratio is offered for an esophoria at near which is not due to a low amplitude of accommodation or to toxicity, the correction is similar to that employed for cases of low amplitude. A bifocal which reduces the total accommodative effort may also reduce the esophoria. A survey of the graphic analysis of such a case will show a correction midway between the P.R.A. and N.R.A. findings which would tend to balance the blur point prism findings and should compensate for the phoria.

(1) This add may also be determined by adding the two findings and dividing the sum by two.

D. Esophoria at Far

1. *With Esophoria at Near and Hypertonic Accommodation*

a. Morgan (1954) stated that if the distant phoria was less than the near one, corrective prism can be worn; but if more than the near one, prism would create problems by reversing the fusional needs at near.

b. An esophoria at far may be due to latent and uncorrected hyperopia, particularly if the ACA ratio is normal or high. Such cases usually also reveal either an esophoria at near or a very low exophoria at near. If the ACA ratio is low, the excess accommodation cannot produce an esophoria at near. These premises are illustrated in Figure XXI-12.

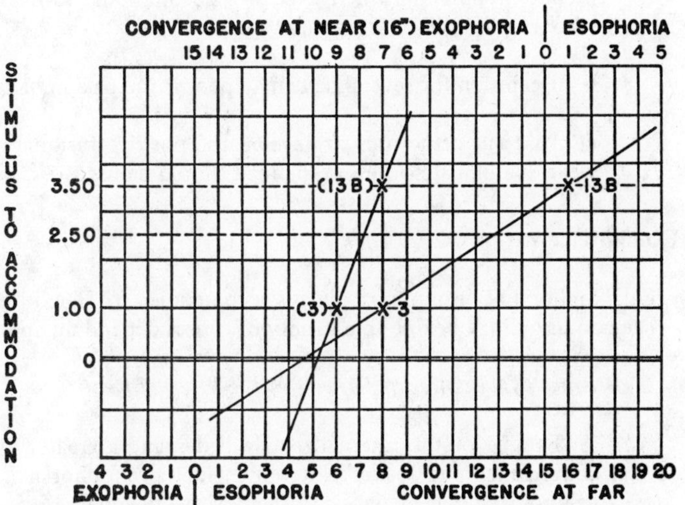

Figure XXI-12 – Effects upon near phoria of ACA ratio in uncorrected or latent hyperopia. *(3)* distant phoria in low ACA ratio; line *(3), (13B)* slope of ACA in low ratio; *3* distant phoria in high ACA ratio; *13B*, near phoria in high ACA ratio; line *3, 13B* slope of ACA in high ratio. Note: Findings are shown at actual level of accommodative stimulation which prevails when hyperope of 1.00 D is uncorrected.

c. Attempts to alter the phoria or to build up base-in prism reserve by orthoptics are not ordinarily successful in such cases. The best correction is to determine the existence of the latency and supply extra plus power. Where this plus cannot be accepted for distance because of blurring the vision, a bifocal will assist at the nearpoint. Upon occasion, prism base-out, which relieves the fusional divergence effort, may provide comfort if the accommodative effort which is being used is not a source of discomfort in itself.

(1) If the esophoria at far did not reduce the base-in reserve at far, it was probably due to the accommodative effort and needed plus lenses (Kratz, 1959). Base-out prism would not be accepted.

2. *With Esophoria at Near not Associated with Excess Accommodation*

a. Where the ACA ratio shows that the esophoria at far and near is not due to hypertonic accommodation, the esophoria may be anatomic or neurologic. Usually the esophoria is manifested at both near and far.

b. Orthoptics designed to alter the phoria is ineffective. The negative fusional convergence may be increased by training to reach a reserve limit commensurate with the criteria of comfort. If myopia accompanies the esophoria, care must be taken not to increase the esophoria at near with full myopic correction, although as noted earlier, Flom and Takahishi found that the esophoria reduced to its original amount after the minus correction had been worn a while.

3. *Esophoria at Far With High Exophoria at Near*

a. This is basically an exophoric problem. The high nearpoint exophoria requires an excessive use of positive fusional convergence to achieve nearpoint single vision. If the eyes are in use for prolonged periods at the nearpoint, the residual contraction of the muscles and the constant supply of positive fusional innervation persist to the farpoint because the momentary dissociation of the test is insufficient to exhibit full relaxation of the fusional effort. Consequently an esophoria is revealed at the distance, comparable to the pseudo-myopia, at which excessive accommodative effort might develop in the hyperope who was engaged in severe near work.

b. Occlusion for several days may permit the true imbalance to be exhibited at far.

c. Base-out orthoptics to develop the positive fusional convergence or base-in for constant wear to eliminate or lessen the load should be used.

E. Exophoria at Far

1. Exophoria at far is almost always accompanied by an exhibition of exophoria at the nearpoint. The condition may be due to a variety of causes depending upon other indications.

2. *Because of Weakness or Fatigue of the Internal Recti*

a. Fatigue of the internal recti will demand a greater innervation for the same amount of convergence end result. Not only will the exophoria at far and near be revealed, but the nearpoint of convergence and the positive fusional reserve will be deficient.

b. A lower ACA ratio will be exhibited than actually exists because the convergence response will be deficient in comparison to the accommodative response for the same innervation. However, the fusional reserve may be deficient because of excessive dependence upon the fusional convergence due to less accommodative-convergence.

c. Occlusion will rest the fusional convergence with an exhibited restoration of the fusional reserve and perhaps a decrease of the exophoria at far.

(1) Since the exophoria at far may not be due to fatigued internal recti, the exophoria may also increase at far after occlusion due to dissociation.

d. The fatigue should increase with use of the internal recti so that the symptoms should be more severe and the deficiencies greater if the eyes are retested at different periods of the day. Systemic disorders may be the cause of the condition.

3. *Because of the ACA Ratio*

a. If the ACA ratio is high, it is unlikely that the exophoria at near will be high. However, if the ACA ratio is high or even normal and an exophoria at far is the disturbing factor, it may be possible to assist the imbalance at far, if orthoptics or prism are not feasible, by altering the stimulation to accommodation. Additional minus will induce excess accommodation which will add to the accommodative-convergence and assist the fusional convergence. Such over-correction is only practical if no pseudomyopia or latent hyperopia is prevalent and if the amplitude is sufficiently high to bear the burden.

b. If the ACA ratio is low, the exophoria at near will be large in amount. If the fusional reserve is adequate, no difficulty may be experienced, but if it is inadequate, either base-out treatment for the fusional reserve or base-in prescription to relieve the load is indicated. Changes in the refractive sphere will not assist the convergence to any great extent.

4. *With an Undeveloped Accommodation*

a. If accommodation is not used, as in high ametropias, little accommodative-convergence will be employed. Such cases will depend entirely or mainly upon fusional convergence and will exhibit very large exophorias at near. The major corrective procedure is that of correcting the ametropia and teaching the patient the use of accommodation. When that has been accomplished, the matter of lateral imbalance may present itself in an entirely different aspect.

5. *In Presbyopia*

a. In advanced senility, no effort is made to accommodate. Consequently, no accommodative-convergence is supplied and the burden rests essentially with the fusional convergence. A large exophoria is revealed. The patient may be taught to use the convergence by base-out visual training or prism base-in may be prescribed in the bifocal segment.

(1) As presbyopia develops, excessive accommodative innervation may be supplied to gain a focus and the accommodative-convergence may increase resulting in a decreased exophoria at near without the reading add. When the add is applied, the accommodative effort is decreased sharply and the accommodative-convergence is reduced accordingly so that the exophoria tends to appear to increase. Since with the application of the add, the fusional convergence must carry the major burden, it may be necessary to develop the fusional reserve by base-out visual training. This procedure is frequently known as *bifocal reconditioning.*

(2) To determine whether elderly people require prism, Wick (1960) recommended that prisms of 6 to 8 pd be introduced with the base in various directions before the eyes while the patient observed a nearpoint target. If the patient continued with single vision, no prism was needed. But if the targets separated and drifted apart, a need may be considered. Lesser amounts of prism could be next tried until the limiting amount was determined.

VIII. DETERMINATION OF THE LATERAL PRISM

A. The chief criteria for determining the amount of lateral prism are those of Percival and Sheard.

B. Percival's premise for lateral prism has been noted earlier. It is the prism which just allows his criteria to be fulfilled.

1. The Negative Fusional Reserve (N.F.R.) and the Positive Fusional Reserve (P.F.R.) added together comprise the Total Fusional Reserve (T.F.R.).

a. The results can be attained by the following three different formulae:

(1) *For exophoria*

(a) PFR –1/3 TFR

[1] A negative answer indicates prism base-in; a positive answer indicates no prism.

(b) NFR –2/3 TFR

[1] A positive answer indicates prism base-in; a negative answer indicates no prism needed.

(c) 1/3 the larger (either PFR or NFR) –2/3 the lesser (either the PFR or NFR)

[1] A positive answer indicates prism base-in; a negative, no prism.

(2) *For esophoria*

(a) NFR –1/3 TFR

[1] A negative answer indicates prism base-out; a positive answer indicates no prism.

(b) PFR –2/3 TFR

[1] A positive answer indicates prism base-out; a negative, no prism.

(c) 1/3 the larger (PFR or NFR) –2/3 the lesser (PFR or NFR)

[1] A positive answer indicates prism base-out; a negative, no prism.

2. Examples:

a. *Exophoria:* NFR equals 12 and PFR equals 18

(1) PFR – 1/3 TFR = 18 – 1/3 (30) = 8, no prism

(2) NFR –2/3 TFR = 12 –2/3 (30) = –8, no prism

(3) 1/3 PFR –2/3 NFR = 1/3 (18) –2/3 (12) = –2, no prism

b. *Esophoria:* NFR equals 3, PFR equals 12

(1) NFR + 1/3 TFR = –3 + 1/3 (15) = 2 prism base-out

(2) PFR –2/3 TFR = 12 – 2/3 (15) = 2 prism base-out

(3) 1/3 PFR –2/3 NFR = 1/3 (12) – 2/3 (3) = 2 prism base-out

C. Sheard's criteria for prism correction may be expressed as: the required fusional vergence overcoming the demand must be twice the demand, or the formula is written as follows:

1. *2/3 the phoria – 1/3 the compensating fusional reserve* = the prism needed

a. The compensating fusional reserve is base-out duction to blur for exophoria and base-in duction to blur for esophoria.

b. If the answer is plus, prism is needed; if minus, no prism is needed.

2. Examples:

a. 9 Δ exophoria, 12 Δ for No. 16A
2/3 (9) –1/3 (12) = +2.0 pd of base-in needed for exophoria.

b. 3 Δ esophoria, 8 Δ for No. 17A
2/3 (3) –1/3 (8) = – 1-1/3, no prism needed

3. Allen (1960) expressed the Sheard criteria in the formula: $\frac{\text{phoria x 2} - \text{compensating duction}}{3}$

D. Sheard and Percival Rule applied to Lens Change

1. If the ACA ratio permits, an attempt to alleviate the discrepancy may be attempted by altering the convergence through the accommodative-convergence by changing the stimulus to accommodation.

a. *Graphical Method*

(1) After the prism correction is determined, it is equivalent to a change in convergence demand at that distance.

(a) Base in prism moves the demand point to the right of the original position and base out moves it to the left.

(2) A line is drawn through this new demand point parallel to the true slope of the zone.

(3) A vertical line is drawn from the original demand point to this new line.

(4) The point of intersection is extended horizontally to the stimulus to accommodation ordinate at the left of the graph.

(5) The difference between the dioptric value of this horizontal line and the initial accommodative level stimulus line is the spherical power needed, being minus if above the original stimulus line and plus if below it.

b. *Formula method*

(1) In the following equations P equals the prism change needed according to Sheard's method, G equals the ACA ratio or gradient, and S equals the change in power of the lens.

(a) $S = \frac{P}{G}$ Since P is determined by 2/3 phoria –1/3 Compensating Duction,

(b) then, $S = \frac{\text{2/3 phoria} - \text{1/3 Comp. Duction}}{G}$

(c) If Comp. Duction was base-out, use plus; if base-in, use minus.

(2) The above formula may be applied to Percival's method, although subject upon occasion to large lens differences beyond practical considerations.

(a) By Percival's criterion, P = 1/3 greater duction –2/3 lesser duction

(b) Then, $S = \frac{\text{1/3 greater duction} - \text{2/3 lesser duction.}}{G}$

(c) The signs agree, as in Sheard's calculation above, with the needed prism base.

E. Maxwell regarded 16 pd as the normal value for the base-out to break finding and used the break to determine a prismatic Rx for exophoria, as follows:

1. Rx for exophoria at near = 1/5 (16 pd minus base-out to break)

F. Maddox offered the following rule for distance:

1. Rx for exophoria at far = 1/2 exophoria.

G. **Thorington** offered the following rule for presbyopes:

1. Rx for exophoria at near = exophoria – 10 pd

H. **Turville** (Lindsay, 1949)

1. Where exophoria is manifested on the infinity balance chart and the two charts approach each other or fuse, the amount of prism which restores the charts to the relatively normal position in regard to each other is found to be wearable. In esophoria, the patient's descriptions of what he sees are usually too unreliable, although the use of polaroid and two chart sections, or a septum mirror and two chart sections, with the uppers reversed in esophoria, may help to determine as accuarte results.

I. **Marton** (1952)

1. Marton charted perceptual scotomas, or areal suppressions with fine test objects on the perimeter or tangent screen. The amount of lateral prism which removed the suppression area was maintained to be prescribable.

J. **Giles** (1965)

1. Giles comments that Landolt desired 2/3 of the range in reserve for comfort. Giles agrees with Landolt's 2/3 for the PFR but believes only 1/3 of the NFR is sufficient. He gives the following specific rules:

a. Correct 1/3 of the distance exophoria and 1/4 of the near exophoria.

b. Use 1/2 of the distant esophoria but seldom correct the near esophoria.

(1) Use ½ the amount of extra plus needed to restore a normal near exo for non-presbyopes and more add for presbyopes.

c. Correct the full exo for distance in myopia.

d. For myopia and esophoria, prescribe on the basis of 1/3 the distance Negative Fusional Reserve.

K. The author has mentioned the use of a subjective determinant for the prescription of vertical prism and has used the same basis for prescribing prism laterally, particularly at the farpoint.

L. **Allen** (1960)

1. Allen gives the following additional rules:

a. If the patient has considerable exophoria at far and near, base-in for near is satisfactory; if considerable esophoria at far and near, base-out wear is satisfactory.

b. If the patient is nearly orthophoric at far with considerable exophoria or esophoria at near, a special near Rx with prism is indicated or a special add for near may be determined by the following proportions:

(1) $$\frac{\text{Prism Needed}}{\text{ACA Ratio}} \quad \text{or} \quad \frac{\text{Prism Needed x 2.5}}{\text{phoria at 40 cm.} - \text{phoria at 6 m} + 15}$$

(a) Esophoria is written as positive and exophoria as a negative value.

c. Since the fusional reserve is measured by the blur point, it must be measured carefully using fine type.

M. Summary

1. Of the above rules, the Sheard criterion is most widely employed.

a. Allen emphasizes that the Sheard criterion is only a guide but indicates a safe amount of prism if not in excess of 3 PD for each eye.

2. Certain principles do seem to be in agreement in regard to the correction of exophoria.

a. Orthoptics to develop the fusional reserve seem satisfactory to non-presbyopes with the exceptions previously noted.

b. The extent of the hyperopic state is usually under-corrected, when prism base-in is prescribed.

3. If the exophoria varies from far to near, but is larger at near than at far, the prismatic correction for far will usually prove satisfactory for near also.

4. If the exophoria at far is greater than that at near, and the distant correction is not satisfactory for near, separate amounts of prism for both near and far may be needed in separates Rx's. Likewise, if the exophoria is evident only at near, prism in a separate Rx or in the segment of a bifocal only may be used.

5. A mechanical limit based upon weight, appearance and the distortion produced by prisms is found in the prescription of prisms. Usually this limit is set at 6 pd for each eye, although some state it at 4 pd and others as high as 10 pd for each eye. (Note: See Emmes report above, however.)

6. Neill (1963) pointed out that contact lenses in young people reduced esophoria in hyperopes due to lowered accommodative demand and reduced exophoria in myopes due to increased accommodative demand.

7. Morgan and Allen both mentioned that anti-reflection coatings helped the wearing of prisms.

8. Base-in prisms make red objects appear nearer than blue, while base-out creates the reverse effect due to chrome stereopsis. The wearer should be cautioned to be careful at night when other clues are absent (Allen, 1960).

9. If one eye was higher than the other (hyper-eye) and fixation was at 15 inches, a 2 mm. discrepancy would require an added compensatory rotation of 0.3°, equivalent in prism to: dioptric power of the spectacles at 14 mms. from the eye x 0.13 (Glazer, 1955).

N. The effects of long wear

1. Carter (1963) reported an adaptation effect after long wear of prisms in which the patient often exhibited the same phoria and fixation disparity that was measured prior to the wearing of the prism. Ogle and Prangen (1953) and Ellerbrock and Fry (1941) reported this in vertical discrepancies, and Carter found it also for lateral ones, both base-in and base-out.

a. Carter predicated a shift in the near heterophoria as a change due to a shift in proximal convergence. The newly corrected myope showed esophoria because he was used to using excess fusional convergence and now added accommodative-convergence. Later the patient learned to readapt and revealed exophoria again. Similarly, the newly corrected presbyope showed exophoria at first because the add relaxed the excessive accommodative-convergence which he was accustomed to using. The adaptation for distance and changes for near were proximal changes, reflex in character, induced by fusional convergence as a conditioned reflex, more effective for far and for exo rather than eso, and usually presented in the absence of asthenopia.

(1) Individuals lacking this adaptation phenomena will obtain comfort from prism which reduces the fusional demand. Those who have it will reveal after wearing prism the same phoria as before.

(2) Presence of asthenopia with the phoria usually indicates a lack of this adaptive process and prism should be prescribed.

b. Carter (1963) found no special problems with patients who have worn prism for years. Small changes from time to time were likely to be found but were not due to the prism. If the adaptation phenomena showed up, prism should not have been increased to compensate for it.

(1) 2 PD in any direction appears the limit before some spatial distortion is present.

(2) More relief is gained from vertical prism than from base-out, and the least relief is gained from base-in.

(a) This does not seem consistent with the fact that most clinicians report that base-in prism is more acceptably worn than base-out.

(3) Plondre and Howell (1965) reported the results obtained from the prescription of lateral prisms for both esophoria and exophoria. Relief from headaches and neck tension was most predominant.

(a) Patients noticed the ground slanting downward with prism base-out and upwards with prism base-in.

(b) A "pulling" sensation is noted as the muscles relax.

(c) A phoria was found upon follow-up examinations. This was ascribed to further relaxation of the muscles, but Carter's explanation (See above) is called to the reader's attention.

(d) 1/3 to 1/2 the amount of the phoria was used for determining the amount of correction prism.

(e) Roy (1956-1958) reported some beneficial results of vertical prism prescribed for a wide variety of asthenopic symptoms, particularly neck tension, brow and forehead tension, headaches, and even migraines.

IX. SYNDROMES

A. The earliest and still classical classifications of function upon which diagnostic import is laid is the Duane-White classification of convergence and divergence malfunction. Although derived from and still applied to strabismus conditions rather than phoria problems and implying in its application that the older concept of phorias as latent strabismus is essentially predominant, the original syndromes have been modified by Tait who applied them to the more recent concepts of the accommodative-convergence relationships (Tait, 1951).

1. *The Duane-White Syndromes are as follows:*

a. *Convergence Insufficiency*

(1) Slight exophoria at far

(2) Marked exophoria at near

(3) The Pc of Convergence 3 or more inches removed

(4) May be accommodative or non-accommodative in origin and may be secondary to divergence excess

(5) Tait comments that this condition is merely one exhibiting a deficient ACA ratio.

b. *Convergence Excess*

(1) Orthophoria or moderate esophoria at far

(2) Esophoria at near

(3) If due to accommodative excess, may be an undercorrected hyperope, an overcorrected myope, or a beginning presbyope

(4) May not be due to accommodative excess and may be complicated by divergence deficiency

(5) Tait considers this type a definitely excessive ACA ratio.

c. *Divergence Insufficiency*

(1) Primary

(a) Esophoria at far up to 8 Δ

(b) Esophoria at near

[1] A normal ACA according to Tait.

(2) Secondary

(a) over 8 Δ esophoria at far

(b) a higher esophoria at near

[1] Excessive ACA ratio

(3) May be secondary to convergence excess

d. *Divergence Excess*

(1) Marked exophoria at far

(2) Equal or less exophoria at near

(a) If the Pc of Convergence is normal, it is a primary type.

(b) If the Pc of Convergence is deficient, it is a secondary type.

(3) Depending on the amplitude of fusional convergence, this may be an excess ACA ratio.

B. Kratz (1954) commented that varied ophthalmological opinion was found as to just what constituted convergence excess, insufficiency or divergence excess, or insufficiency. The tonic position of convergence at far (orthophoria, esophoria, or exophoria) was the starting point and combines, as indicated by Tait, with either a supernormal, subnormal or normal convergence function for the new finding.

1. Kratz considered the various categories as merely expressions of the position of the Neumueller zone according to accommodative effort.

a. The zone can move to the left at infinity with normal relative convergence at near, or if tonic convergence insufficiency exists, the tonic position at far is exophoria.

b. The zone can move to the left at near with the far normal, exhibiting a functional convergence insufficiency with a low near point of convergence.

c. All fusional findings may be low exhibiting a narrowing of the zone.

C. The classification is not a satisfactory one except from a surgical standpoint. It postulates a totally separate divergence and convergence function, which has not as yet been confirmed, and draws up differentiating classifications by ignoring the ACA relationship. Based on the import of the graphical systems, particularly the work begun by Sheard, the later attempts at analysis of the function of convergence are in greater conformity with the view expressed by Scobee that esophoria and exophoria are merely different manifestations affecting the same function.

1. Michaels (1953) commented on convergence insufficiency:

a. If it exists as a clinical entity, no clear cut standard techniques for diagnosing convergence insufficiency are described.

(1) The best indication is the nearpoint of convergence with adduction findings as auxiliaries.

b. No clear cut relation is established between the nearpoint of convergence and the phoria at far, and that with the phoria at near is insignificant.

c. Three different methods of diagnosis based on the nearpoint of convergence, the phorias and the adduction findings are not comparable and do not give similar results.

d. The correlation between the nearpoint of convergence and the adductor in all groups is of equal extent but not high enough to select all cases of remote near point of convergence or inadequate adductor findings.

e. No significant signs, symptoms, or significant relations to comfort or acuity are given.

f. Michaels doubts that a condition of lowered convergence ability may even exist.

X. TABLES OF EXPECTEDS

A. Non-graphical methods of analysis have chiefly been based upon comparisons of individual test results to "norms" or "expecteds." These methods grew from the realization that the consideration of the individual findings as special entities to be corrected each by itself had proved unfruitful and that, as implied in the graphical considerations, the various tests were merely symptoms of a basic condition for which syndromes might be derived.

B. Optometric Extension Program

1. One of the more widely exploited systems has been that formulated by the Optometric Extension Program, a graduate educational organization of optometrists. The system of analysis originally derived from the outline of procedure delineated by Sheard, and to a great extent upon the original Sheard graphical analysis applied in syndrome form. However, while the original tenets were simply performed and developed, the system has now digressed markedly from the elementary principles which help form the cohesive tenets of the entire development of both graphical and syndrome analysis as standardly employed and understood.

a. The *basic premises* might be summarized by stating the following:

(1) Accommodation and convergence functions are interrelated through their association.

(2) A zone of play between functions exists (probably indicative of relative convergence) which permits some extension of one without influencing the other.

(3) Discomfort is produced by unequal extensions of one function in comparison to the other which reduces this zone of play and by association is reflected in the performance of the non-extended function.

(4) By comparison to a table of expecteds, the fluctuations of each function may be noted to be in accord with the function at fault, so that if certain findings are low, the others are automatically higher.

(5) Certain key findings may be grouped together into syndromes which have characteristic appearances.

2. Certain expecteds have been accepted as standards, together with certain findings for which no expecteds are offered but which are classified according to an assumption that there should be 2.50 D. of accommodation associated with 15 pd of convergence in non-presbyopic subjects.

3. The cause and effect of ocular abnormality is heavily oriented towards the influences of environmental factors as the sole or overwhelmingly major contribution towards the resultant status. While no clear cut data rule out the value of environmental factors (see Chapter I), neither are there sufficient acceptable data which substantiate the concept promulgated to the total or nearly total exclusion of hereditary, anatomical, and purely chance influences. Since classical definitions and many basic premises of physiological optics are often either totally re-defined or completely ignored, the explanation of the conceptual background of the method would require almost a complete text in itself, an obvious impossibility in this work. The interested reader is referred to the several available texts which are totally devoted to the subject.

4. Besides, the system has an ingrained potentiality for complexity in that, as Hebbard (1952) noted, a system which employs ironclad standards for determination of tests *inherently variable by method* is forced to classify each patient if any test does not meet the standard. This in turn leads to an increasing category of classifications, as has happened in the program under consideration.

5. Michaels (1955 and 1956) analyzed the approach in great detail. The potential of doubt, expressed above, in considering a fixed, rigid set of norms as a diagnostic method was indicated in the following single example from this work.

a. If a diagnosis depends upon comparison of a phoria to the fusional reserve, a statistical norm (rather than a rigidly arbitrary one) is needed to help decide if the problem is a high exophoria or a low fusional reserve.

b. Haines's data, recalculated by Michaels for the Optometric Extention Program tests No. 10 (the Adduction at Far) and No. 11 (Abduction at Far) give the following results:

(1) **TABLE XXI-2**

Test	Mean	Ave. Deviation	S.D.	N
No. 10	*22.26Δ*	*± 6.11Δ*	*7.63*	*443*
No. 11	*9.24Δ*	*± 1.46Δ*	*1.82*	*443*

c. Test No. 10 is low if less than 22.26 PD by 1 PD according to the OEP. Converted to a Z score, *such a deviation would occur by chance* approximately 45% of the time.

(1) If part of the symptom of a B-type case equals 11 – 16B and of a C-type case, 10 – 16B, then if the plus power were cut because the low No. 10 made a C-type case of the data, the examiner could be wrong, by chance, almost as often as he was right.

d. To be considered statistically significant, the No. 11 finding would have to deviate ±15 PD for a 5% level of confidence or ±19.5 PD for a 1% level of confidence.

C. A large number of investigators have published data dealing with the normals or expecteds for the various tests. Working with statistical methods, they have attempted to establish findings which would include a statistically approved number of cases and have determined standard deviations of the results. A typical distribution of the phorias and ACA relationship is indicated in Figure XXI-13 and XXI-14, as found by Tait (1951). Scobee and Green (1951) found that 95% of a group between the ages of 17½ and 30 revealed phorias at far of from 4 esophoria to 4 exophoria, and the same limits included the same percentage of a similar group aged 18 to 35 in a later study. Different test methods also revealed different results as has been noted, and thus Scobee and Green reported that at 40 cms., the mean for a Von Graefe test was 3 Δ with a standard deviation of ±5.2 Δ, while with the screened Maddox rod, the mean was 5.9 Δ with a S.D. of ±5.8 Δ. Haines (1938, 1941) established certain minimums in a lengthy comprehensive study (see Table XXI-3), and Shepard (Haines, 1938, 1941) likewise determined standards and attempted to establish a basis for judging the accuracy of the findings and procedures themselves. Hirsch (1948) also found a median finding of 3 to 4Δ for the Von Graefe at near, confirming Scobee and Green's findings. Emmes (1949) found the gradient to be 3 with a ±1.64 S.D.

D. Morgan's system

1. Morgan (1944b) compared the expecteds of different investigators and found that, on the whole, and considering the difference in technique and groups included, the similarities were marked. He evolved a table from all these which considered the grouping of the whole around the mean and which considered the number of subjects included within the standard deviation.

2. Morgan listed the tests, the means, and the standard deviation in Table XXI-4.

a. The various means and S.D. included at least 58% of the subjects for the lowest range (Negative Relative Convergence) to 87% for the highest range (the Binocular Cross Cylinder).

3. It can be seen from the above that while it is possible for a subject to vary from any one

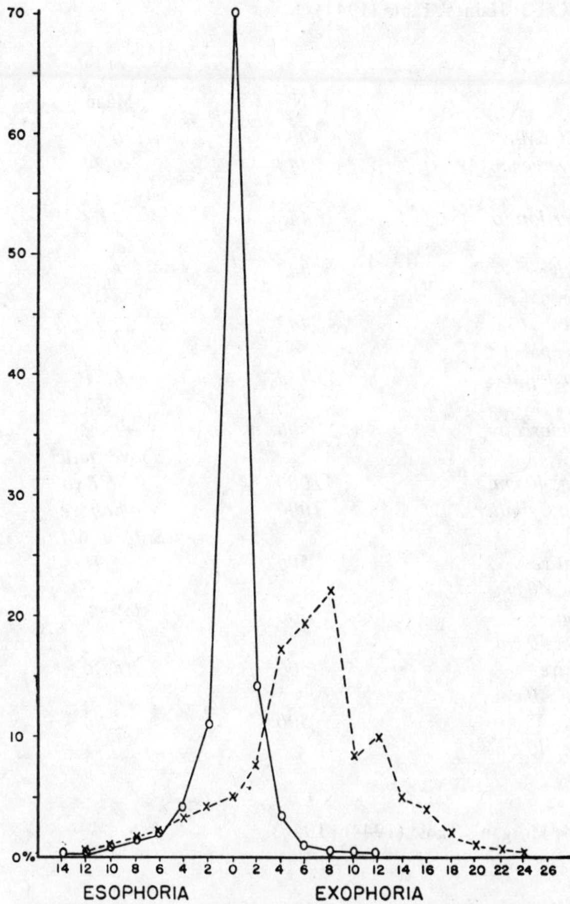

Figure XXI-13 – Percentage Distribution of Heterophoria in 4,880 Ocularly Comfortable Subjects (Tait). Solid line represents phoria test at distance; dotted line represents phoria test at near-point (13 inches).

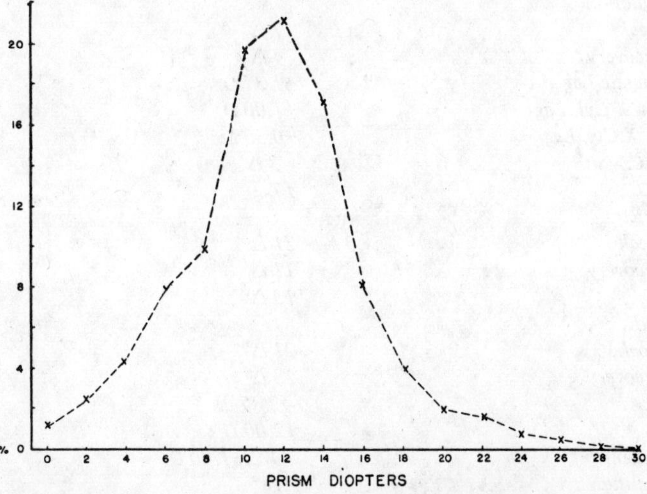

Figure XXI-14 – Percentage Distribution of Accommodative Convergence in 4,793 Ocularly Comfortable Patients (Tait).

TABLE XXI-3: Haines' Table (1941)

Tests	N	Mean	Mean Dev
Lateral Phoria, 6M	*1000*	*0*	*±1.00*
Negative Convergence 6M	*443*	*9.24*	*±1.46*
Negative Reversion to Fusion, 6M	*443*	*4.63*	*±1.42*
Positive Relative Convergence, 6M	*443*	*8.71*	*±2.13*
Positive Total Convergence, 6M	*443*	*22.26*	*±6.11*
Positive Reversion to Fusion, 6M	*443*	*6.31*	*±2.86*
Dynamic Retinoscopy, 40 cm.	*900*	*+1.02 above static*	*±0.41*
Lateral phoria, 40 cm.	*1000*	*4.85 Exo*	*±3.25*
Fused Crossed Cylinder, 40 cm.	*1000*	*+.44 above Subj. at 6M.*	*±0.43*
Negative Relative Convergence, 40 cm.	*500*	*14.91*	*±3.22*
Negative Total Convergence, 40 cm.	*500*	*22.44*	*±2.84*
Positive Relative Convergence, 40 cm.	*500*	*16.30*	*±2.94*
Positive Total Convergence, 40 cm.	*500*	*22.86*	*±5.41*

TABLE XXI-4: Morgan's Table (1944b; 1946)

Test	Mean	S.D.
Phoria	*1 Δ Exo*	*±2 Δ*
Adduction		
Blur	*9 Δ*	*±4 Δ*
Break	*19 Δ*	*±8 Δ*
Recovery	*10 Δ*	*±4 Δ*
Abduction		
Break	*7 Δ*	*±3 Δ*
Recovery	*4 Δ*	*±2 Δ*
Dynamic Lag	*+1.37 D.*	*±0.37 D.*
Mon. X Cyl. Lag	*+1.00 D.*	*±0.50 D.*
Bin. X Cyl. Lag	*+0.50 D.*	*±0.50 D.*
F.S.C.	*−3 Δ*	*±5 Δ*
P.R.C.	*17 Δ*	*±5 Δ*
P.F.R.		
Break	*21 Δ*	*±6 Δ*
Recovery	*11 Δ*	*±7 Δ*
N.R.C.	*13 Δ*	*±4 Δ*
N.F.R.		
Break	*21 Δ*	*±4 Δ*
Recovery	*13 Δ*	*±5 Δ*
P.R.A.	*−2.37 Δ*	*±1.12 D.*
N.R.A.	*+2.00 D.*	*±0.50 D.*
Gradient	*−4 Δ/+1.00 D.*	*±2 Δ*
Amplitude	*Age**	*±2.00 D.*

** Amplitude from Donders' or Duane's tables.*

finding without great significance, the percentages of inclusion are sufficiently high so that the departure of the findings from the normal range of all the tests would be very significant and even departure from a large proportion of tests would be worthy of consideration.

4. The concept that the tests might vary together depends upon verification by calculation of a *coefficient of correlation* between the tests.

a. A perfectly positive correlation of +1 would indicate that the tests were influenced by the same factors in the same manner. A perfectly negative correlation of –1 would indicate that they were influenced by the same factors in exactly the opposite manner. The predictability of the results of one test based upon another is expressed by the square of the coefficient. If the correlation between the two tests were ±0.7, then the predictability would be $(0.7)^2 = 0.49$, or about half. That is, a prediction of the results of one test based upon the results of another would be correct about half the time. *It is obvious that a correlation coefficient of at least .71 is required to exceed the laws of chance.* A correlation coefficient of +0.8 equals a 64% likelihood. As the number of patients involved in the study increases, a +0.8 is considered good.

b. Morgan (1944; 1946) found the following table of coefficients between the various tests and data of the ordinary clinical routine:

TABLE XXI-5

	5	*14B*	*14A*	*13B*	*16A*	*17A*	*16B br*	*16B rec*	*17B br*	*17B rec*	*20*	*21*	*Gr*	*Age*
14B	*+.7*													
14A	*+.6*	*+.8*												
13B	*0*	*0*	*–.3*											
16A	*+.4*	*+.3*	*+.3*	*+.2*										
17A	*0*	*0*	*0*	*0*	*0*									
16B br	*0*	*0*	*0*	*0*	*+.7*	–								
16B rec	–	–	–	–	–	–	*+.5*							
17B br	*0*	*0*	*0*	*0*	*0*	*+.5*	*0*	*0*						
17B rec	–	–	–	–	–	–	*0*	–	*+.6*					
20	*–.5*	*–.3*	*–.4*	–	*0*	*+.5*	*0*	–	*+.3*	–				
21	*+.5*	*+.4*	*+.4*	*0*	*+.5*	*0*	*+.4*	–	*0*	–	*–.5*			
Gradient	*0*	*0*	*0*	*0*	*0*	*0*	*0*	–	*0*	–	*0*	*0*		
Age	*+.4*	*+.5*	*+.4*	*+.2*	*0*	*0*	*0*	–	*0*	–	*–.7*	*+.4*	*0*	
Amp Acc.	*–.5*	*–.6*	*–.6*	*–.3*	*0*	*0*	*0*	–	*0*	–	*+.8*	*–.4*	*0*	*–.8*

(1) – denotes correlation of less than 0.2.

c. Table XXI-6 gives the rank of correlation of any two tests in order from the highest to the lowest (Morgan, 1948, 1964).

d. A study of the correlations indicates quite readily that only a few tests have a coefficient so high that any prediction can be made of one of them from the behavior of the others. Also it is significant that the correlation between the gradient, expressive of the accommodative-convergence relationship, and all other tests is 0, except when the near phoria is used in its determination. This indicates that any calculation based upon the influence of the relation of accommodation and convergence in the tests compared is a purely empirical calculation which is not based upon the implications of the relationship. The comparison of the dynamic skiametry to a lag of accommodation based on the phoria, or of the cross cylinder findings to phoria determined lags, is dependent upon an assumption, based upon the accommodative-convergence relationship, which the above correlations do not verify.

(1) The gradient is reliable but not exactly valid because less than 1.00 D. of accommodation is revealed, while the subject actually uses less than 2.50 D. of accommodation for 16 inches. Convergence is therefore not altered in respect to 1.00 D. of actual accommodative change.

TABLE XXI-6

Coefficient of Correlation	Square of Coefficient	Tests
+0.8	*64*	*Bin. X Cyl. and Mon. X Cyl.*
+0.8	*64*	*P.R.A. and Amplitude*
−0.8	*64*	*Age and Amplitude*
+.07	*49*	*Mon. X Cyl. and Dynamic*
+0.7	*49*	*P.R.C. and P.F.C. (break)*
−0.7	*49*	*Age and P.R.A.*
+0.6	*36*	*Bin. X Cyl. and Dynamic*
+0.6	*36*	*N.F.R. break and recovery*
−0.6	*36*	*Mon. X Cyl. and Amplitude*
+0.5	*25*	*N.R.A. and Dynamic*
+0.5	*25*	*Mon. X Cyl. and Age*
+0.5	*25*	*N.R.A. and P.R.C.*
+0.5	*25*	*N.R.C. and N.F.R. (break)*
+0.5	*25*	*P.R.A. and N.R.C.*
+0.5	*25*	*P.F.R. break and recovery*
−0.5	*25*	*P.R.A. and Dynamic*
−0.5	*25*	*Amplitude and Dynamic*
−0.5	*25*	*N.R.A. and P.R.A.*
+0.4	*16*	*P.R.C. and Dynamic*
+0.4	*16*	*Age and Dynamic*
+0.4	*16*	*N.R.A. and Mon. X Cyl.*
+0.4	*16*	*N.R.A. and Bin. X Cyl.*
+0.4	*16*	*P.F.R. (break) and N.R.A.*
+0.4	*16*	*N.R.A. and Age*
−0.4	*16*	*P.R.A. and Bin. X Cyl.*
−0.4	*16*	*P.R.A. and Age*
+0.3	*9*	*P.R.C. and Mon. X Cyl.*
+0.3	*9*	*P.R.A. and M.F.R. break*
−0.3	*9*	*P.R.A. and Bin. X Cyl.*
−0.3	*9*	*F.S.C. and Bin. X Cyl.*
- 0.3	*9*	*F.S.C. and Amplitude*
+0.2	*4*	*F.S.C. and Age*
+0.2	*4*	*F.S.C. and P.R.C.*

(2) Manas (1952), in a series of similar correlations between the refractive finding and the various tests, also found results comparable to those Morgan reported. As indicated in Morgan's findings, the only reasonable correlation existed between the subjective and tests indicating added plus at near.

5. Because the coefficients of correlation for most tests are so low, it is possible to segregate the tests into groups which are related to each other by virtue of the direction in which they vary. By ignoring the degree of the relationship, it can be observed from the above table that certain tests tend to become higher together when other tests would tend to become lower together. No single test is offered which is reliable enough for diagnostic purposes, nor, due to the low coefficient, will each test vary in the expected manner in every case. However, if the group as a whole varies in a given direction, it may be assumed that the indication is sufficiently significant for diagnostic purposes even if some one test does not agree with the predicted variation.

a. The tests divided into the following three groups (Morgan 1944; 1946):

TABLE XXI-7

A	B	C
abduction	*adduction*	*phoria*
N.R.C.	*P.R.C.*	*F.S.C.*
N.F.R.	*P.F.R.*	*gradient*
P.R.A.	*Bin. Cross Cyl.*	
amplitude	*Mon. Cross Cyl.*	
	dynamic	
	N.R.A.	

b. Group A can be raised or increased by plus sphere, base-out prism, or visual training. Group B can be increased by minus sphere, base-in prism, or visual training. Which method is used in each will depend upon the values of Group C, the age of the patient, judgment, and the availability of the patient for training.

6. *Application of Morgan's calculations*

a. It is obvious that in accommodative fatigue cases, the tests in group B will tend to show higher findings than the normal. If the case is due to actual accommodative insufficiency, the amplitude will also be subnormal. If the potential accommodative ability is normal but accommodative fatigue exists, the amplitude will be normal, but the symptoms of accommodative distress will still be present. The analysis provides a means of determining the non-presbyopic individuals who are suffering from accommodative difficulties.

(1) In a similar manner, if the convergence is at fault, the tests of group A will tend to be higher than normal.

(2) Since no tests correlate with the gradient, no attempt is made to determine the status of any of the tests upon the basis of a calculation between a test of accommodative status and one of convergence status dependent upon the accommodative-convergence relationship. The entire basis of the determination of the "high" or "low" position of any test is determined by the simple comparison of the results of the test with the expecteds, which include the mean and the statistically acceptable range of standard deviation.

b. Because the number of individuals included is high enough for statistical significance, Morgan (1944, 1946) established a series of clinical norms which included consideration of their standard deviations.

(1) It will be noted that the norms for dynamic skiametry are given as an amount in excess of the subjective finding. This is in contrast to the accustomed method of presenting the dynamic finding in relation to the static retinoscopy finding. However, Morgan considered that the dynamic finding measured the relative accommodation and was subject to the same influences which affected other tests of relative accommodation. As an objective test of relative accommodation, it was more consistent to compare its results to the same standard to which other tests of the same function were compared, i.e., the subjective, than to the retinoscopy which might have little similarity to the subjective finding.

c. *The table of norms* recommended for clinical purposes can be combined with the trend classification of the tests to present the following condensed guide (Table XXI-8).

d. *Use of the Expecteds*

TABLE XXI-8 (Table of Norms)

Tests	Norms	Range	Group
No. 8 Phoria at far	*1 exo ± 1*	*ortho to 2 exo*	*(C)*
No. 9 Adduction	*9 ± 2*	*7 to 11*	*(B)*
No. 10 Convergence–break	*19 ± 4*	*15 to 23*	*(B)*
Convergence–recovery	*10 ± 2*	*8 to 12*	
No. 11 Abduction–break	*7 ± 2*	*5 to 9*	*(A)*
Abduction–recovery	*4 ± 1*	*3 to 5*	
No. 5 Dynamic Skiametry	*+1.37 ± 12*	*1.25 to 1.50*	*B*
No. 14A Mon. C.C.	*+1.00 ± 25*	*.75 to 1.25*	*B*
No. 14B Bin. C.C.	*+ .50 ± 25*	*.25 to .75*	*B*
No. 13B Phoria at near (Fus. Sup. Conv.)	*3 exo ± 3*	*ortho to 6 exo*	*(C)*
No. 16A Pos. Rel. Conv.	*17 ± 3, or no blur*	*14 to 20, or no blur*	*B*
No. 16B Pos. Fus. Res.–break	*21 ± 3*	*18 to 24*	*B*
Pos. Fus. Res.–recovery	*11 ± 4*	*7 to 15*	
No. 17A Neg. Rel. Conv	*13 ± 2, or no blur*	*11 to 15, or no blur*	*A*
No. 17B Neg. Fus. Res.–break	*21 ± 2*	*19 to 23*	*A*
Neg. Fus. Res.–recovery	*13 ± 3*	*10 to 16*	
No. 20 Pos. Rel. Acc	*–2.37 ± .62*	*–1.75 to –3.00*	*A*
No. 21 Neg. Rel. Acc	*+2.00 ± .25*	*+1.75 to +.225*	*B*
Gradient	*4 exo ± 1 above No. 13B*	*3 to 5 exo above No. 13*	*(C)*
No. 19 Amp. Accom.	*Age*	*±2.00 D.*	*A*

(1) It must be remembered that the norms for tests 5, 14A, 14B, 20 and 21 are values for lens power *above or in addition* to the subjective.

(2) The value for the gradient is the amount of exophoria found above the original nearpoint phoria value. If 13B is 6 pd of exophoria and the gradient test shows an exophoria of 10 pd, the gradient value is recorded as 4 pd, which is normal by the above table.

(3) While indications are given for classification of the farpoint tests, Morgan did not indicate these tests specifically in his groupings. The analysis can apparently be made from the nearpoint tests alone.

(4) The value stated for the dynamic skiametry is the value determined at the point known as high-neutral.

e. *Procedure*

(1) The tests are recorded in agreement with the instructions given above. The values are compared to the range of expecteds. Values exceeding the upper limits of the range are noted as *high,* while those below the lower limits are noted as *low.*

(a) The Adduction, Abduction, Positive Fusional Reserve and Negative Fusional Reserve tests, which include both a break and recovery value, are noted as single tests. If either of the components of the test, the break or the recovery, is abnormal, the test as a whole is noted as abnormal.

(2) When the findings have been noted as either high or low, the groups as a whole are indicated. If most of the A group is high, the entire classification is considered high. If most of the B group is low, the entire classification is so noted. If the tests within a group are at variance or not indicative, the classification is negative.

(a) If neither the A or B groups are predominantly high or low, the case is a simple refractive case without nearpoint problems.

(b) If the results show the classes to fall $\frac{A}{B}$, *convergence* difficulty is indicated.

[1] This fraction is used to indicate the A group as high and the B group as low.

(c) If the results show the classes to fall $\frac{B}{A}$, *accommodative* fatigue is indicated.

(3) The Gradient

(a) The gradient falls within neither class and is useful as an indication of the status of the accommodation-convergence relationship. If it is low, it obviously indicates little dependence upon accommodative-convergence; if high, great dependence upon it.

(b) The gradient can be used to divide either accommodative or convergence fatigue cases into three categories, each depending upon the status of the gradient. However, this subdivision is not so much indicative of the causes of the complaint as a guide to the methods of correction to be applied. This application is treated below.

(c) The accommodative-convergence can be calculated as follows: (See also Chapter VII.)

[1] The calculated gradient = P.D. in cms. – .4 (phoria – F.S.C.).

[a] F.S.C. is the fusional supplementary convergence (the near phoria).

[2] Accommodative-convergence = (P.D. in cms.) (2.5) – (phoria at far) + (F.S.C.)

f. *Correction*

(1) Accommodative Fatigue

(a) The obvious correction for accommodative fatigue is to reduce the burden of the accommodation. Since the A group can be raised by either the application of base-out prism, plus add, or visual training, the easiest solution is to prescribe a plus add for near which does not lower the B data significantly. The question of whether this additional power can also be accepted at far must be determined by the examiner upon the basis of the actual cause of the complaint, whether the patient will tolerate blurring of his vision at distance, and the personal factors connected with the correction, such as the amount of time it will be worn, the characteristics of the function to which the glasses are assigned by the wearer, and so forth. The examiner will have some indication of the excess power above the subjective for maximum acuity which still permits tolerable distant acuity. However, it may be necessary to provide separate corrections for both far and near or bifocals.

(b) Determination of the effect of the extra plus at the farpoint is only part of the problem, however. While it is desirable to reduce the burden upon the accommodation, this must be accomplished at near with as little interference with the habitual convergence habits as is possible. It is in this regard that the gradient test becomes indicative.

(c) *Indications of the gradient.*

[1] If the gradient is *low,* little accommodative-convergence is used, and the extra plus should not interfere greatly with the convergence. The determination will also depend upon other tests, but not to the degree involved with a normal or high gradient. If the gradient is *normal* or *high*, the convergence may be handicapped by the extra plus. The decision to prescribe the plus will then depend upon the actual values of the tests dealing with fusional convergence.

[a] If the extra plus markedly reduces the amount of accommodative-convergence, the fusional or supplementary convergence must be increased to secure fixation at the nearpoint. The employment of this fusional convergence will tend to show an increase of the phoria at near, which would be the gradient, and also tends to decrease the Positive Fusional Reserve value. The added plus would, therefore, increase the demand and at the same time decrease the reserve. Also it would reduce the Positive Relative Convergence in relation to the Negative Relative Convergence. Thus, by both Sheard's and Percival's criteria, the added plus might create a problem of fusional convergence.

[b] The decision to prescribe the plus would depend upon the gradient, plus the values of the original nearpoint phoria, and the Positive Relative and Negative Relative Convergence findings. If these tests indicate a potential source of discomfort due to convergence, it might be well to either reduce the plus power or to provide prism base-out exercises with it thereby having to increase the reserve of positive fusional convergence.

(d) *The amount of plus.*

[1] As already indicated, the amount of plus given depends upon the distance acuity and the gradient indications. However, some basic amount must be determined as a starting point, which can be modified, if necessary, as the above indications require. The basic amount is readily determined by noting the excess above the upper limits of the norms found in the tests of plus add: the dynamic skiametry, monocular, and binocular cross cylinder findings.

[a] If the dynamic skiametry showed +2.00, the dissociated cross cylinder +1.75, and the binocular cross cylinder +1.25 above the subjective, the excesses of each above the upper limits of their respective norms of 1.50, 1.25, and 0.75 would be an extra +0.50. If the three disagreed, a range would be indicated.

(e) A type of accommodative problem was reported by Wardale (1961) which did not exhibit a typical syndrome. These consisted of relatively young people between the ages of 13 and 21 who complained of blur at reading, headache, and fatigue. They exhibited an esophoria at near, but the indicative indication seemed to be a tendency to hold the print closer than necessary. Few manifested any great hyperopia or a reading acceptance above the distance correction.

Wardale found that a +0.50 D. provided relief in many cases, but the Rx was always only for near, as no spastic accommodation for distance was revealed.

[1] The question remains as to whether the esophoria was a result of excessive accommodation or of hyperactive convergence. If the latter, the problem might lie more in the field of a convergence difficulty than an accommodative one.

(2) Convergence Fatigue

(a) Convergence fatigue may be handled from the standpoint of visual training, prism base-in, or minus lenses. Visual training is the more customary procedure. The choice would depend upon the phoria and the gradient. For example, if the phoria were orthophoria and abduction finding was low, prism base-in would be contraindicated. Likewise, the choice between a minus add and visual training might depend upon the phoria value and the gradient again. If the gradient was high, the minus value (or reduction of plus value) might induce an extra accommodative-convergence to assist the convergence. Such a procedure would depend upon indications of sufficient amplitude and low plus acceptance values in the dynamic skiametry and the binocular and monocular cross cylinder tests. If the gradient is low, this procedure would be of little help, and the positive fusional reserve would need to be increased by visual training, or the demand would need to be decreased by prism base-in.

(3) Prism Application

(a) If an accommodative case reveals a high gradient and the application of plus is deemed inadvisable unless some method of assisting the convergence is attempted, visual training may be given the patient to develop the reserve of fusional convergence. In many instances, visual training will not be practical, either because of difficulty in maintaining the visits required or because an immediate agent for relief must be provided. Prism base-in may then be prescribed with the additional plus power. This prism may be determined by either the methods previously described for lateral imbalances or by adding a sufficient amount to reduce the increase revealed in the gradient to a normal disparity. That is, if the gradient proved to be 7 pd, exceeding the upper limits of the expected by 2 pd, the prescription of 2 pd base-in with a +1.00 lens, with which the gradient is taken, would leave the fusional convergence in the same status in which a normal gradient would have left it. If less plus is prescribed, the prism may be reduced proportionately.

(b) From Sheard's and Percival's systems, it will be observed that only small amounts of prism will produce noticeable changes in the relation of the fusional demand and reserve so that the average patient may require very limited amounts to restore comfort.

(c) In convergence cases the amounts of prism may be required to be larger if the convergence is badly in need of assistance. Some patients will develop fairly large breakpoints by means of visual training exercises but will not increase the blur point or fusional range to the amount required. Such cases may require prism prescriptions despite visual training.

7. *Orthoptics or Visual Training*

a. Purposes

(1) Orthoptics or Visual Training as applied to the binocular case may be used for many purposes other than merely altering either the implications of the findings determined by Morgan's or the graphical method of analysis. These varying purposes have been summarized by Hofstetter (1949) as follows:

(a) To train the patient to make more reliable and valid observations and reports

(b) To teach the patient to tolerate ocular or visual conditions which are either not subject to correction or which are unavoidably induced by the use of the ophthalmic correction

(c) To develop perceptual skills for special needs

(d) As a psychological measure

(e) To develop motor functions otherwise not adequate for normal vision.

(2) Morgan (1947) and Flom (1954) discussed the correction of anomalies by considering their causation as either sensory, integrative, or motor. Eskridge (1965) expanded their classification by adding a division to the anomalies for diagnostic implications leading towards potential visual training as follows:

(a) *Anomalies of the sensory processes*

[1] These are due to pathology, ametropia, amblyopia, eccentric fixation, or reduced amplitude of accommodation.

(b) *Anomalies of the integrative processes*

[1] These are due to aniseikonia, suppression, or anomalous correspondence.

(c) *Anomalies of perception*

[1] These are due to anomalies in the brain or to an uncritical observer.

(d) *Motor anomalies*

[1] These are chiefly motor restrictions, latent or manifest deviations, problems of the accommodative-convergence ratio, or anomalies of the fusional movements.

(e) Eskridge emphasized that a disorder of prior rank must have been corrected before treatment of a malfunction of the next rank was attempted. That is, an anomaly in the (A) group should have been corrected before an alleviation of an anomaly in (C) or (D) was attempted.

b. Effectivity

(1) Morgan (1947) conducted a series of investigations of the results of orthoptic training upon the different functions and findings utilizing three groups, one given intensive training, one given less intensive training, and a third acting as a control group. He found that certain responses were readily available by all methods of training, while others were not possible by any means. Every known system of orthoptics application was used. The following findings were divided into three groups

ranking, in order, those most amenable to training from the easiest to the most difficult to affect.

(a) *Easiest to alter*

[1] Positive Fusional Reserve of Convergence (16B)

[2] Positive Relative Convergence (16A)

[3] Adduction (10)

[4] Negative Fusional Reserve (17B)

[5] Positive Relative Accommodation (20)

[6] Negative Relative Convergence (17A)

[7] Abduction

(b) *Alterable to a limited degree*

[1] Negative Relative Accommodation (21)

[2] Added plus to perceptible blur at far

[3] Nearpoint phoria (13B)

[4] Phoria at far (8)

[5] Amplitude of Accommodation (19)

[6] Monocular Cross Cylinder (14A)

[7] Binocular Cross Cylinder (14B)

(c) *Not significantly alterable*

[1] Ophthalmometer (2)

[2] Static skiametry (4)

[3] Subjective to best visual acuity (7A)

[4] Dynamic skiametry (5, 6)

[5] Gradient (15A, 15B)

(2) Fry (1943) and Hofstetter (1945) expressed much the same opinions in regard to the findings, when graphically expressed in terms of the five fundamental variables.

(a) *The width of the zone* is readily varied by training.

[1] As the width is expressed by the relative convergence lines made up of the positive and negative relative convergence and accommodation findings, it will be noted that these findings agree with their classification, in the main, in Morgan's determination preceding this section.

(b) *The slope of the zone is not alterable.*

[1] Although the gradient and the ACA ratio had been considered as not alterable, recent investigators, such as Schapero and Levy (1953), Manas (1955), Morgan and Peters (1951), Flom (1960) and others, indicated that the ratio changed with age and with other influences. Similarly, the slope, while considered fixed throughout its median range, shows variations at either end.

(c) *The height of the zone,* as expressed by the amplitude of accommodation, is alterable to only a limited degree.

[1] The true amplitude may not actually be alterable, but the finding determined by clinical procedure, which is interpreted to express the amplitude, is somewhat affected, within narrow limits, by training.

(d) *The position of the zone* is alterable only to a limited degree.

[1] This agrees with Morgan's conclusion about the far phoria which establishes the position.

(e) Findings outside the zone, such as duction breaks, are readily alterable.

(f) An increase in the zone at one stimulus position results in corresponding increases at all levels of accommodation.

(g) Validity and reliability of findings are all improved by training.

(3) Hofstetter (1954) indicated how various types of visual training may be related to the accommodation-convergence graph (Figure XXI-15).

(a) Arrows labeled *a* represent binocular minus lens training at various levels of convergence.

(b) Arrows labeled *b* represent binocular plus lens training at various levels of convergence.

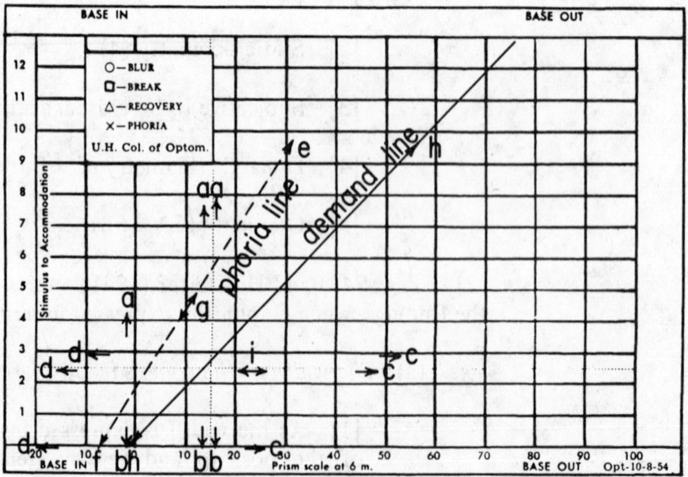

Figure XXI-15.

(c) Arrows labeled *c* represent base-out training at various levels of accommodation.

(d) Arrows labeled *d* represent base-in training at various levels of accommodation.

(e) Arrows labeled *e* represent monocular minus lens training..

(f) Arrows labeled *f* represent monocular plus lens training.

(g) The double-headed arrow labeled *g* represents accommodative rock.

(h) The arrow labeled *h* represents binocular pushups.

(4) In a study of intermittent exotropia, Heath and Hofstetter (1952) expressed the opinion that the zone might not actually be changeable and that the results sometimes attained might be due to other functions not directly measured in the routine examination.

(5) Ellerbrock (1953) indicated that the stereoscope itself can be graphed so that the prismatic effects for different levels of accommodation could be used to indicate training procedures (Figure XXI-16).

(a) If a slope of exophoria or esophoria is drawn on the graph, the intersection of these slopes with the broken lines in Figure XXI-16 will be the starting points of training with targets of different displacement. The move for esophoria will be from far to near and for exophoria from near to far, as the arrows indicate.

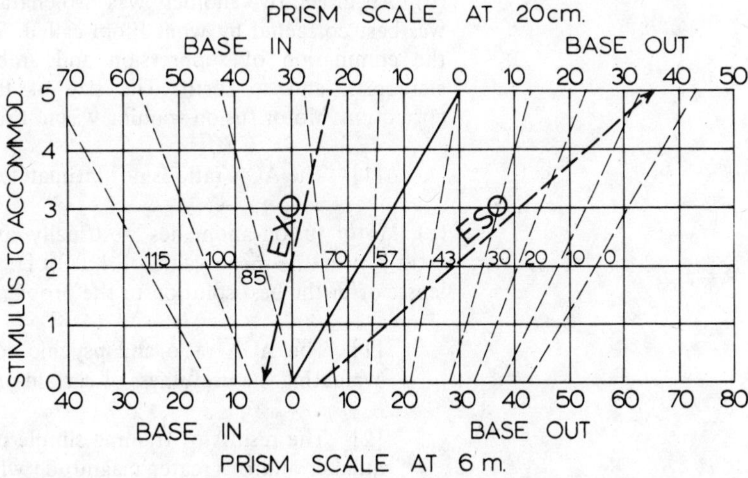

Figure XXI-16 – The prismatic effects produced by targets having different separations are given above. For these data, the lenses were assumed to have a power of +5.00 D., with the optical centers 85 mms. apart. The line connecting the zero positions of the two scales is the normal demand line of accommodation and convergence for an interpupillary distance of 60 mms.

(6) In another study, Morgan (1947) found that visual problems were segregated, from an orthoptic standpoint, into three classifications.

(a) If the fault lay in the sensory mechanism, the best correction was by means of lenses.

(b) If it lay in the motor mechanism, best results were obtained by training on devices designed to increase motility.

(c) If it lay in the integrative mechanism, resulting in limited stereopsis or suppression, best results were secured by training on fusion and stereoscopic devices.

(d) According to the location of the fault, correction of one factor will result in improvement in the others.

(e) In connection with this segregation, Nicholls (1950), working with aviation problems, commented that, contrary to assumed opinion, little relation was demonstrated between integrative function, such as stereopsis, and the expression of motor function, such as phorias. Nicholls actually reported no true relation between the state of phorias, the duction limits, and stereoscopic ability, with the exception of vertical phorias over 1 Δ in amount.

(7) In a later study than that of Morgan's, Flom (1954) found similar results in the main. He summarized the use of the zone of clear binocular single vision in relation to its application to the analysis of the cause of disturbances of binocular vision.

(a) A sensory malfunction, usually characterized by a small zone of fusion, was best corrected by lenses (as noted by Morgan and others) or whatever therapy was best suited to remove the sensory disturbance.

[1] The ACA ratio is not involved in this process.

(b) An integrative anomaly was also characterized by a small zone of fusion but was best corrected by what Flom called "qualitative orthoptics." This included the elimination of suppression and amblyopia, development of fusion and stereopsis, and so forth. The size of the zone often increased with such correction. Motor fusion training was not required in many cases.

[1] The ACA ratio is not intimately related to this type of anomaly.

(c) Motor fusion anomalies are usually corrected best by orthoptics if the ACA ratio is near the mean value of 4/1.00 D. If the ratio is low or high, prisms and lenses offer the best solution to the problem.

[1] The ACA ratio and psychic convergence need to be considered in evaluating the usefulness of certain procedures.

[2] The results of training simple motor fusion anomalies were generally quicker and of greater magnitude when the motor mechanism was trained immediately and directly than by the method of training various primary and secondary skills in the order of their presumed development.

(d) The nearpoint of convergence and the positive side of the zone appear to be the most trainable. The negative side of the zone is only slightly affected, and the phorias and ACA do not appear to be amenable to training by orthoptics (although later studies show it amenable to other influences and varying at the ends of the slope).

(e) The PRA was the most frequently noted invalid finding, and apparent increases may not represent a true change in this value.

(8) *Fatigue*

(a) Much emphasis has been placed upon the role of fatigue in the accommodative and convergence functions, even to the delineating of cases as accommodative or convergence fatigue problems. Insofar as fatigue affects the functions, Weber (1950) reported the following conclusion concerning the actual effect of use upon various ocular performances.

[1] Acuity was not diminished at either near or far by fatigue, expressed as working-day fatigue.

[2] The speed of accommodation was not affected nor the strength of the extraocular muscles.

[3] A slight recession of the amplitude of accommodation and the ability to sustain accommodation was found in only certain subjects.

[4] As previously discussed in the chapter on *History,* ocular fatigue must be of the focal cerebral type.

(b) Stein and Hofstetter (1951) testing subjects after twelve continuous hours of viewing television, likewise found no change in ACA variables, asthenopia, light reflexes, phorias at far or near, ductions, accommodative amplitudes, or similar findings.

XI. OLDER PATIENTS

A. The zone in presbyopia

1. Hofstetter (1948) commented that the use of the range of accommodation to assist in determining the proper add was predicated upon the assumption that only the amplitude of accommodation was the limiting factor in the determination. However, if the ACA ratio and other factors became directly involved, contradictory results were sometimes apparent by use of the range as the sole criterion. In an actual study of the habits of prescribing the adds actually used in clinical practice, Hofstetter (1949) concluded that certain indefinable criteria seem to have been employed, since the adds actually prescribed did not agree with precisely either the Duane or Donders' tables, or other rules postulated for the purpose.

a. The range could fulfill the assumption of perfectly balanced positive and negative relative accommodation only if total presbyopia existed. Lederer (1948) attempted to explain the value of the range in determining changes in the add by advocating that while accommodation lagged behind its demand point, and thus should not have been extended sufficiently to warrant small changes in add as often as such changes seemed to be required, the range did serve as a criterion because each change of 0.25 D. in the add effected a shift of 5 cms. in the range.

2. It is obvious that if an add is used, the demand upon accommodation is lessened. Consequently, the amount of accommodative innervation, and concurrently, the amount of accommodative-convergence is lessened. Since the total convergence demand is the same as before an add was applied, the lessened accommodative-convergence must be supplanted by additional

fusional convergence. Thus, the indication of fusional convergence used, the phoria at near, is generally increased in the exophoric direction; the positive fusional reserve is correspondingly decreased; and the negative fusional reserve tests also usually show an increase.

a. Such cases will fall into the convergence difficulty category if analyzed by Morgan's method, even though the presbyopia is the obvious source of difficulty.

3. The changes of function with age seemed to be predominantly as follows (Hirsch, Alpern and Schultz, 1948):

a. Tonic convergence is increased slightly with age.

b. Fusional supplementary convergence (the near phoria) is slightly decreased.

c. The accommodative-convergence decreases slightly.

(1) Morgan and Peters (1951) found no decrease in accommodative-convergence with age, but Kephart and Oliver (1952) and also Fry (1959) found some (see also Chapter VII).

4. It is also possible to determine the problem by graphical analysis.

a. Since the lowered amplitude will lower the entire height of the zone, to even zero in total presbyopia, and since the vertical separation of the findings is decreased, it is advisable to use a graph in which the separations are based upon 5 Δ and 0.50 D. spacings, as shown in Figure XXI-17.

b. A new demand line for the add is constructed by using the point on the ordinate which corresponds to the stimulus to accommodation for the stimulus to accommodation line and the point on the abscissa which corresponds to the nearpoint testing distance for the

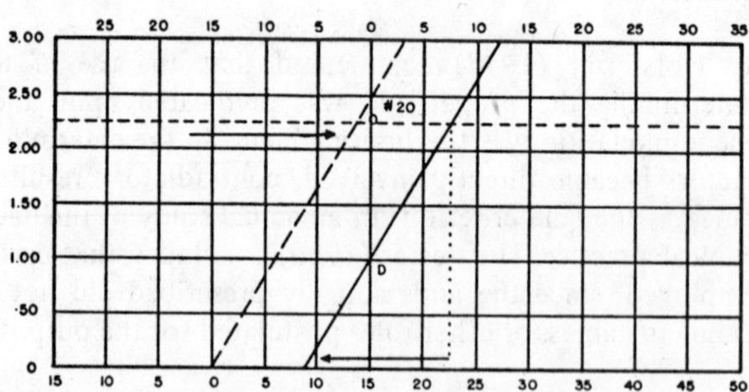

Figure XXI-17 – Graph Adapted To Presbyopia. Oblique dashed line represents original non-presbyopic line of demand; solid line represents parallel line of demand at 40 cms. with a +1.50 add in place. Height of zone shown as horizontally dashed line, determined by positive relative accommodation finding, 20. Range through the add is seen to be from 75 to 26 cms. (expressed by lower arrow). Range through distance Rx is from infinity to 45 cms. (upper arrow). As two arrows overlap, no intermediate add is indicated. D represents point of demand with add; 20 finding = –1.25 D.

stimulus to convergence line. At the intersection of these two lines, the new demand line is drawn parallel to the original demand line.

(1) For example, if a +1.50 D. add is used at 40 cms., the new stimulus to accommodation line is found at 1.00 D. of accommodation on the ordinate, while 15 Δ on the bottom abscissa or 0 Δ on the top one represents the convergence stimulation (Figure XXI-17).

c. The range which the add permits can be shown on the graph by marking the positive relative accommodation findings taken through the add straight above the newly noted demand point. This establishes the maximum accommodative line. The number of prism diopters which is represented on this line at the point where the new demand line intersects it represents the nearpoint of the range, while the number of prism diopters at the intersection of the new demand line and the zero stimulus line represents the farpoint of the range. The value of these prism diopter indications in linear amounts, when read from the lower abscissa, was given by the following table (Abel, 1951):

(1) **TABLE XXI-9**

Prism Diopters on Lower Convergence Abscissa	Approximate Linear Distance in cms. from Center of Rotation of Eyes
0	*infinity*
6	*100*
12	*50*
15	*40*
20	*30*
23	*26*
26	*23*
30	*20*
35	*17*
37.5	*16*
40	*15*
43	*14*

(2) If the add is changed, a new demand line is required, and new ranges are determinable.

(3) The original demand line, without the add, and the new demand line, with the add, can be compared at the upper and lower limits of the zone. If the upper limits of the original demand line does not touch or overlap the lower limit of the new demand line, an area which neither fulfills will exist at that point, and this area will be blurred indicating the need for an intermediate add or trifocal (Figure XXI-17).

d. The ACA ratio, which should not alter, is determinable by extending the phoria line up to the 2.50 D. stimulus to accommodation position. Also, the new demand line and phoria line can be compared to the relative convergence lines and the need for altering the add or assisting the convergence demonstrated by using Sheard's or Percival's criteria in regard to this line, just as was used in regard to the original lines in the non-presbyope. The effect of the ACA ratio in this regard is evident by noting the differences in relation to these limits of the demand position when the add is modified by a small amount in a high and low ACA ratio (Figure XXI-18 A & B).

(1) An extremely high ACA ratio will also restrict the minus lens to blur add below the upper limits of the zone as expressed by the amplitude. Likewise, since the ability to accommodate is lowered by the decreased amplitude, the patient may sometimes be unable to induce extra accommodative-convergence in the base-out test, particularly if the ratio is low, and a break will occur before a blur is noted.

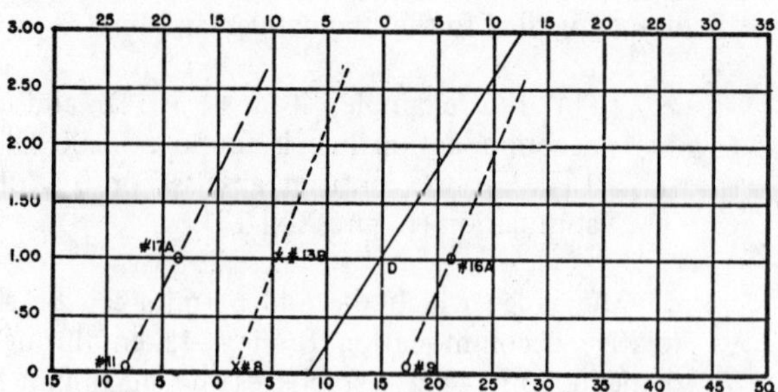

Figure XXI-18A – Slope of low ACA ratio, compared to limits of zone, in Presbyopia. D represents demand point with +1.50 add, and oblique solid line is new demand line developed from that point. Near phoria taken with add. It will be noted that the phoria compared to the pos. fus. res. (both measured from D) do not meet Sheard's criteria.

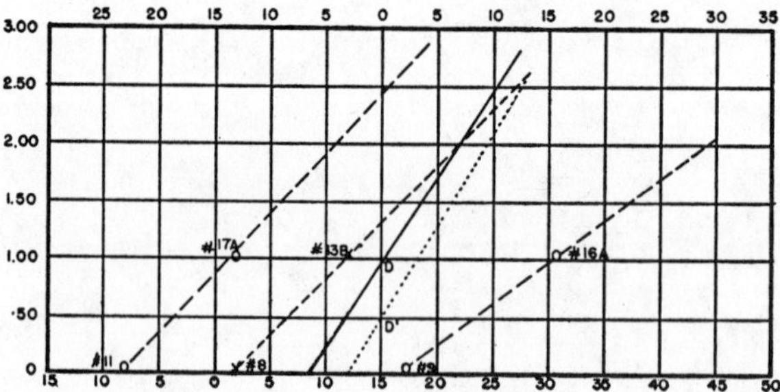

Figure XXI-18B – ACA Graph in Presbyopia in high ratio. Add and other symbols same as above. Note that if the new demand line is altered by changing the add, another demand line (dotted line) is formed. The relationship between the phoria line and the pos. fusional reserve line is altered sharply. In the above graph, the relationship from D meets Sheard's criteria for comfort, but if an extra + .50 is supplied, the relationship as measured from D′ no longer meets Sheard's criteria. In Figure XXI-18A, a change of .50 D., in either direction, alters the relationship only slightly.

(2) Ellerbrock and Zinnecker (1952) commented that where the ACA ratio was high and the fusional reserve low, a trifocal, by virtue of lesser inhibition to accommodative-convergence, was helpful. When the high ACA ratio was accompanied by a high exophoria, more difficulty was encountered than when a high esophoria was accompanied by a high ACA ratio.

(3) Other aids for the problem of a low fusional reserve in relation to the new demand line are as follows:

(a) The use of large segments decentered inwards to create base-in effect at near

(b) Prism segments in the bifocals

(c) Separate reading corrections incorporating base-in effect

(d) Fusional base-out training

B. The Aged

1. Wick (1960) divided the older patients into categories determined by age.

a. From 40 to 60 he called late maturity; from 60 to 75, senescence; from 75 and upwards, senility. Above 50, treatment may be considered geriatric.

b. He quotes Thewlis (1919):

(1) "The object of treatment of diseases in senility is to restore the diseased organ or tissue to the state normal to senility, not to the state normal to maturity."

c. Besides the vascular and accommodative changes expected in advanced age, older patients may exhibit poorer light adaptation due to the consistently constricted pupil. The norms for the really elderly have not been determined with exactitude, although the chapter on Visual Acuity reports some normals for the aspect. Lowered muscular tonus and response is more or less expected, and the increased exophoria, recessed PP of Convergence, and lowered ductions in all directions have been mentioned by many clinicians.

(1) Of 100 subjects from age 60 to 91, for example, 83% possessed visual acuity of 20/20 or better; 11% of 20/25; and 6% from 20/30 to 20/50. Fletcher (1949) found that glare resistance tests were passed by 6 out of 7 at the age of 20, were failed by 1 out of 3 at the age of 30 to 40, while 9 out of 10 failed them at the ages of 60 to 70, and all failed them above the age of 70.

2. Besides the normal physical alterations expected due to aging, the major effects are psychological. Bab (1961) discussed the psychological problems of aging in detail.

a. "Old age" means a stagnancy of development with actual retrogression and with the accompaniment of disease, including not only general diseases but those common to advanced years. The mental attitude, influenced by experience, and the developments of maturity are changed by certain psychological and somatic factors.

(1) The isolation and retirement accompanying old age, predicated upon the change in income, and social value concept of retirement from earning a living, the loss of husband or wife, the loss of friends and a decreased connection with long-established affiliations leads to an "inner-directed" attitude. The gradual dimunition of somatic faculties, i.e., slowing of movements, the quicker approach of fatigue, a lessening of faculties, the deterioration of memory and the inability to learn new subjects (leading to a negative attitude towards anything new) further strengthens withdrawal from outward associations.

(2) The resultant anxiety, really an anxiety of further isolation from the outside world and increased boredom, is increased by either pain or discomfort or by the lessening of function of vision or hearing. Such losses predicate further decrease in information, entertainment, hobbies, and associations, and suffering becomes dominant.

b. No specific routine of handling is particularly effective, such as, psychoanalysis, hypnosis or a blunt "nothing can be done" attitude. The last, particularly, may result in utter despair. Actually, hope is needed. The best therapy is that which will turn the patient away from malignant anxiety toward a benign inner freedom.

c. Bab proposed that it should be realized that to be blind is different from the fear of becoming blind. Activity of the patient should be encouraged and the will of the patient strengthened as much as possible. Anxiety should be relieved as much as possible, not, of course, by offering non-realistic and unattainable hopes of cure, but by establishing faith of the patient in the doctor (his presence assuring the patient of an outlet for his accompanying or causative neuroses) and in religion or philosophy. The condition and situation should be explained in detail with the positive aspects emphasized.

d. Not only should whatever possible effects and devices be used to assist the relief or discomfort of pain or abet the defect (as magnifiers for poor vision), but the essential fear of isolation should be attacked by educating and helping the patient use his time, e.g., walks, radio (if T.V. is not feasible), hobbies, visits from friends, and talking books (records).

3. It may be repeated for it is important that the clinician remember that the objective with the elderly is not to attempt to restore the function to the normal, as assumed for all ages, but to restore the function to the normal for that age group. This criterion is exceedingly important when combined with Wick's comment that the objective in cases over 65 years of age is to rarely change the habitual visual patterns, no matter how inconsistent with the patterns of younger normals. The refractionist who has suddenly introduced cylinders to such a patient, or prescribed prisms (except where definite diplopia has become manifest) is well aware of the significance of Wick's statement.

a. Wick (1960) pointed out that the less complicated the nearpoint lens the easier it is for the patient to adjust to it at a later age. Morgan also emphasized that older people get the best results with the least disturbing and simplest correction. If a lens was used which might have affected the habitual visual orientation – even changes in base curve are questionable, not to mention cylinders at different powers and axes – the potential effects should have been explained beforehand to the patient. It is preferable that changes be small, and Wick estimated that up to 1.00 D. of spherical change would be accepted fairly readily.

(1) The working distance, the P.D., the seg height, and all such details should be precisely measured and changed as little as possible from the previously accustomed criteria. If a change is needed, such as moving the working distance closer to enable greater magnification from a stronger add, the change should be fully explained and demonstrated, and the examiner should be certain it is understood fully before making it.

XII. GENERAL CONSIDERATIONS

A. **Symptoms and small ametropias** (Bridgman, 1956; Nathan, 1957)

1. Symptoms are frequently not in proportion to the error found. Minor changes in correction or minor adjustments seem to produce benefits apparently out of proportion to the changes.

a. Small ametropias of 0.50 D. or less often indicate marked symptoms which are relieved by correction. Yet the aberrations of the eye and so forth, in themselves, exceed 0.50 D. and the depth of focus varies up to 0.50 D. without stimulating accommodation. Many subjects reveal up to 1.25 D. of perceptual tolerance, that is, accommodation can be varied that much without a subjective realization of blur.

2. Much of the dominant therapeutic effect may be considered as "general" while the "visual" effects are minimal or non-existent. Lancaster indicated that if relief was immediate, it was

probably due to the relief of anxiety and improved confidence. Nathan (1957) believed that the great majority of low ametropia sufferers actually suffered from neuroses due to the fear of impaired vision or blindness. An anxiety status was relieved by spectacles as an "eyestrain" cure. This fear was especially apparent in myopes. Since "eyestrain" implied an increasing impairment or potential precursor of blindness, and lenses may have expanded vision, the wearing of spectacles may have saved the vision for later. Other causes of the neuroses may have been a distaste for the task, general physical debility, or the need for occupational spectacles.

a. The anxiety state may result in an onset of fatigue after only a slight exertion. History may be vague, but if the neuroses are deeply seated, the history itself will be a neurotic history.

b. Bridgman (1956) described even poor readers as examples of neurosis or maladjustment. Poor readers often exhibited many adjustment problems, such as defensive behavior, aggressive reactions, recessive and withdrawal behavior, and self-consciousness. Often a high degree of parental maladjustment was found. The poor reading may be part of a broader pattern of maladjustment, and once established, the two amplify and reinforce each other.

(1) The poor visual performance may come first in some cases, but not in many. Treatment of the adjustment problem is often better than emphasis on remedial training, which re-emphasizes inadequate performance around which the current problems are centered.

(2) However, orthoptics, visual training, or remedial reading training may often achieve results through the application of attention and concern, and increase confidence by indirect mechanisms. The effect of the enthusiasm of the trainer upon the trainee is hard to evaluate. The orthoptist should take advantage of these factors.

3. Care must especially be taken not to leap to conclusions that small differences found from previous corrections are responsible for the symptoms. Often such differences could be found by the same examiner upon successive examinations. Sloane (1954) compared examinations of 21 adolescents, all refracted on the same day and under identical conditions by three ophthalmologists. In only one instance were identical findings disclosed, although the differences were small in all cases.

a. A fluctuation of results with repeated refractions by the same examiner upon the same patient were reported by Humphriss (1958). The variation was 0.25 D., usually in the cylinder. Humphriss believed this may have been due to changes in the size of the pupil.

(1) It is equally likely, of course, that the differences found by the same examiner are results purely of errors inherent in the techniques, questioning, and response variations found from day-to-day between the examiner and the patient.

B. The Refractive Failure (Stillerman, 1965)

1. Stillerman (1965) divides the problem of "refractive failure" into two categories – those due to errors in the science of refraction, or the refractionist's skill as a "doctor"; and those due to errors in the art of refraction, or the refractionist's skill as a "human being." In the first instance, the refractionist failed to analyze the functional needs of the patient or erred in dealing with certain objective, physical, or scientific aspects. In the second instance, he ignored or miscalculated the subjective, psychological, emotional, non-scientific and/or functional problems of the patient.

2. In dealing with the first category, the potential errors should be dealt with in the order listed below, from the first towards the succeeding ones, as each one is found to be non-indicative. In dealing with the second, much skill and understanding, as well as emotional control on the refractionist's own part, may be required.

3. *Errors in the science*

a. *Check the order blank against the record and the Rx against the order blank.* If correct check the following:

(1) The optical centers and interpupillary distance

(a) If correct, prismatic effect and errors are ruled out.

(2) The height of the bifocal, the position of the segs (whether equal position for both eyes, etc.)

(3) The fit of the frame, the pressure points, and if the shape interferes with the range of vision.

b. *Check the visual acuity at far*

(1) Use a +0.25 and a –0.25 D. sphere; then a +0.50 and a –0.50 D. sphere before the Rx at both the chart and at a window for greater distance.

c. *Check the near acuity*

(1) Note the history for difficulties with glasses, and, if not working, for other nearpoint needs.

(2) Recheck the near acuity, the range, and the extent of the field:

(a) The add may be too strong as the patient's idea of his working distance may be wrong. It is best to check with appropriate targets at similar circumstances, such as at a desk.

(3) Check the effectivity of the lenses, the position of the frame (particularly in strong lenses), and the vertex distances.

d. *Note the major changes from the old Rx*

(1) Note the changes in the sphere, the cylinder, and the prism

(a) Avoid sizable changes in size or distance and shape.

(2) Check for tint

(a) This should be included in the new if present in the old.

(3) Check the interpupillary distance

(a) If a wrong interpupillary distance has been worn for years, do not change.

(4) Note the base curve

(a) A change in base curve will alter the aniseikonic effects.

(5) Note the type of bifocal.

(6) Note whether there is a marked increase in the plus power

(a) Often this will not be accepted without a blur.

(b) The patient should be warned ahead of time, or the Rx should be modified.

e. *Note the following anisometropic problems:*

(1) Whether induced prism and of what amount

(2) Aniseikonia

f. *Note the convergence problems*

(1) Prism may be needed

g. If none of the above is indicated when comparing the old and the new Rx's as a cause of the problem, repeat the refraction.

4. *Errors in the Art*

a. There may have been pre-examination irritations in the office.

b. The doctor's lack of interest or inattention to the history and complaint may irk the patient.

c. The doctor's lack of patience during the subjective examination, for example with a slow patient, may have irritated the patient.

d. An indecisive or compulsive patient may be very precise or finicky in answering. If cut off, and he feels that not enough attention is being paid him, it must be impressed upon him that the examiner can tell if he errs in his answering.

e. It should be noted whether the examiner failed to discuss or warn a patient of anticipated problems. It is exceedingly important that this be done in advance.

f. The chronically dissatisfied patient is characterized by the following:

(1) He is usually accompanied by many pairs of glasses.

(2) The cause may be systemic or emotional.

g. If the patient has an appliance neurosis, he will demonstrate the following:

(1) He is one of those people who cannot wear a hearing aid, a denture or braces, or any of those things.

(2) He usually is very curious, and asks about, contact lenses.

h. If the patient cannot accept the Rx of the retinoscope, do not insist that he accept it.

i. The non-payment of fee (deadbeat syndrome).

(1) It is an axiom among spectacle prescribers that, "glasses that are not paid for, never fit."

A. The appraisal of visual loss for compensation and insurance purposes has been established by official policy of the American Medical Association. The basic determination of loss acuity was derived by Snell and Sterling (Nicholls, 1950) who utilized a series of meshed glass plates of given absorption and diffraction upon a number of subjects to determine the resultant dimunition of acuity. Each plate was estimated to reduce vision by 16.6% and tabulated as follows:

1. Meshed glass loss

TABLE XXI-10

No. plates before eye	Snellen fraction	Fractional loss	% loss	% remaining
1.	*20/40*	*1/6*	*16.6*	*83.4*
2.	*20/65*	*2/6*	*33.3*	*66.7*
3.	*20/100*	*3/6*	*50.0*	*50.0*
4.	*20/160*	*4/6*	*66.7*	*33.3*
5.	*20/250*	*5/6*	*83.4*	*16.6*
6.	*20/400*	*6/6*	*industrial blindness*	

2. The theoretical calculations agree quite closely with the above experimentally determined figures. As the resolving angle is increased arithmetically, the visual efficiency decreases geometrically. Each increase of 1′ of angle represents a decrease in efficiency to .836. For example:

a. **TABLE XXI-11**

Vision	Minutes of angle	Fraction	Percentage
20/40	*2′*	*.836 of 20/20*	*.836 x 100%–83.6%*
20/60	*3′*	*.836 of 20/40*	*.836 x 83.6–69.89%*
20/80	*4′*	*.836 of 20/50*	*.836 x 69.89–58.4%*

B. The recommendations have been revised from time to time. According to the standards established by the Council on Industrial Health of the American Medical Association, as revised in 1955, the following criteria must be met:

1. Central visual acuity

a. *Test*

(1) A Snellen chart using black letters or numbers without serifs, an illiterate E, or a Landolt broken ring chart may be used.

(2) Illumination should be five foot-candles with the chart surface clean.

(3) Test distances should be 6 meters (20 feet), and 36 cms. (14 inches).

(4) The progression of lines should be geometric, with each line 20% larger than the next smaller line and 20% smaller than the next larger line.

(5) Reading should be recorded in terms of the Snellen fraction or the visual angle. At near, a Jaeger point system stating the inches of test distance should be used.

(6) The best acuity with ophthalmic lenses should be noted.

b. *In Aphakia*

(1) Monocular aphakia is to be considered a partial disability. Grant only 50% of the

central visual efficiency of that eye when corrected, if the other eye is better.

(2) If binocular aphakia exists, or if a monocular aphakic eye is used mainly, apply 25% as an added handicap to the efficiency of the eye or eyes.

(a) If the aphakic eye sees 20/40, and 20/40 equals 85% of efficiency, an 85% x 50% equals 43% loss for 1 above, and 85% x 75% equals a 64% efficiency for number 2.

c. *Central visual efficiency* corresponding to central visual acuity *for distance.*

(1) **TABLE XXI-12**

Snellen		Visual Angle	% Central	
Feet	**Meters**	**In Minutes**	**Visual Efficiency**	**% Loss**
20/16	*6/5*	*0.80*	*100*	*0*
20/20	*6/6*	*1.00*	*100*	*0*
20/25	*6/7.5*	*1.25*	*95*	*5*
20/32	*6/10*	*1.60*	*90*	*10*
20/40	*6/12*	*2.00*	*85*	*15*
20/50	*6/15*	*2.50*	*75*	*25*
20/64	*6/20*	*3.20*	*65*	*35*
20/80	*6/24*	*4.00*	*60*	*40*
20/100	*6/30*	*5.00*	*50*	*50*
20/125	*6/38*	*6.30*	*40*	*60*
20/160	*6/48*	*8.00*	*30*	*70*
20/200	*6/60*	*10.00*	*20*	*80*
20/300	*6/90*	*15.00*	*15*	*85*
20/400	*6/120*	*20.00*	*10*	*90*
20/800	*6/240*	*40.00*	*5*	*95*

(a) Lebensohn (1965) commented that a reduction of acuity to 10/40 may show the discrimination has been lessened to two minutes of arc, or halved, but that the visual efficiency is only reduced 15%.

d. *Central visual efficiency* corresponding to central visual acuity *for near:*

TABLE XXI-13

			Visual Angle	Visual	
Snellen	**Jaeger**	**Point**	**In Minutes**	**Efficiency**	**% of Loss**
14/14 (20/20)	*1–*	*3*	*1.00*	*100*	*0*
14/18 (20/26)	*2–*	*4*	*1.25*	*100*	*0*
14/22 (20/32)		*5*	*1.60*	*95*	*5*
14/28 (20/40)	*3*	*6*	*2.00*	*90*	*10*
14/35 (20/50)	*6*	*8*	*2.50*	*50*	*50*
14/45 (20/64)	*7–*	*9+*	*3.20*	*40*	*60*
14/56 (20/80)	*8*	*12*	*4.00*	*20*	*80*
14/70 (20/100)	*11*	*14*	*5.00*	*10*	*90*
14/87 (20/124)			*6.30*	*10*	*90*
14/112 (20/160)	*14*	*22*	*8.00*	*5*	*95*
14/140 (20/200)			*10.00*	*2*	*98*

e. Acuity for far plus the acuity for near = *efficiency of the visual acuity.*

(1) 20/40 = 85% for far; + J3, which = 90% for near = $\frac{175}{2}$ = 82%.

2. The Visual Field

a. *The Test*

(1) $\frac{3}{330}$ size of target with a 7 foot-candle illumination is used. A 6 mm. target in white should be used for aphakics.

(2) The test object should be moved from the periphery towards the center.

(3) Two fields should be taken and should agree within 15°.

(4) The tests should be made in each of the eight meridians, spaced 45° apart.

b. *The efficiency*

(1) The total of the degrees of all eight meridians is added together. Normally, this will total 500.

(2) This is divided by 5. The resultant is the percent of the field and its difference from 100 is the percent of loss.

(a) For example, if all of the meridians had contracted down to 25°, then 8 x 25 would = 200, divided by 5 would equal a 40% field or a loss of 60%

c. *The blind spot*

(1) The extent of enlargement in degrees, multiplied by 8, and then divided by 5, equals the percentage of loss of the blind spot. Its difference from 100% would give the efficiency of the size of the blind spot.

(a) For example, if the field blind spot is enlarged by 5°, multiplied by 8 this would equal 40, then divided by 5 equals 8. The percentage of loss for the blind spot is 8%, or conversely, there is a 92% efficiency.

3. Ocular Motility

a. *The Test*

(1) A tangent screen or perimeter is used and a small test light is moved throughout the eight principal meridians.

(2) The degree of separation of diplopic images, if present, is noted at the 10°, 20° and 30° position from the fixation point in the three superior meridians, and at the 10°, 20°, 30°, and 40° position in the five horizontal and inferior meridians.

b. *Efficiency*

(1) Diplopia within 20° of the central gaze is a 100° loss of efficiency of one eye.

(2) Diplopia between 20 and 30° is a 20% loss; 30 and 40° is a 10% loss of one eye.

(3) The loss of binocular vision without other binocular abnormality is a 50% loss of motility efficiency of one eye.

4. Calculating the visual efficiency of one eye

a. The central acuity efficiency is multiplied by the field efficiency and the total is multiplied by the motility efficiency.

(1) For example, if the central acuity efficiency were 30%, the field efficiency 40%,

and the motility efficiency 70%, we would have 30 x 40 X 70 = 0.084 = an 8.4% total of one eye efficiency.

5. Calculating the binocular efficiency

a. (The percent of efficiency of the better eye x 3) + (the percent of efficiency of the worst eye), all over 4, equals the binocular efficiency.

(1) For example, one perfect eye and one blind eye would be: $\frac{(100 \times 3) + 0}{4} = 75\%$.

(2) If both eyes are diseased or injured, the loss in motility is applied only to the poorer eye. The better eye's efficiency is based only on its percent of central visual efficiency multiplied by the percent of the field efficiency.

(3) A total binocular efficiency under 10% can be considered blindness.

REFERENCES

Abel, C.: Graphical Analysis of Clinical Findings. L.A. Coll. of Optometry Extension, Received, 1951.

Allen, M.J. (1960): Prescription of Prism for Lateral Imbalance. J.A.O.A., 32: 379.

Alpern, M. (1950): The Zone of Clear Single Vision at Upper Levels of Accommodation and Convergence. A.A.A.O., 27: 491.

Alpern, M. (1962): Convergence: The Eye by Davson, vol. 3, Occidental Press, N.Y.

Bab, W. (1961): Management of Psychologic Problems in Geriatric Ophthalmology. E.E.N.T., 40: 40.

Bannon, R.E. (1943): Diagnostic and Therapeutic Use of Monocular Occlusion. A.A.A.O., 20: 345.

Bannon, R.E. (1955): Physiologic Factors in Multifocal Correction. A.A.A.O., 32: 57.

Bridgman, C.S. (1956): The Optometrist and Psychological Factors in Visual Work. A.A.A.O., 33: 341.

Burman, B. (1956): A Simplified Graphic Representation of Clinical Findings in Accommodation Convergence Analysis. A.A.A.O., 33: 283.

Carter, D.B. (1963): Effects of Prolonged Wearing of Prism. A.A.A.O., 40: 265.

Carter, D.B. (1968): Notes On Fixation Disparity, J.A.O.A., 38: 1103.

**Cholerton, M. (1947): The Critical Fusion Frequency of Flicker as an Index of Fatigue. Some Recent Advances in Ophthalmic Optics. Trans. R.H.L. Jubilee Congress.*

**Council on Industrial Health, A.M.A. (1955): Estimation of Loss of Visual Efficiency, Revised, 1955. Arch. Oph., 54: 462.*

**Council on Industrial Health, A.M.A. (1958): Guides to the Evaluation of Permanent Impairment; The Visual System, J.A.M.A., Sept. 27.*

**Curcio, M.: The Qualitative Estimation of Central Vision. Penn. St. Coll. of Optometry Alum. Bull.*

Duke-Elder, W.S. (1963): Textbook of Refraction, 7th ed., C.V. Mosby Co., St. Louis.

Ellerbrock, V.J. (1949): Experimental Investigation of Vertical Fusional Movements. A.A.A.O., 26: 327, 388.

Ellerbrock, V.J. (1950): Tonicity Induced by Fusional Movements. A.A.A.O., 27: 8.

Ellerbrock, V.J. (1953): The Prescription of Visual Training by A Graphical Method. A.A.A.O., 30: 559.

Ellerbrock, V.J. & Fry, G.A. (1941): The Aftereffect Induced by Vertical Divergence. A.A.A.O., 18: 450.

Ellerbrock, V.J. & Zinnecker, K.S. (1952): Effect of Multifocal Lenses on Convergence. A.A.A.O., 29: 82.

Elvin, F.T. (1954): The Results of Prescribing the Vertical Prism from the Turville Test. A.A.A.O., 31: 308.

Emmes, A.B. (1949): A Statistical Analysis of Accommodative-Convergence Gradient. A.A.A.O., 26: 474.

Emmes, A.B. (1968): Prismatic Correction Of A Large Progressive Hypertropia, A.A.A.O., 45: 771.

Eskridge, J.B. (1963): Criteria for Determining the Need and Amount of Ophthalmic Prisms Corrections. A.A.A.O., 40: 332.

Eskridge, J.B. (1965): Diagnosis in Opthoptics. Opt. Weekly, 56 (36): 32.

Fletcher, E.D. (1949): Visual Problems in Motor Vehicle Operation. Night Vision and Age. Optometric Extension Program, 3, nos. 5 & 6.

Flom, M.C. (1954): The Use of Accommodative Convergence Relationship in Prescribing Orthoptics. The Penn. Optometrist, 14 (3):

Flom, M.C. (1960): On the Relationship Between Accommodation and Accommodative Convergence. III. Effect of Orthoptics. A.A.A.O., 37: 619.

Flom, M.C. (1963): Treatment of Binocular Anomalies of Vision. Vision of Children. Chilton Books, Phila.

Friedenwald, J.S. (1952): Diagnosis and Treatment of Anisophoria. Arch. Oph. 36: 343.

Fry, G.A. (1937): An Experimental Analysis of the Accommodation-Convergence Relation. A.A.A.O., 14: 402.

Fry, G.A. (1939): Further Experiments on the Accommodation-Convergence Relation. A.A.A.O., 16: 325.

Fry, G.A. (1943): Fundamental Variables in Relationship between Accommodation and Convergence. Opt. Weekly, 34: 153, 183.

Fry, G.A.: Unpublished Ohio State Notes on Analysis. Received 1945.

Fry, G.A. & Kehoe, J.C. (1940): An

Empirical Method of Determining the Vertical Prismatic Effect at the Reading Distance. A.A.A.O., 17: 543.

*Giles, G.H. (1947): The Practice of Orthoptics. Hammond, Hammond & Co., Ltd., London.

Giles, G.H. (1965): The Theory and Practice of Refraction, 2nd ed., Chilton Books, Phila.

Glazer, W.H. (1955): Problems of the Hyper-Eye. O.J.R.O., 42 (2): 35.

Haines, H.F. (1938): An Experimental Analysis of the Factors Affecting the Relationship between Accommodation and Convergence. The Ohio State Univ.

Haines, H.F. (1941): Normal Values of Visual Functions and Their Application to Case Analysis. A.A.A.O., 18: 1.

Heath, G.G. (1959): The Use of Graphic Analysis in Visual Training. A.A.A.O., 36. 337.

Heath, G. & Hofstetter, H.W. (1952): The Effect of Orthoptics on the Zone of Binocular Vision in Intermittent Exotropia. A.A.A.O., 29: 12.

Hebbard, F.W. (1952): Consistency of Clinical Data. Opt. Weekly, 43: 1011, 1269, 1597.

*Hebbard, F.W. (1961): Case Analysis. The O-Eye-O. Vol. 4.

Hirsch, M.J. (1948): A Clinical Investigation of a Method of Testing Phorias at 40 cms., A.A.A.O., 25: 492.

Hirsch, M.J. (1963): The Refraction of Children in Vision of Children, Chilton Books, Phila.

Hirsch, M.J., Alpern, M. & Schultz, H.L. (1948): The Variation of Phoria with Age. A.A.A.O., 25: 535.

Hofstetter, H.W. (1945): The Zone of Clear Single Binocular Vision. A.A.A.O., 22: 301, 361.

Hofstetter, H.W. (1948): The Accommodative Range Through the Near Correction. A.A.A.O., 25: 275.

Hofstetter, H.W. (1949): The Function of Visual Training in Optometric Practice. The O-Eye-O, 18 (2).

Hofstetter, H.W. (1949): A Survey of Practices in Prescribing Presbyopic Adds. A.A.A.O., 26: 483.

*Hofstetter, H.W. (1950): The A.M.A. Method of Appraisal of Visual Efficiency. A.A.A.O., 27: 55.

Hofstetter, H.W. (1954): Optometric Contributions in Accommodation and Convergence Studies. J.A.O.A., 22: 431.

*Hofstetter, H.W. (1955): An Illustrative Case Analysis Involving Accommodation and Convergence Findings. A.A.A.O., 32: 94.

Hofstetter, H.W. (1968): A Revised Schematic For Graphical Analysis Of The Accommodative Convergence Relationship, Canadian J.O., 30 (2): 49.

Humphriss, D. (1950): How Much Shall I Give? South African Optometrist, 17: 7.

Humphriss, D. (1958): Periodic Refractive Fluctuations in the Healthy Eye. B.J. Phys. Opt., 15: 30.

Hurst, W.A. (1964): The Determination of the Near Point Working Distance of the Public School Child. J.A.O.A., 35: 610.

Knoll, H.A. (1960): Temporary Asthenopia Following A Cylinder Axis Change – A Case Report. A.A.A.O., 37: 32.

Kratz, J.D. (1954): A Consideration of Convergence and Divergence Anomalies. A.A.A.O., 31: 170.

Kratz, J.D. (1959): An Interpretation of the Blur Findings. J.A.O.A., Jan. 30: 401.

*Lebensohn, J.E. (1953): Anisophoria, Anisometropia and the Final Prescription. A.J. Oph. 36: 643.

Lebensohn, J.E. (1955): Nature of Innervational Hyperphoria. A.J. Oph., 39: 654.

Lebensohn, J.E. (1965): A Chronology of Ophthalmic Progress. A.J. Oph., 59: 883.

Lederer, J. (1948): The Theory of Incomplete Accommodation. Australasion J. Opt., April.

*Lesser, K. (1934): Fundamentals of Procedure and Analysis in Optometric Examination.

Lindsay, J. (1949): Prescribing Prisms. Optics.

*Lopez, R.B. (1953): A Discussion of Ocular Syndrome. O.J.R.O., 40 (24): 39.

*Maddox, E.E. (1893): The Clinical Use of Prisms and the Decentering of Lenses, 2nd ed. John Wright & Co., Bristol, England.

Manas, L. (1950-1952): Relation of Refractive Error to Optometric Tests. Opt. Weekly, 41: 1323, 1473; 42: 703, 991, 1755; 43: 581, 1725.

Manas, L. (1955): The Inconsistency of the ACA Ratio. A.A.A.O., 32: 304.

Marlow, F.W. (1932): The Technique of the Prolonged Occlusion Test. A.J. Oph., 19: 194.

Marlow, F.W. (1924): Relative Position of Rest of Eyes and Prolonged Occlusion. A.J. Oph., 7: 484.

Marton, H.B. (1951): Some Problems of Heterophoria. B.J. Phys. Opt., 8: 100.

Michaels, D.D. (1953): A Clinical Study of Convergence Insufficiency. A.A.A.O., 30: 65.

Michaels, D.D. (1955): Some Problems of Binocular Vision. A.A.A.O., 32: 409.

*Michaels, D.D. (1955 and 1956): Optometric Diagnosis. Opt. Weekly, 46: 935, 1103, 1281, 1445, 1765, 1931; 47: 589, 635, 689, 1923, 2061, 2231.

Morgan, M.W. (1944a): The Clinical Aspects of Accommodation and Convergence. A.A.A.O., 21: 301.

Morgan, M.W. (1944b): Analysis of Clinical Data. A.A.A.O., 21: 477.

Morgan, M.W. (1947): An Investigation of the Use of Stereoscopic Targets in Orthoptics. A.A.A.O., 24: 411.

*Morgan, M.W. (1950): Comparison of Clinical Methods of Measuring Accommodative-Convergence. A.A.A.O., 27: 385.

Morgan, M.W. (1954): The Prescribing of Prism. The Calif. Optometrist, August-Sept.

Morgan, M.W. (1960): Anomalies of the Visual Neuromuscular System of the Aging Patient and Their Correction in Vision of the Aging Patient, Chilton Books, Phila.

*Morgan, M.W. (1964): The Analysis of Clinical Data. Opt. Weekly, Orig. Opt. Weekly, 1948, 39: 1811, 1843.

*Morgan, M.W. (1968): Accommodation and Vergences. A.A.A.O., 45: 417.

Morgan, M.W. & Peters, H.B. (1951): Accommodative Convergence in presbyopia. A.A.A.O., 28: 3.

Nathan, J. (1957): Small Errors of Refraction. B.J. Phys. Opt., 14: 204.

Neill, J.C. (1963): Contact Lenses for Young People, in Vision of Children. Chilton Books, Phila.

Neumueller, J.F. (1946): The Correlation of Optometric Binocular Measurements for Refractive Diagnosis. A.A.A.O., 23: 235.

Nicholls, J.V.V. (1950): Heterophoria and Depth Perception in Aviation. A.J. Oph., 33: 1497, 1775, 1891.

Ogle, K.N. (1956): Stereoscopic Acuity and the Role of Convergence. J. Opt. Soc. America, 46: 269.

Ogle, K.N.; Martens, T.G.; Dyer, J.A. (1967): Oculomotor Imbalance In Binocular Vision and Fixation Disparity, Lea & Febiger, Phila.

Ogle, K.N. & Prangen, A. de H. (1953): Observations On Vertical Divergence And Phoria, Arch. Oph., 49: 313.

Parks, M.M. (1958): Isolated Cyclo-Vertical Muscle Palsy. Arch. Oph., 60: 1027.

Pascal, J.I. (1949): Hyperphoria – Paretic or Comitant. Opt. World, 37 (10): 20.

Percival, A. (1928): The Prescribing of Spectacles. J. Wright, Bristol, England.

*Pitts, D.C. & Hofstetter, H.W. (1959): The Manned-Line Graphing of Zone of Clear Single Binocular Vision. J.A.O.A., 31: 51.

Plondre, A.R. & Howell, W.H. (1965): Lateral Heterophoria: Symptoms, Measurement and Treatment. J.A.O.A., 35: 811.

Posner, A. (1951): The Prescribing Prisms for Hyperphoria. A.J. Oph., 34 (2, Pt. 1): 197.

Pratt, C.B. (1962): The Variation in Phorias With Time After Dissociation and Magnitude of Convergence. A.A.A.O., 39: 257.

Roy, R.L. (1956): Headaches and Binocular Stress. Opt. Weekly, 47: 815.

Roy, R.L. (1958): Symptomotology of Binocular Stress. Opt. Weekly, 49: 907.

**Schapero, M. (1955): The Characteristics of Ten Basic Visual Training Problems. A.A.A.O., 32: 337.*

Schapero, M. & Levy, M. (1953): The Variation of Proximal Convergence with Change in Distance. A.A.A.O., 30: 403.

Scobee, R.G. (1952): The Oculorotary Muscles, 2nd ed. C.V. Mosby Co., St. Louis.

Scobee, R.G. & Green, E.L. (1951): Further Studies in the Relationship Between Heterophoria and Prism Vergence. A.J. Oph., 34: 401.

Sheard, C. (1923): A Dozen Worthwhile Points in Ocular Refraction. A.J. Phys. Opt., 4: 443.

Sheard, C. (1930): Zones of Ocular Comfort. A.A.A.O., 7: 9.

Sheard, C. (1931): Ocular Discomfort and Its Relief. E.E.N.T., July.

Shepard, C.F. (1941): The Most Probable "Expecteds." Opt. Weekly., 32.

Sloan, L.L.; Sears, M.L. & Jablonski, M.D. (1960): Convergence-Accommodation Relationships. Arch. Oph., 63.

Sloane, A.E.; Dunphy, E.B.; Emmons, W.V.; Gallagher, J. (1954): A Comparison of Refraction Results in the Same Individuals. A.J. Oph., 37.

Snell, A.C. (1953): Relation of Headache to Single Binocular Vision and Functional Monocularity. Arch. Oph., 51.

Snell, A.G. & Lueck, I.B. (1965): Presbyopia. Refraction, I.O.C., 5: 2.

Stein, H. & Hofstetter, H.W. (1951): Effect of Prolonged Television Viewing on Certain Optometric Findings. A.A.A.O., 28: 10.

Stillerman, M.L. (1965): The Refraction Failure. Refraction, I.O.C., 5: 2.

Tait, E.F. (1951): Accommodative Convergence. A.J. Oph., 34: 8.

Textor, R.T. (1949): Clinical Indications for Prescribing Prisms. A.A.A.O., 26: 12.

**Tiffin, J. (1948): Eyes for the Job. J. of N.Y. State Opt. Assoc. 15: 2.*

Tubis, R.A. (1954): An Evaluation Of Vertical Divergence Tests On The Basis Of Fixation Disparity, A.A.A.O., 31: 12.

Walsh, R. (1946): The Measurement and Correction of Hyperphorias in Refractive Cases. A.A.A.O., 23: 9.

Wardale, P.J. (1961): Near Vision Additions for Non-Presbyopes. Oph. Opt., 1: 3.

Weber, R.A. (1950): Ocular Fatigue. Arch. Oph., 43: 2.

Wick, R.E. (1950): Geriatrics and Optometry. A.A.A.O., 27: 3, 4, 5.

Wick, R.E. (1960): Management of the Aging Practice in Optometric Practice. In Vision of the Aging Patient, Chilton Books, Phila.

Wick, R.E. (1963): Management of the Young Patient in Optometric Practice. In Vision of Children, Chilton Books, Phila.

Problems of Aphakia 22

I. PROBLEMS OF CORRECTED APHAKIA

A. Refractive

1. *Hyperopia* (Cowan, 1949)

a. *12.6 Diopters of curvature hyperopia* is the average for the emmetropic aphakic.

(1) For each 3 mm. of axial length the dioptric value becomes 4.00 D. instead of 3.00 D. per mm. as in the normal eye, provided the lens is placed on the anterior principal focus.

(2) The principal points, which were at 1.505 and 1.631 mm. behind the cornea, now coincide at the vertex of the optical zone of the cornea. The principal planes of the corrected eye lie between the correcting lens and the eye.

(3) The nodal points, which were 7.13 and 7.256 mm. behind the cornea, now coincide in one point, located 7.8 mm. behind the cornea for the uncorrected eye. The nodal points of the corrected system lie 4 mm. closer to the cornea than in the phakic eye.

(4) The anterior principal focal distance is 23.214 mm. instead of 16.74 mm.

(5) The retinal image tends to be formed 31.014 mm. behind the cornea or 7.014 mm. behind the actual retina itself.

b. The Rx is +9.75 D. at the anterior principal focus of the eye.

(1) The Rx is +10.75 D. at a position 14 mm. in front of the cornea.

c. *Estimate of the resultant error* (Leahy, 1955)

(1) The error may be calculated by the formula: *+11.00 plus ½ the error prior to the cataract*

(a) For a 10.00 D. myope prior to cataract: +11.00 + ½(−10) = +6.00.

(b) For an 8.00 D. hyperope prior to cataract: +11.00 + ½(+8) = +15.00.

(2) The removal of the crystalline lens neutralizes approximately 24.00 D. of myopia.

(a) Batra (1967) refracted 100 cases that were emmetropic prior to cataract surgery and found the following results in the post-surgical refraction:

[1] Ninety-three percent of the cases needed a spherical correction between +9.00 and +11.00.

[2] Eighty percent of the cases exhibited astigmatism of from +1.00 to +2.00 D.

[3] Ninety-one percent of the cases revealed the astigmatism against-the-rule.

[4] The average case could be corrected by a +10.00 to +11.00 sphere combined with a +1.50 to +2.00 D. cylinder against-the-rule.

2. *Direction of the visual axis*

a. The shift in the location of the principal points changed the orientation of the visual axis (Cowan, 1949, 1953).

(1) The eye must turn 2° farther out to place the image on the fovea.

(2) Angle kappa disappears and the visual axis coincides with the center of the pupil.

(a) This may cause the eye to converge for near to an extra extent equivalent to 5° further than previously required (Stimson, 1957).

3. *Aberrations of the cornea* were most noticeable (Cowan, 1953).

a. The crystalline lens usually assists in neutralizing the corneal aberrations.

b. Surgery induces optical irregularities of the cornea and increases or creates astigmatism.

c. An irregular pupil may result from the surgery.

4. *Greater sensitivity to glare* and excess light becomes evident.

a. The absorption credited to the crystalline lens is absent.

(1) The eye becomes more sensitive to the increased transmission of violet and ultraviolet wavelengths.

(a) A transitory bluish vision may become apparent following exposure to a bright light.

5. *Acuity*

a. 20/20 vision with a cataract spectacle lens may be only 20/25 true vision.

b. If the vision is truly 20/20, the increased magnification will frequently permit a recording of 20/10.

B. Magnification

1. *Image size increases* approximately 30% (Cowan, 1953).

a. The increase is larger if the eye was previously myopic than if it was emmetropic and larger if emmetropic than if hyperopic.

(1) The retinal image size is 23.21/16.74 (the relative anterior principal foci) which equals 1.38x, but at 14 mm. in front of the cornea, the magnification actually becomes 1.33x (a 33% increase in size).

2. The aphakic eye actually has four different kinds of images, when size of the image is considered (Pascal, 1954).

a. The clearly focused retinal image of the emmetrope, prior to surgery, may be given the value of 1.00.

b. The blurred retinal image of the aphakic eye has the relative value of 0.96.

c. The optical image of the aphakic eye, located behind the retina, has the relative value of 1.35.

d. The clear corrected image of the aphakic, on the retina, has the relative value of 1.30.

3. The formula for magnification due to the power factor may be expressed as follows:

a. $P = 1 \div (1 - V_o h)$

(1) V_o is the vertex power of the lens in diopters and h is the distance of the spectacle lens from the effective optical center of the crystalline lens in meter.

(a) For example: given a +11.00 D. lens, 14 mm. before the cornea, and allowing 5.7 mm. from the cornea to the center of the crystalline lens, or a total of 19.7 mm. from correcting lens to center of crystalline lens.

[1] $P = 1 \div [1 - (11)(0.0197)] = 1 \div (1 - 0.217) = 1 \div 0.793 = 1.28\text{x M.}$

b. *If the error is axial,* the magnification of the ophthalmic lens is the same as for emmetropia.

c. *If the error is refractive or curvature,* the magnification depends on whether the cornea, curvature of the crystalline lens, or index of the lens is the chief agent.

(1) If the ametropia is refractive, the magnification will increase with the degree of plus and decrease with the degree of minus needed. The percent of change is equal to the power of the lens needed in diopters multiplied by the distance of that lens from the "seat" of the refractive ametropia.

(a) If it lies on the cornea, only the shape factor will influence the magnification.

(b) If the seat is the curvature or index of the crystalline lens, the magnification compared to the emmetropic eye will be 0.5% per diopter.

(2) If refractive but half corneal and half lenticular, one of the following may occur:

(a) Magnification will vary for axial cases from 26% for a –5.00 lens to 00 for a +5.00 lens.

(b) Magnification will vary for curvature cases from 36% for a –6.00 D. lens to 5% for a +6.00 D. lens.

(c) The only prospect of equalizing aniseikonia where one eye is inoperable and the other is highly hyperopic is with spectacles (Obrig, 1944).

4. Even when both eyes are aphakic and the magnification is binocular, the patient requires several weeks before the previous size adjustments are forgotten. In the interim, false orientation is exceedingly troublesome, particularly since most aphakics are elderly people who are least adaptable.

5. In addition to the central magnification, *peripheral magnification of the field* also occurs, so that an ordinary visual field of 48° tends to cover the retinal area usually covered by a 62° field, a magnification of 1.3x.

C. Pincushion Distortion (Spherical Aberration)

1. Straight lines become curves and the linear world becomes one consisting of parabolas.

2. Verticals change and writhe as fixation changes from one point to another.

a. The aphakic spectacle wearer learns to hold the eyes motionless and to move his head.

(1) Ordinary spectacles provide a central area of undistorted view through 12 mm. of the lens, while aspheric spectacles extend this area to 26 mm.

3. If the wearer looks at his feet, all straight lines curve away like a spiral staircase.

4. With the eyes centered in the lens in the primary position, peripheral lines form a symmetrical pincushion.

a. If the gaze is depressed, the curves at the bottom tend to straighten but those overhead tend to dip deeper.

5. A change in the vertex distance from the normal 10 mm. for aphakic spectacles by 5 mm. will tend to alter this distortion by 27 to 30%.

a. The distortion is reduced by moving the lens farther from the eye, but other effects of the cataract lens are worsened.

D. Limitations of the Field

1. The *Jack-in-the Box* or *Roving Ring Scotoma* (Welsh, 1966, 1967).

a. If a –12.00 D. lens, 44 mm. in diameter, is placed before the aphakic eye, the margins will exhibit 26.4 Δ (22 x 1.2 Δ), according to Prentice's formula.

(1) As 1 Δ approximately equals .573°, the amount of bending at the peripheral edge will be 13.2°.

(2) A peripheral ray of light at an angle of 62° incidence will miss the eye entirely (Fig. XXII-1).

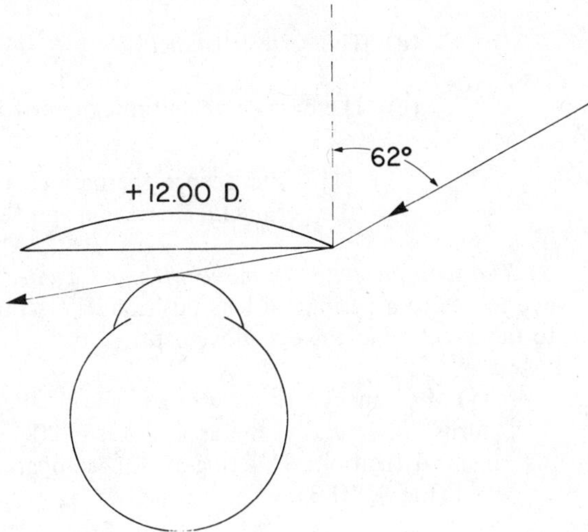

Figure XXII-1 – Illustrating how a peripheral ray at an angle of 62° is bent by a strong lens so as to miss entering the eye altogether (after Welsh).

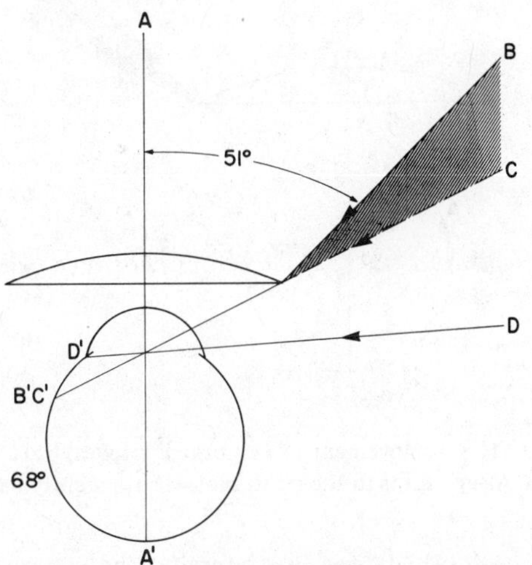

Figure XXII-2 – Another means of illustrating the ring scotoma (after Stimson). The visible field of 52°, from A to B is magnified by the strong lens to occupy 62° on the retina from A′ to B′. Area of the field from C to D occupies retinal peripheral area C′ to D′. Area of field B to C is not represented on retina, forming scotoma.

b. *A circular blind area will begin at about 51° and extend to about 64°.*

(1) The range of useful view will extend from about 35 to 55° with a scotoma of 12 to 18° completely surrounding the field in a ring (Fig. XXII-2). The actual range will depend upon the following factors:

(a) The effective power at the periphery of the lens

(b) The size of the lens

(c) The size of the pupil

(d) The vertex distance

(e) The base curve and thickness of the correction lens

[1] The deeper the base curve, the larger the total field but the greater the peripheral aberration and the smaller the useful field.

c. *The scotoma tends to move with an "against motion"* to the motion of the eye. As the eye moves to a peripheral lens position, the scotoma moves to a more central one opposite to the direction of the eye movement.

(1) For an eye fixing straight ahead, the blind area begins 51° laterally. If the eye turns 30° laterally, the area moves in 20°, and the blind area now begins 32° from the central fixation. This ring at 32° is apparent whether the motion is up, down, in, or out (Fig. XXII-3).

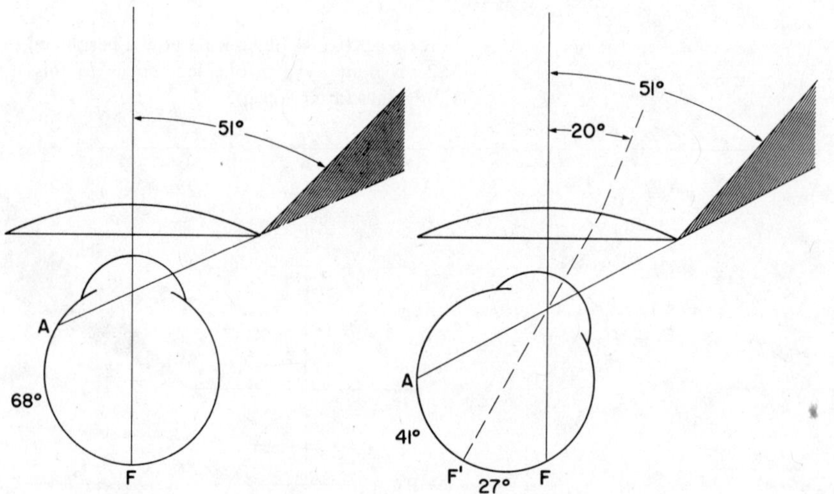

Figure XXII-3 – Movement of eye bringing fovea, F, to position, F', and bringing ring scotoma closer to fovea. As eye turns to the right, scotoma apparently moves opposite to eye.

(a) To see 30° laterally, the eye must actually turn 42° because of the bending action of the periphery of the lens.

(b) As the shift varies with the extent of rotation of the eye, and since it completely encircles the field, it is known as the *"Roving Ring Scotoma."*

(2) When the patient sees an object, and turns his eye towards it, the scotoma may move a sufficient distance inwards to occlude it. Upon shifting his eye from it, the scotoma again shifts and the object becomes visible again. This produces what has become known as the "Jack-in-the-Box" phenomena (Fig. XXII-4).

d. Although an aspheric lens tends to reduce the width of the scotomatous ring, the wide field of so-called panoramic vision cannot be secured with either spheric or aspheric cataract lenses by means of eye movements. Panoramic vision requires rapid head turning to keep the object within the useful field.

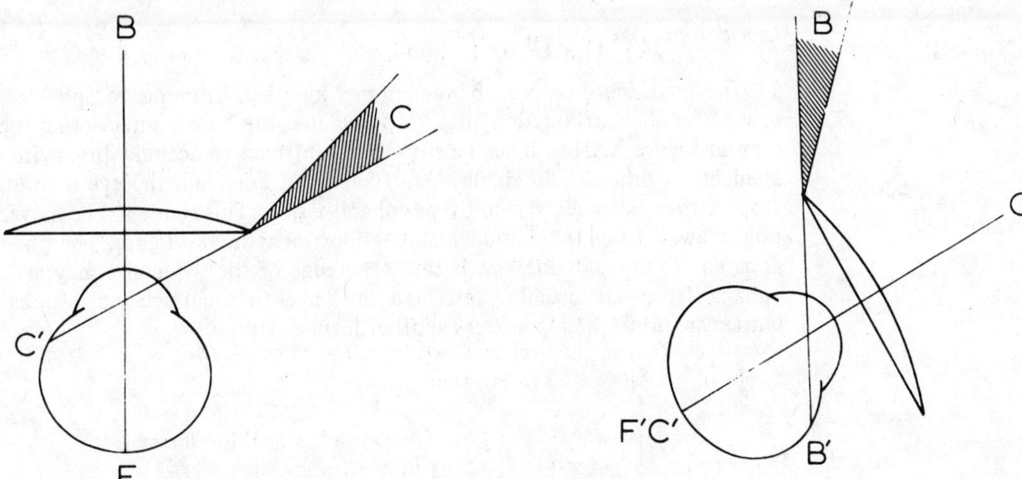

Figure XXII-4 – Jack-in-the-box phenomenom. As head and eye turn towards an object previously invisible in the ring scotoma, scotoma courses across retinal field from C′ to F, and objects lying in the field between B and the scotoma become visible and invisible, popping in and out of view.

2. *Errors in Field Charting*

a. Since the real field covers a greater expanse of retina due to the magnification of the lenses, a 30% "instrument" error would reveal a constricted field.

(1) The non-corrected aphakic field would appear larger than normal due to a slight shift of the nodal points back. The corrected eye would have a smaller field due to the shift of the nodal points forward.

(2) The relative sizes of the normal, uncorrected, and corrected fields are shown in Figure XXII-5.

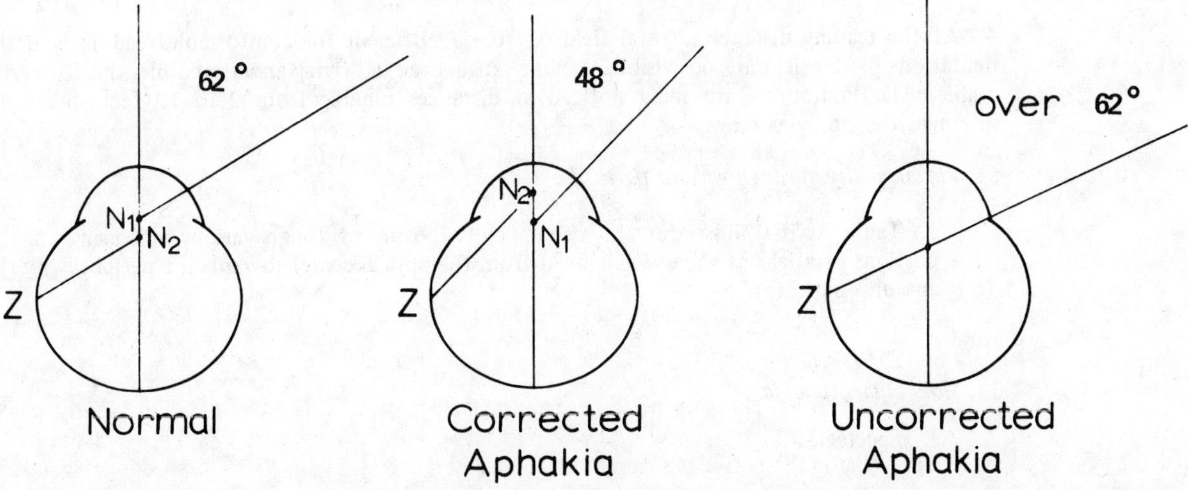

Figure XXII-5 – Relative Angular sizes of projected visual fields from identical retinal points, z, under described circumstances. As the aphakic correction magnifies the retinal image, the larger retinal area projects to a smaller real field, and the measured blind spot size in the aphakic may represent a much enlarged retinal blindspot.

b. The useful field of vision may be so limited that serious neurological and ocular diseases ordinarily apparent by field charts may escape clinical notice (Troutman 1963).

3. *Quasi-scotoma* (Welsh, 1967) .

a. The quasi scotoma is a phenomenom which is not unique to aphakic corrections but is caused by the introduction of a stop-like aperture barely intersecting the line of sight. As seen in Figure XXII-6, if such a stop barely intrudes to occlude direct vision of a light, a star at night, or other bright single small fixation objects, and the eye is rotated away from the stop, it then becomes visible by peripheral vision. This is due to the movement of the nodal points away from the occluder and is illustrated in the figure. The phenomenom is more apparent to the aphakic eye because the edge of the spectacles may act as the stop, since aphakic lenses are usually prescribed smaller than usual spectacle lenses are, and often in lenticular form, which produces another form of stop.

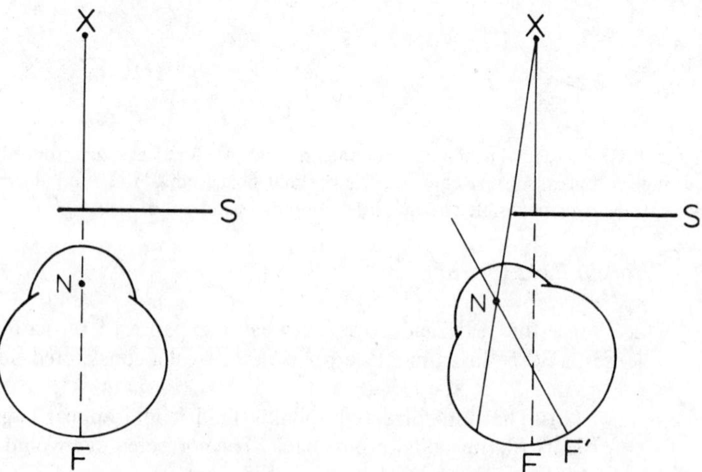

Figure XXII-6 – Pseudo-scotoma. The rotation of the eye away from the edge of a stop, S, which blocks a ray from object X, to fovea F, enables a beam to be bent into the eye from a more peripheral course and thus render X visible.

4. At the reading distance, a total field of 70° is sufficient for comfortable reading, and the limitations of the field are not visible. At long range, even in driving an automobile, the 70° is still usable. The limitations are most noticed at distances ranging from 2 to 10 feet, the usual intermediate and living ranges.

5. *Visual acuity through various parts of a cataract lens.*

a. Table XXII-1 illustrates the visual acuity possible through various increasing angular portions of a lens as the eye is moved from the optical center towards the periphery by the amounts indicated.

E. Fusion

1. *Monocular Aphakia*

a. Spectacles

(1) Aniseikonia of 30% ordinarily prevents fusion, although fusion of the central field is reported possible and existent.

(a) The problem is not merely due to the magnification but also to the varying prismatic effect in varying portions of the periphery of the lenses.

(b) Tests and measurements of the phorias are often variable and unreliable.

(c) Both prism prescription or muscle surgery are often unsuccessful (Cowan, 1953).

[1] Goar (1955) disagreed and claimed that fusion sufficient for good usage did occur.
[2] He believed one danger of permitting cataracts to become hypermature was that the continued expanse of occlusion may lead to a further weakening of previously existing fusion.

Table XXII-1

Types of Lens	central 10°	next 15°	next 15°	next 15°	outer 35°
Regular	*20/20*	*20/40*	*20/80-*	*blind*	*motion*
Aspheric A	*20/20*	*20/30+*	*20/60+*	*blind*	*motion*
Aspheric B	*20/20*	*20/25*	*20/40*	*blind*	*motion*
Contact Lens	*20/20*	*20/20*	*20/20*	*20/30–*	*20/30-20/40*

b. Contact Lenses

(1) Fusional problems such as suppression may be related to the length of time of occlusion.

(a) Many tests of fusion attempted upon monocular aphakics have neither accurately described nor measured the situation. Imbalances tend to decrease with the wear of contact lenses.

[1] Cowan did not feel that the results with contact lenses were as good as claimed, but Rosenbloom (1953), Foley (1954), Spaeth and O'Neill (1960) and Goar (1955) reported cases of successful binocularity using them.

(2) Prismatic problems are automatically reduced or eliminated with contact lenses.

(3) *Dominancy*

(a) If the aphakic eye is the dominant one, the contact lens is usually well accepted, but if it is the non-dominant one, the patient tends to rely upon the non-aphakic dominant eye even if acuity is not quite so good.

(4) *Nearpoint*

(a) The phakic eye accommodates as an object is brought nearer, while the aphakic eye requires a +2.50 add for 16 inches. Even at 20 feet, the phakic eye accommodates 1/6 diopter.

(b) As the object approaches the nearpoint, the image in the phakic eye is smaller but clearer, while that of the aphakic eye is larger but blurred.

[1] The aniseikonia increases.

[2] The prismatic imbalance increases.

[a] In cases where the patient requires a spectacle correction for the phakic eye, the contact lens power for the aphakic eye should be such that a spectacle lens of similar power in the vertical meridian to that worn before the phakic eye can be required to be worn over the contact lens on the aphakic eye. This would eliminate vertical imbalance problems at near caused by the distance correction when the patient turns the eyes down to the nearpoint portion of the bifocal lens.

[b] As seen below, such a combination might produce a telescopic effect which would alter the original aniseikonia. If the aniseikonia were increased, the added problem thus induced would offset the gain in vertical balance.

[3] Ogle et al. (1958), felt that this still did not preclude fusion.

(c) *Progressive addition lenses,* such as the Omnifocal and Varilux, were excellently suited for cases of aphakia, according to Koetting (1968).

[1] For monocular cases, the progressive range would help to alleviate, within a limited area, the objections of inequality of clarity between the aphakic and phakic eye, as the fixation progressed from far to near.

[2] Koetting quoted Brenns as having found ready acceptance of such lens types by aphakics wearing contact lenses for distance.

[3] The shape of the pupil, whether round or keyholed, did not indicate a difference in percentage of acceptance of the progressive addition. However, Koetting reported that those with keyhole pupils required +0.50 D. more addition than did those with round pupils.

[a] It may be conjectured that the keyhole pupil interfered with precise fixation through the relatively smaller near field of the lens, and that the additional plus power enabled the wearer to use portions of the intermediate power area for near vision.

(5) *Magnification differences* are the chief problem.

(a) These need to be equalized as much as possible.

(b) Theoretically, a thin contact lens as compared to a thin spectacle lens reduces magnification from 28% to about 5.5 to 9.0% (Dyer and Ogle, 1960). If the shape factor is added, the magnification of the contact lens averages 11% (Troutman, 1963). Ogle, Burian, and Bannon (1958) report a mean residual error of 9%.

(c) The reduction or elimination of the magnification by a contact lens depends on the following factors:

[1] The refractive state of the aphakic eye prior to the cataract extraction

[2] Error of the phakic eye

[3] The effect on the power of the cornea of the surgery

[4] Whether 1 and 2 are axial, refractive, or both

[5] The factors involved in the design of the contact lens

(d) Axial ametropia

[1] If a spectacle lens is placed at the anterior focal point of the eye, the magnification is the same as if the eye were emmetropic despite its actual error.

[a] For the myopic eye, the magnification can be increased 1½% per diopter when moved to the cornea.

[b] For the hyperopic eye, the magnification is decreased by the same value.

[2] If both eyes use contact lenses, the principal results are as shown in Table XXII-2.

[a] Percent magnification due to power factor only of the retinal image relative to that of the retinal image of an emmetropic eye, for eyes of various axial ametropias after cataract extraction and after the total refractive state has been corrected by corneal contact lenses (Ogle, 1950):

Table XXII-2

Refractive State	Magnification %	Refractive State	Magnification %
+6	*-2.5*	*-1*	*+10*
+5	*-1*	*-2*	*+11.5*
+4	*+1*	*-3*	*+13*
+3	*+3*	*-4*	*+15*
+2	*+4.5*	*-5*	*+17*
+1	*+6*	*-6*	*+18*
0	*+8*		

[3] If one eye uses a contact lens and the other a spectacle, the shape factor table must be added (see Chapter VIII on Aniseikonia).

(e) If the refractive ametropia is half corneal and half lenticular, the aniseikonia for various corrections for axial and refractive states in contact lenses are as follows:

[1] If ametropia is equal for both eyes:

[a] Axial – 15% in high myopia to 2% in high hyperopia

[b] Refractive – 10% regardless of amount

[c] ½ axial, ½ refractive – 9% for –5.00 to 7% for +6.00.

[2] Emmetropia in both eyes:

[a] 13% if no lens before the phakic eye; 10% if a zero lens is placed before the phakic eye.

(6) *Probability of Fusion*

(a) Residual aniseikonia is rarely eliminated, and approximately 9–11% remains at best.

[1] $\frac{\text{larger focal length}}{\text{smaller focal length}} - 100 = \%$ magnification

(b) Large size differences still permit fusion of small objects, near the point of fixation, due to the larger size of Panum's areas near the macular region.

[1] Outside these regions disparity increases rapidly to the periphery.

[a] An aniseikonia of 3% would cause objects farther than 4 to 5° of arc to be outside of Panum's area, and only that small area of the frontal plane would remain within the region of single binocular vision (Troutman, 1963).

[b] Aniseikonia of 2% or less would result in a defect of the optical relationships and a loss of the field of stereopsis, although a one degree field of central stereopsis might still be revealed éven with an aniseikonia of 10% (Troutman).

[c] A difference of 0.75% to 1½%, prevalent in 3 to 5% of the population, still produces subjective symptoms.

(c) If visual acuity is 20/20 or better, the threshold is 0.25 to 0.5%.

[1] The threshold increases as acuity decreases.

[2] Three to four times the threshold is considered significant.

[3] Differences of 5 to 6% rarely result in binocularity.

(d) Since peripheral images play an important part in fusional movements, it is difficult to reconcile unilateral aphakia and fusion. A form of suppression or replacement may occur which is not readily detectable.

(e) *Effects of Dominancy*

[1] If the aphakia is in the dominant eye and that is the eye that is occluded, the patient is likely to be unhappy. It may be necessary to permit use of the dominant eye upon occasion.

[2] If the non-dominant eye is the aphakic one, occlusion is accepted more readily. However, even in this instance the eye should be allowed to see part of the time, as with a nearpoint Rx.

[3] If the aphakic eye had 20/40 vision or less and the non-aphakic eye had 20/70, the patient probably preferred the non-aphakic eye (Leahy, 1955).

[a] The aphakic eye must be at least two lines better than the other eye to make a cataract lens acceptable, if the non-cataractous eye has visual acuity poorer than 20/70.

[4] One method used is to correct the phakic eye for far and the aphakic eye for near.

(f) *Nearpoint*

[1] Since total absence of accommodation exists in the aphakic eye, prismatic effects of the Rx and the add for one eye while the other accommodates present a fusional problem.

[a] Lubkin et al. (1960), got stereopsis with 12 prism diopters of base-in if both eyes had 20/20 vision. They added two to four Δ for the nearpoint and held the print high enough to center them in the lenses of the separate near Rx's. While they got stereopsis, comfort was not always present.

c. *Spectacle Lens combinations*

(1) Attempts have been made to equalize the resultant size differences in monocular contact lens applications by the use of either size difference lenses in spectacles or by constructing a Galilean telescope with the spectacle as the objective and the contact lens as the ocular (Boeder, 1938).

(a) The use of a size element in the spectacles before the eye is often not acceptable because of cosmetic reasons, the weight of the lenses, or the complexity of the optics required.

(b) The use of the Galilean telescope requires two contact lenses instead of one along with a complex optical refractive arrangement before the phakic eye.

(2) Enoch (1968) successfully applied a clinical technique utilizing a minifying telescope before the aphakic eye. This technique is described as follows:

(a) Since eikonometers are not readily available, arbitrary size differences of 6-8% are selected. Boeder recommended that a size difference closer to 9% be used.

(b) This correction does not attempt to fully correct the aniseikonia but merely to bring the patient within a range permitting fusion.

(c) The lesser the size difference for which correction is made, the lesser the lens power is required, the lesser the weight of the unit, and the lesser is the amount of slab-off prism needed in most instances.

(d) The angular magnification, M, may be expressed in terms of the refractive power, (F), of the focal length, (f), with the subfix (–) representing a minus element, and (+) representing a plus element. The arrow indicates direction of course of light.

[1] $f_{(+)} = - f_{(-)} \vec{M}$; ($\vec{M} = - \frac{F_{(-)}}{F_{(+)}} = - \frac{f_{(+)}}{f_{(-)}}$) for magnification.

[2] $- f_{(-)} = f_{(+)} \overleftarrow{M}$; ($\overleftarrow{M} = - \frac{f_{(-)}}{f_{(+)}} = - \frac{F_{(+)}}{F_{(-)}}$) for minification.

[3] $f_{(+)} = - f_{(-)} + d$ (d = difference in focal length between units)

[a] d is used as the difference in vertex distance between the spectacle lens and the contact lens.

[4] To compute for the required minifying correction with the reverse telescope:

$$\text{[a] } F_{(+)} = \frac{1 - \overleftarrow{M}}{d} \text{ or } F_{(-)} = \frac{F_{(+)}}{\overleftarrow{M}} \quad (\overleftarrow{M} = \text{minification \%}).$$

[5] Rounding off the results to 0.12 D. may introduce errors of ±2% and change the required vertex. Enoch has derived a table of common possibilities to avoid this error.

(e) Enoch's Table of Sample Solutions in 0.12 D Steps:

[1] Table XXII-3

Aphakic Minification %	Vertex D. mm.	F(+) D.S.	F(-) D.S.	Phakic Magnification %
12.3	15.4	8.00	9.12	14.1
11.8	15.7	7.50	8.50	13.3
11.1	15.8	7.00	7.87	12.5
11.2	13.9	8.00	9.00	12.5
10.3	15.9	6.50	7.25	11.5
10.0	11.1	9.00	10.00	11.1
9.7	13.8	7.00	7.75	10.7
9.4	15.8	6.00	6.62	10.4
8.7	13.4	6.50	7.12	9.6
8.7	16.6	5.25	5.75	9.5
8.6	10.7	8.00	8.75	9.4
8.3	15.1	5.50	6.00	9.1
8.1	11.7	7.00	7.62	8.9
8.0	13.9	5.75	6.25	8.6
7.9	10.9	7.25	7.87	8.6
7.7	12.9	6.00	6.50	8.3
7.6	16.2	4.62	5.00	8.1
7.4	11.9	6.25	6.75	8.0
7.2	15.4	4.75	5.12	7.9
7.2	14.6	4.87	5.25	7.7
7.1	11.0	6.50	7.00	7.7
6.9	14.0	5.00	5.37	7.4
6.9	10.2	6.75	7.25	7.4
6.6	12.7	5.25	5.62	7.1
6.7	9.5	7.00	7.50	7.1
6.3	11.6	5.50	5.87	6.8
6.1	15.7	3.87	4.12	6.5
6.0	10.6	5.75	6.12	6.5
5.9	14.7	4.00	4.25	6.3
5.8	9.8	6.00	6.37	6.2
5.7	13.8	4.12	4.37	6.1
5.6	9.1	6.25	6.62	6.0
5.6	13.1	4.25	4.50	5.9

(3) The negative correction is placed in the spectacle frame and the positive element is added to the power of the contact lens.

(a) If the computed $F_{(+)}$ component is added to the correction, as determined in the spectacle plane, and the vertex distance is then allowed for movement back to the cornea for the sum of the two, an error is then created in both values. The correction should first be modified for the corneal position, and then the computed telescopic value added to it.

(b) Enoch recommended identical base curves and lens thicknesses for both eyes in the spectacle lenses to minimize size differences induced by the spectacle lens factors and the employment of frames with rocking pads and cable or riding bow temples for accurate placement of the lenses before the eyes.

(c) Flat-top bifocals with possible slab-off prisms are recommended to correct for vertical induced prism due to both off axis viewing and displacement of the contact lens in the downward gaze.

(4) Both spectacles and contact lenses must be prescribed at the same time. As the contact lens not only acquires added plus power in being moved from the spectacle to the corneal plane, but also the addition of plus power for the telescopic effect, the resultant lenses frequently approach or exceed +20.00 D.

(5) Errors

(a) Errors may also result while evaluating the resultant refractive state with the telescope in place.

(b) The spectacles are adjusted for proper vertex distance since small adjustments in this distance often improve resolution.

(c) The contact lens component is the correction combined with an add for the telescopic element. By noting its conjugate in space without the spectacle, by either retinoscopy or the push-up test, the value of $F_{(+)}$ may be checked.

(d) Centration problems due to the movement of the heavy plus contact lens and the effects of iridectomy, and lid aperture may affect the results.

[1] If needed for centering, larger corneal lenses scleral lenses, or lenses with toric back curves for corneal astigmatism, may be used.

[2] The corneal lenses are fitted on K in an attempt to limit movement, and a black magic marker, to which the eye is insensitive, is used to block out iridectomy zones which cause poorer imagery.

(e) The differences in power produce prismatic effect upon looking through the spectacle plane.

[1] The flat-top bifocal is therefore fitted rather high.

[2] A priori estimates of the slab-off prism needed are not satisfactory due to motion of the high power contact lens which occurs when looking downward. An estimate of the prism needed at the nearpoint can be made.

[a] A single vision lens of the same base curve as the bifocal to be used can be prescribed first, pending completion of the contact lens fitting. Vertical prism can be measured through this by means of a nearpoint Maddox Rod technique through that portion of the lens corresponding to the reading position, since the bifocal will add little if any prismatic effect. The contact lens fitting should be fairly well along, and if the findings are not precisely stable from time to time, a value in the midpoint of the various findings should be chosen.

(6) *Summary of technique*

(a) Refract in the usual manner.

(b) Fit a rocking pad frame with cable or riding bow temples and determine the vertex distance from a medium minus element in the frame to the contact lens plane.

(c) Determine the aniseikonia, or use 6-8% (Boeder, 9%).

(d) Consult the tables for the desired minification and vertex distances to find $F_{(+)}$ and $F_{(-)}$.

[1] Fit $F_{(-)}$ in the spectacle plane as a single vision lens. Add $F_{(+)}$ to the refractive Rx computed for the spectacle plane.

(e) Place the required Rx for the phakic eye in the spectacle plane and note the lens between that and the $F_{(-)}$ which is thickest.

[1] Choose the thickest lens thickness for both lenses within reason.

[2] Employ a base curve which matches that of the intended bifocal to be used.

(f) Use a large contact lens with a lenticular zone or a scleral lens.

(g) Dispense both the contact lens and the spectacles at the first fitting.

[1] Adjust the vertex distance to the correct values.

[2] Check the power of the contact lens as previously described. Adjust the add, $F_{(+)}$, to its proper value and then the vertex distance for best acuity.

(h) Determine the off-axis prism needed for the reading height as previously described.

(i) A flat-top bifocal with the same base curve as the single vision lens and the same thickness is prescribed when the fitting is well along. The seg is fitted high, and slab-off prism as indicated is included.

(j) At selected times, the vision, fusion, stereopsis thresholds, muscle balance and, if possible, remaining size error are re-evaluated. Care for precise centration of the contact lens during such tests must be taken.

(k) If muscle surgery is needed, it should precede the fitting of a scleral lens. If needling is needed, it should precede the fitting of the telescopic device.

2. *Binocular aphakia*

a. Many binocularly aphakic patients do not acquire good binocular vision through spectacles that correct aphakia due to the fixation angles and the prismatic effects of the lenses. Goar maintained that such patients did get fusion, however.

(1) At near many aphakics already have a weak convergence, and this is accentuated by the base-out prism effect of the strong plus lenses.

(2) Added to the prismatic effect, the loss of angle kappa results in the need for

about as much convergence effort for the distance fixation as was formerly used for the nearpoint (Stimson, 1957).

F. Clear near vision with only the distance Rx.

1. *The factors allegedly involved* (Bettman, 1950).

a. The effect of the *added plus of the periphery.*

(1) This factor can be disproved by centering the visual axes through the optical centers of the lenses.

b. Spectacles *moved away from the eye* will alter the vertex.

(1) This factor can be disproved by holding the lenses strictly in place.

(a) A +10.00 D. lens is increased 0.10 D. per 1 mm. of movement.

c. *Magnification of the Rx*

(1) A 30% increase in magnification such as an aphakic Rx produces will enable a patient with J2 acuity to read the J1 line.

(2) However, Rosenbloom (1953) and Bettman (1950) reduced the magnification by using contact lenses and still found an increased ability to read at near.

d. *Sharper acuity*

(1) Since most aphakics may be able to see as well as the 20/10 line at far, due to the magnification, they probably can see better than the J1 line, if it were accurately focused.

e. Selection of *certain rays of the caustic* or interpretation of the diffusion circles

f. *The pinhole effect* produced by the small pupil

(1) Pupils do vary in size, yet acuity for aphakia does not vary with the change of pupil size. Also, many aphakics have oval pupils.

g. *The corneal power* may be changed by the lid pressure, the external muscle compression, or ciliary compression.

(1) Even when the lid is held off the eye, and the ciliary and the muscles are paralyzed, and the cornea is measured through a keratometer to note any change, as Bettman did through a half-silvered mirror, the increase in near acuity with a distance correction is usually still apparent.

h. *Changes in the vitreous face*

(1) No such change has been observed.

i. *The contraction of the ciliary or extra-ocular muscles* may lengthen the eyeball.

(1) *Paralysis* of the ciliary or the extraocular muscles does not interfere with the ability to see at near.

j. *The retina is pulled forward.*

(1) This, theoretically, should increase the problem of seeing at near rather than abet it.

2. *The factors that are apparently involved*

a. In some cases, acuity can be shown to be clear at both the farpoint and the nearpoint at the same time when letters or a grid are used as the fixation objects.

(1) *Chromatic aberration*

(a) Since the aphakic eye has an increased sensitivity to violet and ultraviolet rays, the eye is apparently myopic when fixed at the distance for the ultraviolet band.

(2) *Increased spherical aberration*

(a) *Spherical aberration* of the cornea is ordinarily neutralized by the lens. With the absence of the crystalline lens, the caustic of the aphakic eye becomes longer and narrower.

(b) If the pupil is rather small, the caustic is reduced in size, but the pinhole effect of the pupil then helps the acuity.

(c) If the pupil is large, the caustic is increased in size.

(3) The corrected *aphakic eye is weaker* than the normal eye.

(a) A weaker optical system has a greater depth of focus.

(4) *Aphakic acuity at far* is often good enough so that it is *slightly over-corrected* in plus for an acuity of 20/20.

(a) Often the refractor is farther from the eye than the eyewire of the resultant spectacle.

(b) The deeply back-curved lenses of the spectacles are often farther at the pole of the lens than the measured vertex.

b. Of the apparently involved factors, it is likely that the caustic, chromatic aberration, over-correction, and magnification are the chief ones responsible.

II. REFRACTION OF THE APHAKIC (Mann, 1961)

A. Time

1. Refraction can begin two weeks after surgery and should be repeated at weekly intervals.

a. A +12.00 D. lens can be held before the eye and the patient allowed to view the examiner's face.

b. An early refraction is affected by low intraocular pressure, lowered corneal transparency, with or without folds in Descemet's membrane, and similar changes in the structure.

c. Vision may be improved with a correction, but the axis and the cylinder of the astigmatism will change remarkably.

(1) Elenius and Karo (1968) reported that of 40 eyes showing astigmatism with-the-rule ten days after surgery, 34 showed astigmatism against-the-rule three months after surgery. In 6 eyes, the with-the-rule astigmatism persisted. In 22 other eyes, against-the-rule astigmatism was observed at both intervals.

(2) The axis of the weakest meridian at the tenth day was distributed across the whole scale from 0 to 180 degrees. At the end of the third month, the axis distribution was concentrated about the vertical meridian as reported by others.

(3) The astigmatism reduced from an average of 3.1 D. at the third month to 2.6 D. at the sixth month, but the axis remained within 1°.

(4) Large postoperative changes in power were associated with large shifts in the position of the axis.

d. The Rx should be ordered only when two successive refractions at a weekly interval agree.

(1) However, no Rx should be ordered before six to eight weeks after the operation, although Kirsch recommended a temporary Rx at four weeks.

e. The refraction may continue to change for from three to six months and then usually remains constant. Kirsch (1965) usually allowed at least two and a half months before finding a permanent correction.

B. Technique (Kirsch, 1965; Mann, 1961).

1. The keratometer is used to indicate the astigmatic error.

2. Retinoscopy is used with plus cylinders as this allows a lesser plus sphere to be used in the back cell (Leahy, 1955).

3. Subjective

a. *The Fixed Frame Technique*

(1) A +10.00 D. may be permanently fixed in a spectacle frame. This frame is fitted to the face and the refractor placed in front of it.

(a) This requires lesser powers in the refractor, and therefore does not affect the vertex as much.

(b) The vertex is known with the fixed spectacle frame.

(c) The pantoscopic tilt of the frame is already established at approximately ten degrees.

[1] An average frame may be tilted from 15 to 20°, although Stimson considered 7 to 12° as normal.

[a] Tilt will change the spherical power and induced cylinder power in accord with the formulae:

(i) New spherical power = $F\ 1 + \frac{\sin^2 0}{3}$

(ii) Induced cylinder = F tan ^{2} 0, where F is the power in the meridian tilted and 0 is the angle of tilt.

[2] A +10.00 D. lens, for example, tilted 10° has an induced power of +10.00 D. sph. + .31 D. cyl. axis 180.

[3] The same effect is experienced when the optical center is displaced so that the line of sight passes through a peripheral portion of the lens.

(d) The true effectivity of strong lenses is established.

[1] For example, if a +10.00D., which is composed of a combination of a +13.00D. and a –3.00D., is used in the trial frame, the actual effective power may be 10.55D.

(2) If the total examination is done on a refractor alone, it usually is about one diopter too strong. In such cases it is always best to finish the final refraction in a trial frame.

b. *Trial Frame Technique*

(1) The trial frame must be perfectly level and the PD of the patient correctly placed.

(2) Introduce pantoscopic tilt.

(a) Keep the lower edge as close to the face as possible, as the line of sight must often be directed below the horizon.

(3) Start with lenses estimated from the pre-cataract eye.

(a) A +10.00 D. for emmetropia before the aphakia is commonly used.

(b) The power may be estimated from the known refractive state prior to the onset of cataracts as previously described.

(4) The vertex from the back cell to the eye must be determined accurately.

(a) It must be remembered that as the distance from the eyes is increased, all the aberrations increase and the field of view diminishes.

(b) The distance may be measured by special devices for the purpose, or a stenopaic slit may be placed in the back cell and a measuring rule may be passed through the slit until it touches the lid. The distance from the lid to the point at which the stenopaic slit intercepts the rule will indicate the vertex distance.

(c) The strongest plus lens should be placed in the back cell as close to the lashes as possible without touching (9 to 10 mm.).

[1] Since many trial sets are composed of symmetrically shaped lenses, and their forms do not match the actual forms of the finished spectacle lenses, it is suggested that the lenses in the trial frame be made to follow the form of the finished lenses which usually have a –3.00 D. back curve. The strong lens in the back-cells, therefore, will consist of a composite of

two lenses. For example, a +10.00 lens is actually made up of a +13.00 D. and a –3.00 D. lens with the minus curve of the –3.00 closest to the eye, and the strong convex curve of the +13.00 away from the eye, towards the test chart.

[2] As noted before such a combination does not actually total +10.00 D., and the approximate effectivity of the combination of all lenses in the trial frame should be known.

(d) If the finished correction can be placed at precisely the same distance from the eye as the trial frame is, the vertex distance need not be measured.

(5) Introduce cylinders in the front cells.

(a) Use a cross cylinder to check the power and the axis.

[1] If the ophthalmometer indicates a cylinder power which appears to be high, use a 0.50 D. cross cylinder.

[2] If it appears to be lower, use a 0.25 D. cross cylinder.

4. *The Near Rx*

a. Add spheres for the working distance.

(1) Usually, less power is needed than the equivalent working distance power.

(a) For example, if the patient is reading at 13 inches, a +3 will not be required, but a +2.50 or even a +2.00 will give acuity practically as good.

[1] This overcorrection is due to the total high plus near power in relation to the vertex distance. In a normal correction, an add of +2.50 combined with the usual range of distance corrections would change little in effective power, i.e., with changes of distance from the lens to the eye. However, the near vertex power of a typical aphakic lens might measure +14.50 D. and would gain rapidly in effective power depending upon lens distance from the eye.

(b) If the distance power is very strong, the add should be kept weak.

[1] This is particularly true when binocular Rx's are prescribed due to the prism base-out effect of the strong plus lens. The rule should be followed particularly if the distance PD is 68 mm. or over.

[2] In using progressive addition forms of lenses (Omnifocal and Varilux), Breuns (1966) found that 54% of the successful cases of aphakic contact lens wearers using such lenses were overfitted in plus by +0.25 to +0.50 D. Koetting (1968) also used mostly adds of +2.75 and +3.00 D. Since these apply to cases corrected for distance with contact lenses while the immediately preceding rules apply to spectacle only corrections, the statements are not contradictory. It can be conjectured that the wearers of the progressive additions might be using part of the intermediate area of the lens for close work and hence required the extra plus to reach usual nearpoint focus.

(c) If acuity, however, is less than 20/40, then stronger adds may be used to increase the acuity until best vision is reached.

(d) The profile of the lens will also affect the effectivity of the lens for the nearpoint.

[1] As the convexity of the front curve is increased, the lens power required for near becomes weaker.

[2] Do not alter the profile radically from the trial lenses giving the best Rx.

5. *Convergence* (Mann, 1961)

a. The problem lies in a possible dire combination of muscle imbalances and prismatic effects of the strong lenses.

(1) Patients with convergence deficiencies may do better with a separate near Rx which has prism base-in incorporated.

(a) If there was considerable exophoria at far, the lenses were decentered by altering the PD inward to help compensate (Kirsch, 1965). However, the lenses were decentered as little as possible (Volk, 1965) since displacement of the optic axis from the line of sight induced a change in both spherical and astigmatic powers.

(2) After the Rx for each eye is determined, the lenses should be centered and a red glass with a Maddox rod used to measure the heterophoria at far.

(a) The examiner must be certain that the lenses are exactly centered.

(b) Each finding should be checked several times until the examiner is sure of the reading.

(3) The measurement should be repeated and confirmed for the nearpoint.

(a) The lateral phoria at near is usually an exophoria.

(4) The examiner should watch closely to be sure the lenses have neither oblique nor vertical tilt since the effectivity will be changed markedly.

b. If a decentered position is found more acceptable, the Rx is ordered with the separation of optical centers found rather than with the patient's PD.

(1) The power is then rechecked with the lenses in the new position.

(2) If further correction was needed, Linksz (1965) held that neither the prescription of prism nor the use of surgery was usually successful.

III. THE SPECTACLE CORRECTION

A. Precautions in ordering the Rx

1. The lenses should be fitted as closely to the eye as possible, just clearing the eyelash tips.

a. This enlarges the field of view since the same rotation covers a larger angular area of the lens.

b. Magnification is decreased and the eye also looks smaller to others viewing the patient.

c. If the sample frame appears to fit the patient at a distance from the eye other than the trial frame distance, an adjustment for the change in vertex distance should be made.

(1) The approximate formula to estimate the effective power of a known lens for a known vertex is as follows:

(a) $Fe = D \pm \frac{D^2 d}{1000}$, where Fe is the effective power, D is the power of the lens in the frame, and d in millimeters is the difference in the distance of the frame to the trial frame from which the Rx is determined. Plus is used if the position is closer to the eye and minus if it is farther from the eye than the trial frame.

[1] A +11.00 D. lens sits 6 mm. closer than in the trial frame.

[a] effective power $= 11.00 + \frac{(11.00 \times 11.00 \times 6)}{1000} = 11.726$ D.

(b) Another formula is $Fe = \frac{1000}{f \pm d}$ where Fe is the effective power, f is the focal length of the lens, and d is the difference in distance.

d. The closer the lens to the eye, the smaller the diameter needed and therefore a lighter and thinner lens can be prescribed.

2. *Adjust the frame for the pantoscopic tilt.*

a. Most refractors fit or are placed before the eyes in vertical position, whereas the final Rx is usually tilted from at least 7 to 12°.

b. If the trial frame is not placed at a pantoscopic tilt during the refraction, there is an increase or change in both spherical and cylindrical powers, and these can be mathematically computed by formula, as explained earlier (see Section II, B, 3).

(1) The axis of the cylinder, however, is not a constant and varies according to the fixation angle of the eye. Generally, it is at right angles to the angle of vergence.

(a) For example, if the right eye looks up and out, the axis becomes 45°.

(2) If the tilt is oblique, plus cylinders are produced with both sphere and cylinder increased and the plus axis is rotated towards the horizontal.

c. If a vertical position of the lens is altered, as for example the center of the lens is raised or lowered, the same effect as if the lens were tilted is created.

(1) In such a case, a change in the angle of the tilt of the lens is needed to compensate for the vertical change.

(2) Table XXII-4 shows optical center position vs. pantoscopic tilt (A.O.Co. Manual-Optical Considerations in Fitting Cataract Lenses) when line of sight is parallel to temples of spectacles.

3. *The base curve* of the lens should be ordered, if possible, with the peripheral power effect in mind.

a. The profile effect of a trial lens and the change of effectivity for near, if different, should be noted.

(1) Table XXII-5 illustrates the amount of error for different decentrations for a +14.00 D. sphere with a pantoscopic angle of 10°.

(2) The same powered lens at 10° from the optical center would represent the following total powers for different forms as follows:

(a) Biconvex: +16.75 +3.37 cyl.; Plano convex: +14.75 +1.12 cyl.; –3.00 base curve + 14.44 + 0.80 cyl.

(3) A + 10.43 lens power at 40° below the center of the lens indicates the following powers for the following constructions:

(a) A biconvex = +12.01 D. sphere combined with a +6.19 D. cylinder axis 180.

(b) A planoconvex = a + 10.27 D. sphere combined with a +2.09 D. cylinder axis 180.

(c) A –3.00 base curve = a +10.00 D. sphere combined with a +1.01 D. cylinder axis 180.

(d) A –6.00 base curve = a +9.93 D. sphere combined with a +.59 D. cylinder axis 180.

[1] A –3.00 base curve is the best spherical equivalent lens at 30° from the center.

(4) **Table XXII-4**

Pantascopic Angle (degrees)	**Distance in mms. of O.C. below line of sight**
0	*+ 0*
5	*+2.2*
10	*+4.5*
15	*+6.8*
20	*+9.3*

(5) **Table XXII-5**

Decentration down in mms.	**plano convex**		**–3.00 base**		**aspheric**	
0	*+0.31*	*– .26*	*+0.21*	*– .20*	*–0.01*	*–0.05*
3.0	*+0.51*	*– .42*	*+0.58*	*– .46*	*+0.19*	*–0.15*
6.0	*+0.99*	*– .75*	*+1.40*	*–1.03*	*+0.81*	*–0.53*
9.0	*+1.81*	*–1.31*	*+2.80*	*–1.98*	*+1.91*	*–1.23*

b. Volk (1965) noted that strong plus lenses spheres had large amounts of oblique power excess and oblique astigmatism in which the meridianal power exceeded the transmeridianal power. Besides blur, there was severe pincushion distortion. Objects were enlarged and elongated in the meridianal direction and displaced towards the viewer. Visual acuity at the margins was less than one-tenth of that through the center. Objects moving across the lens changed shape, size, distance and speed, and if fixation was maintained and the head or the head and the eye moved, blurring and distortion occurred.

c. The –3.00 base curve is the lens of choice for powers less than 10.50 D. and for cylinders less than –1.50 D. Minus cylinder lenses serve better in regard to the strong, astigmatic, aniseikonic effects.

(1) The flatter lens base curve, such as the –3.00 D. base curve, also provides less weight, improves the appearance, and reduces the size of the ring scotoma, thereby enlarging the absolute field.

(2) If a minus cylinder lens, that is, one with the cylinder on the back surface, is being used, the patient should be retested in the trial frame with a minus cylinder placed in the back cell of the trial frame. The minus curve of the cylinder should face the eye.

4. *Centering*

a. The interpupillary distance should be as exact as possible.

(1) The alteration of the interpupillary distance to induce prismatic effect for the correction of weak convergence should not be forgotten, however.

b. The marked variations in power of the lens off the optical center should be kept in mind.

c. It must be remembered that in strong lenses, each mm. is equivalent to .10 prism diopters or more of prismatic effect.

d. The matter of centering the optical center so that the optic axis of the lens passes through the center of rotation of the eye insofar as can be determined, is again emphasized here, where the large errors induced by misalignment of strong lenses for aphakic corrections are of the utmost importance. Fuller's discussion of the subject, as well as a technique for ascertaining such alignment, has been given in section IX, D, 7, of Chapter XXVI, Single Vision Lenses.

5. *Power*

a. Never make an aphakic correction too weak in plus.

(1) It is generally better to correct the vision for good room vision.

6. *The Near Correction*

a. The top of the bifocal segs should be kept close to the distance optical center since the distance, distortion, and power variation limits use to the upper portion of segments.

(1) A flat top, or similar type, provides a better area of use. Jump is not important.

(2) The segs need to be decentered for prism, more than normally used because the distance already provides a heavy base-out effect.

(a) Table of seg insets for each eye, based on a –3.00 base spherical lens and center of rotation distance of 27mms. (Am. Opt. Co. Bulletin):

Table XXII-6

Rx	**+10.00**		**+12.00**		**+14.00**		**+16.00**	
Reading Distance	**13″**	**16″**	**13″**	**16″**	**13″**	**16″**	**13″**	**16″**
Distance PD								
56	*3.5*	*2.9*	*3.9*	*3.3*	*4.4*	*3.7*	*5.0*	*4.2*
60	*3.7*	*3.1*	*4.2*	*3.5*	*4.7*	*4.0*	*5.3*	*4.5*
64	*4.0*	*3.4*	*4.4*	*3.8*	*5.0*	*4.2*	*5.7*	*4.8*
68	*4.2*	*3.6*	*4.7*	*4.0*	*5.3*	*4.5*	*6.0*	*5.1*
72	*4.5*	*3.8*	*5.0*	*4.2*	*5.6*	*4.8*	*6.4*	*5.4*

b. If the patient is not used to bifocals or if a very strong addition is needed in cases of very poor visual acuity, it is better to prescribe separate Rx's for far and near. Also, separate Rx's will serve better if one eye is to be used for far vision and the other for near vision, or if there is a desire to make the generally occluded eye useful on some occasions in cases of monocular aphakia.

(1) Likewise, if the convergence problem is too great for the patient to overcome, separate Rx's will allow the near prescription to be decentered to eliminate as much prism base-out effect as possible.

7. *Tint*

a. Most aphakic lenses come in a mild shade of tint to help with the increased ultraviolet transmission and the greater pupil size when an iridectomy has been performed.

b. A form of the Pulfrich phenomenon is possible if the tint is increased greatly or one eye is partly cataractous and absorbs a good portion of the light.

(1) Unequal intensities of view in both eyes usually result in spatial disparity.

(2) This can be tested by placing a tint before one eye and swinging an arc or a metronome.

(a) If the swing is circular toward and away from the patient, the intensity should be equalized for both eyes. If one eye permits a higher transmission, it may need a darker tint than the other.

8. *Final verification of the prescription before ordering*

a. The trial frame with all the lenses in it which gave the best acuity can be placed on the Vertometer and the final combined effective Rx read from the instrument.

9. *Lens choices*

a. Most lenses today are *lenticular,* and some are made of *plastic* for lighter weight. These latter gain not only in lessened weight but also in thinness and still give an effective field.

(1) As noted earlier, due to the magnification, the field of view in a lenticular cataract lens is limited. A rotation of the eye of 30° does not cover a magnified field of 30°. A lenticular section of 40° is needed for a 30° field.

(a) Davis and Clotar (1956) listed the following comparisons of several types of cataract lenses in Table XXII-7.

[1] For a +12.00 D. sphere with a useful diameter of 47 mm., aberrations of the 30° peripheral bundle are considered.

b. Since the chromatic aberration was less in aphakia, both in the transverse and longitudinal meridians (Stimson), crown and flint combinations were used more freely.

c. Both plastic and glass aspheric lenses are now generally used.

(1) The clear field is generally increased to 26 mm. from the usual 12 mm.

(2) At the time of printing, only the Volk Catraconoid Aspheric lens provided a bifocal form of aspheric cataract lens with aspheric effect at the near seg.

[a] **Table XXII-7**

Lens	Color	Power	Astigmatism	Approx. Wgt. In Grams	Thickness In MM.
Regular -3.00 B.C.	*.30*	*+.90*	*+1.90*	*16.2*	*7.0*
Doublet with 1.616 glass (-3.00 B.C.; 34 mm. spot)	*.11*	*-.30*	*+.15*	*21.5*	*7.5*
Doublet with 1.70 glass (34 mm. spot)	–	*-.30*	*+.20*	*24.7*	*7.0*
Flat with 1.616 glass (34 mm. spot)	*.10*	*-.15*	*+.15*	*24.8*	*7.5*
Corrected cemented lenticular	*.11*	*-.30*	*+.15*	*17.7*	*5.5*
Style E uncorrected (30 mm. spot)	*.30*	*+.90*	*+1.90*	*11.1*	*4.6*

(a) In the construction of aspheric cataract lenses with a single continuous surface, Davis (1959) found that in regard to the chief aberrations (curvature of the field, astigmatism, and lateral color) such lenses were restricted in design. As the tangential curve in one meridian was influenced by the sagittal curve of the other meridian if the tangential curvature was set for any two points in the field, the sagittal was predetermined and a compromise was chosen. To hold down lateral color, a tangential blur, the tangential error was kept to a minimum allowing the sagittal to increase. A –3 or –4 D. base curve was least sensitive to this stop position. Aspheric lenses showed less cylinder at 30° from center.

(b) Conoid lenses use an ellipsoid surface on the front and a spherical or toric back surface. These reduce in power both meridionally and transmeridionally, but more so the former. With an appropriate ellipsoid eccentricity, the power reduction and surface astigmatism developed as necessary to correct oblique power errors, oblique astigmatic errors, and distortion (Volk, 1961 and 1965).

[1] The range of powers is from +7.50 D. to +24.00 D., and the back surfaces is –3.00 D. if no ocular astigmatism exists. If ocular astigmatism exists, the back surface is toric and straddles the –3.00 D. Front curves vary in 0.25 D. steps.

[2] The bifocal is a straight top and is between both lens surfaces proportional to the axis of the front surface of the ellipsoid which, lying in front of the segment, corrects for near as well as for far. The adds are variable up to +5.00 D. The segs are 22 mm. wide, placed 3 mm. below the optical centers and decentered 1.75 mm. nasalward. A large depth of focus is obtainable so that both the punctum proximum and the punctum remotum are extended.

[3] Visual acuity is slightly less peripherally than centrally. Distortion is reduced. The reading area is wider and clearer. The field of view is wider and prismatic effect is less. The lenses are thinner than ordinary spherical lenses.

[a] The visual acuity falls at the margin due to the chromatic aberrations and the astigmatic variation from an ideal lens surface.

(c) The following is a chart showing the differences in thickness at the apex, in mm., between ordinary spherical lenses and conoid lenses of same power and diameter. Conoid lenses are thinner by the amount shown.

[1] **Table XXII-8**

Diopters			**Lens**		**Diameter**		
Base Curve	38	40	42	44	46	48	50
11.00	0	0	.1	.1	.2	.2	.2
12.00	0	0	.1	.1	.2	.2	.2
13.00	0	0	.1	.2	.2	.2	.3
14.00	0	0	.1	.2	.2	.3	.5
15.00	.1	.1	.1	.2	.2	.3	.5
16.00	.1	.2	.2	.4	.5	.7	.9
17.00	.3	.4	.5	.7	.8	1.1	1.4
18.00	.3	.4	.5	.7	.9	1.2	1.7
19.00	.4	.5	.7	.9	1.2	1.5	3.3
20.00	.6	.8	.9	1.3	1.7	2.5	3.7

d. Catmin magnifying lenses are also used upon occasion. These are really a reversed telescope and are used essentially in attempts to secure binocularity when monocular aphakia exists. They are exceedingly uncosmetic.

10. *Choice of frame*

a. *Simply shaped lenses of small size* and of shapes in which the maximum and minimum diameters are not too different are best since these reduce the thickness considerably. If necessary, the DBL should be increased to compensate for smaller lens sizes.

(1) In certain frames with relatively square shapes, the addition of two to three PD of prism with base-up OU to the blank tended to give thinner lenses in the usable portion (Volk, 1965). The primary position of the level should be mainly on the ocular side and any regrinding done on the ocular side.

11. *Verification of the finished correction*

a. *Vision* should be checked with the *finished Rx in place.*

(1) The power should be verified by fitting the frame as close as possible to just clear the lashes.

(a) When the frame is moved close or farther, if vision improves, the power needs to be modified accordingly.

(b) The lenses may be rotated while one eye is occluded.

(c) A variation in the axis of only 3° will often noticeably affect the vision.

b. *The lenses should be rotated one at a time* with one eye occluded.

(1) A variation in the cylinder axis as little as 3° may often noticeably affect the visual acuity.

c. *The frame should be twisted so that one lens center is above the other* by about 2 mm. and then below the other by the same amount.

(1) This allows for the vertical centering or the cylinder axis being incorrect and discovered.

d. *The lenses should be tilted forward and backward.*

(1) The optical effect of the pantoscopic angle has been previously discussed.

e. *The lenses should be moved in a plane* before the eye—up, in, down, and out.

(1) If the pupil is not before the optical center of the lens, the variation will improve vision as the optical center is aligned.

(2) If on the optical center, movement will introduce peripheral changes in power.

(3) This test must be done monocularly since if one eye is off the optical center and one on, the binocular movement will not have a specific indication.

(a) This test often reveals the difference in the monocular interpupillary distance, and for aphakics it is advisable that the interpupillary distance be measured by some monocular method of measurement.

(b) Again, it must be reiterated that the interpupillary distance may be deliberately decentered in order to help convergence.

f. *The cross cylinder* should be used before the finished correction to recheck the cylinder axis and power.

g. *A provisional lens system for aphakia may be used.*

(1) These are temporary corrections made up in a final frame which fit the patient accurately.

(2) The patient is refracted through this temporary correction and the changes that are required are noted.

(3) The final lens is made on the same profile including the power changes.

12. *Situations in which the correction may not be satisfactory*

a. The vertex distance, the tilt of the lens, and the centering may not be correct.

b. The correction may have been ordered too soon and the refraction may still be changing as the cornea heals.

c. The profile of the lens may vary from the trial lenses.

d. Physiological factors may be involved, such as:

(1) Tunnel vision
(2) Distortion of the periphery
(3) Displacement of orientation
(4) Too limited a field
(5) The need to hold the eye fixed and move the head

e. It must be remembered in the fitting of aphakic lenses, the first lenses fitted will be compared to the vision prior to surgery. The later lenses fitted will be compared to the earlier ones and will therefore imply a constant improvement. For this reason, it is sometimes advantageous to defer the fitting of the first lenses for some time or to permit the first lenses to be fitted by someone other than the final examiner.

IV. CONTACT LENSES

A. As with the spectacle lenses, enough time must elapse for the cornea to have taken on a fixed curve before contact lenses are fitted. Kirsch (1965) recommended at least two and half months after surgery.

B. The Physical Fit

1. The lenticular form is satisfactory if a round pupil or an iridectomy which is concealed by the upper lid is the situation.

a. If the lens falls low on the cornea and the lid overlaps, it can be raised by a minus edge treatment.

b. If the lid does not overlap, the lens must be fitted more tightly in order to help it center.

(1) The K findings can be split to as much as one-half the astigmatic difference, even with a large lens.

(2) The size of the lens is generally fairly large, and the optical zone is also generally fairly large.

(3) As with spectacles, the contact lens can be overplussed somewhat to give the best vision at the room distance. Since most patients will require a pair of spectacles for reading, the spectacles can have a little minus in the upper portion, besides a bifocal in the other, to improve the acuity for driving, the theater, and other extreme distance locations.

C. The Optical Properties

1. With a contact lens, the field of vision is almost normal since most peripheral aberrations are essentially eliminated.

2. Magnification is reduced so that it is a better Rx for monocular aphakia.

a. In myopia up to –6 D., contact lenses on both eyes seemed to be best (Ogle et al., 1951).

b. In hyperopia up to +5 D., one contact lens and one spectacle seemed to be best (Ogle et al., 1951).

c. Six percent of residual aniseikonia remained in unilateral aphakia corrected by contact lenses (Budd and Mackinson). Others, as noted earlier, have indicated as much as 9% remains.

(1) Ogle considered a haptic lens a better correction for this purpose than a corneal one.

3. Stone (1968) makes the following comparison between haptic and corneal contact lenses as applied to aphakia:

a. *Binocularity*

(1) Haptic

(a) The lens manually depresses the eye, significant if unilateral.

(b) Hyperphoria is induced.

(c) The weight is on the temporal and upper part of the eye; the lens may rotate.

(d) The lens rides slightly outward, and may induce exophoria and excyclophoria.

(2) Corneal

(a) The lens usually rides low and induces prism base down effect.

(b) Hyperphoria is varying in degree.

b. *Size*

(1) Magnification is 2.46% more than for the corneal for +15.00 D. power.

c. *Photophobia*

(1) The diameter of the effective entrance pupil of the haptic is 3% larger than for the corneal admitting 9% more light.

d. *In Unilateral Aphakia*

(1) Haptic lenses provide a poorer cosmetic appearance, a larger retinal image size, induced hyperphoria, exophoria, excyclophoria, and admit more light to the eye.

(2) Corneal lenses cause a possibly variable vertical phoria; apical types (large flat corneals) create a larger image than standard corneals.

e. *In Binocular Aphakia*

(1) Haptics interfere with fusion because of exophoria or cyclophoria; on corneals because of possible variable phorias; apical types interfere least.

4. Even the contact lens wearer will require, however, spectacles for many other occasions, such as upon first arising, upon retiring, and upon such instances as the contact lens does not serve.

V. REHABILITATION

A. It is generally found that most of the difficulty in adjusting to aphakic spectacles lies in the fact that little explanation of the problems which will occur is made to the patient, either pre-or postoperatively. If loaner lenses of 10.00 or 12.00 D. powers, which need not necessarily provide good vision but yet serve to illustrate the problems, are provided the patient immediately, and if daily therapy in which the problems are explained and the patient is helped and taught to feed himself, to move about, to perform the acts of hygiene, and to do other things in general such as hanging clothes, playing cards, are introduced, Liddy, et al. (1967), found that patients adjusted much more easily. They conducted sessions for four days, each session lasting 45 minutes, in which the first day most of the activities were mainly sedentary and included practicing reaching for objects, picking up objects, and filling a cup with water. The second day, the first day's lessons were reviewed and exercises involving moving from room to room were introduced. The third day, the previous lessons were again reviewed, motility again stressed, and how to go up and down stairs, how to get in and out of a bathtub and how to open and close doors were taught. On the fourth day, outdoor activities such as walking about the grounds, and stepping up and down curbs, were taught. They found that patients given this training adjusted far more readily to the wearing of cataract spectacles than otherwise. It is recommended that cataract patients be given full explanations of the problems which they might encounter so that they realize that these problems are typical of cataract lenses. Also, they should be encouraged by understanding that others have learned to adjust to them and to perform natural activities with them. The training can perhaps be performed by either the refractionist or the refractionist's assistant prior to or when the final lenses are being prescribed.

REFERENCES

American Optical Co.: Optical Considerations In Fitting Cataract Lenses.

Batra, D.V. (1967): Refraction in Aphakia. Indian J. Opt., 1: 14.

Bettman, J.W. (1950): Apparent Accommodation in Aphakic Eyes. A.J. Oph. 33: 921.

Boeder, P. (1938): Power and Magnification Properties of Contact Lenses. Arch. Oph., 19: 54.

Breuns, E. (1966): Die Kombination von Kontakt Linse and Varilux bei Aphakie. 2nd Varilux Int. Symp., Essen, Germany. (Cited by Koetting, 1968).

Cowan, A. (1949): Aphakia. A.J. Oph. 32: 419.

Cowan, A. (1953): Monocular Aphakia. Arch. Oph. 50: 16.

Davis, J.K. (1959): Problems and Compromises in the Design of Aspheric Cataract Lenses. A.A.A.O., 36: 279.

Davis, J.K. & Clotàr, G. (1956): An Approach to the Problem of a Corrected Curve Achromatic Cataract Lens. A.A.A.O., 33: 279.

Dyer, J.A. and Ogle, K.N. (1960): Correction of Unilateral Aphakia with Contact Lenses: Report of seven cases. A.J. Oph. 50: 11.

Elenius, V. & Karo, T. (1968): Changes in Refractive Power of the Cornea After Cataract Extraction. E.E.N.T., 47: 54.

Enoch, J.M. (1968): A Spectacle-Contact Lens Combination Used As a Reverse Galilean Telescope in Unilateral Aphakia. A.A.A.O., 45: 231.

Foley, J. (1954): Orthoptics Investigation in Unilateral Aphakia. B. Orth. J. 11: 3.

**Goar, E.L. (1953): Correspondence, Monocular Aphakia. Arch. Oph. 50: 779.*

Goar, E.L. (1955): The Management of Monocular Cataracts. Arch. Oph. 54: 73.

Goar, E.L. (1957): Contact Lenses in Monocular Aphakia. Arch. Oph. 58: 159.

**Halass, S. (1966): Aniseikonia, A Survey of the Literature. A.A.A.O., 43: 505.*

Kirsch, R.E. (1965): Aphakic Refraction. Refraction., I.O.C., 5 (2).

Koetting, R. (1968): Some Results in Fitting Aphakics With Progressive Addition Lenses Opt. Weekly, 59 (7): 43.

**Kornzweig, A.L., Feldstein, M. and Schneider, J. (1957): The Eye in Old Age. A.J. Oph., 44.*

Leahy, B.D. (1955): The Management of Aphakia. A.J. Oph. 39: 67.

Liddy, B. St. L., Carr, R., McCullock, C. (1967): Aphakic Rehabilitation. A.J. Oph., 63: 1743.

Linksz, A. (1965): Optical Complications of Aphakia. – Complications After Cataract Surgery, I.O.C., part II., 5 (1).

Lubkin, V., Stollerman, H., and Linksz, A. (1960): Stereopsis in Monocular Aphakia with Spectacle Correction. A.J. Oph. 61: 273.

**Mann, Wm. A. (1961): Optical Correction of Aphakia. Cataract Surgery and Ophthalmology, I.O.C., 1 (3).*

Obrig, T.E. (1944): Modern Ophthalmic Lenses and Optical Glass. Chilton Books, Phila.

Ogle, K.N. (1950): Researches in Binocular Vision. Sanders Co., Phila.

Ogle, K.N., Burian, H.M., and Bannon, R.E. (1958): On the Correction of Unilateral Aphakia with Contact Lenses. Arch. Oph. 59: 652.

Pascal, J.I. (1954): Image Magnification in Corrected Aphakia. E.E.N.T. 33: 290.

Rosenbloom, A. (1953): The Correction of Unilateral Aphakia with Corneal Contact Lenses. A.A.A.O., 30: 536.

Spaeth, P.G. and O'Neill, P.M. (1960): Functional Results with Contact Lenses in Unilateral Congenital Cataracts, High Myopia, and Traumatic Cataracts. A.J. Oph. 46: 635.

Stimson, R.L. (1951): Optical Dispensing. C.V. Mosby Co., St. Louis.

Stimson, R.L. (1957): Lenses For Aphakia. B.J. Physiol. Optics, 14: 78.

Stone, J. (1968): Optical Comparisons Between Haptic and Corneal Lenses For Aphakia. A.A.A.O., 45: 528.

Troutman, R.C. (1963): Artiphakia and Aniseikonia. A.J. Oph., 56: 602.

Volk, D. (1965): Aspheria Ophthalmic Lenses. Refraction, I.O.C., 5 (2).

Volk, D. (1961): Conoid Cataract Lenses For the Correction of Aphakia. A.J. Oph., 51: 615.

Welsh, R.C. (1966): Spectacles For Aphakia. Chas. Thomas & Sons, Springfield, Illinois.

Welsh, R.C. (1967): Defects of Vision Through Aphakic Lenses. B.J. Oph. 51: 306.

**Wick, R.E. (1960): The Management of the Aging Patient in Optometric Practice, (M.J. Hirsch and R.E. Wick, ed.), Chilton Books, Philadelphia.*

23 Visual Correction With Contact Lenses

I. INTRODUCTION

A. Spectacle lenses and contact lenses differ in the manner in which they correct ametropia. The spectacle lens corrects ametropia by imaging a distant object at the far point of the unaccommodated eye. It is bounded on both surfaces by air and is positioned at a finite distance from the cornea. The eye rotates behind the lens so that the line of sight is directed through peripheral regions of the lens. The contact lens, on the other hand, is positioned at the surface of the cornea. It is immersed in tear fluid and corrects the refractive state by bathing the cornea in tear fluid to neutralize most of its refractive power. It provides the eye with a new anterior refracting surface of such power as to produce a near emmetropic system. The lens rotates with the eye so that most of the time, the line of sight is directed through the central region of the lens.

B. The visual correction provided by a contact lens is a function of the optical properties of both the contact lens and the fluid media present between the contact lens and the cornea. The plastic and fluid components combine to form the *contact lens-fluid lens system.*

II. THE CONTACT LENS-FLUID LENS SYSTEM

A. Optical Model

1. The CL-FL system may be conveniently described as consisting of a thick contact lens and a thin fluid lens bounded by air on both surfaces. It is as if each lens were suspended in air in serial fashion before the cornea (Bennett, 1963; Sarver, 1963a) (Figure XXIII-1).

a. The thin fluid film that covers the anterior surface of the lens may be disregarded. Although it must be unbroken and of uniform thickness to provide a good optical surface, it contributes no significant power to the system.

2. The back vertex power of the CL-FL system is equal to the back vertex power of the contact lens in air (F_{CL}) plus the thin lens power of the fluid lens in air (F_{FL}) (Sarver, 1963): $F_{system} = F_{CL} + F_{FI}$. --- (1)

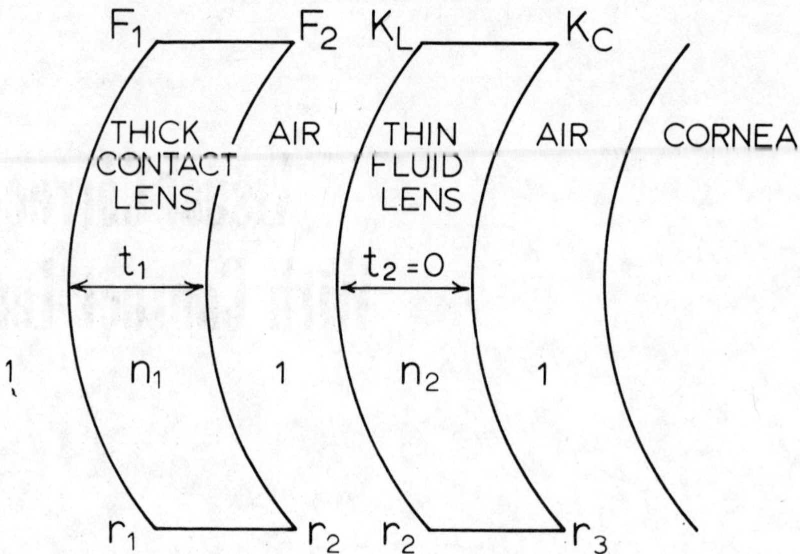

Figure XXIII-1– The "Contact Lens – Fluid Lens System" with each component separated by a thin layer of air.

a. So long as the fluid lens is very thin, as it is with corneal lenses (Sarver, 1962), and minimal clearance scleral lenses, (Bier, 1957) the equation (1) is clinically accurate.

3. *Contact lens power*

a. The *back vertex power* of the contact lens in air is given by the following equation:

$$F_{CL} = \frac{F_1}{1 - cF_1} + F_2 \qquad (2)$$

(1) Where F_{CL} is the back vertex power of the contact lens in air, F_1 and F_2 are the powers of the anterior and posterior lens surfaces respectively, and $c = t_1/n_1$.

b. The *thickness* of the contact lens must be taken into account because it contributes a significant amount of plus power to the total power of the contact lens (approximately +0.25 diopters per 0.1 mm. of lens thickness for lenses of refractive index 1.490).

c. The *curvature of the posterior lens surface* was variously termed the base curve (Mandell, 1965), the optic zone radius (Mandell, 1965), or the central posterior curve, (Girard, 1964). It was specified in millimeters radius of curvature and/or "diopters" K reading (D.K.). The power of this posterior lens surface must not be confused with its K reading.

(1) If the radius of the posterior lens surface is 7.67 mm, its K reading is 44.00 K.D.

$$\left(K = \frac{1.3375 - 1}{.00767} = 44.00 \text{ D.K.}\right).$$

(2) The power of this surface in air is –63.89 diopters $\left(F_2 = \frac{1 - 1.490}{.00767} = -63.89 \text{ D.}\right)$.

(3) The K reading of this surface can be converted to its power in air by using the constant –1.452. (See Table 1 for derivation)

$$(F_2 = K \times -1.452 = 44.00 \times -1.452 = -63.89 \text{ D.})$$

Table XXIII-1

Table of optical constants for converting the surface value of a plastic contact lens (n = 1.490) (From Mandell, 1965, p. 328).

To Convert from	to	Multiply by
Contact Lens surface power in air	*Contact lens surface power in fluid*	$C_1 = 0.314$
K reading of contact lens surface	*Contact lens surface power in air*	$C_2 = 1.452$
K reading of contact lens surface	*Contact lens surface power in fluid*	$C_3 = 0.452$

Derivation:

$$C_1 = \frac{n_{fluid} - n_{plastic}}{n_{air} - n_{plastic}} = \frac{1.336 - 1.490}{1 - 1.490} = 0.314$$

$$C_2 = \frac{n_{air} - n_{plastic}}{n_{air} - n_{keratometer}} = \frac{1 - 1.490}{1 - 1.3375} = 1.452$$

$$C_3 = \frac{n_{fluid} - n_{plastic}}{n_{air} - n_{keratometer}} = \frac{1.336 - 1.490}{1 - 1.3375} = 0.456$$

d. The *curvature of the anterior lens surface* is such as to satisfy the relationship given by equation (2).

(1) For example:

(a) Given: Base curve = 44.00 D.K.; $F_{CL} = -2.00$ D.; $t_1 = 0.20$ mm.; $n_1 = 1.490$; Find r_1

(b) $F_2 = 44.00 \times -1.452 = -63.89$ D.;

(c) $$F_1 = \frac{F_{CL} - F_2}{1 + \frac{t}{n}(F_{CL} - F_2)}$$

$$= \frac{-2.00 - (-63.89)}{1 + \frac{.00020}{1.49}(-2.00 + 63.89)}$$

$$= 61.38 \text{ D.}$$

(d) $$r_1 = \frac{n - 1}{F_1} = \frac{0.490}{61.38} = 0.00798 \text{ m}$$

$$= 7.98 \text{ mm.}$$

e. The curvature of the anterior lens surface can be calculated with great ease by using thin lens optics and adding a correction factor for lens thickness to the radius so determined.

(1) The correction (Braff, 1959-63; Sarver and Kerr, 1964; Mandell, 1964) factor, k, is given by the expression, $k = \frac{n-1}{n}(t_1)$. When n = 1.490, $k = 0.329\ t_1$.

(a) The correction factor is derived by taking the partial derivative of r_1 with respect to t_1 in an expanded expression of equation (2), with F_{CL} and F_2 held constant. The result is $\frac{\delta r_1}{\delta t_1} = \frac{1-n}{n}$ and therefore $\Delta r_1 = \frac{1-n}{n}\Delta t_1$. Thus, an incremental change in r_1 is related to an incremental change in t_1 by the expression $\frac{1-n}{n}$ when lens power and base curve are held constant.

(2) For example:

(a) Given: Base curve = 44.00 D.K.; F_{CL} = −2.00 D.; t_1 = 0.20 mm.; n_1 = 1.490; Find r_1

(b) $F_2 = -63.89$ D.

(c) $F_1 = F_{CL} - F_2 = -2.00 - (-63.89) = +61.89$ D.

(d) $r = \frac{n-1}{F_1} = \frac{0.490}{61.89} = 0.00791$ m. = 7.91 mm.

(e) $r_1 = r + kt_1 = 7.91 + 0.329 \times 0.20 = 7.91 + .07 = 7.98$ mm.

(3) Contact lens radius-power tables (Mandell, 1965) facilitate this calculation.

4. *Fluid lens power*

a. The fluid lens surfaces are formed by, and therefore equal to, the curvature of the contact lens base curve and anterior corneal surface respectively.

b. The thin lens power of the fluid lens in air is equal to the difference between the K reading of the contact lens base curve and the K reading of the cornea, that is: $F_{FL} = K_L - K_C$ --- (3)

c. Unlike the surface power of the contact lens in air, the surface power of the fluid lens in air *is* given by its keratometer value. That is to say, a fluid lens surface with a keratometer value of 44.00 D.K. also has a power of 44.00 D. in air. The reason lies in the simple fact that the refractive index of tear fluid (n_2 = 1.336) is essentially the same as the refractive index used to calibrate the keratometer (n = 1.3375) and the ophthalmometer (n = 1.336).

(1) If the contact lens base curve is the same as the corneal curvature, the power of the fluid lens is plano.

(a) Example: Base curve, 43.00 D.K.; Corneal K Reading, 43.00 D.K.; Fluid lens power, plano.

[1] $F_{FL} = K_L - K_C = 43.00 - 43.00 = 0$

(2) If the contact lens base curve is steeper than the corneal curvature, the power of the fluid lens is plus.

(a) Example: Base Curve, 44.00 D.K.; Corneal K reading, 43.00 D.K.; Fluid lens power, +1.00 D.

[1] $F_{FL} = K_L - K_C = 44.00 - 43.00 = +1.00$ D.

(3) If the contact lens base curve is flatter than the corneal curvature, the power of the fluid lens is minus.

(a) Example: Base Curve, 42.00 D.K.; Corneal K Reading, 43.00 D.K.; Fluid lens power, –1.00 D.

$$[1]\quad F_{FL} = K_L - K_C = 42.00 - 43.00 = -1.00 \text{ D.}$$

d. One of the major advantages of specifying the base curve of a contact lens and the curvature of the cornea in K "diopters" is that it gives the surface powers of the fluid lens in air, and thus facilitates the calculation of the contact lens prescription.

B. Power of the CL-FL system

1. To fully correct a given refractive state the CL-FL system must image a distant object at the same position in space as that occupied by the secondary focal point of the correcting spectacle lens. That is to say, the power of the CL-FL system must be equal to the eye's refractive state at the plane of the cornea (Figure XXIII-2).

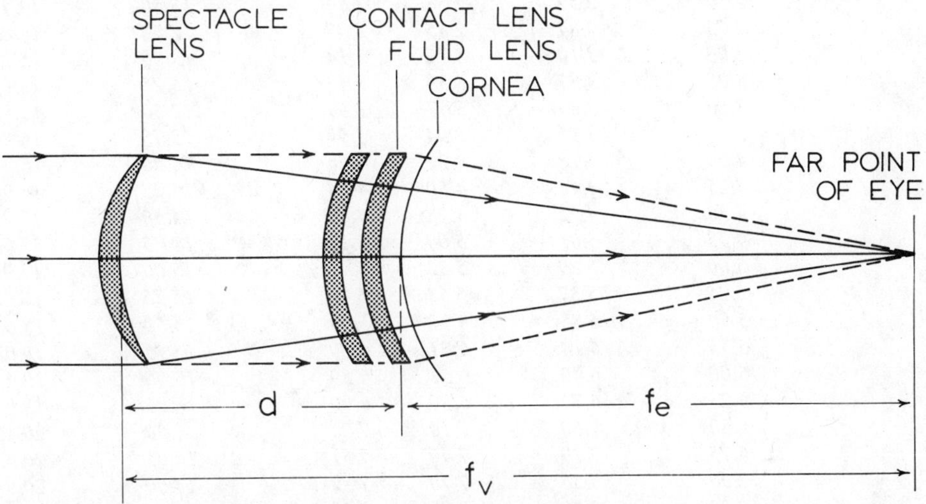

Figure XXIII-2 – To fully correct a given refractive error the CL-FL system must image a distant object at the same position in space as that occupied by the secondary focal point of the correcting spectacle lens.

a. The refractive state at the plane of the cornea is given by the equation

$$Fe = \frac{F_v}{1 - dF_v} \quad \text{------------------------------ (4)}$$

(1) Where Fe is the effective power at the plane of the cornea in diopters, F_v is the back vertex power of the spectacle lens in diopters, and d is the distance of the spectacle lens from the cornea in meters.

(a) Example: Spectacle refraction, –7.00.; Vertex distance, 11 mm.; Effective power at the plane of the cornea, –6.50 D.

$$[1]\quad Fe = \frac{-7.00}{1 - .011\,(-7.00)} = -6.50 \text{ D.}$$

b. Tables 2a and 2b give the values of Fe for various values of F_v and d.

Table XXIII-2a

Effective Power of Plus Spectacle Lenses at the Corneal Plane for Vertex Distances of 11, 13, and 15 Millimeters.

Spectacle lens power F_v	Vertex distance 11mm	13mm F_e	15mm	Spectacle lens power F_v	Vertex distance 11mm	13mm F_e	15mm
0.25	0.25	0.25	0.25	10.25	11.55	11.83	12.11
0.50	0.50	0.50	0.50	10.50	11.87	12.16	12.46
0.75	0.76	0.76	0.76	10.75	12.19	12.50	12.82
1.00	1.01	1.01	1.02	11.00	12.51	12.84	13.17
1.25	1.27	1.27	1.27	11.25	12.84	13.18	13.53
1.50	1.53	1.53	1.53	11.50	13.17	13.52	13.90
1.75	1.78	1.79	1.80	11.75	13.49	13.87	14.26
2.00	2.04	2.05	2.06	12.00	13.82	14.22	14.63
2.25	2.31	2.32	2.33	12.25	14.16	14.57	15.01
2.50	2.57	2.58	2.60	12.50	14.49	14.93	15.38
2.75	2.84	2.85	2.87	12.75	14.83	15.28	15.77
3.00	3.10	3.12	3.14	13.00	15.17	15.64	16.15
3.25	3.37	3.39	3.42	13.25	15.51	16.01	16.54
3.50	3.64	3.67	3.69	13.50	15.85	16.37	16.93
3.75	3.91	3.94	3.97	13.75	16.20	16.74	17.32
4.00	4.18	4.22	4.26	14.00	16.55	17.11	17.72
4.25	4.46	4.50	4.54	14.25	16.90	17.49	18.12
4.50	4.73	4.78	4.83	14.50	17.25	17.87	18.53
4.75	5.01	5.06	5.11	17.75	17.61	18.25	18.94
5.00	5.29	5.35	5.41	15.00	17.96	18.63	19.35
5.25	5.57	5.63	5.70	15.25	18.32	19.02	19.77
5.50	5.85	5.92	5.99	15.50	18.69	19.41	20.20
5.75	6.14	6.21	6.29	15.75	19.05	19.81	20.62
6.00	6.42	6.51	6.59	16.00	19.42	20.20	21.05
6.25	6.71	6.80	6.90	16.25	19.79	20.60	21.49
6.50	7.00	7.10	7.20	16.50	20.16	21.01	21.93
6.75	7.29	7.40	7.51	16.75	20.53	21.41	22.37
7.00	7.58	7.70	7.82	17.00	20.91	21.82	22.82
7.25	7.88	8.00	8.13	17.25	21.29	22.24	23.27
7.50	8.17	8.31	8.45	17.50	21.67	22.65	23.73
7.75	8.47	8.62	8.77	17.75	22.06	23.07	24.19
8.00	8.77	8.93	9.09	18.00	22.44	23.50	24.66
8.25	9.07	9.24	9.42	18.25	22.83	23.93	25.13
8.50	9.38	9.56	9.74	18.50	23.23	24.36	25.61
8.75	9.68	9.87	10.07	18.75	23.62	24.79	26.09
9.00	9.99	10.19	10.40	19.00	24.02	25.23	26.57
9.25	10.30	10.51	10.74	19.25	24.42	25.68	27.07
9.50	10.61	10.84	11.08	19.50	24.82	26.12	27.56
9.75	10.92	11.17	11.42	19.75	25.23	26.57	28.06
10.00	11.24	11.49	11.76	20.00	25.64	27.03	28.57

Table XXIII-2b

Effective Power of Minus Spectacle Lenses at the Corneal Plane for Vertex Distances of 11, 13, and 15 Millimeters.

Spectacle lens power F_v	Vertex distance 11mm	13mm F_e	15mm	Spectacle lens power F_v	Vertex distance 11mm	13mm F_e	15mm
− 0.25	−0.25	−0.25	−0.25	−10.25	− 9.21	− 9.04	− 8.88
− 0.50	−0.50	−0.50	−0.50	−10.50	− 9.41	− 9.24	− 9.07
− 0.75	−0.74	−0.74	−0.74	−10.75	− 9.61	− 9.43	− 9.26

Table XXIII-2b continued.

Spectacle lens power F_v	Vertex distance 11mm	13mm F_e	15mm	Spectacle lens power F_v	Vertex distance 11mm	13mm F_e	15mm
– 1.00	–0.99	–0.99	–0.99	–11.00	– 9.81	– 9.62	– 9.44
– 1.25	–1.23	–1.23	–1.23	–11.25	–10.01	– 9.81	– 9.63
– 1.50	–1.48	–1.47	–1.47	–11.50	–10.21	–10.00	– 9.81
– 1.75	–1.72	–1.71	–1.71	–11.75	–10.41	–10.19	– 9.99
– 2.00	–1.96	–1.95	–1.94	–12.00	–10.60	–10.38	–10.17
– 2.25	–2.20	–2.19	–2.18	–12.25	–10.80	–10.57	–10.35
– 2.50	–2.43	–2.42	–2.41	–12.50	–10.99	–10.75	–10.53
– 2.75	–2.67	–2.66	–2.64	–12.75	–11.18	–10.94	–10.70
– 3.00	–2.90	–2.89	–2.87	–13.00	–11.37	–11.12	–10.88
– 3.25	–3.14	–3.12	–3.10	–13.25	–11.56	–11.30	–11.05
– 3.50	–3.37	–3.35	–3.33	–13.50	–11.75	–11.48	–11.23
– 3.75	–3.60	–3.58	–3.55	–13.75	–11.94	–11.66	–11.40
– 4.00	–3.83	–3.80	–3.77	–14.00	–12.13	–11.84	–11.57
– 4.25	–4.06	–4.03	–4.00	–14.25	–12.32	–12.02	–11.74
– 4.50	–4.29	–4.25	–4.22	–14.50	–12.51	–12.20	–11.91
– 4.75	–4.51	–4.47	–4.43	–14.75	–12.69	–12.38	–12.08
– 5.00	–4.74	–4.69	–4.65	–15.00	–12.88	–12.55	–12.24
– 5.25	–4.96	–4.91	–4.87	–15.25	–13.06	–12.73	–12.41
– 5.50	–5.19	–5.13	–5.08	–15.50	–13.24	–12.90	–12.58
– 5.75	–5.41	–5.35	–5.29	–15.75	–13.42	–13.07	–12.74
– 6.00	–5.63	–5.57	–5.50	–16.00	–13.61	–13.25	–12.90
– 6.25	–5.85	–5.78	–5.71	–16.25	–13.79	–13.42	–13.07
– 6.50	–6.07	–5.99	–5.92	–16.50	–13.97	–13.59	–13.23
– 6.75	–6.28	–6.21	–6.13	–16.75	–14.14	–13.75	–13.39
– 7.00	–6.50	–6.42	–6.33	–17.00	–14.32	–13.92	–13.55
– 7.25	–6.71	–6.63	–6.54	–17.25	–14.50	–14.09	–13.70
– 7.50	–6.93	–6.83	–6.74	–17.50	–14.68	–14.26	–13.86
– 7.75	–7.14	–7.04	–6.94	–17.75	–14.85	–14.42	–14.02
– 8.00	–7.35	–7.25	–7.14	–18.00	–15.03	–14.59	–17.17
– 8.25	–7.56	–7.45	–7.34	–18.25	–15.20	–14.75	–14.33
– 8.50	–7.77	–7.65	–7.54	–18.50	–15.37	–14.91	–14.48
– 8.75	–7.98	–7.86	–7.73	–18.75	–15.54	–15.08	–14.63
– 9.00	–8.19	–7.86	–7.93	–19.00	–15.72	–15.24	–14.79
– 9.25	–8.40	–8.26	–8.12	–19.25	–15.89	–15.40	–14.94
– 9.50	–8.60	–8.46	–8.32	–19.50	–16.06	–15.56	–15.09
– 9.75	–8.81	–8.65	–8.51	–19.75	–16.23	–15.72	–15.24
–10.00	–9.01	–8.85	–8.70	–20.00	–16.38	–15.87	–15.38

2. For a compound spectacle lens (sphero-cylinder) the power of each principal meridian is referred to the plane of the cornea. The respective effective powers are then combined into a compound lens prescription.

a. Example: Spectacle refraction, –7.00 = –3.00 axis 180; Vertex distance, 11 mm.

(1) From Table XXIII-2: F_v at 180 = –7.00 D., F_e at 180 = –6.50 D.

F_v at 90 = –10.00 D., F_e at 90 = –9.00 D.

b. The lens power (prescription) required to fully correct the refractive state at the plane of the cornea is thus –6.50 = –2.50 axis 180.

c. When fitting a contact lens, the power of the CL-FL system must be –6.50 = –2.50 axis 180 to fully correct the refractive state.

III. THE SPHERICAL CONTACT LENS PRESCRIPTION

A. The spherical contact lens prescription can be determined by calculation, by refraction techniques, or by a combination of both.

B. Short method of calculation

1. This is the method most commonly used to convert the spectacle lens prescription into a spherical contact lens prescription. It has the advantage of being simple and generally yields satisfactory results.

2. *The calculation is made as follows:*

a. The spectacle lens prescription is recorded in minus cylinder form.

b. The spherical component of this prescription is referred to the plane of the cornea.

(1) The contact lens is specified with this power when the lens is fitted "on K", i.e., the base curve of the contact lens is equal to the flat keratometer reading of the cornea.

(2) The plus power of the lens is increased 0.25 diopters (minus power decreased 0.25 diopters) for each 0.25 D.K. that the base curve is flatter than K.

(3) The plus power of the lens is decreased 0.25 diopters (minus power increased 0.25 diopters) for each 0.25 D.K. that the base curve is steeper than K.

c. Example:

Spectacle Rx –7.00 ◯ –3.00 axis 180; Vertex distance = 11 mm; Corneal K reading = 42.00 at 180, 44.50 at 90; Contact lens base curve, 42.25 D.K.

(1) The spherical component of the prescription is –7.00 D. Referred to the plane of the cornea it becomes –6.50 D.

(2) Since the base curve of the contact lens is 0.25 D.K. steeper than the flat corneal K reading, the minus power is increased 0.25 D., thus the power of the contact lens is specified as –6.75 D. (–6.50 + [–0.25] = –6.75 D.)

3. *Solution using the optical model is as follows:*

a. The power of the CL-FL system must be -6.50 D. to correct the refractive state in the primary principal meridian.

b. The power of the fluid lens in air in this meridian is +0.25 D. ($F_{FL} = K_L - K_C = 42.25 - 42.00 = +0.25$D.).

c. The required contact lens power is thus –6.75 D. ($F_{CL} = F_{system} - F_{FL} = -6.50 - (+0.25) = -6.75$ D.).

4. The short method of calculation is confined to the lens power requirements in the primary principal meridian of the eye's dioptric system. In applying this method of calculation, it is assumed that the power of the fluid lens in the secondary principal meridian is such as to provide the additional correction needed in this meridian. When this assumption is incorrect, an astigmatic refractive state remains uncorrected. This latter error is termed residual astigmatism and is discussed later in this chapter.

C. Long method of calculation

1. The procedures employed in the long method of calculation are the same as those employed in the short method of calculation but they are applied to both principal meridians of the CL-FL system rather than just one meridian.

a. The optical cross method is convenient to use when calculating the contact lens power required to correct the refractive state in each principal meridian.

b. Using the previous example, the solution is developed in Figure XXIII-3. It will be noted that a spherical contact lens with a base curve of 42.25 D.K. and a back vertex power of –6.75 D. fully corrects the refractive state in both principal meridians of the eye.

Figure XXIII-3

K_L: 42.25 (at 90), 42.25 (at 180) – K_C: 44.50 (at 90), 42.00 (at 180) = F_{FL}: –2.25 D (at 90), +0.25 D (at 180)

Power of the fluid lens:

$$F_{FL} \text{ at } 90 = K_L - K_C = 42.25 - 44.50 = -2.25\text{ D}$$
$$F_{FL} \text{ at } 180 = K_L - K_C = 42.25 - 42.00 = +0.25\text{ D}$$

F_e: –9.00 D (at 90), –6.50 D (at 180) – F_{FL}: –2.25 D (at 90), +0.25 D (at 180) = F_{CL}: –6.75 D (at 90), –6.75 D (at 180)

Power of the contact lens:

$$F_{CL} \text{ at } 90 = F_e - F_{FL} = -9.00 - (-2.25) = -6.75\text{ D}$$
$$F_{CL} \text{ at } 180 = F_e - F_{FL} = -6.50 - (+0.25) = -6.75\text{ D}$$

Figure XXIII-3 – Long method of calculating the contact lens power using optical crosses. Given: spectacle prescription: –7.00 –3.00 axis 180; vertex distance: 11mm.; corneal K readings: 44.50 at 90, 42.00 at 180; contact lens base curve: 42.25 D.K.

c. The CL-FL system thus corrects the sphero-cylindrical refractive state by virtue of the fact that the fluid lens cylinder corrects the astigmatic component of the refractive state.

2. The long method of calculation is simplified by employing the sphero-cylindrical prescription (Rx) of the various components, thus equation (1) becomes Rx system = $Rx_{CL} + Rx_{FL}$ ----- (5)

a. The contact lens power of the previous example is calculated by substracting the Rx of the fluid lens in air from the correcting spectacle Rx referred to the plane of the cornea, thus:

(1) Rx system	–6.50 ⊂ –2.50 axis 180
$-Rx_{FL}$	–(+0.25 ⊂ –2.50 axis 180)
Rx_{CL}	–6.75 D. Sph.

b. The Rx of the contact lens in air (–6.75 D. Sphere) plus the Rx of the fluid lens in air

(+0.25 ⊃ −2.50 axis 180) combine to form the Rx of the CL-FL system (−6.50 ⊃ −2.50 axis 180) and thus supply the lens power needed to correct the refractive error.

(1) In this example the result obtained using the short method of calculation is the same as the result obtained using the long method of calculation. This is not always the case as will be demonstrated in the section on residual astigmatism.

c. When the calculated contact lens prescription (Rx_{CL}) results in a sphero-cylinder, the equivalent sphere is prescribed as the power of the spherical contact lens.

D. The contact lens prescription by refraction

1. The contact lens prescription cannot be determined solely from the spectacle lens prescription. It can be determined by refracting through a contact lens of known base curve and power.

2. The contact lens base curve is determined by measuring the curvature of the cornea and/or by observing the fit and performance of a series of diagnostic contact lenses on the eye. It is normally selected to fulfill the fitting needs of the eye rather than the power needs (although the latter is possible).

3. Once the base curve has been chosen, a diagnostic contact lens having the selected base curve and a known back vertex power is placed on the eye and a refraction is performed. The base curve establishes the power of the fluid lens. The refraction determines the prescription that must be added to the power of the diagnostic contact lens to correct the refractive state.

4. This method of determining contact lens power is especially useful when the corneal K readings are unknown or cannot be accurately measured (i. e. keratoconus).

5. Example:

a. Diagnostic contact lens: Base curve 44.00 D.K.; Power −2.00 D.

b. Refraction over contact lenses: −1.00 D. sphere

c. The power of 44.00 D.K. base curve contact lens required to correct refractive error is −2.00 + (−1.00) or −3.00 D. diopter sphere.

E. The contact lens prescription by refraction and calculation

1. If the refraction is performed through a diagnostic contact lens having a base curve other than the one to be prescribed for the patient, the final contact lens power must be altered because the final fluid lens prescription is being altered.

2. Example:

a. Diagnostic contact lens: Base curve, 44.00 D.K.; Power, −2.00 D.

b. Refraction over contact lenses: −1.00 D. sphere

(1) Power of 44.00 D.K. base curve contact lens required to correct the refractive error is −3.00 diopter sphere.

(2) If a 44.50 D.K. base curve is prescribed, the power of the fluid lens is increased +0.50 D.; therefore, the power of the contact lens must be increased by −0.50 D. to keep the power of the CL-FL system constant. The power of the contact lens required is −3.00 + (−0.50), or −3.50 D. sphere.

(3) If a 43.50 D.K. base curve is prescribed, the power of the fluid lens is increased –0.50 D.; therefore, the power of the contact lens must be increased by +0.50 D. The power of the contact lens required is –3.00 + (+0.50), or –2.50 D. sphere.

F. Clinical results in determining the contact lens prescription

1. Determination of the contact lens prescription by the three methods described, namely (1) the short method of calculation, (2) the long method of calculation, and (3) by refraction, frequently produced disparate results (Sarver, 1968).

a. The power of spherical corneal contact lenses was determined by Sarver (1968) by each of the three methods for a group of 119 patients and compared to the spherical lens power that gave the patient best visual acuity after he had adapted to wearing the lenses.

(1) The short method of calculation resulted in the smallest error in determining the best spherical contact lens power. The mean error was –0.01 D. with a standard error of ±0.33 D.

(2) In the long method of calculation, the mean error was –0.10 D., but the lens power was a little too high in plus. The standard error was about the same as with the short method of calculation, namely ±0.31 D.

(3) The mean error by refraction through a diagnostic contact lens was +0.06 D. with a greater standard error (±0.41 D.) than resulted with either method of calculation. Tearing by the novice patient doubtless contributed to the greater variability in lens power determination by this method.

2. The disparate lens powers resulting from these three methods of determining the contact lens prescription and variations from the best spherical lens power are due to errors of measurement and to false assumptions underlying the calculations.

a. *Refraction*

(1) An error in measuring the refractive state of the eye will result in a similar error when this information is used to calculate the contact lens power.

b. *Keratometry*

(1) Errors in corneal keratometry (especially the flatter K reading) may result in an improper calculation of contact lens power.

(a) An overcorrection of a myopic refractive state (undercorrection of a hyperopic refractive state) may result if the cornea is steeper (shorter radius of curvature) than the K reading assigned to it, while an undercorrection may result if the cornea is flatter than the K reading assigned to it.

(b) Furthermore, the nature of keratometry is such that even if a given keratometer reading is valid it may not accurately describe the curvature of that small portion of the cornea through which the line of sight passes.

c. *Vertex distance*

(1) Errors in measuring the vertex distance are not clinically significant when the refractive state is small but become increasingly significant as the refractive state is increased.

(a) A 2 mm. error in vertex distance results in a contact lens power error of about 0.25 D. when the spectacle plane refractive state is ± 12.50 diopters.

(2) This error can be avoided when the contact lens prescription is determined by refracting through a diagnostic contact lens having a back vertex power that is within a few diopters of the power required to correct the refractive state.

d. *Assumptions*

(1) Calculations used to determine the contact lens prescription were based on the assumptions that the CL-FL system was a centered optical system and that light from an object of regard exhibited normal incidence upon the sytem. When the contact lens was tilted or decentered, as was frequently the case for certain lens designs, the vergence properties of the system were altered (Westheimer, 1961; Sarver, 1963a,b).

IV. RESIDUAL ASTIGMATISM

A. Residual astigmatism was an astigmatic refractive state that was present when a contact lens was placed upon the cornea to correct an existing ametropia (Mandell, 1965). It was a common visual problem among contact lens patients (Bailey, 1961a) and frequently reduced correctable visual acuity from 20/20 to 20/25 or less. Residual astigmatism with spherical contact lenses was generally *physiological* but was also *induced* by the lenses.

1. *Physiological residual astigmatism* was caused by any or all of the following (Bailey, 1961b; Bennett, 1963; Mandell, 1965):

a. That portion of the anterior corneal surface cylinder that is not neutralized by the fluid lens.

b. The difference in curvature of the principal meridians of the posterior corneal surface.

c. The difference in curvature of the principal meridians at interfaces of the crystalline lens.

d. Tilt of the crystaline lens.

e. Variability of the refractive index of the cornea, crystalline lens, or vitreous.

f. The oblique incidence of light upon the cornea.

g. An eccentric position of the fovea in relation to the visual axis.

h. Mal-alignment of the various elements that constitute the optical system of the eye.

i. Some irregularity in the shape of the macular area.

2. *Induced residual astigmatism* was a product of the contact lens itself. It was caused by the tilt or decentration of the lens (Tocher, 1962; Sarver, 1963b), toric anterior and/or posterior surface of the contact lens (Korb, 1960), and warping or flexure of a thin contact lens (Bailey, 1961b).

B. Incidence of residual astigmatism

1. Bailey reported on the measured residual astigmatism of 105 subjects fitted with spherical corneal contact lenses. He found that 83% of the sample showed at least half a diopter of residual astigmatism in one or both eyes.

2. Sarver (1969) tabulated the measured residual astigmatism of 204 subjects fitted with spherical

corneal contact lenses. The mean value for the sample was –0.23 D. axis 90 ± 30 degrees with a standard deviation of ± 0.30 D. The range was from 0.75 D. with-the-rule to 1.25 D.against-the-rule. 34% of the eyes showed 0.50 D. or more of residual astigmatism.

C. Calculation of residual astigmatism

1. Residual astigmatism is calculated by subtracting Δ K from the total astigmatism of the eye referred to the plane of the cornea, where Δ K is the difference between the K readings of the two principal corneal meridians.

   a. Δ K is often incorrectly called the corneal astigmatism. It is a measure of anterior corneal surface toricity, but the index of refraction of the cornea is greater than the index used to calibrate the keratometer. Decentration of the corneal apex and/or tilt of the anterior corneal surface with respect to the line of sight results in an oblique astigmatism that constitutes part of the corneal astigmatism. This component of corneal astigmatism is not measured with the keratometer.

2. Although Δ K is the difference between the two K readings of the cornea, it is actually the amount of anterior corneal surface cylinder that is neutralized by the fluid lens and is therefore equal to the cylinder power of the posterior fluid lens surface in air. The latter is a minus cylinder with axis along the flat meridian.

   a. Example:

      (1) Subjective Rx, plano = –2.00 axis 90

      (2) Corneal K readings, = 43.00 at 90 and 44.00 at 180

      (3) Calculated residual astigmatism = total astigmatism – Δ K

      (4) CRA = (–2.00 axis 90) – (–1.00 axis 90) = –1.00 axis 90

3. The long method of calculating contact lens power provides the calculated residual astigmatism.

   a. Example:

      (1) Spectacle Rx = –7.00 = –3.00 axis 90

      (2) Vertex distance = 11 mm.

      (3) Corneal K readings = 44.00 at 180, 42.50 at 90

      (4) Contact lens base curve = 43.00 D.K.

      (5) Referred to the corneal plane the spectacle Rx is –6.50 = –2.50 axis 90.

      (6) By the long method of calculation the *required contact lens power* is –7.00 = –1.00 axis 90, computed as follows:

Rx system	–6.50 ⊃ –2.50 axis 90
$-Rx_{FL}$	–(+0.50 ⊃ –1.50 axis 90)
Rx_{CL}	–7.00 ⊃ 1.00 axis 90

(7) If a spherical contact lens is prescribed, the power would be specified as the spherical equivalent of the calculated prescription or –7.50 D.

(8) The calculated residual refractive error is +0.50 = –1.00 axis 90.

(9) The calculated residual astigmatism is –1.00 axis 90.

4. Several investigators (Kratz & Walton, 1949; Carter, 1963; Sarver, 1969) have calculated the residual astigmatism of independent samples with very similar results. Their findings are summarized in Table XXIII-3. The mean calculated residual astigmatism was about –0.50 axis 90.

Table XXIII-3

Investigator	N	Mean	Mode	S.D.	Range
Carter[18]	*100*	*0.50 D atr*	*0.50 D atr*	*±0.41 D*	*0.50 D wtr 2.00 D atr*
Kratz & Walton[19]	*295*		*0.50 D atr*		
Sarver[17]	*408*	*0.51 D atr*	*0.75 D atr*	*±0.45 D*	*0.75 D wtr 2.00 D atr*

Distribution of calculated residual astigmatism reported by three investigators. (atr: against-the-rule, wtr: with-the-rule)

D. Prediction of residual astigmatism

1. It has been stated (Bailey, 1961c) that the residual astigmatism that will be present with a spherical contact lens can be predicted with an accuracy which will vary primarily with the degree of error made by the clinician either with the keratometer or in his refraction. The implication in this statement is that the calculated residual astigmatism is probably the best value to use in predicting the residual astigmatism that will be measured with the contact lens in situ.

2. The author, (Sarver, 1969) in a study of 408 eyes, found the measured residual astigmatism to be significantly smaller than the calculated residual astigmatism. The results of this study are shown in Figures XXIII-4 and 5.

a. The mean difference between the calculated and measured residual astigmatism is relatively small for calculated values between 0.25 D. with-the-rule and 0.50 D. against-the-rule. In this range, errors of measurement readily obscure the differences that become more apparent with larger calculated values.

b. The measured residual astigmatism is related to the calculated residual astigmatism by the linear regression equation $y = 0.274x + 0.086$, where y is the measured residual astigmatism and x is the calculated residual astigmatism. For clinical use this equation can be simplified to $y = 0.3x$.

c. The values given by the above equation are within ± 0.25 D. of the measured residual astigmatism for 68% of the eyes and within ± 0.50 D. for 98% of the eyes.

(1) Example:

(a) If the calculated residual astigmatism is –1.50 axis 90, the measured residual astigmatism would be predicted to be between zero and –1.00 axis 90 at a very high level of confidence ($y = 0.3x \pm 0.50$ D.)

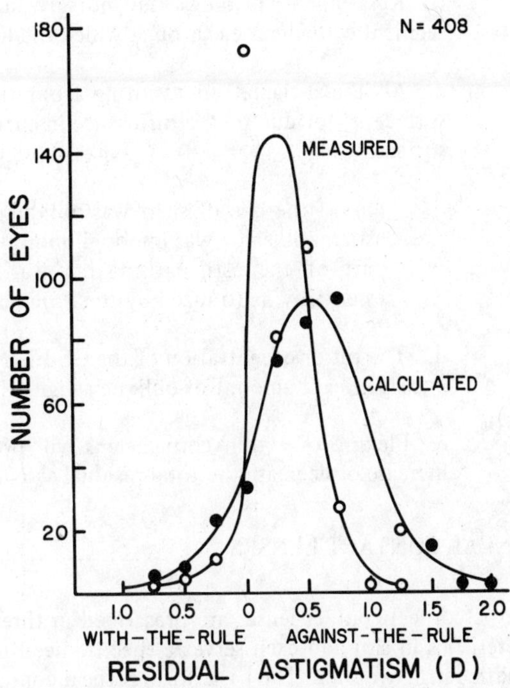

Figure XXIII-4 – Distribution of calculated and measured residual astigmatism (from Sarver, 1969).

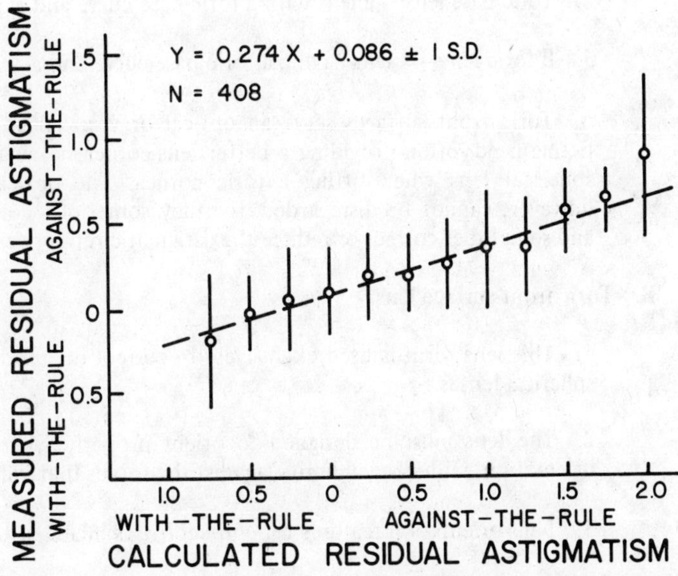

Figure XXIII-5 – Calculated vs. measured residual astigmatism with the mean and plus and minus one standard deviation of measured values plotted for each calculated value (from Sarver, 1969).

3. A number of reasons can be given to account for the difference between the calculated and measured residual astigmatism.

   a. Errors of measurement in refraction or K readings probably produce a random difference.

b. Keratometer readings may not give a valid description of the corneal toricity for the segment of the cornea through which the line of sight passes.

c. All the astigmatism resulting from the incidence of light upon the anterior corneal surface is not due to the difference in curvature between the two principal meridians of this surface.

(1) If the line of sight was oblique to this surface, as it frequently was, an additional astigmatic error was imposed upon the refractive state of the eye (Sarver, 1963b). This part of the astigmatism that was produced by the anterior corneal surface, and essentially neutralized by the fluid lens, was not measured with the keratometer.

d. The tilt or decentration of the CL-FL system relative to the line of sight produces a small but significant amount of oblique astigmatism.

e. Flexure of a thin corneal lens will produce an induced residual astigmatism that may increase or decrease the total residual astigmatism.

V. TORIC CORNEAL CONTACT LENSES

A. Toric corneal contact lenses are prescribed in three basic forms. Each has unique cylindrical power characteristics in situ and each serves a specific need in fitting the toric cornea and/or in correcting an astigmatic refractive state. The basic toric corneal contact lens forms are as follows:

1. Toric front surface lens – a lens with a spherical base curve and a toric front surface.

2. Toric base lens – a lens with a toric base curve and a spherical front surface.

3. Bitoric lens – a lens having a toric base curve and a toric front surface.

4. Toric front surfaces serve an optical or visual need. Toric back surfaces serve a physical or fitting need, often providing a better lens-cornea bearing relationship than that obtainable with a spherical lens when fitting a toric cornea. The optical properties of the back toric surface, however, cannot be disregarded, for they sometimes contribute to the astigmatic refractive state and sometimes correct or reduce the astigmatic refractive state.

B. Toric front surface lens

1. This lens form is used exclusively to correct the residual astigmatism that may be present with spherical lenses.

2. The lens must be designed to orient properly when in situ and to maintain its meridional orientation, within small limits, against the forces that will act to rotate the lens.

3. Lens orientation features for *corneal lenses* included the following factors (Mandell, 1965):

a. Prism ballast

b. Truncation, single or double

c. Prism ballast and truncation

d. Metal ballast

e. A scleral flange

f. Toric secondary curves

4. The *scleral lens* has excellent orientation properties and lends itself well to the application of a front surface cylinder.

5. The cylindrical power of the lens is the same on the eye as it is when measured (in air) with a lensometer, because all of the cylinder is on the anterior lens surface.

6. Theoretically the sphero-cylindrical prescription of this lens form can be determined by the long method of calculation.

a. Example:

(1) Spectalce Rx = –2.00 ⊃ –1.50 axis 90

(2) Corneal K readings = 43.50 at 90, 44.00 at 180

(3) Base curve of contact lens = 43.50 D.K.

(4) The contact lens power is given by equation (5), thus

Rx_{system}	–2.00 ⊃ –1.50 axis 90
$-Rx_{FL}$	–(0 ⊃ –0.50 axis 90)
Rx_{CL}	–2.00 ⊃ –1.00 axis 90

(5) This lens has a spherical base curve and a toric front surface and, if properly oriented on the eye, will theoretically correct the refractive state.

7. It was previously pointed out that the residual astigmatism could be predicted only with an accuracy of ± 0.50 D. and ± 20 to 30 degrees in axis. It was, therefore, more accurate to determine the sphero-cylindrical prescription of this lens form by refracting through a spherical diagnostic contact lens of known base curve and power.

8. The meridional orientation of the lens must also be taken into account so that the axis of the front surface cylinder will be the same as the axis of the residual astigmatism. A prism ballast lens, for example, will generally rotate up 10 to 15 degrees nasally. If the measured residual astigmatism of the right eye is –1.00 axis 90, the cylindrical power is ordered –1.00 axis 75 to 80 degrees. Lens rotation of 10 to 15 degrees will place the cylinder axis at or near 90 degrees.

9. Greater accuracy was achieved, when correcting residual astigmatism, by the use of a technique in which the *location of the base of the prism ballasted lens was determined before* the cylindrical power was added to the front surface of the lens (Borish, 1960, 1962a, 1963, 1968). The technique briefly encompassed the following steps:

a. A spherical ballasted lens of desired prismatic power is first fitted to the eye to achieve maximum wear so that the effects of lid pressure, tearing, squinting, and other influences of adaptation or discomfort upon the orientation of the base of the lens are eliminated.

(1) Borish (1968) used 3/4 to 1 Δ for lenses larger than 9.2 and power greater than –1.00 D., and 1¼ to 1½ Δ for plus lenses or those of lower minus power, or for lenses smaller than 9.2 in powers less than –1.75 D. For powers over –1.75, the lesser prism diopter often provided sufficient ballast even in small lenses.

(a) Of prime interest is the fact that the ballast depends upon the amount of plastic present at the base of the lens. Thus, in small lenses, although the prismatic effect remains the same, optically speaking, the ballasted effect is often less than in larger lenses, or missing.

(b) Similarly, low prismatic amounts provide greater ballast in minus lenses of the same optical value than in plus lenses. In the latter, the center of gravity of the plus lens, as can be seen by drawing a profile, often remains relatively closer to the center of the lens than in an equivalent minus lens.

[1] Consequently, truncating the base of a plus lens helps the ballasting effect by moving the center of gravity closer to the bottom of the lens, while truncating the apex often fails to assist the ballast. In a minus lens, truncation of the base actually diminishes the ballasting effect of the lens.

b. The base of the lens is marked by a thin line covering the area of the peripheral curves of the lens as a segment of a line from the edge of the lens towards the center. This mark should be in a medium not soluble in the tears, such as marking ink or plastic marker.

(1) When the base has been consistently oriented in the eye (as full or advanced wearing time is attained), the position of the base can be reliably read by the following technique.

(a) A 0.12 spectacle trial case cylinder is marked with red crayon or marking pencil so that the axis of the cylinder (designated on the rim or edge of the lens) appears as a red line bisecting the spectacle trial lens.

(b) A trial frame is placed on the patient's face and the lens cell accurately centered before the patient's eye with the contact lens in the eye.

(c) The spectacle trial lens, bearing the red line, is placed in the trial cell before the eye, and the axis is rotated until this line is either coincident with or parallel to the line on the contact lens which indicates the position of the base.

(d) The position of the base can then be read from the protractor of the spectacle trial frame.

[1] This reading, plus 180°, indicates the base position for addition of the cylinder, when determined.

[a] For example, if the red line of the spectacle lens is parallel to the line indicating the base of the contact lens at 110° on the protractor, the base rides at 110 +180, or 290°.

(2) In some cases the base will vary within a given number of degrees. Since the power of a cylinder varies only slightly, especially in lower powers, up to 10 to 15°, the midpoint of such a range will often prove satisfactory unless the cylinder power needed is excessive.

c. The cylindrical power needed for correction of the residual astigmatism is also measured through the ballasted spherical contact lens. Frequently, the resultant residual astigmatism varies slightly from that found through a non-prismatic spherical lens, possibly due to the obliquity of the surfaces of a prismatic lens (which seems to induce some slight minus cylinder fortunately at a 90° [or base-apex] axis).

(1) The contact lens may be returned for addition of the cylinder, where the

laboratory has the facilities for so doing, or a duplicate lens bearing the cylinder may be ordered to replace the spherical one.

(a) All physical characteristics of the lens should be identical with that of the sperical one as changes in any aspect may change the orientation of the new lens.

(2) It should be noted that not only is the power of the cylinder and its axis ordered, but also the position of the base of the lens is designated.

(a) An order might read: add +0.50 sph. –0.75 cyl axis 100 to enclosed lens. Base rides at 280°.

[1] It was usual that, after a minus cylinder was determined, added plus sphere would also be found (Borish, 1963; 1966).

d. If the resultant cylinder axis falls at an oblique position, from 30 to 60 or 120 to 150 degrees, the lens after cylinder addition will often fail to orient as it did prior to cylinder addition. If the physical configuration of a prismatic lens, base down, and a simple cylinder axis 45°, are combined mentally into one lens, the reason is apparent. The final physical configuration bears little resemblance to the weight distribution of the lens prior to the addition of the cylinder. In such cases, special edging, or large amounts of prism were needed (Borish, 1962b). Similarly, if the base does not orient in the lower quadrant, but fixes at an oblique position or rotates widely, and the cylinder is in the vertical position, the resultant lens will not orient as expected. The measures necessary to correct such problems fall largely within the province of fitting techniques rather than in this chapter.

e. The use of the cross-cylinder for disclosing the presence of astigmatism, as described in the chapter dealing with Subjective Techniques, was found satisfactory and repeatable for testing residual astigmatism through a contact lens (Borish, 1962a, 1963).

(1) After the cylinder is determined, the eye should be fogged with added plus sphere, and then unfogged to best acuity. It will be found that in many cases, a resultant sphero-cylindrical combination often equivalent to a plus cylinder is found. The previous simple sphere actually represented the correction of the spherical equivalent of the eye.

C. Toric base lens

1. The toric base spherical front surface lens is used to fit the toric cornea but introduces a cylinder into the CL-FL system that cannot be disregarded.

2. The cylindrical power of this lens is a function of the toricity of the posterior lens surface, the index of refraction of the lens, the index of refraction of the media in contact with the lens, and the orientation of the lens.

3. The toricity of the contact lens base curve is commonly stated in terms of ΔK_{CL}, where ΔK_{CL} is the K reading difference between the curvatures of the toric back surface. Thus, if the radii of curvature of a toric base lens is 7.50 mm. (45.00 D.K.) in one principal meridian and 7.85 mm. (43.00 D.K.) in the second principal meridian, the base curve is said to have two diopters of toricity. The cylindrical power of this surface, however, is *not* two diopters. As previously pointed out, the power of a contact lens surface is equal to the K reading of the surface times a constant (See Table 1). Similarly, the difference in power between two meridians of a contact lens is equal to the difference in K readings of these meridians times a constant.

4. The cylinder power of a toric back surface lens of refractive index 1.490 can be summarized as follows:

a. The cylinder power of a toric back surface lens *in air* is equal to ΔK_{CL} x 1.452. This is a minus cylinder with axis along the flat meridian.

b. The cylinder power of a toric back surface lens *on the eye* is ΔK_{CL} x 0.456. This is a minus cylinder with axis along the flat meridian.

(1) Note: The cylinder induced by these back surfaces may require correction by an added minus cylinder with its axis parallel to the steep meridian of the lens.

c. The cylinder power of a toric back surface lens *on the eye* is equal to .314 times the cylinder power of this lens as measured *in air* with the lensometer.

d. Example:

(1) A toric base spherical front surface lens (n = 1.490) is fitted to an eye having an against-the-rule corneal toricity. The K readings of the contact lens base curve are 45.00 D.K. and 43.00 D.K.

(2) The cylinder power of the lens in air is –2.90 ([43.00 – 45.00] x 1.452).

(3) The cylinder power of the lens of the eye is –0.90 D. ([43.00 – 45.00] x 0.456).

(4) If the eye manifests a residual astigmatism of about –1.00 axis 90 degrees with a spherical contact lens, and if this toric base lens orients on the eye with its flat meridian vertical, the induced cylinder will correct the residual astigmatism.

(5) If the eye manifests no residual astigmatism with a spherical contact lens, this toric base lens will induce a measured residual astigmatism of +1.00 axis 90 degrees and should be rejected in favor of a bitoric lens.

5. This lens form thus provides a proper prescription for correcting the ametropia when the residual astigmatism manifested with a spherical contact lens is equal to about one half of the ΔK_{CL}, and the flat meridian of the lens orients along the axis of the minus cylinder that corrects the residual refractive state present with a spherical contact lens. The fitting characteristics of a toric base lens could sometimes be *compromised and changed* in the interest of providing a *better optical correction* of the refractive state (Sellers, 1967).

D. Bitoric corneal contact lenses

1. The bitoric corneal contact lens is used to fit the toric cornea. The power characteristics of this lens form can be used to fully correct an ametropia, including induced residual astigmatism and/or physiological residual astigmatism. The prescription can be determined by calculation or by a combination of calculation and refraction.

2. The bitoric prescription may be calculated by the long method of calculation.

a. Example: Spectacle Rx: –1.00 ⊃ –2.00 axis 180; Corneal K reading: 43.00 at 180 and 46.00 at 90.

b. If the base curve is fitted "on K" in both principal meridians, the power of the fluid lens is zero and the required power of the bitoric contact lens is equal to the spectacle Rx referred to the plane of the cornea, namely –1.00 ⊃ –2.00 axis 180.

c. If the base curve is fitted other than "on K", say 42.50 at 180 and 45.00 at 90; the usual calculation is made:

Rx_{system}	–1.00 –2.00 axis 180
$-Rx_{FL}$	–(–0.50 ⊃ –0.50 axis 180)
Rx_{CL}	–0.50 ⊃ – 1.50 axis 180

(1) To correct the refractive state the lens must orient with its flat meridian horizontal. If the lens rotates on the eye, a residual astigmatism will be induced and visual acuity will diminish.

3. Inherent in this calculation is the assumption that the physiological residual astigmatism is equal to the difference between the spectacle lens cylinder and the corneal Δ K. Since this assumption is frequently false, the calculation may result in an improper bitoric prescription.

4. It is not unusual to encounter a patient whose refractive state is corrected with a spherical contact lens but whose corneal toricity is such as to require a toric base curve lens to achieve an optimum lens cornea bearing relationship. If a spherical contact lens corrects the refractive state, the back surface of the fluid lens contributes all the necessary cylinder power. Because this cylinder is formed by the cornea, it does not change in axis or power as the spherical lens rotates on the eye.

a. The spherical lens can be replaced with a bitoric lens without introducing any additional cylinder into the CL-FL system (Sarver, 1963c). This is achieved by placing a cylinder on the front surface of the contact lens of such magnitude and axis as to neutralize the back surface cylinder when the lens is on the eye. The front surface cylinder corrects the residual astigmatism *induced* by the back surface cylinder.

b. Expressed in meridional powers this relationship becomes $F_s + K_s = F_f + K_f$ -------(6) where F_s and F_f are the back vertex power of the bitoric contact lens in the steeper and flatter meridians respectively, and K_s and K_f are the K readings of the contact lens base curve in the steeper and flatter meridians respectively.

c. Example: A spherical contact lens with a base curve of 42.00 D.K. and back vertex power –2.00 D. corrects the refractive error of a given eye. A lens with a toric base of 42.00 D.K. and 45.00 D.K. respectively provides an optimum lens cornea bearing relationship.

(1) The back vertex power required in the 42.00 D.K. meridian is –2.00 D.

(2) The back vertex power required in the 45.00 D.K. meridian is –5.00 D. ($F_s = F_f + K_f - K_s = -2.00 + 42.00 - 45.00 = -5.00$ D.).

(3) The lens is ordered with a base curve of 42.00 D.K. and power –2.00 D. in the flatter meridian, and 45.00 D.K. and power –5.00 D. in the steeper meridian. With a lensometer this lens will measure –2.00 ⊃ –3.00 axis along the flatter meridian. On the eye it will have the power effect of a –2.00 D. spherical contact lens.

(a) *Cylinder power in air*

[1] The back surface cylinder equals (42.00 – 45.00) x 0.456 = –1.35 axis 90.

[2] The front surface cylinder is ground +1.35 axis 90 so that total lens cylinder equals –3.00 axis 90.

(b) *Cylinder power in situ*

[1] The back surface cylinder equals (42.00 – 45.00) x 0.456 = –1.35 axis 90.

[2] Since the front surface cylinder is + 1.35 axis 90, the total cylinder of the lens in situ is zero.

(4) The lens can rotate on the eye without producing a change in the cylinder power of the system.

(5) The power of this bitoric lens can be calculated without knowledge of the corneal K readings and without assumptions about physiological residual astigmatism.

5. When physiological residual astigmatism is present, the bitoric lens prescription is first calculated to have spherical power effect in situ. This compensates for the induced residual astigmatism. The additional cylinder power needed to correct the physiological residual astigmatism is then added to the prescription of the above bitoric lens. This approach, employing a combination of calculation and refraction through a spherical contact lens, increases the accuracy of the bitoric contact lens prescription.

VI. VISION WITH CONTACT LENSES

A. It was previously stated that spectacle lenses and contact lenses differed in the manner in which they corrected ametropia. The optical properties of the two systems differed in many significant respects and made the visual world of the contact lens wearer quite different than the visual world of the spectacle lens wearer (Westheimer, 1962). The patient's visual response to a given lens system was strongly influenced by the visual acuity he achieved with the system, but his response could not be evaluated solely in terms of Snellen acuity. Optical properties of the lens system, other than focal power, affected his total visual response. Some achieved better vision with spectacle lenses, others with contact lenses.

B. Aberrations

1. Westheimer (1961) pointed out that the aberrations of a visual aid could only be discussed in the context of the use of the device in association with the eyes. The eyes rotate behind spectacle lenses but contact lenses rotated with the eyes. Most of the aberrations associated with the wearing of spectacle lenses, especially strong spectacle lenses, were significantly reduced with contact lenses. The reason lay in the simple fact that the small bundle of rays entering the pupil and passing through the center of rotation of the eye passed through or near the center of a contact lens but frequently passed through peripheral portions of a spectacle lens. Among these aberrations were oblique astigmatism, distortion, coma, and curvature of the field.

2. Contact lenses in air have more spherical aberration than spectacle lenses because they have a relatively high curvature for their aperture (Westheimer, 1961). The peripheral aberration of the cornea ordinarily reduces the peripheral aberration of opposite type of the periphery of the crystalline lens. On the eye, the contact lens increases the resultant aberration of the eye by replacing the aspherical corneal surface with its spherical surface as the interface of greatest refractive power. Millodot (1969) demonstrated that visual acuity was not adversely affected by this spherical aberration when contact lenses were worn under conditions of high luminance. As the luminance level was reduced and the pupil dilated, however, visual acuity with contact lenses decreased more rapidly than with spectacle lenses.

C. Accommodation

1. When a patient whose ametropia is corrected with contact lenses views a near object, he must accommodate a different amount than would be necessary if his ametropia was corrected with spectacle lenses. The ocular accommodation, or more precisely the stimulus to accommodation, required to view a near object through these two lens types has been calculated and compared by several investigators (Alpern, 1949; Westheimer, 1962; Bennett, 1963; Mandell, 1965; Stone, 1968). The myope viewing a near object will accommodate *more* when his ametropia is corrected with contact lenses than when it is corrected with spectacle lenses. The hyperope will, under the same conditions, accommodate *less* with contact lenses than with spectacle lenses (Figure XXIII-6).

2. When spectacle lenses are replaced with contact lenses, the frontal plane containing the correcting lens is shifted from a finite position in front of the cornea to a position at the surface of the cornea. This change in lens position is primarily responsible for the change in the stimulus to accommodation. The greater the shift in position, the greater the change in accommodative stimulus for a given shift in lens position.

3. These facts have a number of *clinical implications.*

a. The *myope* who is fitted with contact lenses may experience asthenopia or "focusing" difficulty when doing close work. This is observed frequently among college students. The symptoms generally subside as the patient adapts to the greater accommodative stimulus.

b. The *myope who is approaching presbyopia* will experience vision difficulty when reading with a full contact lens correction due to the increased demand on accommodation.

c. The *hyperope who is approaching presbyopia* will experience less difficulty when reading with a full contact lens correction than with the equivalent spectacle lens correction.

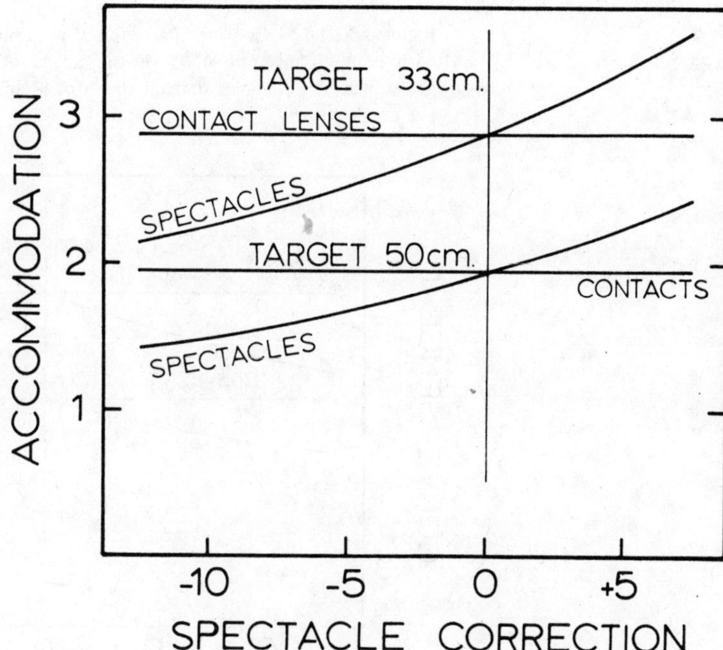

Figure XXIII-6 – Ocular accommodation required when patient with the spectacle ametropia shown on the abscissae of the graph views a target 33.3 cm. and 50 cm., respectively, in front of the spectacle plane (14 mm. in front of the corneal vertex) when wearing spectacle lenses and contact lenses (from Westheimer, 1962).

D. Convergence

1. The convergence (in prism diopters) required for an emmetrope to bifixate a near object is equal to the dioptric distance from the object to the centers of rotation of the eyes multiplied by the subject's interpupillary distance in centimeters.

2. The convergence required for an ametrope to bifixate a near object when wearing contact

lenses is the same as that required of the emmetrope, because the lenses rotate with the eyes and the lines of sight remain relatively well directed through the centers of the lenses.

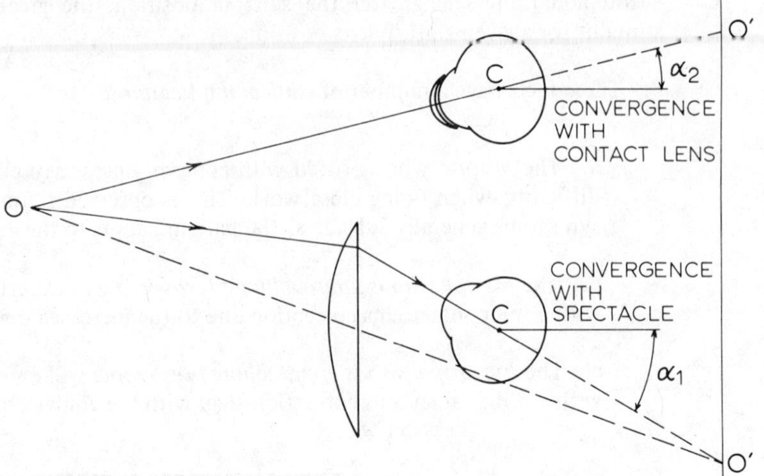

Figure XXIII-7 – Convergence required with plus spectacle lens (α_1) is greater than with contact lens (α_2). O′ is the image of O as formed by the spectacle lens positioned at a distance d from the corneal apex. C is the center of rotation of the eye.

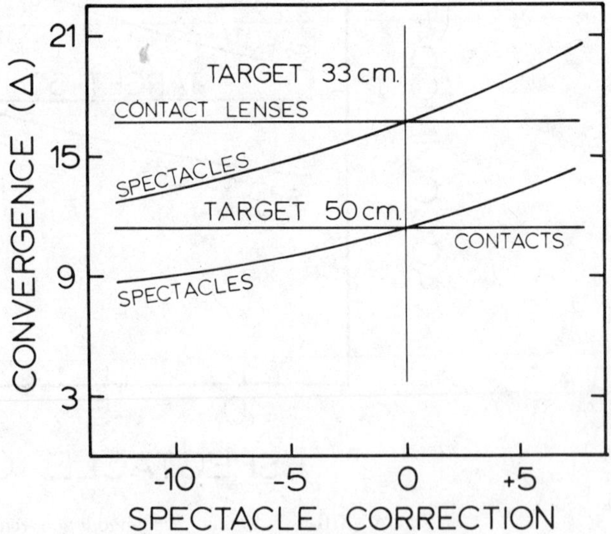

Figure XXIII-8 – Convergence in prism diopters that has to be exerted by patient (P.D. 65 mm.) with the spectacle ametropia shown on the abscissae of the graph, when viewing a target 33.3 cm. and 50 cm., respectively, in front of the spectacle plane when wearing spectacle lenses and contact lenses (from Westheimer, 1962).

3. When an ametrope wearing spectacle lenses centered for his distance P.D. fixated a near object, the amount of convergence required was not only a function of his interpupillary distance and the distance of the object, but was also a function of the refracting power of the spectacle lenses (Figure XXIII-7) (Alpern, 1949). As the myope converges to bifixate a near object, his lines of sight depart from the centers of his spectacle lenses and encounter increasing amounts of base-in prismatic

effect. The spectacle wearing hyperope encounters base-out prismatic effect as he converges to bifixate a near object. Thus, to bifixate a given object at a distance less than infinity, the bespectacled myope converges less than the emmetrope (or the contact lens wearer) while the hyperope wearing spectacles converges more than the emmetrope (or the contact lens wearer).

4. The convergence required to bifixate a near object when wearing spectacle lenses and when wearing contact lenses has been calculated by a number of investigators (Alpern, 1949; Westheimer, 1962; Bennett, 1963; Stone, 1968). Figure XXIII-8 clearly shows that the myope who discards his spectacle lenses in favor of contact lenses must converge more to bifixate a given near object while the hyperope will converge less under the same conditions.

E. Accommodation / convergence ratio

1. The myope must accommodate more and converge more when fixating a near object with contact lenses compared to spectacle lenses.

2. The hyperope will accommodate less and converge less when fixating a near object with contact lenses compared to spectacle lenses.

3. Stone (1967; 1968) and Bennett (1963) have shown that the ratio between accommodation and convergence was almost the same with contact lenses as with spectacle lenses, provided that the contact lenses remained centered, the spectacle lenses were centered for distance vision, and the spectacle lens vertex distance was approximately half the distance between the spectacle lens and the eye's center of rotation.

F. Prism in contact lenses

1. A prism contact lens may be considered as consisting of a thin afocal miniscus prism separated by air from a refractive portion. The prismatic power, at any point on the lens, may be calculated approximately by applying Prentice's rule to the refractive component and adding this to the prism component of the lens. For example, a lens of +5.00 D. power combined with a 1.5 Δ prism (base down) and riding 2 mm below the line of sight would have an effective prism of 2.5 Δ base down. (Mandell, 1967).

2. The effective prismatic power of an afocal prism contact lens increases toward the apex of the prism. Thus a plano prism contact lens positioning low on the cornea will have greater prismatic effect than would be measured at the geometric center of the lens.

3. A given amount of prism in a contact lens is as effective as the same amount of prism in a spectacle lens (Bailey, 1966). Immersing the lens in tear fluid on the eye does not significantly alter the prismatic effect. Vertical position of the lens and tilt of the lens will alter the prismatic effect to a small degree.

4. For near targets the prismatic effect of a contact lens is greater than that of a spectacle lens because, for near viewing conditions, the deviating effect of a prism increases as the prism is moved closer to the center of rotation of the eye.

G. Magnification

1. When an ametrope observes a distant object through corrective lenses, the previously blurred retinal images not only come into sharp focus but also undergo a change in size. This change in image size was termed *spectacle magnification* and was defined as the ratio of the retinal image size in the corrected ametropic eye to that in the uncorrected eye, having reference to an object at infinity (Bennett, 1963; Emsley, 1963). Spectacle magnification was a product of the *power* and *shape* factors of the correcting lens (Morgan and Peters, 1948).

a. The power factor is given by the expression $1/(1 - hF_v)$, where h is the distance between the posterior lens surface and the entrance pupil (in meters), and F_v is the back vertex power of the lens (in diopters).

b. The shape factor is $1/(1 - dF_1)$, where d is the reduced thickness t/n and F_1 is the power of the anterior lens surface (in diopters). When the lens is very thin, as it frequently is with contact lenses, the shape factor may be disregarded.

2. Mandell (1965) used the term *magnification of correction* in preference to the term *spectacle magnification* because it better expressed the concept of magnification with any type of corrective lens, including spectacle lenses and contact lenses. The two terms were synonymous.

3. The magnification of correction (MC) is readily calculated when a given ametropia is corrected with a spectacle lens and when it is corrected with a contact lens having the same effective power as the spectacle lens. The spectacle lens alters the size of the retinal image more than the contact lens, due primarily to its position at a finite distance from the cornea.

4. For a given eye, the relative change in magnification resulting when a spectacle lens is replaced with a contact lens is given by the ratio of the magnifications of correction for the two lens types.

a. Example:

(1) MC with a spectacle lens.

(a) $F_v = -7.50$ D. sphere.

(b) $F_1 = +3.50$ D.

(c) t = 0.6 mm.

(d) Vertex distance = 13 mm. ∴ h = 16 mm.

(e) $$MC_s = \frac{1}{1 - hF_v} \times \frac{1}{1 - dF_1}$$

$$= \frac{1}{1 - (.016 \times -7.50)} \times \frac{1}{1 - (\frac{.0006}{1.5} \times 3.50)} = 0.89$$

(f) The clear image is thus 11% smaller than the blurred image.

b. MC with a contact lens having the same effective power at the cornea as the −7.50 D. spectacle lens.

(1) $F_v = -6.87$ D.

(2) t = 0.15 mm.

(3) n = 1.49

(4) Base curve fitted "on K" at 43.50 D.K.

(5) $F_1 = 55.71$ D. by calculation

(6) h = 3 mm.

(7) $$MC_c = \frac{1}{1 - hF_v} \times \frac{1}{1 - dF_1}$$

$$= \frac{1}{1 - (.003 \times -6.87)} \times \frac{1}{1 - (\frac{.00015}{1.49} \times 55.71} = 0.98$$

(8) The clear image is thus 2% smaller than the blurred image.

c. MC ratio

(1) $$\frac{MC_c}{MC_s} = \frac{0.98}{0.89} = 1.10$$

(2) The retinal image with the contact lens is thus 10% larger than the retinal image with the spectacle lens.

5. Westheimer (1962) calculated the magnification of correction for a series of spectacle lenses and for a series of contact lenses having the same effective power at the corneal plane (Figure XXIII-9). He also calculated the MC ratio (contact lens/spectacle lens magnification ratio) to show the change in image size that occurred when a given spectacle lens correction was replaced with a contact lens correction.

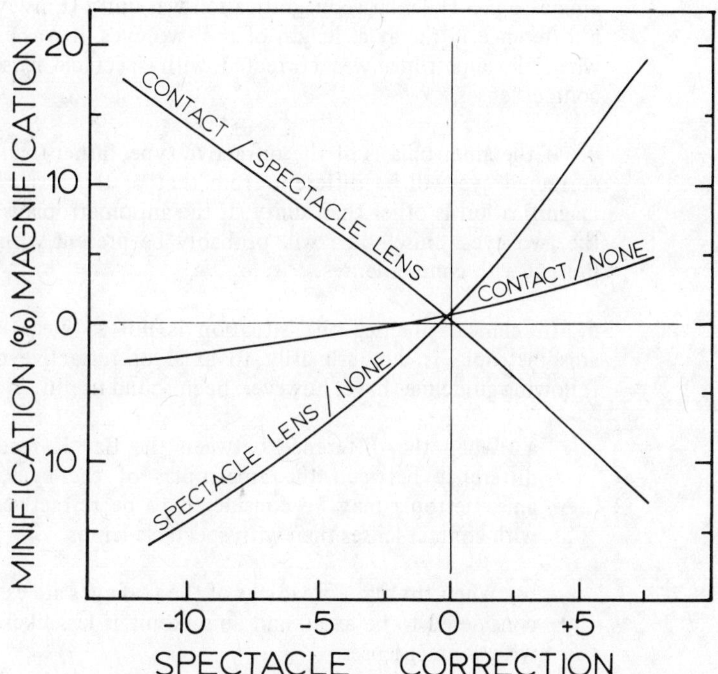

Figure XXIII-9 – Magnifications of spectacle lens correction compared to unaided vision, contact lens correction compared to unaided vision, and contact lens correction compared to vision with the spectacle lens correction. Spectacle lenses have the powers and thicknesses of the orthogon series (Bausch and Lomb Incorporated). The contact lenses are fitted on K for 43.50 D. and have thicknesses of average values. Abscissae: spectacle ametropia in diopters. Effectivity has been allowed for so that all points on a vertical line refer to the same ametropia (from Westheimer, 1962).

6. Contact lenses increase the size of the retinal image for the myope and reduce the size of the retinal image for the hyperope relative to the image formed with spectacle lenses.

H. Anisometropia

1. Contact lenses often afford a means by which to cope with the primary problems associated with the spectacle lens correction of unequal ametropias in the two eyes. These problems include induced heterophorias and aniseikonia (See Chapter VIII).

a. Heterophorias are induced when the eyes rotate away from the optical centers of unequal spectacle lens corrections and encounter disparate amounts of prismatic effect.

b. Aniseikonia is a product of the unequal magnification of the two spectacle lenses, differences between the two eyes (dioptric and possibly neural), and perceptual influences (See Chapter VIII).

2. When contact lenses of unequal powers center and rotate with the eyes, no heterophoria is induced. A significant heterophoria is not induced even if the lenses sag or decenter because the displacement from the line of sight is seldom more than a millimeter or two. An exception may occur in the correction of unilateral aphakia where a one millimeter gravitational drop of the lens will induce 1.5 Δ of vertical phoria for a +15.00 D. contact lens.

3. Knapp stated, and Ogle (1950) demonstrated, that if the (spectacle) correcting lens was placed before the eye so that the second principal plane coincided with the anterior focal point of the axial ametropic eye, the size of the image on the retina would be the same as though the eye were emmetropic. The relative magnification was unity (Emsley, 1963). If the anisometropia was due to a difference in the axial length of the two eyes, it was unlikely that aniseikonia would be present when the ametropia was corrected with spectacle lenses but probably would be present with contact lenses.

4. If the ametropia is of the refractive type, rather than axial, the size of the retinal image of the corrected eye will be different from that of the image were the eye emmetropic. The relative magnification is other than unity. If the anisometropia is due to a difference in the focal power of the two eyes, aniseikonia will probably be present with spectacle lenses, but is not likely to be present with contact lenses.

5. In clinical practice the situation is not so clear cut, and we cannot know whether the anisometropia is due primarily to axial or refractive differences between the two eyes. The following guidelines have, however, been found useful:

a. When the difference between the flat K reading of the two eyes approximates the difference between the ametropias of the eyes, and is in the expected direction, the anisometropia may be considered to be refractive. Aniseikonia is less likely to be present with contact lenses than with spectacle lenses.

b. When the flat K readings of the two eyes are essentially equal, the anisometropia may be considered to be axial, and aniseikonia is less likely to be present with spectacle lenses than with contact lenses.

c. Although a formal study is not available to confirm the reliability of these guidelines, eikonometer measurements of numerous clinical patients examined in the Contact Lens Clinic of the School of Optometry of the University of California have given promising results.

6. When the axis or amount of astigmatism is significantly different between the two eyes, meridional aniseikonia is likely to be present with spectacle lenses because astigmatism is a

refractive anomaly. Contact lenses are a most favorable form of correction under these conditions. The thin, toric fluid lens induces very little meridional aniseikonia, and since the contact lenses reduce the magnification of correction to an amount approaching unity, meridional aniseikonia is essentially eliminated.

I. Aphakia (See also Chapter XXII)

1. *Spectacle lenses versus contact lenses*

a. *Spectacle lenses* may provide the aphakic patient with good visual acuity but they leave much to be desired as a device for restoring good vision. High plus spectacle lenses, positioned at a finite distance in front of the cornea, produced a number of undesirable visual effects (Benton and Welsh, 1966).

(1) Objects in space appear magnified as much as 25% or more.

(2) Objects appear closer and the patient makes errors in spatial judgements.

(3) Vision blurs when the patient directs his gaze through the periphery of the lens due to peripheral power gain and oblique astigmatism.

(4) False orientation results from several lens aberrations.

(5) The rapidly increasing prismatic effect away from the optical centers of the lenses produces an annular scotoma.

(6) An object visible within the peripheral field of the lens disappears when the patient turns his eyes to fixate it through the periphery of the lens. This produces the well known Jack-in-the-box phenomenon.

b. *Contact lenses* are superior to spectacle lenses in restoring nearly normal vision.

(1) The magnification of objects is reduced from about 25% to about 8% or 10%.

(2) Spatial judgment is greatly improved with the reduction in magnification and the elimination of several aberrations.

(3) The visual and fixation fields are restored to near normal size and configuration (Welsh, in Girard, 1964).

2. *Monocular aphakia*

a. Although some patients with monocular aphakia have been reported to achieve single binocular vision with spectacle lenses (Berens et al., 1933), they were the exception rather than the rule. The great difference in image size and the heterophoria induced with eye rotations normally elicits an intolerable diplopia.

b. Contact lenses are far more effective than spectacle lenses in restoring single binocular vision for the patient who has one aphakic eye and good vision in the contralateral eye. Since the difference in image size was still significant (5% to 10%) it was not surprising that such patients often failed to meet strict criteria for normal binocular vision (Rosenbloom, 1953; Burian and Bannon, 1958). Most such patients are subjectively comfortable and quite pleased with their single binocular vision, in spite of the fact that central suppression and reduced stereopsis can often be demonstrated.

if necessary, by the judicious selection of contact lens/spectacle lens combinations (Boeder, 1938; Burian and Bannon, 1958). The interested reader is referred to the above references for a detailed treatment of this topic (see also Chapter XXII).

d. The monocular aphake will frequently experience diplopia when he begins wearing his contact lens. The diplopia diminishes in frequency and subsides after a period of a few days to a week. The diplopia is understandable in the light of existing conditions.

(1) The stimulus to fusion was disrupted by the developing cataract and post-surgical visual state of monocularity.

(2) The induced aniseikonia is not conducive to a good quality of fusion.

(3) The high plus contact lens moves vertically with each blink and induces a variable vertical phoria.

3. *The contact lens prescription*

a. Determining the contact lens prescription for the aphakic eye by the method of calculation often leads to error. The reason lies in the simple fact that a small error in vertex distance measurement results in a significant error in contact lens power. For a spectacle plane refraction of +15.00 D, a two millimeter error in vertex distance measurement results in a contact lens power error of about 0.67 D. (See Table 2).

b. The power of the contact lens is determined with greater accuracy by using a contact lens fitting set of high plus powers (+12.00 D to +15.00 D). Refraction is performed through a contact lens having the appropriate base curve and the results are added to the back vertex power of the contact lens employed. The added lens power is relatively small and vertex distance errors are no longer significant.

c. Care must be taken to measure the *back vertex power* and not the *front vertex power* of the high plus fitting lens since these two power parameters can differ by as much as 1.00 D for a +15.00 lens of the usual thickness (Figure XXIII-10). The back vertex power can be measured directly by using a contact lens holder (available with new model lensometers) that positions the posterior lens surface in the plane of stop. When this is not available, the graph of Figure XXIII-10 can be used to convert the measured front vertex power to back vertex power.

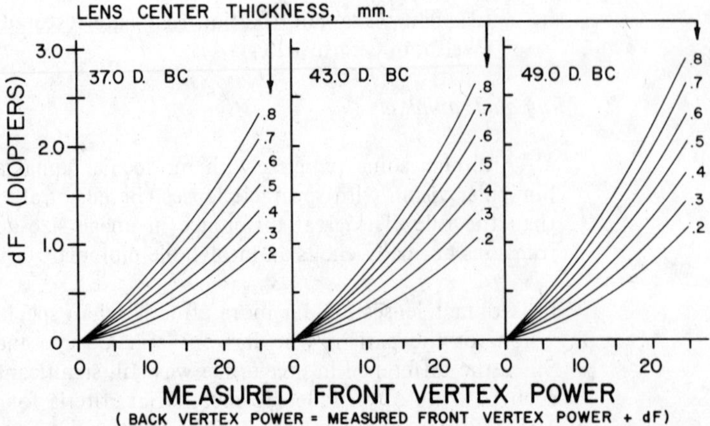

Figure XXIII-10– Back vertex power in diopters for contact lenses (n=1.490) of various base curves (expressed in diopters K reading) and lens thicknesses (in mm.). The front vertex power measurement, shown on the abscissae, is obtained by placing the anterior lens surface against the 6.5 mm. aperture stop of a lensometer or vertometer. The back vertex power of the lens is equal to the measured front vertex power plus df.

J. Keratoconus

1. Of all patients whose vision anomalies are amenable to correction with contact lenses, none are so dependent upon this lens form for vision improvement as the patient with keratoconus. Spectacle lenses can provide good visual acuity only in the very early stages of the developing conus. As the condition progresses, astigmatism increases in magnitude and becomes more irregular, and spectacle lenses are no longer effective in providing good visual acuity. A rapid increase in astigmatism is one of the early signs of keratoconus and a cause for further investigation.

2. When contact lenses are applied in keratoconus the fluid lens neutralizes 90% of the anterior corneal surface toricity and irregularity. Visual acuity ranging from 20/70 to 20/400 with spectacle lenses is generally restored to between 20/20 and 20/40 with contact lenses. The limitation on the visual acuity attainable with contact lenses is more dependent upon corneal transparency than upon corneal surface regularity. Corneal transparency is reduced by the structural changes that accompany the stretching and thinning of the cornea and by the typical recurrent apical erosions produced by a contact lens that bears heavily upon the central region of the conus. A significant additional vision benefit derived with contact lenses is the elimination of multiple ghost images that are present with spectacle lenses.

3. The contact lens prescription cannot be accurately calculated for the patient with keratoconus because the keratometer readings are generally invalid. The lens power must be determined by the method of refraction. Moderate to strong minus power is usually required for keratoconus and diagnostic contact lenses should be designed accordingly.

K. Blur with contact lenses

1. Although contact lenses provide a number of visual advantages over spectacle lenses, especially when they are used to correct such visual anomalies as aphakia, keratoconus and various types of high refractive states, they may also cause certain visual disturbances that are unique with contact lenses. The blurred vision produced by contact lenses has various causes. These causes must be differentiated if clear vision is to be restored.

2. *Residual refractive state*

a. A residual spherical and/or astigmatic refractive state will obviously affect visual acuity and should be carefully measured by refraction, if the wearer reports constantly blurred vision.

b. When the *residual refractive state is a sphero-cylinder,* altering the power of the spherical contact lens by an amount equal to the spherical equivalent of this residual error will often improve visual acuity.

c. When the *residual astigmatism exceeds* an amount that is subjectively acceptable by the patient (generally about 0.75 diopters), a contact lens form that provides a meridionally oriented cylindrical correction must be prescribed.

(1) Although .75 of residual astigmatism is given as a limiting amount, no actual amount can be designated as the error indicating the need for correction. Some cases exhibit difficulty in attaining satisfactory vision with lesser amounts, while some will tolerate greater amounts. Individual preferences or tolerances of the extent of blur which each finds acceptable tend to influence this. In general, as the age level of the patient increases, the amount of residual astigmatism which elicits a demand for correction drops below .75 D.

3. *Flare*

a. Flare is a type of blur that is characterized by the presence of a secondary image that appears to radiate out from the object of regard. This image may be relatively intense or quite dim depending upon the conditions that produce the flare effect.

b. When a portion of the bundle of rays from an object of regard entered the pupil after passing through the secondary curve of the lens or through the liquid meniscus bordering the edge of the lens, the rays were deviated so that a second image of the object was observed at a position in space displaced from the object (Mandell, 1965).

c. Flare is generally caused by a lens with an optic zone diameter that is smaller than the pupil diameter. It may also be experienced when the optic zone diameter is large enough but the lens decenters in a manner to produce the effect. Flare may thus be constant or intermittent. It is generally more apparent under conditions of reduced illumination such as driving at night, viewing a movie, or dining by candlelight.

(1) It appears to be more readily tolerated when constant and in a consistent position than when intermittent and variable in position.

d. Flare is not experienced by all corneal lens wearers who have large pupils. Patients with pupil diameters in excess of seven millimeters can even wear small diameter lenses without being annoyed by flare. One study (Sarver, 1966) showed that periodic blur, flare, and edge reflections were more prevalent among patients fitted with small diameter lenses than among those fitted with larger diameter lenses, but the presence of flare, with small diameter lenses, could not have been predicted solely on the basis of pupil diameter.

e. Flare is eliminated or made more tolerable by altering the lens design to improve lens centration or to permit the use of a larger optic zone diameter or both.

4. *Lens warpage and flattening*

a. It is not unusual for a thin corneal contact lens to become warped, distorted, or flattened with appropriate alterations in vision. High minus lenses with thin centers underwent these changes most readily (Salvatori, 1961; Morrison et al., 1965). Contact lens hydration (Gordon, 1965) and/or the release of internal stresses, developed in the plastic during the manufacturing process (Arner, 1967), appeared to be the primary causes of subsequent changes in lens curvature. Pressures exerted by materials in the contact lens case or through rough lens handling may also be contributing causes. The author has seen several corneal lenses turned inside out by excessive digital pressure exerted while applying wetting solution.

b. Alterations in lens curvature do not change the power of the contact lens in air because the front and back surface radii change about equally. The power of the CL-FL system *is changed*, however, because front surface curvature changes are about 3 times as effective as back surface curvature changes in altering the power of the system.

c. When a lens "flattened" it generally flattened aspherically, with the central region of the lens becoming flatter and paracentral regions becoming steeper (Koetting, 1966). The effect on vision thus depended on lens position and centration.

d. When a flattened lens centers before the pupil the CL-FL system increases in minus power. This effect may partly explain why myopes remain corrected for longer periods of time with contact lenses than with spectacle lenses. The author has seen myopes become overcorrected by as much as one and a half diopters by lens flattening.

(1) This same effect may result in reduced visual acuity when a contact lens is lost and subsequently replaced. Although the new contact lens has the same power and base curve as the original lens, the original lens had gradually flattened, thus imparting

more minus to the power of the CL-FL system so that it kept pace with the increasing myopia. The power of the new CL-FL system is not sufficient to correct the myopia and reduced visual acuity is reported by the patient. A new lens of greater minus power restores good visual acuity.

5. *The anterior tear film and anterior lens surface*

a. The thin film of fluid present on the anterior lens surface does not significantly alter the power of the CL-FL system. It does, however, play an extremely important role in providing clear vision, since it imparts perhaps forty diopters of vergence to the incident light bundle. It must be clear, unbroken, and of uniform thickness. It must be rapidly restored to this same physical state following each blink and must remain relatively stable between blinks. If these conditions are not fulfilled, the wearer will experience blurred vision. He may report filmy or hazy vision, halo, fog, or blur. This blur may be constant or intermittent. It may occur when placing the lenses on the eyes, early in the wearing period, or later in the wearing period.

b. The anterior lens surface must be hydrophylic to support a thin uniform tear film. Methylmethacrylate resin, the hard plastic generally used to manufacture contact lenses is a hydrophobic solid with a contact angle of 60 degrees (Hind and Szekely, 1959). Water beads up as droplets on such a surface. The contact angle must be reduced to zero to make the lens surface hydrophylic. When the contact angle is zero the lens is completely wetted.

(1) The incomplete surface wetting of a contact lens, that causes the patient to experience blurred vision, is readily observed with the slit-lamp biomicroscope. The uniform layer of tear fluid is seen to be replaced by a very thin film of fluid that rapidly evaporates, following each blink, to leave a dry, oily, irregular appearing lens surface. In some instances large portions of a dry lens surface are seen to be covered with droplets of tear fluid.

c. Improper wetting of the lens surface was caused by the deposit or accumulation of ocular secretions and foreign substances in and on the surface of the lens (Hind and Szekely, 1959). This was due to poor personal hygiene, inadequate lens cleaning, hydration and wetting, excess stimulation of the sebaceous lid glands due to poorly finished lens surfaces and/or edges, and the presence of a tear fluid supply that is not sufficient to sustain immersion wetting of the lens (Szekely and Krezanoski, 1960).

6. *Physiological effects on vision*

a. A transparent cornea is a major requisite for clear vision. To remain transparent the cornea must be in a state of relative dehydration (Adler, 1965). When contact lenses were worn, they may have interfered with the normal dehydrating mechanism by altering the osmolarity of the tear fluid and/or by reducing the supply of oxygen available for corneal tissue respiration (Langham, 1952; Smelser, 1952; Smelser and Chen, 1955; Hill and Fatt, 1964; Adler, 1965). The resulting tissue hydration produced a turgescent cornea and visual symptoms of haze, cloudiness, or halo that persisted for a period of time following removal of the contact lens (Kinsey, 1952; Smelser and Chen, 1955).

b. The changes that accompany corneal hydration with contact lens wear include the following:

(1) An increase in corneal thickness by as much as 10% (Harris and Mandell, 1969).

(2) An increase in corneal curvature (i.e. steeper K readings).

(3) Corneal clouding in a region corresponding to the center of the lens position. This

is readily seen by direct observation when using sclerotic scatter type of illumination with the slit-lamp.

(4) Epithelial and/or endothelial edema, most readily observed by direct and indirect retro-illumination with the slit lamp biomicroscope.

(5) Epithelial staining due to cell desquamation.

c. Blur may also be caused by the stagnation of tear fluid and the formation of a collection of bubbles in the retro-lens space. This occurs when tear fluid interchange is restricted and bubbles collect in an area of corneal clearance. The bubbles adhere to the corneal epithelium and produce dimple staining. Blurred vision occurs when the bubble formation is centrally located on the cornea.

d. When the etiology of blur is physiological, good vision is restored by appropriate attention to the fit and performance of the contact lens rather than to the power of the CL-FL system.

REFERENCES

Adler, F.H. (1965): Physiology of the Eye, Clinical Application, 4th ed., The C.V. Mosby Co., St. Louis.

Alpern, M. (1949): Accommodation and Convergence with Contact Lenses, A.A.A.O., 26: 379.

Arner, R. (1967): The Dimensional Stability of Corneal Contact Lenses as a Function of Fabrication Technique, J.A.O.A., 38: 202.

Bailey, N.J. (1961a): Residual Astigmatism With Contact Lenses, Part I, Incidence, O.J.R.O., 98: 30.

**Bailey, N.J. (1961b): Residual Astigmatism With Contact Lenses, Part III, Possible Sites, O.J.R.O., 98: 31.*

**Bailey, N.J. (1961c): Residual Astigmatism With Contact Lenses, Part II, Predictability, O.J.R.O., 98: 40.*

Bailey, N.J. (1966): Prism in a Contact Lens, J.A.O.A., 37: 44.

Bennett, A.G., (1963): Optics of Contact Lenses, 3rd Edition, Assoc. of Dispensing Opticians, Nottingham Place.

Benton, C.D. Jr., and Welsh, R.C. (1966): Spectacles for Aphakia, Springfield, C. Thomas.

Berens, C., Connolly, P.T., and Kern, D. (1933): Certain Motor Anomalies of the Eye in Relation to Prescribing Lenses, A.J. Oph., 16: 210.

Bier, N. (1957): Contact Lens Routine and Practice, 2nd edition, Butterworth, London.

Boeder, P. (1938): Power and Magnification Properties of Contact Lenses, Arch. Oph., 19: 54.

Borish, I.M. (1960): Cylinder Lenses. Bulletin No. 4, Indiana Contact Lens Co., Marion, Indiana.

Borish, I.M. (1962a): Procedure For Fitting Ballasted Cylinder Lenses and High Riding Bifocals. Bulletin No. 8, Indiana Contact Lens Co., Marion, Ind. Rev. ed: (1968) The Penn. Optometrist, XXVIII, 21.

Borish, I.M. (1962b): Contact Lens Centering. J. Ill. Opt. Assoc., 20 (3).

Borish, I.M. (1963): Review of 500 Cases of Residual Astigmatism Corrected by Front-Surface Ballasted Contact Lenses. Paper presented 1st Annual Symposium on Contact Lenses, Ohio State University.

Borish, I.M. (1966): Refracting For Residual Astigmatism. The Penn. Optometrist, XXVI: 11.

Burian, O., and Bannon, R. (1958): On the Correction of Unilateral Aphakia With Contact Lenses, Arch. Oph., 59 (8): 639.

Braff, S.M. (1959-1963): Power Determination for Contact Lenses, in Encylcopedia of Contact Lens Practice, South Bend, Indiana, International Optics Pub. Corp., 2: Chap. 32., p. 27.

Carter, J.H. (1963): Residual Astigmatism of the Human Eye, Opt. Weekly, 54 (27): 1271.

**Contact Lenses Clinic, School of Optometry, University of California, Berkeley, Calif.*

Emsley, H.H. (1963): Visual Optics, 5th ed., London, Hatton Press, 1.

Girard, L.J. (1964): ed., Corneal Contact Lenses, The C.V. Mosby Co., St. Louis.

Gordon, S. (1965): Contact Lens Hydration: A Study of the Wetting-drying Cycle, Opt. Weekly, 56 (14): 55.

Harris, M.G., and Mandell, R.B. (1969): Contact Lens Adaptation: Osmotic Theory, A.A.A.O., 46: 196.

Hill, R.M., and Fatt, I. (1964): Oxygen Deprivation of the Cornea by Contact Lenses and Lid Closure, A.A.A.O., 41: 678.

Hind, H.W., and Szekely, I.W. (1959): Wetting and Hydration of Contact Lenses. Contacto, 3: 65.

Kinsey, V.E. (1952): An Explanation of the Corneal Haze and Halos Produced by Contact Lenses, A.J. Oph., 35: 691.

Koetting, R.A. (1966): Interpreting Corneal Contact Lens Base Curve Changes, Opt. Weekly, 57: 9.

Korb, D.R. (1960): A Preliminary Report on Toric Contact Lenses, Opt. Weekly, 51: 2501.

Kratz, J.D. and Walton, W.G. (1949): A Modification of Javal's Rule for the Correction of Astigmatism, A.A.A.O., 26: 295.

Langham, M.E. (1952): Utilization of O_2 *by the Component Layers of the Living Cornea, J. Physiol. (Lon.), 117: 461.*

**Luneberg, R.J. (1970): Analysis of the Physical and Optical Fit of Contact Lenses. Opt. Weekly, 61 (41): 912-918.*

Mandell, R.B. (1964): A Simplified Method to Calculate Front Surface Radius of Contact Lenses, A.A.A.O., 41: 102.

Mandell, R.B. (1965): Contact Lens Practice: Basic and Advanced, C. Thomas, Springfield.

Mandell, R.B. (1967): Prism Power In Contact Lenses, A.A.A.O., 44: 573.

**Mandell, R.B., Polse, K.A. (1970): Contact Lenses Worn All Day the First Day, Contacto 14 (3): 16.*

**Mandell, Polse and Fatt (1970): Corneal Swelling Caused by Contact Lens Wear, 83: 3. Arch. Oph. 83 (1): 39.*

Millodot, M. (1969): Variation Of Visual Acuity With Contact Lenses, Arch. Oph., 84: 461.

Morgan, M.W. Jr., and Peters, H.B. (1948): The Optics of Ophthalmic Lenses, Berkeley, Univ. of Calif.

Morrison, R.J., Kaufman, and Cerulli (1965): Base Curve Changes of Polymethylmethacrylate Contact Lenses, A.A.A.O., 42: 17.

Ogle, K.N. (1950): Researches in Binocular Vision, W.B. Saunders, Phila.

Rosenbloom, A. (1953): The Correction of Unilateral Aphakia With Corneal Contact Lenses, A.A.A.O., 30: 536.

Salvatori, P. (1961): The Effect of Hydration Upon Corneal Radius, J.A.O.A., 32: 644.

Sarver, M.D. (1962): Fluid Lens Power Effect With Contact Lenses, A.A.A.O., 39: 434.

Sarver, M.D. (1963a): Calculation of the Optical Specifications of Contact Lenses, A.A.A.O., 40: 20.

Sarver, M.D. (1963b): The Effect of Contact Lens Tilt Upon Residual Astigmatism, A.A.A.O., 40: 730.

Sarver, M.D. (1963c): A Toric Base Corneal Contact Lens With Spherical Power Effect, J.A.O.A., 34: 1136.

Sarver, M.D. (1963d): Verification of Contact Lens Power, J.A.O.A., 34: 1304.

Sarver, M.D. and Kerr, K. (1964): A Radius of Curvature Measuring Device for Contact Lenses, A.A.A.O., 41: 481.

Sarver, M.D. (1966): Comparison of Small and Large Corneal Contact Lenses, A.A.A.O., 43: 633.

Sarver, M.D. (1968): Unpublished study, Contact Lens Clinic, University of Calif. School of Optometry.

Sarver, M.D. (1969): A Study of Residual Astigmatism, A.A.A.O., 46: 578.

Sellers, E. (1967): Some Practical Observations on the Fitting of Toric Corneal Contact Lenses, Paper read before Contact Lens Section, A.A.A.O., Chicago.

Smelser, G.K. (1952): Relation of Factors Involved in Maintenance of Optical Properties of Cornea to Contact Lens Wear, Arch. Oph., 47: 328.

Smelser, G. and Chen, D.K., (1955): Physiological Changes in Cornea Induced by Contact Lenses, Arch. Oph., 53: 565.

Stone, J. (1967): Near Vision Difficulties in Non-presbyopic Corneal Lens Wearers, The Contact Lens, 1: 14.

Stone, J. (1968): The Effect of Contact Lenses on Heterophoria and Other Binocular Functions, The Contact Lens, 1: 5-8, 26, 32.

Szekely, I.J., and Krezanoski, J.Z. (1960): Hygienic Contact Lens Care and Patient Comfort, A.A.A.O., 37: 572.

Tocher, R.B. (1962): Astigmatism Due to the Tilt of a Contact Lens, A.A.A.O., 39: 3.

**Welsh, R.C. (1967): Defects of Vision Through Aphakic Spectacle Lenses That Are Correctable by Contact Lenses, in Girard, Corneal and Scleral Contact Lenses, Mosby, St. Louis.*

Westheimer, G. (1961): Aberrations of Contact Lenses, A.A.A.O., 38: 445.

Westheimer, G. (1962): The Visual World of the Contact Lens Wearer, J.A.O.A., 34: 135.

24 Low Vision Aids

I. LOW VISION DEFINED

A. Most state and federal laws pertaining to blind persons define legal blindness, for various official purposes, as a distance visual acuity rating in the better eye with best ophthalmic correction which is no better than 20/200, or as a defect in the visual field so that the widest diameter of vision subtends an angle no greater than 20°.

1. For educational purposes, the partially-seeing child is considered to be one who has a distance visual acuity of 20/70 to 20/200 in the better eye with best ophthalmic correction, and who can use vision as his primary channel of learning.

a. Limitations of these definitions include the following:

(1) The failure to consider near or reading vision, or any defects within the peripheral visual field which do not result in a contraction of the field itself but block out certain areas.

(2) The inability to give a true indication of the individual's visual efficiency from a behavioral and functional point of view.

2. From a functional viewpoint, the low vision patient is one whose visual problem interferes with the performance of routine but undemanding visual tasks related to his daily pattern of living.

3. *Travel vision* is defined as vision of 3/200 or better where the peripheral field of vision is at least 50° in the widest diameter.

B. Classification of visual impairment for rehabilitation services is outlined in the Rehabilitation Codes of the U.S. Office of Vocational Rehabilitation which includes an evaluation of central visual acuity at far and near point, visual field, ocular motility, color vision, and binocular function.

C. A *functional classification system* for the visually impaired individual by Genensky (1970) differentiated between the functionally blind and the functionally sighted patient in relation to his ability to read and write, to identify familiar objects, and to travel safely in an unfamiliar environment.

1. He further classified the functionally sighted patient group into those who are unable to maneuver in an unfamiliar environment, and those who are unable to read and write.

II. HISTORICAL OVERVIEW

A. The principle of the Galilean telescope was utilized for high myopia by Gustavus Adolphus in 1631, and by the Jesuit priest, F. Eschinardi, in 1667. He proposed a telescope with 2.11X.

B. In 1637, René Descartes was the first to design an afocal magnifying lens; the first actual low vision aid, based on the Cartesian principle, appears to have been made by J. Gregory in 1663.

C. In 1695, Christian Huygens in his *Dioptrica* specified the precise rule to be used for the adjustment of a telescope to the refractive state of the eye.

D. In 1786, H. Dixon introduced a reflecting telescope using two spherical mirrors mounted in a spectacle frame with the distance between mirrors variable, thereby accommodating various refractive anomalies.

E. In 1900, Allvar Gullstrand designed the first aspheric glass lenses for the correction of spherical aberration. They were known as Katral lenses and were designed for the correction of aphakia.

F. In 1908, Moritz von Rohr was the first to suggest the use of a corrected doublet eyepiece for telescopic lenses with magnifications of 1.3X and 1.8X. The design required a fixed separation of the objective and eyepiece lenses with slip-over plus lenses to accommodate different working distances and slip-over lenses attached to the eyepiece for the refractive correction.

G. In 1930, William Feinbloom designed a meridional magnifying telescopic unit having a power of 1.8X in the horizontal meridian and 1.3X in the vertical meridian in an attempt to provide normal localization of objects seen through telescopic lenses.

H. In 1936, Joseph Dallos suggested the use of a contact lens for the eyepiece of a telescopic spectacle; the objective of the system consisted of an ophthalmic plus lens.

1. Feinbloom (1933) described the design characteristics of a series of telescopic and microscopic lenses.

III. PREVALENCE OF LOW VISION

A. Historical Aspects

1. In 1932, the first study of causes of blindness in children was undertaken by the Committee on Statistics of the Blind, a project jointly sponsored by the National Society for the Prevention of Blindness and the American Foundation for the Blind.

a. The committee developed a standard classification for causes of blindness and for visual acuity measurements.

2. In 1962, the Model Reporting Area for Blindness Statistics was organized under the sponsorship of the National Institute of Neurological Diseases and Blindness of the U.S. Public Health Service (Goldstein and Goldberg, 1967).

3. Information regarding both the prevalence of low vision and the characteristics of the low vision population is quite incomplete.

a. Between 1830 and 1930 each decennial census has endeavored to provide information on the number and characteristics of blind persons in this country. These data were not reliable due to difficulties in defining and identifying blind persons.

b. There was also a failure to establish a definition of low vision that would consider not only visual but also functional and behavioral aspects of the problem.

B. Present Status Incidence of Low Vision

1. United States census data, showing population growth from 1940 to 1960, revealed the following trends by age groups:

a. Under 20 years of age, the population increased more than 50%.

b. Between ages 20 and 64, there was an increase of 20.8%.

c. Age 65 and over, an 83.3% increase was recorded.

2. Refined methods of reporting coupled with an increased population resulted in an increased number of low vision patients. This increase can be attributed to the following factors:

a. Greater life expectancy associated with a greater incidence of ocular and systemic degenerative disorders

b. Increased literacy of aging persons

c. Unwillingness of many to accept poor vision as a required part of old age

d. Society's demand for visual efficiency as a vital factor in competing successfully in business, technology, and leisure time activities

3. In a geriatric study Ford (1970) reported on the incidence of non-institutionalized persons in the United States considered to be blind or unable to read newsprint as being twenty-four in 1,000 in the age range 65-74, and ninety-six per 1,000 over age 75.

4. It has been reliably estimated by the National Society for the Prevention of Blindness (1969) that there are about 400,000 legally blind people in the United States. (Over 50% of these individuals are over the age of 60.)

a. Sloan (1960) states that approximately two-thirds of those individuals classified as legally blind can be helped by the prescription of a low vision aid.

(1) A larger group (3.6 per 1,000) is not usually counted in statistics on the prevalence of blindness because these individuals are able to read letters smaller than the 20/200 Snellen letter standard, yet they too have impaired vision sufficient to require a low vision aid.

(2) These data indicate that the number of persons who can be helped by reading aids are seven times the number classified as blind. This number totals approximately 1,000,000.

5. Based on an estimated 30,000 new cases of legal blindness a year, Riley (1969) estimated the number of cases in each low vision category in the United States.

a. **TABLE XXIV-1**

Degree of Partial Sight	Incidence	Prevalence
Light perception & projection	3,000	30,000
Less than 5/200	5,000	50,000
5/200 but less than 10/200	3,000	30,000
10/200 but less than 20/200	5,000	50,000
20/200	8,000	80,000
Restricted field	2,000	20,000
Unknown	2,000	20,000

b. Of significance is the estimate that approximately two-thirds of the legally blind have sufficient residual vision to benefit by some type of low vision aid.

6. The most recent survey on the number and characteristics of persons six years and over with visual impairments show an estimated 5,029,000, 969,000 of whom cannot read ordinary newsprint, and 310,000 of whom cannot identify features of friends and/or moving objects (U.S. Dept. of Health, Education and Welfare, Public Health Service, 1968).

7. Comparisons of age distributions of total and new cases of legal blindness are described in Figures XXIV-1 and XXIV-2.

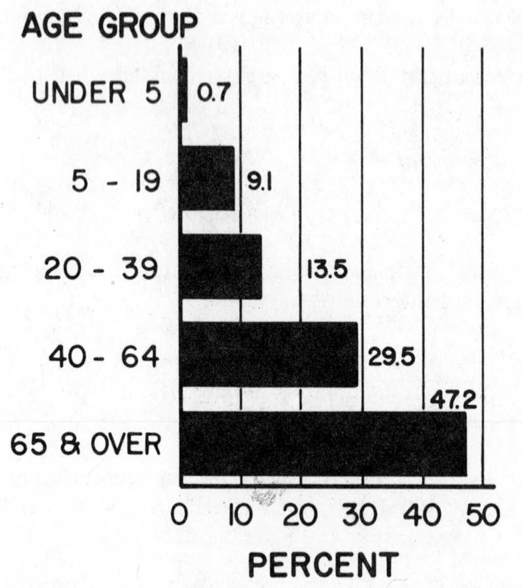

Figure XXIV-1 – Distribution of total cases of legal blindness by age group, United States, 1962.

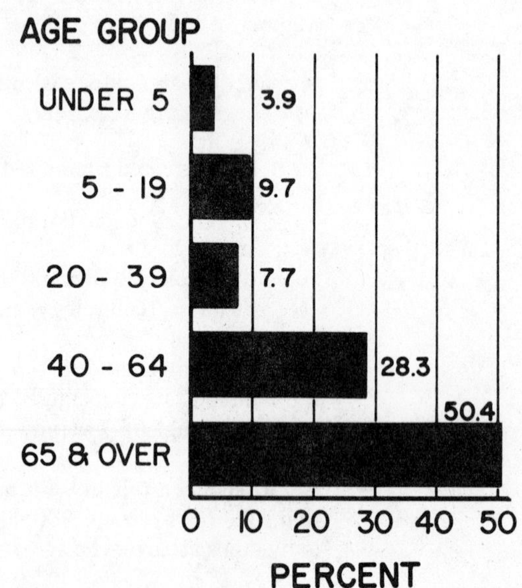

Figure XXIV-2 – Distribution of new cases of legal blindness by age group, United States, 1962.

8. Scott (1969) summarized studies presenting data on incidence of low vision by classifying the nearly one million blind people in the United States into four groups:

a. *The aged blind* are all people over 65 years of age who are blind according to the currently accepted administrative definition of blindness. This includes over two-thirds of all blind persons.

b. *Non-aged unemployable adults* whose characteristics, including blindness, either place them out of the labor force, or tend to make employment extremely difficult. This group includes blind people who have little education and women for whom employment is not normally expected (10 to 15 percent).

c. *Adults* who are potentially employable, most of whom are males and have no major handicap other than blindness (10 to 15 percent).

d. Blind *children* who represent two to three percent of the total blind population.

IV. ETIOLOGICAL FACTORS

A. The Standard Classification of Causes of Blindness, developed by the Committee on Statistics of the Blind, was first published in 1933 (Berens, 1933) and revised in 1940 (Kerby, 1940).

B. Classification of blindness is based on:

1. The *site and type* of vision-impairing affection.
2. The *etiology* or underlying cause of this affection.

a. Figure XXIV-3 presents total cases of legal blindness by site and type of eye infection.

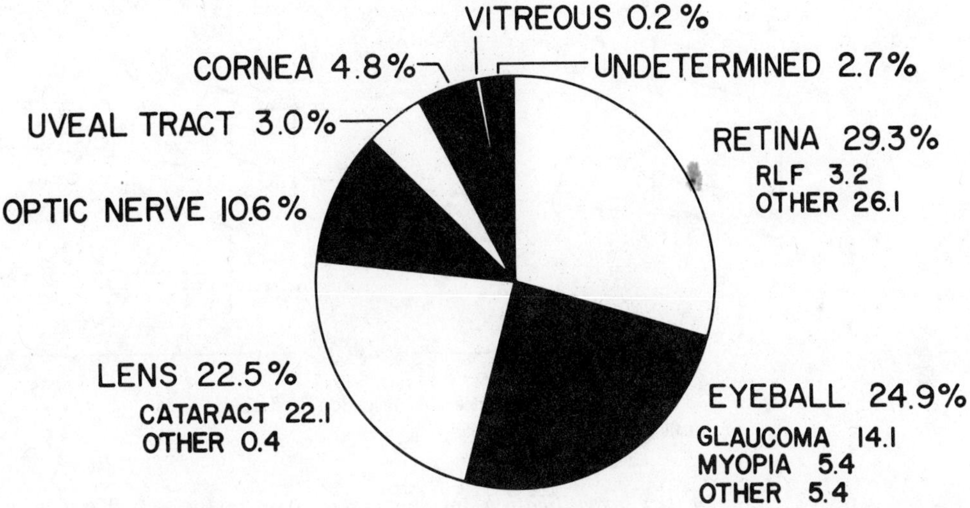

Figure XXIV-3 – Total cases of legal blindness by site and type of eye affection United States, 1962 (per cent of estimated total cases).

C. Lebensohn (1958) estimated that about 60% of the partial vision in children was of prenatal origin; infectious diseases accounted for over 20%; while accidents for about 10%.

D. Godber (1962) classified low vision by site of affection (cornea, lens, uveal tract, retina, optic nerve, vitreous); by etiology (infectious diseases, trauma, poisonings, tumors, prenatal influences); and by clinical entity (macular lesions, cataract, glaucoma, optic nerve, and diabetic retinopathy).

E. Low vision patients can be divided into the following three groups (Lederer, 1956):

1. Patients who have irregular astigmatism, conical cornea, or corneal deformity where vision becomes distorted as a result of irregular refraction.

2. Patients with partial opacification of the ocular media resulting from cataracts or corneal opacities.

3. Individuals who have diseases, injuries, or congenital malformations of the inner eye.

F. A small but significant number of persons have low vision as a result of lesions in the optic tract radiations and in the cortex.

V. FACTORS INVOLVED IN LOW VISION CARE

A. Magnification

1. The *object of magnification* is to produce an image which subtends a larger visual angle than that subtended by the object itself.

2. *Relative distance magnification* is achieved by decreasing the distance from the eye to the object viewed. The angular size of the object at a distance "p" (expressed in cm.) relative to its size at 40 cm. can be computed as follows:

a. $Md = \frac{\tan \alpha^1}{\tan \alpha^2} = \frac{40}{p}$ (40 cm. is here assumed to be the average reading distance) (see Figure XXIV-4)

b. Short fixation distances necessitate accommodation for clear vision. If accommodation is not available, auxiliary lenses must be used.

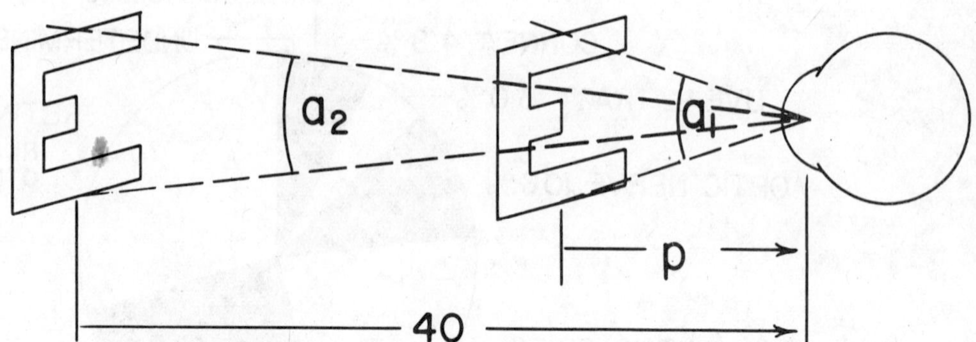

Figure XXIV-4 – Relative distance magnification is defined as tan a_1 / tan a_2 with the distance of fixation for tan a_2 fixed at 40 cm.

3. *Relative size magnification* involves an increase in the actual size of the object viewed. A standard of 10 point type is used to specify the relative magnification resulting from the use of large size print.

a. $Ms = \frac{\tan \alpha^1}{\tan \alpha^2}$ (where α^2 is the angular size of 10 point style and α^1 is the angular size of enlarged type)

b. Relative size magnification is also produced by projection systems in which case

$$Ms = \frac{\text{Image Distance}}{\text{Object Distance}}$$

4. *Angular magnification*

a. Unlike lateral and axial magnification, which are based on linear distances measured parallel and perpendicular to the axis of an optical system, angular magnification is dependent upon the angular sizes of the object and image about a reference point. Since magnifiers are used with an eye, the reference point usually is one of the eye's cardinal points.

b. By definition the angular magnification represents the ratio of the angular size of the image seen through the lens to the angular size of the object seen without the lens, the object in both cases being at the same distance from the eye.

(1) For maximum magnification this distance is equal to the algebraic sum of the anterior focal length of the lens (f) and the distance of the lens from the eye (z).

c. This magnification is given by the mathematical relationship:

(1) In Figure XXIV-5 z and p are the distances of lens and object from the entrance pupil. f equals the focal length of the lens. F = dioptric power of the lens.

(2) $M_0 = 1 + zF$

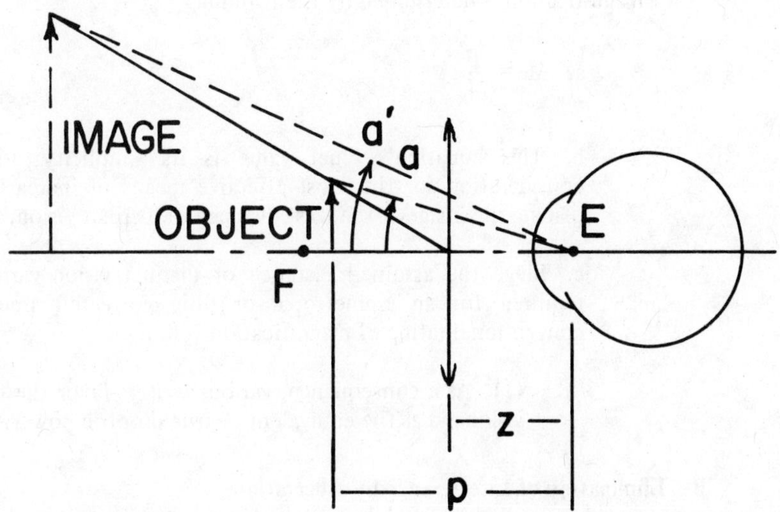

Figure XXIV-5 – Essential schema for computing angular magnification of a lens before an eye.

d. Magnification is limited by variation of the distance of the object from the lens and of available accommodation. For in-focus imagery, the distance of the object image cannot be less than the nearpoint, the shortest distance in which accommodation can take place.

e. Due to the variability of accommodation, two other methods also have been used to compute angular magnification.

(1) These methods use as a reference point for the viewing or working distance what is commonly called "minimal distance of distinct vision," a historic carry over from the angular magnification of microscopes.

(a) This distance has been assumed to be 10 inches or 25 cm.

(b) Each 4.00 D. is equivalent to one diameter of magnification (IX).

(c) Similarly, if 16 inches or 40cm. isused as the assumed unit, then each +2.50 D. equals one diameter of magnification.

5. When dealing with low vision lenses, two effects contribute to the final total magnification.

a. The bringing forward of the object from the reference distance closer to the eye ($\tan \alpha^1 / \tan \alpha^2$).

b. The interposing of a lens between the eye and the object brought closer to the eye ($M = 1 + zF$).

c. The total magnification thus produced is the product of a and b:

(1) $Me = (p \times F)$

(a) p is the reference distance in meters and F the power of the lens; this formula assumes that the object is at the anterior focal point of the lens.

6. If the object is located in the focal plane of the lens and is 25 cm. from the eye, effective magnification is determined by the formula:

a. $Me = \frac{F}{4}$

b. This equation's chief value is its simplicity; its chief limitation is the lack of consideration for the most effective means of increasing the size of the retinal image by placing the image at the least distance of distinct vision.

c. Since the assumed distance of distinct vision varies, and since no accommodation is required for an emmetropic or fully corrected ametropic eye, the usefulness of the conventional rating of magnification is limited.

(1) As a consequence, various writers favor the designation of the power of the low vision aid as the equivalent or true dioptric power.

B. Elimination of Interference by Aberration

1. A contact lens provides a spherically ideal anterior surface of the refracting media of the eye. Its use in low vision is as follows (Rosenbloom, 1969):

a. To eliminate or modify the effects of corneal irregularities as in keratoconus, irregular astigmatism, or corneal scarring.

b. To provide improved visual function, including field of view, over that obtained with the ophthalmic lens counterpart, as in aphakia, high myopia, and high astigmatism.

c. To produce magnification as the ocular component of a telescopic system.

d. To serve as a limiting aperture which will increase visual function and efficiency in patients with certain types of ocular pathology.

2. A stenopaic slit or a multiple pinhole spectacle reduces illumination and provides for the transmission of central pencils of light only.

C. Control of Light

1. Light must be direct, of sufficient intensity, and introduced at such an angle as to avoid glare.

2. Older persons need greater illumination for reading than younger people.

a. Guth, Eastman, and McNelis (1956) found that persons over 60 years of age need about twice as much light for a given task as persons 17 to 20 years of age.

b. According to Fonda (1965), ideal illumination is determined by the patient's requirements in relation to his ocular disorder, the size of type he is able to read, and the work to be performed.

3. Light falling perpendicular to a surface varies inversely to the square of the distance from the light source.

a. A 100-watt bulb, 1 foot from the illuminated surface, produces 100 foot-candles of illumination; at a distance of 10 feet, the illumination is 1 foot-candle.

4. As the illuminated surface is tilted away from the perpendicular, the illumination is reduced directly as the cosine of the angle with the perpendicular through which the surface is tilted.

a. If an illuminated surface located 1 foot from a 100-watt incandescent bulb is tilted 45° from the direction of the light, the illumination is 100 x 0.70 or 70 foot-candles.

b. The illumination on the same surface, 2 feet from the 100-watt bulb and tilted 45° from the direction of the light, is 25 x 0.70 or 17.5 foot-candles.

c. Hence, the distance and position of a light source from the illuminated surface is as significant as the power of the light source itself.

D. Patient Motivation

1. The following findings are especially significant:

a. The age and onset of the visual loss, whether congenital or acquired in origin.
b. The extent to which the patient is dependent or independent in his life style.
c. Vocational and avocational aspirations.
d. Social-emotional factors in patient's readiness to accept his visual aid.
e. Cosmetic aspects of lens design.
f. Mobility involving both mental orientation and physical locomotion.

(1) Mental orientation (Lowenfeld, 1950) refers to the individual's ability to recognize his surroundings and their temporal or spatial relation to himself.

(2) Locomotion refers to the individual's physical ability to move from place to place.

(3) Both are essential for mobility and do not function separately.

2. The well-motivated low vision patient has clearly defined visual needs; he frequently states specific goals to achieve.

VI. TYPES OF LOW VISION AIDS

A. Nonspectacle magnifiers

1. *Hand-held magnifiers* designed as simple double-convex and plano-convex reading lenses are available in virtually all sizes and power (from +4.00 D. to +20.00 D.).

a. The distance between eye and lens is quickly varied depending upon reading distance and magnification needed.

b. In the lower magnifying power, i.e., 1.5X (+6.00 D.) or 2X (+8.00 D.), these units are considered satisfactory from an optical standpoint, but in higher powers, as in 8X (+32.00 D.) or 10X (+40.00 D.) the aberrations, particularly astigmatism by oblique incidence, become so severe that the usable field of view is restricted to an angular diameter of approximately 30°, which covers only a few millimeters of reading material.

(1) One of the limitations of the hand magnifier is its increasing weight with greater power. One means for overcoming this is the use of the Fresnel lens.

(a) The Fresnel lens is a lens with a surface consisting of a concentric series of simple lens sections or zones of the same power, thereby effecting the optics of a simple, large diameter, short focal length lens without the incumbent thickness.

(2) The introducton of high quality lightweight Fresnel lenses in membrane thickness and press-on form for ophthalmic use represents a unique approach (Kopash, 1970).

2. *Loupes* are available in monocular and binocular form and are placed in front of, or in conjunction with, the patient's spectacles.

3. *Stand Magnifiers*

a. Stand magnifiers with *fixed object to lens distance* are used with the eye close to the lens to provide a large field and minimal aberrations.

(1) The amount of accommodation needed depends upon the eye-to-lens distance.

(2) For some patients, single binocular vision can be achieved if the material is held at a convenient reading distance.

b. Focusable stand magnifiers, with *variable object-to-lens distance,* permit variation in magnification and correction for moderate degrees of ametropia.

(1) The Sloan series of focusable stand magnifiers have equivalent powers of 19.00 D., 23.00 D., 29.00 D., 37.00 D., and 53.00 D. (Sloan and Jablonski, 1959).

(2) Such aids have been modified to include a light source in the unit which provides uniform, adequate illumination over the viewing surface. This is especially important since it is very difficult in short viewing distances to achieve proper illumination.

c. Plano-convex magnifiers have a one-piece glass construction consisting of an upper convex curve and a lower flat surface which rests on the printed page.

(1) The advantage is that focus is fixed, and the design increases and distributes the light evenly on the page.

(2) These aids can be used in conjunction with either spectacles or nonspectacle magnifiers to increase magnification and brightness of an object.

d. Fonda (1965) listed the following five indications for a handheld or stand magnifier:

(1) Visual fields constricted to 10° or less.

(2) An auxiliary lens for reading small type.

(3) An interim correction when the decision to prescribe spectacles for certain patients is difficult.

(a) If progress is favorable, spectacles can then be prescribed.

(4) Correction of choice for patients with a hand or head tremor, such as is associated with Parkinson's disease, multiple sclerosis, and cerebral palsy.

(5) Visual loss is extensive, and the potential for correction limited.

(a) Psychologically, the patient realizes that some assistance, although very limited, is possible.

4. *Pinhole spectacles* improve vision for patients with opacities of the ocular media and corneal irregularities when macular function is adequate.

a. They are also useful for determining the potential vision of patients in instances where retinoscopy is not possible.

b. The pinhole design in contact lenses provides improved visual function, wearability, and cosmetic appearance.

5. The *reading slit or Typoscope* is a black masking device with a rectangular opening through which one or more lines of type are exposed at a time. The increased contrast between the lines being read and the surrounding areas is especially helpful for patients with developing cataracts.

a. This reading aid is also useful in adaptive training for it provides improved continuity in reading and in progression from line to line (Lebensohn, 1952).

6. *Projection magnifiers* involve the principle of opaque magnification by the formation of an enlarged image of an opaque object on a screen.

a. Since an image is formed on a translucent screen, viewing distance is varied and permits maximum use of relative distance magnification along with relative size magnification achieved from projection.

b. Limitations in magnification, range, illumination, image contrast, and portability are so extensive that these units are no longer being manufactured.

7. Using a prototype model of a *closed circuit TV* system with a variable magnified image, Genensky (1970) reported successful results for reading and writing with 50 legally blind people.

a. Two 9" TV monitor cameras were used with linear magnification of 1.6X to 6.4X and of 2.6X to 16X respectively.

B. Spectacle Magnifiers

1. *High plus reading lenses,* either in single vision or in bifocal form, range in power from approximately +4.00 to +20.00 Diopters.

a. The lens construction includes one-piece design (Ultex A type), fused bifocal construction, and cement segment designs.

b. According to Fonda (1970), binocular reading additions, ranging in power from +4.00 to +14.00 Diopters, represent the preferred method for correcting low vision patients who possess binocular vision.

(1) In most cases, the bifocal segments required decentration and/or the incorporation of base-in prism.

(2) Where no distance prescription is required, half-eye glasses are well-suited since the lenses are smaller, thinner, lighter in weight, and adaptable to base-in power effects.

(3) Since less than 20% of the patients with vision poorer than 20/60 possess single binocular vision, the need for binocular correction is infrequent.

c. A mathematical method for prescribing high plus reading additions ("microscopic" lenses) was described by Brazelton (1969).

d. Zettel (1964) discussed methods for computing near point reading additions and reported successful results achieved on 458 patients over fifty years of age who were prescribed high adds ranging in power from +3.00 to +10.00 Diopters.

e. High plus reading additions represent a frequently prescribed low vision aid; they provide a larger field, greater depth of focus, are conventional in appearance, and simple in design.

f. The use of a thin "membrane" O.S.G. (Fresnel principle) prism which can be pressed onto the bifocal segment allows the addition of base-in prism without decentration.

2. The *telescopic lens* in its simplest form is of the Galilean type consisting of two lenses, a minus ocular and a plus objective, mounted coaxially and separated by a distance equal to the sum of the focal lengths (see Figure XXIV-6).

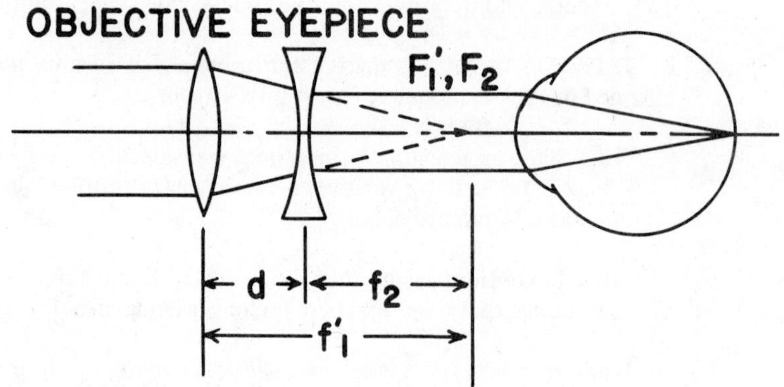

Figure XXIV -6 – Construction of a Galilean telescope. The components are a plus lens objective and minus lens eyepiece positioned so their respective secondary and primary focal points coincide.

a. This form is advantageous in securing a moderately flat field tolerably free from astigmatism.

b. The anterior focus of the plus lens coincides with the posterior focus of the minus lens.

(1) As a consequence, the rays are parallel upon entering and leaving the telescope.

(2) There is no focus, and the unit is known as afocal.

c. The spectacle form power or magnification ranges from 1.5X to 4.0X.

d. Magnification for near is determined by dividing the dioptric power of the reading addition by 4 and then multiplying this by the magnification of the telescopic unit (2.5X with a spectacle addition of +8.00 D. = 2.5 X 2 = 5.0X).

(1) Telescopic spectacles are preferred when maximum reading distance is essential (e.g., 2.2X in the telescopic spectacle with +8.00 D. addition = 4.4X and use at a working distance of 12.5 cm.; by contrast a +18.00 D. sphere = 4.5X and provides a working distance of 5.5cm.).

e. The use of low reading caps also provides intermediate near vision in approximately a 10 to 16 inch range.

(1) Significant results using a 3.5X reading binocular telescope in bifocal form for binocular vision at a 16″ working distance were reported by Feinbloom (1967).

f. Small compact telescopes, designed in powers from 2.5X to 4.0X and mounted in the upper portion of a carrier lens, have been prescribed successfully. By tilting his head slightly downward, the patient is able to utilize the telescopic lens at periodic intervals for improved distance vision.

g. Ready-made telescopic units, such as prism monoculars, binocular sport glasses, and clip-on telescopes, are frequently found useful for the patient who requires magnification of distance objects for short periods of time.

3. In the *contact lens-telescopic system,* a spectacle lens of positive power is used as the objective, and a contact lens of minus power as the eye piece (see Figure XXIV-7).

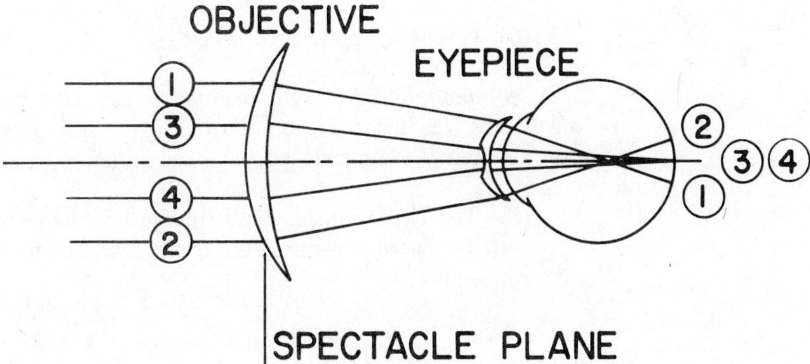

Figure XXIV-7 – Bivisual contact-spectacle telescopic. System is in focus with or without objective lens.

a. The chief advantages of this design are an increased field of view resulting in greater wearability than its counterpart in a spectacle system, lightness in weight, and more conventional appearance.

b. Variations in magnification can be produced by the manipulation of three variables – power of the contact lens, power of the spectacle lens, and the vertex distance between the two.

c. Ludlam (1960) reviewed the history of contact lens-telescopic systems, described the optical and design characteristics of different contact lens-telescopic systems, and reported results on four successful patients who wore minimal clearance scleral lens-telescopic systems for six to eighteen months.

d. A thorough evaluation of the design characteristics and clinical fitting procedures involved in prescribing a contact lens-telescopic system is presented by Mandell (1965).

(1) From a clinical standpoint, the contact lens-telescopic systems, as described by Mandell, rarely have proved successful for regular wear.

4. A *microscopic spectacle* is a magnifying or a lens system of short focal length for near viewing, designed to provide a flat field of view comparatively free from aberrations.

a. It may consist of a single lens (spheric or aspheric), doublet, or triplet design.

b. *Microscopic lenses* extend the magnification range for reading and are available in magnification from 2X to 20X. The purpose of the microscopic lens is twofold:

(1) Primarily, a collimation of the light from an object at near to obtain relative distance magnification.

(2) Secondarily, an enlargement of the retinal image by means of the angular magnification of the lens.

c. Bechtold (1953) listed the following factors as considerations in microscopic lens design:

(1) Correction of aberrations especially astigmatism by oblique incidence

(2) Working distance

(3) Field of view

(4) Number of optical elements

(5) Thickness and weight of magnifiers

(6) Cosmetic appearance

d. A *compound microscopic spectacle* may also be obtained by placing an additional convex lens (reading cap) over the telescopic spectacle units. Ranges of magnification up to approximately 9X are achieved.

(1) The chief clinical disadvantage lies in the progressively restricted field of view with increased magnification, bulkiness, unconventional, and, for many, undersirable appearance.

(2) As the magnification increases, the field properties as they relate to reading distance, field of view, and depth of field deteriorate and result in greater difficulties in space perception.

e. *Aspherical lenses* are generally ground on glass or casted plastic and have a spherical surface on the inside and an aspherical surface on the outside. The spheric surface is ground with the same radius of curvature in all meridians; the radii of the aspheric surface vary with the weaker surface toward the periphery of the lens.

(1) The advantages of such lenses are that they eliminate curvature of the field marginal astigmatism, distortions, and reduce chromatic spherical aberrations.

(2) The lenses are also less conspicuous and, in plastic, are light and virtually adaptable to any frame size. Although plastic scratches more easily than glass, this has rarely been a problem. These lenses range in power from 6X to 12X.

f. Improved performance can be achieved by a *doublet system.* Spherical and chromatic aberrations, coma, curvature of field, and marginal astigmatism are reduced by these designs.

g. *Triplet lenses* involve a central bi-convex element of ground glass surrounded by concave lenses made of glass with a higher index of refraction. Both lens designs can be prescribed either as large diameter, or a bifocal lenses.

(1) Cemented doublet and triplet lenses, mounted as a bifocal in a carrier lens, have the following advantages:

(a) Correction can be ground at distance for host element.

(b) There is simultaneous vision for distance and near.

(c) Corrections for aberrations and distortions are excellent to the very edge of the lens.

(d) They are superior when high minus lenses are required for a distance correction.

(2) According to Bechtold (1953), two lens elements are adequate up to 6X; in 8X, 10X, and 12X three lens systems are required for correcting specified aberrations in order to achieve a 60° field of view.

(a) Construction data on a series of wide-angle magnifying spectacles are presented in Table XXIV-2 (Bechtold, 1953).

TABLE XXIV-2. Construction Data and Optical Characteristics of Series of Magnifiers.*

	4x		6x		8x		10x		12x	
Surface powers†										
F_1	– 4.00		– 2.00		– 2.00		Plano		Plano	
F_2	+11.87		+13.87		+13.87		+12.00		+16.00	
F_3	Plano		+ 8.00		+ 8.00		+ 6.00		+ 8.00	
F_4	+ 8.12		+ 4.37		+ 4.37		+ 6.00		+ 8.87	
F_5					+ 8.75		+14.00		+17.75	
F_6					Plano		+ 3.75		Plano	
Thickness (mm.)										
t_1	3.3		4.5		4.5		4.2		4.6	
t_2	4.2		5.8		5.8		4.4		5.8	
t_3					4.4		6.2		6.4	
Diameters (mm.)										
Lens 1	34		34		34		32		32	
Lens 2	40		40		40		34		34	
Lens 3					40		34		34	
Working distance (mm.)	61.7		38.1		25.3		19.9		14.1	
Diameter of object field (mm.)	66		42		36		25		21	
Axial aberrations										
Spherical aberrations	–.06		–.10		–.15		–.23		–.38	
Coma (%)	+.00		–.01		–.02		–.10		–.34	
Longitudinal color (D)	.27		.40		.50		.62		.70	
Field aberrations	60°	30°	60°	30°	60°	30°	60°	30°	60°	30°
Sagittal focus (D)	– .90	– .22	– 1.49	– .36	– 1.61	– .36	– 3.10	– .61	– 4.91	.91
Tangential focus (D)	+ .12	+ .02	– .35	– .08	+ .96	+ .30	– 2.27	– .09	– 5.58	– .61
Mean field curvature (D)	– .39	– .10	– .92	– .22	– .33	– .03	– 2.69	– .35	– 5.25	– .76
Distortion (%)	– 8.8	– 1.0	– 12.6	– 1.5	– 12.3	– 1.5	–15.0	– 1.9	– 13.9	– 1.5
Transverse color (min. arc)	14	7	21	10	28	14	34	17	46	23

* From Bechtold, E. W.: An improved system of wide-angle magnifying spectacles, Optic. J. Rev. 90:35, 1953.

† Powers are true dioptric powers based upon spectacle crown glass (np – 1.523) rather than marked powers of tools based on 1.53 glass.

(b) Reductions in thickness and weight can be achieved only at the expense of limiting the useful field of view (see Figure XXIV-8).

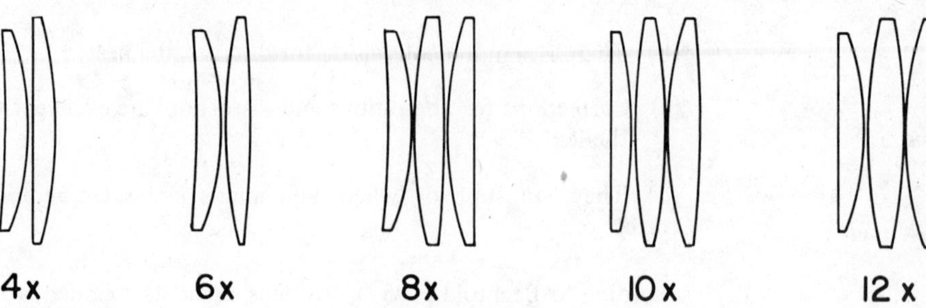

Figure XXIV-8 – Doublet and triplet low vision lens designs (Bechtold).

VII. FACTORS IN EVALUATING LOW VISION AIDS

A. Extent of magnification required to achieve specific visual tasks.

1. With telescopic spectacles, magnifications of 1.5X to 4.0X are available. Greater magnifications are usually impractical because of reduction in field of view, as well as changes in space perception produced.

2. With microscopic lenses, higher magnifications are both practicable and indeed necessary in order to provide the necessary level of correction to enable the typical low vision patient to read book and newspaper print.

3. Most frequently prescribed magnifications for near use extend from 3X to 12X.

B. The focal plane determines the distance or range of clear vision through the low vision aid.

1. For telescopic spectacles, this is located at infinity and range of clear vision extends to approximately 4.0 meters.

2. In microscopic spectacles, the focal point is the nearest possible to the habitual close work and reading distance, although frequently the patient must adapt to abnormally close reading and working distances.

C. The size of the field of view is particularly important in the patient's successful use of the aid; it should be as large as possible and never less than 20° in angular extent (Lederer, 1956).

D. The nature and extent of changes in the patient's space perception produced by the aid.

1. When magnification devices are used, a sudden change is imposed on the visual sense without a corresponding change in the other sense modalities.

2. This spatial-perceptual imbalance can create a significant change in the patient's perception, affecting his judgments in size, direction, and distance.

E. The potential for binocular vision and its incorporation, if indicated, into the low vision aid design.

F. Overall size, weight, appearance, and cost of the low vision aid are factors that will influence the clinical usefulness and acceptance of the aid by the patient.

G. Most important, the examiner should have a thorough understanding of the specific visual requirements or needs of the patient and of his adaptability to, and motivation for, low vision aids.

VIII. EXAMINATION TECHNIQUES AND PROCEDURES

A. Examination techniques and procedures involve four major factors:

1. Case history findings
2. Examination procedure
3. Evaluation of the findings
4. Visual training and after-care

B. Case history findings

1. A good case history will include essential information that will often determine whether or not the patient can be helped, and the appropriate direction the examination should follow. Questioning can reveal the patient's reaction to his visual problem and to his family's attitude.

2. Significant questions in the case history include:

   a. The diagnosis, prognosis, and duration of ocular pathology
   b. Present visual status
   c. Age and educational history
   d. Ability to travel
   e. Type of low vision aids formerly prescribed or now in use
   f. Preferred lighting
   g. Present vocation and future aspirations
   h. Patient's needs and expectations from a low vision aid
   i. The patient's psychological readiness for visual correction

3. Faye and Weiss (1965) posed the following questions for three age groups:

   a. The older patient:

      (1) How long has he been visually handicapped? Has he tried to use visual aids by himself? What is the diagnosis, prognosis, and duration of ocular pathology? What are the patient's goals? Did reading play a large part in the patient's life? How is his general health?

   b. The young adult:

      (1) Is he going to college or into vocational training? Has he been reading print successfully? Does he need visual aids for uses other than reading?

   c. Children:

      (1) Is the disease congenital or acquired? Does he play well with siblings or other children? Does the preschool child hold books and toys close to his eyes? Is the child placed in a regular classroom, sight-saving, sight-conservation, or braille class?

C. Examination procedure

1. The diversity of low vision problems and individual needs require great flexibility in approach.

2. Much of the examination procedure follows a conventional pattern which includes:

a. Visual acuity at far and near

b. Internal and external ocular examination

c. Tonometry and slit lamp biomicroscopy

d. Ophthalmometry

e. Determination of the field of vision

(1) Central field loss study can be carried out on a one meter tangent screen with the fixation target modified by the use of a white ribbon tacked to the upper ends of the screen and stretched to the opposite lower ends to form a cross. The patient is then asked to fixate where the ribbon crosses.

(2) Central fields can also be plotted on the Lloyd's stereo-campimeter with white fixation targets varying from 1 to 5 mm. in size.

(3) Visual field studies often provide qualitative rather than absolute quantitative results.

f. Static retinoscopy

(1) When routine retinoscopy is not possible due to media involvements, "radical" retinoscopy involves moving to whatever working distance and deviation from the optic axis in order to establish a reflex. The working distance must then be calculated and compensated for as in routine retinoscopy.

g. Distance subjective examination including the use of telescopic lenses of varying power and design at far and near point

(1) A sturdy trial frame and trial lenses, pinhole disc, stenopaic slit, hand Jackson Cross-Cylinder (± 0.50 and ± 1.00 D power), and a strong light in a goose-neck lamp for near testing are additional examining equipment.

(2) The variety of test equipment used in subjective refraction is required by the difficulty in securing accurate and reliable responses when vision is impaired.

(3) Diagnostic low vision aids should include telescopic units in large and in reduced aperture design with suitable reading caps; microscopic lenses of large and segment design; appropriate diagnostic control contact lenses; various ready-made binocular and monocular telescopic units; and auxiliary nonspectacle magnifiers of the clip-on and fixed-focus design.

h. Tests of binocular coordination and fusion if feasible

i. Subjective examination at near point including microscopic lens testing

(1) For near refraction, the distance acuity fraction may be used as a guide to selection of the initial trial lens.

(a) Kestenbaum and Sturman (1956) proposed that the denominator of the fraction be divided by the numerator; the resulting number was called "reciprocal of vision" (R.V.) and provided the number of diopters of plus needed to read Jaeger 5 (newsprint); (e.g., 20/80 is 4; 10/70 is 7).

(b) To read J1, the R.V. is doubled.

(2) Sloan (1959) described the special features of near and far visual acuity charts developed at the Wilmer Institute of Johns Hopkins University and states that these optotypes, involving a set of ten letters, provide measures of visual acuity that are comparable to those obtained with Landolt rings.

(a) Table XXIV-3 provides data on the visual angle subtended by the optotypes at 20 feet, 16 and 14 inches.

TABLE XXIV-3. Specifications of Sizes of Optotypes and Number of Characters of Each Size.

Visual Angle in Minutes Subtended For Standard Test Distance* (20 ft., 14 in., 16 in.)	20 ft. (6.1 m.) A	14 in. (35 cm.) B	16 in. (40 cm.) C	Equivalent M Notation (distance in meters at which detail subtends 1′) A	B	C	No. of Characters 20 ft. Chart†
16.0	(20/310) 12.5/200	14/224	40/640	97.5	5.6	6.4	–
12.5	(20/560) 16/200	14/175	40/500	76.5	4.4	5.0	–
10.0	20/200	14/140	40/400	61	3.5	4.0	1
8.0	20/160	14/112	40/320	48.8	2.8	3.2	2
6.25	20/125	14/87.5	40/250	38.2	2.2	2.5	4
5.0	20/100	14/70	40/200	30.5	1.75	2.0	6
4.0	20/80	14/56	40/160	24.4	1.4	1.6	6
3.0	20/60	14/42	40/120	18.3	1.05	1.2	8
2.5	20/50	14/35	40/100	15.25	0.875	1.0	10
2.0	20/40	14/28	40/80	12.2	0.7	0.8	10
1.5	20/30	14/21	40/60	9.2	0.524	0.6	10
1.25	20/25	14/17.5	40/50	7.6	0.44	0.5	10
1.0	20/20	14/14	40/40	6.1	0.35	0.4	10
0.8	20/16	(14/12) 17.5/14	(40/32) 50/40	4.9	0.28	0.32	10
0.65	20/13	(14/9.1) 21.5/14	(40/26) 61.5/40	4.0	0.23	0.26	10

+ These visual angles apply to the component parts of the optotypes, that is, to the width of the lines. The overall dimensions, as in the standard Snellen letters, are five times the above values.
† The near charts have 10 characters on each line.

(3) Since the objective of near correction is usually to read, it should be recognized that acuity per se does not represent or imply reading ability.

(4) For this reason patients are tested with samples of reading material of various sizes typical of book, magazine, and newsprint which can be read at the customary reading distance.

3. Most low vision examinations are carried out at ten feet or less to increase accuracy and sensitivity of patient responses.

a. Acuity should be specified in terms of the Snellen letter read at the test distance in feet (e.g., 10/80, 5/100, etc.).

4. Printed charts (including illuminated charts on a movable stand rather than projector targets) provide improved illumination and contrast control as well as increased flexibility and test distance (see Table XXIV-4 for near visual acuity equivalents).

5. Near testing is carried out at the focal point of the lens or lens combination (disregarding accommodation). Following accurate determination of the magnification or power needed on a standardized test card, realistic reading matter is then substituted for the reading card, such as a newspaper, book, or a magazine.

TABLE XXIV-4. Visual Acuity Equivalents

"x-height" (in mms)[1]	Snellen fraction[2]	Jaeger type designation[3]	Printers' "points"	"Efficiency" (per cent)[4]	Visual angle (in minutes)	Type typical of
.6	20/20	1+	3	100	5.00	Near point test cards
.75	20/25	1	4	95	6.25	Mail order catalogs, Bibles
.9	20/30	2	5	90	7.5	Want ads
1.2	20/40	3	6	85	10.0	Telephone directory
1.5	20/50	5	8	75	12.5	Newspaper text
1.95	20/65	6	9	65	16.25	Adult textbooks
2.1	20/70	7	10	63.5	17.5	Adult textbooks
2.4	20/80	8	12	60	20.0	Children's books (age 9 to 12)
3.0	20/100	10	14	50	25.0	Children's books (age 8 to 9)
3.85	20/130	12	18	40	32.50	Children's books (age 7 to 8)
5.1	20/170	14	24	30	42.50	Large type books
6.0	20/200	17	28	20	50 0	Large type books

[1] "x-height" refers to the vertical height of the lower case "x" in the size of type involved. The table can be extrapolated beyond the limits listed above by measuring the "x-height" of the size of type in question and using the same ratios that can be seen by inspection of the above columns.

[2] When material in question is held 16″ from the eyes.

[3] This system has not been completely standardized. See Fonda, Gerald, *Management of the Patient with Subnormal Vision*, (Saint Louis: the C. V. Mosby Company, 1965), pp. 8-9; 120.

[4] The "efficiency' percent is based on the rating scale adopted by the American Medical Association for use in compensation decisions. See Spaeth, Edmund, "Estimation of Loss of Visual Efficiency," *A.M.A. Archives of Ophthalmology*, Vol. 54, No. 3, Sept. 1955, pp. 462-468.

6. Near acuities should be specified by the test distance in inches and the size of the print read (e.g., 20/50 reduced Snellen at three inches; Jaeger 5 at four inches; 10 point type at eight inches).

7. Lighting is carefully determined in relation to level of intensity and visual need. The patient should be fully instructed as to the specific reading distance and the head-hand-eye fixation requirements.

   a. Some patients may prefer subdued lighting. The quality of illumination (diffuseness, color characteristics, background contrast, presence of glare) is another essential consideration.

8. The use of magnification in low vision examination procedure includes:

   a. Refinement of distance prescription with a low power telescopic lens which will provide a measurable (and qualitative) improvement in visual acuity as a means of verifying and refining the tentative distance correction.

   b. Determination of visual acuity yield with ascending telescopic lens powers involving the use of a full diameter telescope. The use of segment or "bioptic" telescopic lenses is also recommended where appropriate.

   c. Intermediate distance refraction utilizing telescopic lens and low power plus caps which fit over the objective lens.

   d. The near point refraction, utilizing microscopic lenses usually begins with 2X and proceeds with each power increase until a satisfactory level of vision is achieved which will meet the patient's visual needs.

(1) Demonstrate or explain that these lenses have an extremely short depth of focus, possess peripheral aberrations, and have a small usable visual field.

e. Use of non-ophthalmic magnification aids as auxiliary testing units (e.g., head-borne binocular loupe, a fixed-focus magnifying aid).

D. Evaluation of the low vision findings

1. A review of the case history will establish, for the examiner, essential visual needs and expectations. Social, emotional, vocational, avocational, motivational, and educational considerations must enter into any thorough analysis of low vision findings.

2. The most important aspects include the specific need or desire of the patient, his ability to adapt to new situations, his motivation to learn new visual habits, and his understanding of the uses and limitations of the visual aid provided. Additional factors which will affect the decision to prescribe are the patient's age, his temperament, and the duration of his visual impairment.

3. Since low vision prescribing is primarily task oriented, the use of a single aid to fulfill multiple needs is seldom possible. For this reason, multiple aids are frequently used to provide variations in magnification, viewing distance, size of field, and flexibility in use.

E. Visual training and after care

1. Having decided that a patient can benefit from a low vision aid, the patient must be properly trained in its use.

2. Inherent limitations in such factors as working distance, field of vision, and spatial distortions require the patient to learn new motor patterns of coordination involving head, hand, and eye.

3. Adaptive training involves repeated demonstrations, explanations, and continued supervised practice performing visual tasks while wearing the aid in occupational pursuits and at home.

4. Some patients must overcome an inherent psychological resistance to the appearance of "special" low vision designs (Feinbloom, 1958).

5. A fundamental principle is to adjust the environment so that the patient can perform successfully; as he learns to function within this environment, it can be modified towards a more normal one.

a. Frequently, it is useful to start the training with a weaker correction. As the patient succeeds, gradually increase the strength of the correction.

6. The final phase of visual training should involve lenses of appropriate power with material of the type and complexity that is common to daily visual tasks.

7. If the patient shows limited progress during the adaptive training periods, or if his motivation for visual rehabilitation is questionable, the examiner may assume that psychological factors may limit the patient's acceptance of the low vision aid.

a. In some cases, the patient may have lost his visual memory for words. If he has fallen into a pattern of acting like a blind person, he may require the aid of an allied specialist to develop the incentive to read again.

b. Relearning skills in reading, and other adaptive problems, emphasize the necessity for the professional examiner to work closely with social service workers, psychologists, educators, and others who, in their work, may assist the patient in making the necessary adaptation to his new visual role.

8. In determining the proper magnification for a school child, the usual test cards for near may have words that are too difficult or unfamiliar; single letters or numbers may be more adequate. By having the child bring a school book that he is or will be using, accurate prescription determination can be made.

9. A follow-up examination, six to twelve months after aid is dispensed, is essential since some patients experience a decrease in acuity which may be the result of the pathological or aging process present. A change in the low vision aid is frequently needed.

a. In many cases, increased visual activity will result in more varied needs and expectations which, in turn, may require the prescribing of additional types of visual aids.

10. Publications by Bier (1960), Rosenbloom (1958), Maier (1965), and Korb (1969) include more complete details on techniques of low vision aid designs, equipment recommendations, and examples of record forms for low vision analysis.

IX. GUIDEPOSTS IN PRESCRIBING LOW VISION AIDS

A. Clinical results have emphasized the need to be aware constantly that no matter how limited a patient's vision may be, to him that vision and its limitations take on a real significance.

1. If this vision can be improved even slightly, the patient's whole perspective and outlook improve, and the scope of his rehabilitation, both vocationally and avocationally, is broadened.

B. An understanding of the importance of psychic factors is essential in determining whether or not the patient is ready to accept the benefits of a low vision aid.

1. Some patients show a high degree of adaptation to their visual impairment; others may read by braille and show no indication of an interest in reading English symbols; some demonstrate deeply rooted emotional disturbances which may affect their willingness to persevere in the extended training required to adapt successfully to a visual aid.

2. Interdisciplinary cooperation with allied specialists is frequently an essential consideration in planning for the successful rehabilitation of a low vision patient.

C. A good case history will include essential information that will often determine whether or not the patient can be helped and may also indicate the appropriate direction the examination should follow.

1. For each patient a varying pattern of needs emerges based on his individual situation requiring the careful selection of the most appropriate low vision aid(s).

D. The most urgent priority in low vision testing is an accurate determination of the refractive state and the optimum correction to provide best distance acuity.

E. With the exception of corrective lenses, low vision aids are rarely feasible for constant wear.

1. The availability and increasing use of segment telescopes now allow some patients to achieve distance magnification and improved distance acuity with mobility.

F. Always prescribe minimum magnification to meet specific visual needs.

G. A final prescription should be postponed until the patient has demonstrated ability to read again; he should be familiar with the appearance of the visual aid, be able to perform a desired useful task, and demonstrate proficiency in its use.

1. Several appointments on different days are usually best in enabling the patient to achieve both a psychological and an adaptive adjustment to the low vision aid.

H. Use targets for refined testing in adaptive training which relate closely to the patient's vocational and avocational needs and interests.

I. Direct lighting properly placed and of sufficient intensity is essential.

J. Music stands, tilt top tables, or easels may help overcome the inconvenience of the short working distance.

K. Beyond +8.00 D. to +10.00 D., monocular function alone is practicable.

1. In binocular corrections, two clinical approaches to lens design for near use are recommended:

   a. Decentration of each bifocal segment is obtained by dividing the far inter-pupillary distance (PD) in millimeters by the reading distance in inches, plus one (Lebensohn, 1949).

   b. A rule-of-thumb for obtaining base-in prism for each bifocal segment is to decenter 1 mm. or grind 1 prism diopter of base-in prism for each diopter of reading addition (Fonda, 1970).

L. Do not dismiss any patient as hopeless before an adequate evaluation of his low vision status has been carried out.

M. A resource list of materials and services for the low vision patient, including large type books, magnifiers, talking books, projectors, and readers is available from the American Library Association (Mullen, 1968).

1. A manual reporting a complete list of low vision aids and their sources has been compiled by Sloan (1966).

X. THE PARTIALLY SEEING CHILD

A. As defined by Hathaway (1959) and by many state regulations regarding the education of partially seeing children, this group includes children with visual acuity between 20/70 and 20/200 in the better eye with optimum correction, or with other visual deviations which, in the opinion of the vision specialist, require special education.

1. Educationally, they are visually limited children who can use enlarged ink print, or limited amounts of regular print under special conditions as a major mode of instruction rather than braille.

B. The basic educational philosophy in modern programs is based on the concept that these partially seeing children must learn to live in a visually-oriented society.

1. Educational practice today emphasizes not only appropriate grade placement, but also recognition of the range of individual differences that exist among partially seeing children.

C. There are three major types of educational plans in common use for partially seeing children today: the *cooperative plan,* utilizing a special classroom; the *resource room;* and the *itinerant teacher program.*

1. In the cooperative plan, the child is enrolled in a special "sight-saving" class, leaving this class several times a day to join his normally sighted classmates in activities not requiring continued use of the eyes.

2. In the resource room, the child is a member of a regular classroom and has the opportunity to participate with normally seeing children in wholesome competition where he can attain some degree of success, engage in social activities at his own level, and enjoy a sense of group belonging.

a. The itinerant teacher program is designed to provide special educational services in suburban and rural areas.

3. The itinerant teacher, trained in special education procedures, travels from school to school in her area serving not only as a consultant to the regular classroom teacher, but also serving as a supplemental teacher to the partially seeing child, using sight conservation methods, equipment, and supplies.

D. There has been little research on the reading and school achievement of partially seeing children, or on the type sizes considered most appropriate for their instructional materials.

1. With regard to type size, Hathaway (1959) stated that some partially seeing children can read small print more easily than large print, and need to be encouraged to do so. It is only through repeated trials with varying sizes of type that the teacher can determine the one best suited to the child's needs and encourage his use of it.

2. Eakin, Pratt, and McFarland (1961) compared the readability of three sizes of type – 12, 18 and 24 pt. – under the condition of a standard distance of 14 inches, and Nolan (1967) demonstrated that visually limited children read a serif type face (Antique Old Style) faster than a sans serif type face (Metromedium). But he found no significant difference in reading speed between 18 pt. and 24 pt. type sizes.

E. In a most extensive study of school achievement and the effect of type size on a fifth and sixth grade population of over 1,000 visually handicapped children, Birch, Tisdall, Peabody, and Sterrett (1966) found:

1. The typical partially seeing child is of at least average intelligence; yet a significant number in this study were retarded in their educational achievement on an average of two years.

2. Far point visual acuity falls within the 20/70 to 20/200 range for 57.7% of the pupils; better than 20/70 in 28.7%; and poorer than 20/200 in 12.9%.

3. More than half of the vision disabilities of the partially seeing children are accounted for by myopia, hyperopia, cataract and aphakia, and retrolental fibroplasia.

4. No one type size could be considered more appropriate for partially seeing children.

5. Reading speed, comprehension, and degree of visual acuity are not related; a comparison of type size and achievement scores also shows no relationship.

F. In a study by the U.S. Department of Health, Education, and Welfare (1961) of 14,125 legally blind children registered with the American Printing House for the Blind for federal aid in the form of special educational texts and materials, data were reported on the extent of visual loss in relation to the "mode of reading."

1. A review of the data revealed only 24% of the children were reported as totally blind and 16% had light perception.

2. The remaining 60% have residual vision of "a sufficient amount to be of practical use in many phases of their school programs."

3. Approximately 58% read solely by braille; 38% read print; 4% were reported as readers of both print and braille.

G. In a replication of the above study, Nolan (1967) reported data on 18,652 legally blind children and reported no significant differences in findings relating degree of visual loss to "mode of reading."

H. Considerations in planning and in conducting a functional educational program for legally blind children with sufficient residual vision to read printed materials are described by Sibert (1966).

I. The development of visual behavior in low vision children and the use of visual-perceptual training with low vision patients, including outlines of sequential stages and learning experiences to attain higher levels of visual discriminatory ability, were described by Barraga (1964 and 1969).

J. Rosenbloom (1963) reported principles in the visual examination and care of the partially seeing child and enumerated specific research needs in this field. These included:

1. The development of a more educationally functional concept of partial vision in order to more appropriately define and classify children for educational purposes.

2. The need to standardize criteria for use in determining when a child should be admitted to or dismissed from educational programs.

3. The development of visual-perceptual training techniques for increasing in children with severe visual impairments such perceptual skills as accuracy, speed of fusion, binocularity, form, speed, span of recognition.

4. The development of new low vision aids whose design will increase the application, versatility, and acceptability of these aids among children and youth with marked visual impairment.

XI. CLINICAL RESULTS OF LOW VISION STUDIES

A. Feinbloom (1935) presented a summary of prior studies in the low vision field and described the results achieved on 500 low vision patients, 59.5% of whom were aided, 21% of whom were aided but the aid was found to be impractical, and 19.4% of whom could not be benefited.

1. Problems in adaptation to the low vision aid and psychological factors in patient care were also described.

B. Freeman (1954) reported on 175 low vision patients of whom 52% were aided and accepted the low vision aid; 24.5% were offered visual correction but refused to accept it; and 23% could not be helped.

1. In his opinion, the most important factors which determined whether or not an aid was accepted were the skill and experience of the examiner, the personality and outlook on the life of the patient, and the type of adjustment the patient had made to his visual impairment.

C. In a report of 500 patients examined at the Lighthouse of the New York Association for the Blind, Fonda (1955) reported that 48% benefited from the low vision aid.

1. Prescriptions included: one-piece plus magnifying lenses in powers from +8.00 D. to +36.00 D.; doublet microscopes in powers from 8X to 20X; and microscopic bifocals utilizing triplet lens design in 10X and 14X power.

2. Patients with albinism, post-operative aphakia, myopic chorioretinal degeneration, and macular degeneration were most responsive to the aids.

D. A report published by the Industrial Home for the Blind (1957) stated that 68% of a group of 500 patients had been successful in using low vision aids.

1. The results were achieved in patients with high myopia, lens affections, structural anomalies, and glaucoma.

2. Social work and medical examinations were carried out in association with the optometric examination and prescribing of the low vision aids.

E. In reporting an analysis of 365 patients examined over a three-year period, The Cleveland Society for the Blind (Kaine, 1963) indicated that 65% of the patients were fitted successfully with low vision aids. Patients found to be most successful were frequently highly educated, gainfully employed, 11 to 20 years of age, visual loss of congenital origin, and visually impaired for 10 to 14 years.

F. Brazelton, Stamper, and Stern (1970) report on a group of 55 clients of the California Department of Rehabilitation who were given low vision aids. After a period of use from six months to one year, 49 of these patients were still using their aids successfully on the job or in school. The high rate of success was attributed to two factors primarily: specific task oriented prescribing, and generally strong motivation to achieve financial independence or further education.

G. In a survey of 1,800 patients examined over a 14-year period at the Chicago Lighthouse for the Blind, Rosenbloom (1966) reported that approximately 75% of the patients could be benefited by the prescribing of a low vision aid. However, 7.0% did not accept the visual correction. Although fewer in number, congenitally blind individuals had greater success with low vision aids than did the adventitiously blind.

1. Examination of the ocular pathology responsible for the reduced vision revealed that choroidal and/or retinal changes occurred with greatest frequency (60%); 31% of the group suffered from conditions of the optic nerve, primary or secondary, and corneal opacities; while another 9% included congenital or acquired anomalies.

2. A study of the type of ocular pathology, in relation to degree of visual loss, failed to show a significant pattern. Regardless of pathologic type, the most important factors in determining the success in using low vision aids seemed to be the amount of residual vision and the functional field of vision.

a. Patients with less than 3/200 visual acuity, or markedly restricted peripheral fields, related to progressive types of ocular pathology (e.g., diabetic retinopathy, retinitis pigmentosa, advanced glaucoma) are least likely to benefit.

3. Within the *successful outcome groups:*

a. Approximately two-thirds of the patients were prescribed either a microscopic lens ranging in power from 3X to 12X, or a high plus reading addition of from +3.00 D. to +14.00 D. with a median value of +8.00 D. The near vision of over 80% of these patients was improved to the point where magazine and newsprint could be read.

b. Telescopic lenses were prescribed in approximately 15% of the cases:

(1) Small segment telescopes mounted in the upper portion of the prescription carrier lens in plastic provided greater flexibility and have been used successfully, especially with students and young adults.

(2) In selected cases, nonprescription telescopic lenses, designed either as sport glasses or clip-ons, have proved very satisfactory.

4. In a follow-up study (Rosenbloom, 1970), 276 patients were re-examined or interviewed between six months and one year after the low vision aid had been prescribed and dispensed.

a. Approximately 76% of the patients continued to use the visual aid regularly and reported moderately to highly successful results.

b. In approximately 24% of the cases, the patients (over two-thirds of whom were past 60 years of age) had discontinued the use of the low vision aid. In this group, the causes were associated with senile changes, poor health, further visual loss, and lack of interest in, and motivation for, the visual aid.

XII. SOCIAL AND VOCATIONAL REHABILITATION OF THE BLIND AND PARTIALLY SEEING PATIENT

A. Rehabilitation has been defined as the process of restoring the worker to industry, the citizen to society, and the man to himself.

B. At *the national level,* agencies are of two general types: public and private.

1. Scott (1969) identified a total of 793 such agencies; 110 of these agencies are listed as private, and 19 are identified as local public organizations.

2. Public agencies include the Division of Services for the Blind; Rehabilitation Services Administration, U.S. Department of Health, Education, and Welfare; and the United States Library of Congress.

3. National agencies of a private nature include a number of associations: The American Foundation for the Blind, The National Industries for the Blind, The American Printing House, The Howe Press of Perkins School for the Blind, The Hadley School for the Blind, The Braille Institute of America, and publishers of braille and talking book materials (e.g., National Braille Club).

a. There are also special resource agencies providing guide dogs, audio-visual materials, various mechanical and teaching aids, and transcribing services.

C. At the *state level,* most agencies are public in organization. Many states have divisions of rehabilitation organized under either state welfare divisions or state commissions for the blind. Other states, Illinois for example, organize their blind services as a separate agency responsible to the state board of education. All states provide funds that are matched by those of the United States Department of Health, Education and Welfare.

1. Exemplifying an organization at the state level which is independent and private is the Illinois Society for the Prevention of Blindness. This agency, established by Illinois law in 1961, carries out a lay and professional public education program with particular emphasis on sight conservation programs.

D. At the *community level,* various agencies provide a variety of rehabilitation services for blind people (e.g., The Chicago Lighthouse for the Blind and the Illinois Visually Handicapped Institute). These services include sheltered workshops, social services, recreational programs, preschool and college preparatory programs, and a low vision clinic that is inter-disciplinary in its planning and function. There are also agencies offering home teaching for blind, home-bound individuals which are usually part of the State Commission for the Blind programming.

1. Local public organizations at the community level include branch offices of federal programs,

such as the Old-Age, Survivors, and Disability Insurance, and certain publicly supported sheltered workshops for the blind.

2. Other services at the local level include the activities of such fraternal organizations as Lions International and various groups whose primary function is braille transcribing.

E. Scott (1969) lists six types of private agencies serving blind people:

1. *Large multi-functional agencies* offering many services to blind individuals of all ages (e.g., nursery school programs for preschool blind children, recreational programs for blind adolescents, rehabilitation services for blind people of all ages, psychological counseling and casework or group work services, a home teaching service, mobility instruction, a sheltered workshop, and various volunteer and professional services).

2. *General social welfare organizations* which provide services for many people, some of whom may be blind. Goodwill Industries, for example, will often reserve positions for blind people in their shops. Most of these organizations are sheltered workshops in which people with handicaps other than blindness also work.

3. *Small general service agencies for the blind* pattern themselves after the larger multifunctional agencies. Due to the lack of financial and professional resources, the programs of these organizations involving rehabilitation and counseling services are usually modest.

4. *Other blindness organizations* which offer services of a highly particularistic nature such as low vision clinics, summer camps for blind children and adults, and employment services for the blind.

5. There are also *counseling agencies* which usually do not provide any direct services, but exist for the purpose of representing the field, or some segment of it, to the government, to Congress, or to the local community. Such organizations seek to bring about changes within work for the blind by consulting with direct service agencies or by lobbying at the federal and state levels.

REFERENCES

**American Optometric Association, Committee on Visual Problems of Children and Youth (1961): Manual on the Partially Seeing Child. Third rev. ed., St. Louis.*

Barraga, N.C. (1964): Increased Visual Behavior in Low Vision Children. American Foundation for the Blind, New York.

Barraga, N.C. (1969): "Learning Efficiency in Low Vision." J.A.O.A., 40: 807.

Bechtold, E.W. (1953): "An Improved System of Wide-Angle Magnifying Spectacles." O.J.R.O., 90 (22): 35.

Berens, C. (1933): "Standardization of Statistics on Causes of Blindness." Revista de la Asociasion Medica Panamericana, 1, August.

Bier, N. (1960): Correction of Subnormal Vision. Butterworths, London.

Birch, J.W.; Tisdall, W.J.; Peabody, R.; Sterrett, R., School Achievement and Effect of Type Size On Reading in Visually Handicapped Children. Cooperative Research Program of the Office of Education, U.S. Department of Health, Education, and Welfare; Cooperative research project No. 1766; contract no. OE 4-10-028.

Brazelton, F.A. (1969): "Magnification in Microscopic Lenses." A.A.A.O., 46: 304.

Brazelton, F.A.; Stamper, B.; and Stern, V.N. (1970): "Vocational Rehabilitation of the Partially Sighted." A.A.A.O., 47: 612.

Eakin, W.M.; Pratt, R.J.; and McFarland, T.L. (1961): Type Size Research for the Partially Seeing Child. Stanwix House, Pittsburgh.

**Ellerbrock, V.J. (1947): "Report on Survey of Optical Aids for Subnormal Vision." O.J.R.O., 84: 15 (15): 29.*

**Ellerbrock, V.J. (1960): "Partial Vision and Optical Aids. Vision of the Aging Patient. Hirsch, M.J., Wick, R.E., Chilton Books, Phila.*

Estimated Statistics on Blindness and Vision Problems. New York (1966): The National Society for the Prevention of Blindness, New York.

Faye, E.E. and Weiss, S. (1965): "Management of the Low Vision Patient." in Refraction, I.O.C. 5 (2). Little, Brown and Co., Boston.

Feinbloom, W. (1933): "Some New Optical Devices for Subnormal Vision Cases." Opt. Weekly. 24: 1217.

Feinbloom, W. (1935): "Report of 500 Cases of Subnormal Vision." A.J. Opt., 12: 238.

Feinbloom, W. (1958): "Training of the Partially Blind Patient." J.A.O.A., 28: 724.

Feinbloom, W. (1967): "The 3.5 X Reading Binoculars in Spectacle Form for the Partially Blind Patient." Opt. Weekly. 58 (18): 17.

**Filderman, I.P. (1959): "Clinical Procedures for Adapting the Telecon Lens." J.A.O.A., 30: 561.*

**Filderman, I.P. and White, P.E. (1969): Contact Lens Practice and Patient Management. Chilton, Phila.*

Fonda, G. (1955): "Report on Two-Hundred Patients Examined for Correction of Subnormal Vision." AMA Arch. Oph. 54: 300.

Fonda, G. (1965): Management of the Patient with Subnormal Vision. C.V. Mosby Co., St. Louis.

Fonda, G. (1970): "Binocular Reading Additions for Low Vision." Arch. Opt. 83: 294.

Ford, A.B. (1970): "Casualties of Our Time." Science; 167 (3916): 256.

Freeman, E. (1954): "Optometric Rehabilitation of the Partially Blind, A Report on 175 Cases." A.A.A.O., 31: 230.

Genensky, S.M. (1970a): A Functional Classification System of the Visual Impaired to Replace the Legal Definition of Blindness. Santa Monica; The Rand Corporation. Memorandum RM-6246-Rc, April.

Genensky, S.M. (1970b): Closed Circuit TV and the Education of the Partially Sighted. Rand Corp., Santa Monica, March.

Godber, G.E. (1962): "The Blind and the Partially Sighted." Oph., England and Wales 1960; 2 (3): 125.

Goldstein, H. & Goldberg, I.D. (1962): "The Model Reporting Area for Blindness Statistics." The Sight-Saving Review. 32 (2): 84.

Guth, S.K.; Eastman, A.A. and McNelis, J.F. (1956): Lighting Requirements for Older Workers. Illuminating Eng., 51: 656.

Hatfield, Elizabeth M. (1973): Estimates of Blindness in the United States. The Sight-Saving Review, vol. 43, No. 2, pp. 69.

Hathaway, W. (1959): Education and Health of the Partially Seeing Child. Columbia University Press, New York.

**Industrial Home for the Blind, Industrial Home for the Blind Optical Aids Service Survey. New York; IHB, 1957.*

Kaine, P.A. (1963): Low Vision Clinic for Advancing Use of Optical Aids, Vocational Rehabilitation Administration Project No. RD-400. Cleveland Society for the Blind, Cleveland, pp. 23-25.

**Kerby, C.E. (1940): Manual on the Use of the Standard Classification of Causes of Blindness. American Foundation for the Blind, Inc. and the National Society for the Prevention of Blindness, Dec.*

Kestenbaum, A. and Sturman, R.M. (1956): "Reading Glasses for Patients with Very Poor Vision." Arch. Oph., 56: 451.

Kopash, R.: New High Quality Fresnel Lenses for Ophthalmic Use. Publication in preparation.

Korb, D.R. (1969): "A Simplified Procedure for Prescribing Low Vision Reading Lenses." J.A.O.A., 40 (8): 812.

Lebensohn, J.E. (1949): "Practical Problems Pertaining to Presbyopia." A.J. Oph., 32, 32: 22.

**Lebensohn, J.E. (1952): "Interim Management of Incipient Cataract." Quarterly Bulletin, Northwestern University Medical School, 27 (33).*

**Lebensohn, J.E. (1956): Optical Aids for Subnormal Vision. Sight Saving Review 26: 201.*

Lebensohn, J.E. (1958): Newer Optical Aids for Children with Low Vision. A.J. Oph. 46: 813.

Lederer, J. (1956): "The Optometrical Treatment of Subnormal Vision." Australian Opt. 39: (9) September.

**Livingston, J.S.; Justman, J.; Gilbert, H.B. (1955): Sixth Grade Children with Visual Handicaps Enrolled in Sight Conservation Classes. New York; Board of Education of the City of New York.*

Lowenfeld, B. (1950): "Psychological Foundation of Special Methods in Teaching Blind Children." Blindness, ed. by Paul A. Zahl; Princeton University Press.

Ludlam, W.M. (1960): "Clinical Experience with the Contact Lens Telescope." A.A.A.O., 37: 363.

Maier, F.B. (1965): Subnormal Vision – A Clinical Guide to Care of the Partially Sighted. Southern College of Optometry, Memphis.

Mandell, R.B. (1965): Contact Lens Practice: Basic and Advanced. Charles C. Thomas, Springfield.

Mullen, M.M. (1968): Reading Aids for the Handicapped. 5th revision, American Library Association. Chicago.

National Society Prevention of Blindness (1967): Estimated Total Cases and New Cases of Legal Blindness by State. Bulletin of N.S.P.B., New York.

Nolan, C.Y. (1967): "A 1966 Reappraisal of the Relationship Between the Visual Acuity and Mode of Reading for Blind Children." The New Outlook for the Blind. 61: 8, October.

Riley, L.H. (1969): "Low Vision Statistics." J.A.O.A., 40: 820.

Rosenbloom, A.A. (1958): "Principles and Techniques for Examining the Partially Blind Patient." J.A.O.A., 29: 715.

Rosenbloom, A.A. (1963): "The Partially Seeing Child." Vision of Children. Hirsch, M.J. & R. Wick; Chilton, Phila.

Rosenbloom, A.A. (1966): "Subnormal Vision Care: An Analysis of Clinic Patients." Proceedings of the Conference on Aid to the Visually Limited, Washington, D.C.; A.O.A.

Rosenbloom, A.A. (1969): "The Controlled – Pupil Contact Lens in Low Vision Problems." J.A.O.A., 40: 836.

Rosenbloom, A.A. (1970): "Prognostic Factors in Low Vision Rehibilitation." A.A.A.O., 47: 600.

Scott, R.A. (1969): The Making of Blind Men. Russell Sage Foundation, New York.

Sibert, K.N. (1966): "The Legally Blind Child with Useful Residual Vision." The Education For the Blind; December.

Sloan, L.L. (1959): "New Test Charts for the Measurement of Visual Acuity at Far and Near Distances." A.J. Oph., 48: 807.

Sloan, L.L. (1960): Applied Biomedicine: Help for the Visually Handicapped. U.S. Govt. Print. Office. (90th Congress, First Session, Seventh Document no. 55.)

**Sloan, L.L. (1966): Recommended Aids for the Partially Sighted. National Society for the Prevention of Blindness, Inc., New York.*

Sloan, L.L. and Jablonski, M.D. (1959): "Reading Aids for the Partially Blind." Arch. Oph. 62: 465.

U.S. Department of Health, Education and Welfare, Blind Children: Degree of Vision, Mode of Reading. prepared by John Walker Jones, Washington; Government Printing Office 1961. (Bulletin 1961 No. 24.)

**U.S. Department of Health, Education and Welfare, Characteristics of Visually Impaired Persons U.S. July 1963 – June 1964. Series 10; No. 46; Washington; Government Printing Office, August 1968.*

Zettel, J. (1964): "The Care of Low Vision." A.A.A.O., 41: 142.

Ocular Pharmacology 25

I. PRESSURE AGENTS

A. The ophthalmic examiner is naturally concerned with the ocular effects of drugs since many of his patients may be receiving systemic medication which may affect the results of the examination and refraction, or because mydriatics and/or cycloplegics may have been instilled in the patient's eyes. The effect of drugs upon the natural ocular functions as well as upon diseased conditions are, of course, obvious items of interest and attention.

B. The number of drugs which are currently in use is enormous. In addition, new medications are constantly appearing on the market. Therefore a comprehensive consideration of all the drugs which can affect the eye is not possible in a chapter of this size. First consideration will be given to those drugs which are used in treatment of diseases of the eye, their effects, and side effects. Those medications used for conditions not affecting the eye but whose side effects may cause serious ocular problems will be discussed afterwards. Some drugs fall into both categories.

C. Several principles must be considered before taking up the study of the drugs themselves. The most important of these is *drug administration.* Drugs may be given either systemically or topically. In ocular therapeutics, the topical mode of the administration is used much more frequently.

1. *Systemic administration* of drugs in ocular diseases is limited because of the blood aqueous barrier. The existence of this barrier is due to the relatively high impermeability of the intra-ocular capillaries to some components of the blood, as compared to capillaries located elsewhere in the body.

a. Lipid-soluble substances are allowed to pass readily, but water soluble substances have much more difficulty passing, and those which have a molecular weight exceeding 600 do not usually enter at all.

b. However, the permeability can be increased either by inflammatory conditions or by sudden lowering of the intra-ocular pressure by paracentesis of the anterior chamber.

c. The barrier may become so ineffective as to allow even the passage of large protein molecules into the aqueous, which is seen clinically as aqueous flare or Tyndall effect.

2. As already indicated, *topical administration* plays a major role in ocular therapeutics. Several factors are to be considered here.

a. Before any drug can come into direct contact with the eye, it must become dissolved in the tear film layer. Therefore, purely fat soluble substances cannot reach the surface of the eye because of the aqueous tear layer. Also, the normal flow of tears tends to carry medication away from the eye.

b. The cornea is the route of penetration into the eye of any substance which is introduced into the conjunctival sac.

(1) Its penetration is governed by the following factors:

(a) epithelial permeability of the substance,

(b) stromal diffusion,

(c) physico-chemical activity in the stroma of the substance,

(d) absorption of the substance by the limbal blood vessels from the cornea,

(e) endothelial permeability.

(2) The primary site of resistance in absorption into the cornea is the epithelium.

(a) The epithelium allows passage of lipid-soluble substances much more readily than water-soluble substances.

c. Simple diffusion accounts for the main method of travel of substances through the stroma. Water-soluble substances pass through the stroma much easier than lipid-soluble substances.

(1) The endothelium offers little resistance to transfer into the anterior chamber.

d. It can be seen that those substances which have biphasic solubilities – that is, both in water and in lipid – are the ones which will be best absorbed.

e. Detergents or wetting agents are sometimes used to increase the penetration of drugs which would otherwise not be absorbed. Since these have a toxic effect on the epithelium, their use is recommended only when absolutely necessary.

f. It must also be remembered that installation of a drug into the conjunctival sac may be followed by considerable systemic absorption so as to produce disturbing and sometimes possibly even fatal results. The author has observed several cases where severe systematic side effects occurred as a result of the use of topical eye medications.

D. Individual Response

1. Individuals may show wide variation in their responses to drugs. A common example of this is the relative unresponsiveness of the pupils of more heavily pigmented races to mydriatics. Idiosyncratic reactions (unusual responses to drugs) are usually due to some metabolic abnormality which is peculiar to the individual.

2. *Allergy*

a. Some people show allergy to particular drugs. Certain drugs tend to induce allergic reactions more than others. These reactions may be quite severe, indeed even fatal. For instance, penicillin, an extremely useful and usually quite safe drug, may cause death in people who are allergic to it.

E. Combinations of drugs are often used to produce greater effects. This synergism may be merely the sum total of the effects of each or, if their modes of actions are different, may result in a greater net effect (potentiation).

F. Conversely, **antagonism** between drugs may be seen whereby one drug cancels out the effects of the other so that there is no benefit from the drugs. Occasionally, drugs will be used in combinations to minimize the side effects of each other.

II. ADMINISTRATION METHODS

A. Topical administration of drugs may be in the form of aqueous or oily solutions, suspensions, ointments, or creams. They may also be incorporated into filter paper such as fluorescein strips.

1. These medications should have their temperature, pH, and osmolarity adjusted so that they will cause the least amount of irritation to the eye, and discomfort to the patient.

2. Needless to say, any preparation for the eye should be sterile.

3. Prolonged contact of the medication with the eye may be obtained by the use of solutions containing methylcellulose or polyvinyl alcohol.

4. Ointments remain in contact with the eye longer than solutions.

B. Injections about the eye are frequently made. Medications may be introduced subconjunctivally to speed absorption, by-passing the corneal epithelial barrier and passing directly through the sclera which has absorption characteristics similar to that of the corneal stroma.

C. Retro-bulbar injections into the muscle cone are routinely done in many types of intra-ocular surgery. Injection of a local anesthetic has the triple effects of:

1. anesthetizing the globe,
2. paralyzing the four recti muscles and the inferior oblique muscle, and
3. lowering intra-ocular tension.

D. In addition, there may be conditions where it is desirable to place medications near the posterior pole of the eye or the optic nerve to get higher concentrations of the medication than is possible by other routes.

III. TYPES OF EFFECTS

A. It must be remembered that all effects of drugs are mere modifications of normal body responses. Drugs cannot cause any new effects in the body. They either stimulate or interfere with mechanisms which are already present in order to obtain the desired effects. This will be most evident as we study the drugs which mimic the effects of nervous stimulation on the eye.

IV. AUTONOMIC EFFECTORS

A. To best understand the drugs which fall into the class of autonomic effectors, one should be familiar with the effects of the parasympathetic and sympathetic nervous systems on the eye. It is not within the scope of this chapter to review these systems. However, we must recall that the chemical mediator of the parasympathetic system is acetylcholine and this system is called cholinergic, while at effector sites in the sympathetic nervous system the mediator is mainly norepinephrine and hence this system is referred to as adrenergic, (because of its association with the adrenal gland).

1. We can readily divide the autonomic effector drugs into four classes:

a. Parasympathomimetic (cholinergic) drugs which can simulate parasympathetic action either directly or indirectly;

b. parasympatholytic, which block the action of the parasympathetic system;

c. sympathomimetic (adrenergic) which simulate the action of the sympathetic either directly or indirectly, and

d. sympatholytic, which antagonize the action of the sympathetic.

B. Direct Acting Cholinergic Drugs

1. The direct acting parasympathetic drugs mimic the action of acetylcholine, the substance which is produced at all synapses and most effector sites. It is rapidly hydrolyzed by the enzyme cholinesterase. With repeated stimulation, there is repeated release and hydrolysis of the acetylcholine. This quick removal of the released acetylcholine clears the way for the further action of subsequently released acetylcholine.

2. Longer acting parasympathetic drugs are relatively resistant to hydrolysis by cholinesterases.

3. Acetylcholine itself is used in intra-ocular surgery when a quick, intense miosis is desired. It must be instilled directly into the anterior chamber.

4. The most commonly used drug in the cholinergic group is *pilocarpine.* Its important actions are that of constriction of the pupil and of stimulation of accommodation.

a. It is most commonly used in open-angle glaucoma where the stimulation of the ciliary muscles opens up trabecular spaces and increases the facility of out-flow of the aqueous humor. Contraction of the ciliary muscles is also thought to constrict the anterior ciliary arteries as they pass through the belly of the muscle, thereby possibly cutting down on the formation of aqueous humor. This combination of events lowers the intra-ocular pressure and is of utmost importance in treatment of open-angle glaucoma.

b. It is also used in angle closure glaucoma since the miosis it produces pulls the root of the iris out of the chamber angle. This allows a return to the normal aqueous dynamics, provided that peripheral anterior synechiae have not yet formed which would cause permanent adherence of the iris root to the trabecular mesh work.

c. Accommodative esotropia is favorably influenced by pilocarpine, although it has been generally replaced by the anti-cholinesterase inhibitors for this purpose.

d. *Side effects include:*

(1) Induced myopia due to ciliary muscle contraction. In young individuals, this may be disabling. Early presbyopes find it desirable since it does not lower their distance acuity much, but they find that they can again read without a near correction. The effect is not significant in older patients.

(2) Miosis makes vision in dim light difficult, especially when first leaving brightly lit surroundings.

(3) Poor visual acuity due to lenticular opacities may be worsened by miosis.

(4) Continued use may result in a rigid iris which will not dilate. Posterior synechiae may also form.

(5) Allergic reactions in the form of follicular conjunctivitis may necessitate stopping the drug.

(6) Pigmented cysts of the pupillary margin may occur following long usage. They are more commonly seen with the stronger miotics. They clear spontaneously if the miotic is discontinued. The concomitant use of phenylephrine prevents their formation.

5. *Methacholine* (Mecholyl) is a similar drug, whose main value lies in the establishment of the diagnosis of Adie's pupil. A 2.5% solution of this drug will cause miosis in the patient with Adie's pupil, but it will not affect a normal pupil.

6. *Carbachol* is a very powerful miotic. It is usually reserved for those instances where pilocarpine is not effective or where the patient shows an allergic reaction to pilocarpine. It is not well absorbed through the cornea and surface acting agents must be incorporated into the solution to enhance absorption. The surface acting agents produce minimal damage to the corneal epithelium.

C. Cholinesterase Inhibitors

1. These drugs work by destroying the enzyme acetylcholinesterase which normally hydrolyzes acetylcholine. This allows the accumulation of acetylcholine, producing effects of greater intensity and longer duration.

2. *Physiostigmine (eserine)* has been known for over one hundred years. It was the first drug to be used in the treatment of glaucoma. It may be used in either open-angle or angle closure glaucoma. It usually causes severe allergic irritation, if used for prolonged periods.

3. A newer group of anti-cholinesterase agents were developed as an outgrowth of the nerve gases which were produced during World War II. The most popular of these are *DFP* and *Phosophline Iodide.*

a. These two drugs may be used for the treatment of open-angle glaucoma, but must not be used where there are narrow angles since they cause congestion of the ciliary body and may cause angle-closure glaucomà.

b. The latter two anti-cholinesterase agents are also used for the treatment of accommodative squint. Since they stimulate accommodation within the eye without stimulating the synkinesis of convergence, those esotropias which are associated with a high accommodative-convergence to accommodation ratio may be significantly helped and, in some cases, even completely straightened by the use of these drugs.

4. *Side effects:*

a. Those noted for pilocarpine generally hold true, but are usually more marked with these stronger miotics.

b. Retinal detachments may be precipitated in predisposed eyes.

c. Phospholine iodide has been implicated in the formation of cataracts in older patients using the drug.

d. Systemic poisoning may occur. The signs are lacrimation, rhinorrhea, salivation, sweating, bronchial spasms, gastric upset, muscular twitching, convulsions and failure of respiration. The antidote is atropine in large doses.

D. Parasympatholytic drugs

1. The parasympatholytic drugs prevent the entrance of acetylcholine into the effector cells by blocking the action of acetylcholine.

a. This group of drugs causes pupillary dilation and paralysis of accommodation.

(1) The mydriasis and cycloplegia make these drugs useful for doing refractions and ophthalmoscopy.

(2) They are also used in the better eye to lower visual efficiency in the treatment of amblyopia to force the patient to use the amblyopic eye as an alternative to patching.

(3) They are very important in the treatment of anterior uveitis.

(a) Mydriasis prevents the formation of posterior synechiae and may even break those which have already formed, if not too extensive.

(b) Cycloplegia contributes to the comfort of the patient by relaxing the ciliary muscle which goes into spasm in anterior uveitis.

b. These drugs have a deleterious effect on both types of primary glaucoma. Mydriasis may provoke an attack of angle-closure glaucoma, and in open-angle glaucoma will lower the out-flow of the aqueous humour, resulting in increased intra-ocular pressure.

2. *Atropine* is the oldest known and most powerful drug in this category.

a. When instilled into the conjunctival sac, pupillary dilation ensues in about 15 minutes and clinically lasts for about ten to 12 days.

b. Cycloplegia takes about a half hour to occur and clinically persists for three to five days, although, even after two weeks, tests will reveal some of the effects.

c. Enough of this drug may be absorbed into the systemic circulation from the conjunctival sac to cause systemic toxicity which consists of fever, dry skin and mucous membranes, increased heart rate, delusions, unconsciousness, or even death.

d. Severe allergic reactions may occur.

3. *Scopolamine* is very similar in its actions to atropine.

a. However, its effects are more immediately noticeable and persist for only about two days.

b. It causes less allergies than does atropine but still carries the same dangers as atropine in glaucoma patients.

c. Scopolamine is used systemically as a sedative in anesthesia, in Parkinsonism, and in motion sickness. When used systemically, it is liable to cause more mydriasis and cycloplegia than will atropine.

4. *Homatropine* is a synthetic derivative of atropine. It has the same effects as does atropine but is much weaker and of much shorter duration.

5. *Cyclopentolate hydrochloride (Cyclogyl)* is a newer synthetic drug which has gained wide popularity. Its widespread use comes from the fact that it has prompt action and its effects are said to be worn off within six hours, although occasionally they may last up to 24 hours.

6. *Tropicamide (Mydriacyl)* is a synthetic derivative of atropine. It has a rapid onset of action and its effects wear off quickly. It is generally considered to be more efficient as a mydriatic than as a cylcoplegic.

E. Sympathomimetic drugs

1. The sympathomimetic drugs are the two adrenal hormones, adrenalin (epinephrine) and noradrenalin (norepinephrine), and their synthetic derivatives. Norepinephrine is also the chemical mediator at many sympathetic postganglionic nerve endings (effector sites), corresponding to the role of acetylcholine in the parasympathetic system. While norepinephrine is not used frequently in the eye, epinephrine has several valuable uses.

2. *Epinephrine (adrenalin)* has an effect on blood vessels, causing them to constrict.

a. Mild solutions of epinephrine and its derivatives (Visine, Clear Eyes, Vasocon, Prefrin, Zincfrin, Privine) are used in conditions where there is congestion of the conjunctival blood vessels, especially allergic states. Its use results in a transient whitening of the eye along with a period of increased comfort. However, when the effects of the medication wear off there may be a rebound hyperemia of the conjunctival blood vessels. Its prolonged use may result in chronic turgescence of the conjunctiva. Even these dilute solutions may cause mydriasis and angle closure.

b. Stronger solutions are used at the time of surgery to lessen the amount of bleeding on the surface of the eye.

c. Epinephrine has a weak mydriatic effect. Because other drugs have a stronger mydriatic effect than does epinephrine, the latter is not usually used for mydriasis alone. It does have some effect on decreasing the amplitude of accommodation but not enough to be classified as a cycloplegic drug.

d. Adrenalin (Eppy, Glaucon, Epifrin, Epitrate) is used in open-angle glaucoma since it has an immediate effect on decreasing the amount of aqueous which is secreted. This may be related to its effect on the blood vessels in the ciliary body. It has also been shown that after prolonged use an improvement in the aqueous out-flow facility also occurs.

(1) This drug is contra-indicated in angle-closure glaucoma as mydriasis will worsen the attack.

e. Epinephrine is a very potent drug and occasionally enough is absorbed through the conjunctival or nasal lacrimal system to cause alarming symptoms. Fatalities have been recorded from the topical use of the drug. It causes severe discomfort in some people, as burning on installation, palpitations of the heart, and headache.

f. Since epinephrine is a chemically related compound to melanin, its long term use may result in pigmentation of the conjunctiva and cornea.

3. *Phenylephrine (Neo-synephrine)* is an excellent mydriatic with little cylcoplegic effect. It is also used in mild solutions for clearing the conjunctiva.

4. *Hydroxyamphetamine (Paredrine)* is also another effective mydriatic with little cycloplegic action.

5. *Cocaine,* although mainly used as a topical anesthetic, also is sometimes used as a mydriatic. It has its effects by inhibiting the destruction of epinephrine, comparable to the action of the cholinesterases on acetylcholine. Thus the action of the adrenalin is enhanced. Cocaine does not have a mydriatic effect in a sympathectomized eye (Horner's Syndrome). It is usually used in connection with other medications to get a potentiated effect.

F. Symphtholytic drugs

1. While there are a number of symphtholytic agents, their ocular use is still in the investigational stage. They appear to be of value in reducing lid retraction due to thyroid disease.

V. LOCAL ANESTHETICS

A. It must be remembered that all anesthetics are poisons and that local anesthesia must be considered as a carefully controlled selective poisoning of the nerves done in such a way that the nerves regain their function when the medication is stopped. Their mode of action is unknown but it would seem that there is some interference with cellular respiration. If they are absorbed systemically from topical application, there is a marked stimulation of the central nervous system. Fatalities have been recorded from the topical use of these medications.

1. It is worthwhile mentioning that the repeated use of any local anesthetic agent is contra-indicated for the relief of painful corneal conditions, especially abrasions or ulcerations. Because of their toxic effects and interference with corneal healing, a relatively minor lesion which would otherwise be expected to heal promptly could lead to permanent corneal stromal scarring.

2. For many centuries it has been known that the leaves of the cocoa tree had an exhilarating effect when they were chewed. It was not until 1860 that the active principle (cocaine) was identified, and 24 years later the discovery of local anesthesia for use in ocular surgery was announced.

a. *Cocaine,* which is structurally related to atropine, blocks the transmission of impulses in peripheral nerves, eliminating painful sensations. Its application into the conjunctival sac produces numbness in about two minutes which lasts for about ten minutes. Deeper anesthesia is obtained by repeated applications.

b. While cocaine's anesthetic properties are quite strong, it has been largely supplanted by newer synthetic products because of its strong sympathetic stimulation-like effects if absorbed systemically. Its mydriatic effect may be undesirable and produce severely damaging effects on the corneal epithelium.

3. Some of the more recently developed substitutes for cocaine are *benoxinate (Dorsacaine), tetracaine (Pontocaine), dibucaine (Nupercaine),* and *proparacaine (Ophthaine or Ophthetic).*

4. It was discovered in 1899 that *procaine (Novocain)* could be used by injection to produce a regional nerve block without the toxicity of cocaine. Since that time there have been numerous other agents made available, but one of the most currently popular is *lidocaine (Xylocaine).*

a. Much intra-ocular surgery is done under regional nerve block. The patient is awake but sedated.

(1) First the facial nerve is infiltrated to obtain akinesia of the obicularis oculi muscle. The patient is unable to close his lids during surgery, thus preventing him from putting undesirable pressure on the eye.

(2) A retro-bulbar injection is next done. The needle is introduced into the muscle cone through the tissue between the inferior and lateral recti muscles and the

anesthetic agent is then injected. When properly performed, this results in corneal anesthesia, akinesia of the recti muscles and the inferior oblique, and dilation of the pupil as well as a drop in intra-ocular tension.

VI. CARBONIC ANHYDRASE INHIBITORS

A. The first known carbonic anhydrase inhibitor was *acetazolamide (Diamox).* It was first introduced as a diuretic and later noted to cause a decrease in intra-ocular tension in both normal and glaucomatous eyes.

B. These drugs interfere with the enzyme carbonic anhydrase, which catalizes the reaction between water and carbon dioxide forming carbonic acid.

1. We do not have a precise explanation of why they decrease aqueous production.

2. This action does not significantly affect the facility of aqueous out-flow.

3. These drugs do not decrease aqueous formation in the same manner as epinephrine as shown by the fact that the concomitant use of these drugs results in even greater inhibition of aqueous formation.

C. Other members of this group are *methazolamide (Neptazine), diclorphenamide (Daranide),* and *ethoxzolamide (Cardrase).*

1. The major differences between the drugs is their potency, some of the drugs being used in much smaller quantities.

2. They all produce similar side effects, although some patients may tolerate one but not another.

3. Side effects may be severe enough to make discontinuance of the drug mandatory. They include drowsiness, decreased appetite, vomiting, tingling in the extremities, kidney stones, skin eruptions, acidosis of the blood, as well as a decrease in the white blood cell count which may prove to be fatal. They may also cause a dangerous loss of potassium from the body if used for a prolonged period.

4. For these reasons on many occasions patients are not kept on long-term therapy with the carbonic anhydrase inhibitors unless absolutely necessary. Some belief that filtering surgery is preferable to long-term carbonic anhydrase inhibitor therapy is also evident.

5. These drugs, as well as the sulfonamide group of drugs to which they are structurally related, may cause an induced myopia. Upon cessation of the use of this drug, the myopia slowly regresses.

VII. OSMOTIC PRESSURE AGENTS

A. A method for lowering the intra-ocular pressure under emergency conditions is to raise the osmotic pressure of the blood so that fluid is drawn out of the eye. Substances used must be such that they do not diffuse readily into the eye There are three which are currently popular.

1. *Urea* is a safe and effective agent. Administration is by intravenous infusion. It can cause severe headache since it also causes fluid to be drawn from the cerebral spinal fluid. In the inflamed eye, it loses its effectiveness, since the blood aqueous barrier is no longer present against urea.

2. *Mannitol* is a sugar which is not metabolized and works in the same fashion as does urea. It must also be given intravenously. Because of its larger molecular weight the blood aqueous barriers remains intact longer for mannitol than for urea.

3. *Glycerol* is a smaller sugar which can be given orally. The oral administration is more convenient, except that the solution is so sweet that it often causes nausea and/or vomiting. Newer preparations have flavored the glycerol with lemon or lime flavoring to make it more palatable. It is not as effective as urea or mannitol.

4. *Ethyl alcohol,* although not used clinically, also reduces intraocular pressure by raising the osmotic pressure of the blood.

VIII. ANTIBACTERIAL AGENTS

A. Antibacterial agents are widely used in the treatment of ocular infections. They may either have a bacteriocidal action in which the organisms are killed by the antibiotic itself or a bacteriostatic action in which the bacteria is restrained in its growth and reproduction so that the body's own defense mechanisms can be effective.

B. Sulfonamides are chemical antibacterial agents which preceded the development of antibiotics, but are still of considerable value.

1. Two of the drugs commonly used on the eyes are *sulphacetamide (Sulamyd, Vasosulf,* and others) and *sulphafurazole (Gantrisin).*

2. Sulfa drugs are chemically related to the carbonic anhydrase inhibitors and share the same side effects when given systemically. However, when used topically they are well tolerated in the conjunctival sac. Systemic administration may cause a temporary induced myopia.

C. Antibiotics are biologically produced antibacterial agents.

1. Those commonly used for topical application of the eye include *bacitracin, tetracycline, chloramphenicol, neomycin, polymyxin, gramicidin.*

2. *Penicillin* is not recommended for topical use since this may cause sensitization of the patient to the drug and prevent the systemic use of this drug later on when it would be needed.

3. Most of the aforementioned antibiotics are well tolerated in the conjunctival sac. However, neomycin may cause a severe contact dermatitis in sensitive patients.

D. In general, viruses are not susceptible to the action of antibiotics, however, one notable exception is trachoma. This disease can be controlled with the use of sulfonamides, tetracyclines, and erythromycin. This is of particular significance since trachoma is the world's leading cause of blindness.

E. A recently developed drug, *iododeoxyuridine (IDU, Stoxil, Herplex),* is effective in inhibiting the herpes simplex virus in the acute epithelial stages. It does this by interfering in the metabolism of the virus by substitution for thymidine in the formation of its nucleic acids. This course of the disease is shortened and there is thus less likelihood of a disciform keratitis following the acute epithelial phase. However, there is some evidence that recurrences of the disease are somewhat more frequently seen after the use of the drug.

IX. ADRENAL CORTICOSTEROIDS

A. The adrenal cortex secretes a number of potent hormones, collectively known as *corticosteroids.* Among this drug group are cortisone and hydrocortisone which have strong general anti-inflammatory effects on the body as a whole and are indispensable in the treatment of certain eye disorders.

1. Prednisone, prednisoline, and methylprednisoline, triamcinolone and dexamethasone are synthetic derivatives which are more potent and are said to minimize side effects. They are put out

under a variety of trade names by many manufacturers and also in combination with antibiotics and sulfonamides.

2. Corticosteroids have profound effects on the body's metabolism and it is always preferable to administer these topically. For disorders of the anterior segment of the globe, this was possible. However for conditions involving the posterior segment, it is necessary to use systemic administration.

3. The mode of action of the corticosteroids is unknown. They have a powerful anti-inflammatory effect against a wide variety of insults to tissues such as trauma, infection, and allergy. It should be stressed that these drugs are not curative, but suppress the inflammation which the insult causes.

a. Since inflammatory reaction is part of the body's defense mechanism, if these medications are used in the wrong circumstances or without a concomitant use of other necessary medications, they can indeed make the situation worse.

(1) For instance, if used in an infection, there can be a deceptive appearance of improvement while indeed the infective organism is actively multiplying.

(2) Conversely, in self-limited conditions, the effects may be extremely valuable so that significant permanent damage is not done while the disease runs its course.

4. The effects of the corticosteroids in the eye are extremely important. They may limit destruction in the eye so that useful vision is retained rather than being lost.

a. *Beneficial effects in the eye are:*

(1) Inhibition of inflammatory vascularization of the cornea

(2) Decrease in the abnormally increased permeability of the intra-ocular capillaries which are associated with inflammation

(3) Decreased cellular inflammation

(4) Decreased formation of granulation tissue

(5) Decreased fibroblastic activity

b. *Deleterious ocular effects are several*

(1) Corticosteroids will cause a significant increase in intra-ocular pressure in all people who are either heterozygous or homozygous for glaucoma. This effect can occur quite promptly and result in loss of visual field.

(2) The use of corticosteroids worsens the course of active herpes simplex keratitis, possibly resulting in loss of vision or the eye.

(3) Fungal ulcers of the cornea have frequently been reported to have perforated rapidly with the use of the corticosteroids, even when the fungus involved is not usually pathogenic to the cornea.

(4) The prolonged administration of the adrenal corticosteroids has been implicated in the formation of posterior subcapsular cataracts.

(5) Steroids also interfere with wound healing by retarding epithelial and endothelial regeneration and interfere with fibroblast activity in the repair of stromal wounds.

c. The uses of these steroid hormones are varied. They include anterior and posterior uveitis due to many different causes, such as trauma, sympathetic ophthalmia, toxoplasmosis, allergic conjunctivitis, chemical conjunctivitis, and inflammatory vascular diseases.

X. MISCELLANEOUS DRUGS

A. In the past, preparations containing silver and mercury were popular. Some people used these for a protracted length of time and the metals were precipitated out and presented as dark pigmentation on the eye. This was not particularly dangerous but, unfortunately, cases of this dark pigmentation have been confused with malignant melanoma.

XI. SYSTEMIC MEDICATIONS (see also Chapter IX)

A. Systemically administered drugs may also affect the eye adversely. Some medications are life-saving but damage the eye. In these cases, it is desirable to carefully observe the patient from the first sign of ocular side effects so that the drugs may be stopped if possible when these appear.

1. *Ethyl alcohol,* while not usually used for medicinal purposes, does have pharmacological effects. Diplopia occurs due to the esotropia which alcohol can produce. Visual hallucinations are common in the condition known as delirium tremens, which is a withdrawal syndrome. Many alcoholics develop a nutritional amblyopia because they do not partake of an adequate diet.

2. *Methyl alcohol* causes blindness, optic atrophy, and death.

3. Other central nervous system depressants, such as *barbiturates, bromides, antiepileptic medications,* and *tranquilizers,* may cause nystagmus, blurred vision, ptosis, and diplopia.

4. Some of the *phenothiazine tranquilizers* which include Mellaril, Thorazine, Sparine, and Compazine can be stored in the pigment epithelium and cause an irreversible pigmentary retinal degeneration. They also interfere with accommodation and cause oculogyric crises.

5. *Digitalis,* a drug commonly used to stimulate the heart, causes blurred vision, halos, and disturbed color vision, when the patient receives too large a dose.

6. *Chloroquine,* a drug first developed as an antimalarial, has been found to be very useful in systemic lupus erythematosus, a fatal disease. It causes blurred vision and halos due to corneal edema and deposition of crystals of the drug in the corneal epithelium. This is reversible upon cessation of the drug. This drug is also stored in the pigment epithelium and causes an irreversible pigmentary retinal degeneration after large amounts have been taken for a prolonged period of time.

7. Some drugs used for treating *high blood pressure* may cause an interference with accommodation, bringing about presbyopic symptoms in a younger person.

8. Optic neuropathy may be caused by a large number of drugs. This is not a commonly seen complication of drug therapy. Drugs which have been implicated include *chloramphenical, streptomycin, sulfonamides, oral contraceptives, isoniazide* (an anti-tuberculosis agent), and *Vitamin A* (in large overdosage).

9. Many women who have quite successfully worn contact lenses noted difficulty in continuing to wear them after beginning use of *oral contraceptive medication.*

10. *Narcotic* users have blurred vision. Their pupils are miotic.

11. Newly discovered *diabetic patients* or those who have had markedly elevated blood glucose

levels should not have glasses prescribed until good control has been established and maintained for six weeks.

a. Induced myopia is caused by dehydration of the lens by the increased serum osmolarity. Therefore any adult who shows a marked, rapid increase of myopia must be suspected of being diabetic.

b. When diet and medication (either insulin or oral hypoglycemic agents such as Orinase, Diabinese, or DBZ) restore serum glucose to lower levels, a temporary hyperopia occurs, possibly resulting in premature presbyopic symptoms.

B. The above section presents an outline of classes of systemic medications and their possible adverse effects.

1. There are thousands of drugs on the market and many of them are capable of producing ocular side effects.

2. The overall incidence of these, both in absolute numbers and percentage, is surprisingly small in view of the large consumption of medications.

BIBLIOGRAPHY

Bach, M. (1956): Transient myopia after use of acetazoliamide (Diamox). A.M.A. Arch. Ophth. 55, 546-547.

Bellows, J.G. (1934): Surface Anesthesia in Ophthalmology. A.M.A. Arch. Oph. 12, 824-832.

Berliner, R.W. and Orloff J. (1956): Carbonic anhydrase inhibitors, Pharmacol. Rev. 8, 137-174.

Burns, R.P. (1961): Ocular Side Effects of Systemic Medication, Northwest Medicine, Nov.

Duke-Elder, S. (1962): System of Ophthalmology, Vol. VII, St. Louis, Mosby.

Ellis, P.P. and Smith, D.L. (1969): Handbook of Ocular Therapeutics and Pharmacology, St. Louis, Mosby.

Gettes, B.C. (1961): Tropicamide, a new cycloplegic. Arch. Ophthalmol. (Chicago) 65, 632-635.

Goodman, L. and Gilman, A. (1965): Editors, The Pharmacological Basis of Therapeutics, New York, MacMillan.

Gordon, D.M. and Karnofsky, D.A. (1963): Chemotherapy of herpes simplex keratitis. Am. J. Oph., 55, 229-234.

Grant, W.M. (1962): Toxicology of the Eye. Thomas, Springfield, Ill.

Havener, W.H. (1964): Ocular Pharmacology, St. Louis, Mosby, 1966. "Ophthalmology Prescription Handbook," E.J. Browning Medical Publications.

Leibman, K.C.; Alford, P.; Boudet, R.A. (1961): Nature of the inhibition of carbonic anhydrose by acetazolamide and benzthiazide. J. Pharmac. Exp. Ther. 131, 271-274.

Myerson, A. and Thaw, W. (1937): Human Autonomic Pharmacology IX. Effect of cholinergic and adrenergic drugs on the eye. A.M.A. Arch. Oph., 18, 78-90.

Rasgorshek, R.H. and McIntire, W.C. (1955): Cyclogyl, re-evaluation and further studies. A.J. Ophth. 40, 34-37.

Sprague H.B.; White, P.D. and Kellog, J.F. (1925): Disturbances of vision due to digitalis. J. Am. Med. Assoc. 85, 716-720.

Swan, K.C. (1949): Pharmacology and Toxicology of the Cornea. A.M.A. Arch. Oph., 41, 253-275.

26 Single Vision Lenses

I. THE PRESCRIPTION

A. An ophthalmic prescription includes the lens formula, the designation of the frame or mounting, all necessary specifications for the placement of the lenses in the frame and the positioning of the frame on the face.

B. According to custom, the lens formula lists the lens characteristics in the following order: sign of the sphere; power of the sphere; combination sign; sign of the cylinder; power of the cylinder; axis symbol; axis orientation; combination sign; power of the prism; position of the base of the prism. The power of the reading addition is listed under the above. Other special lens characteristics such as the size and style of the multi-focal segment, tint, heat treatment, thickness, base curve, specific brand names, etc., should be listed conspicuously in the vicinity of the other specifications. There is no universal custom followed in arranging the listing of these special characteristics.

1. *The symbols* are abbreviated as follows:

a. For the eyes: right eye, O.D.; left eye, O.S.; both eyes, O.U.
b. For the power signs: + for convex and – for concave.
c. For the combination: ⊃
d. For dioptric power: D.
e. For sphere: S. or Sph., and for cylinder: C. or Cyl.
f. For prism: Pd. or Δ
g. For axis or cylinder: ax or x, and for position of base of prism, either the degree or simply up, down, in, or out.
h. For the reading addition: Add.
i. For the Base Curve: B.C.

2. *The formula* may therefore be illustrated by writing:

O.D. + 1.00 D.S. ◯ –0.50 D. Cyl. ax 175° ◯ 2 Δbase-in.
O.S. + 0.75 D.S. ◯ –0.25 D. Cyl. ax 45° ◯ 1 Δ base-down.
Add: O.U. + 2.00 D.; tint No. 2 or A (according to type of tinted lens and density of the tint).

3. Common usage permits a less formal transcription of the formula: O.D. + 1.00 ◯ –0.50 x 175 ◯ 2 Δ base-in; the designation of the sphere and cylinder, and of the diopter units, etc., being understood. Also, the O.U. is frequently omitted from the designation of the add unless different adds are being prescribed for each eye.

C. A prescription is the designation of an optical system that is intended to relieve certain difficulties of the patient that are related to vision. On occasion the refractionist leaves the completion of the prescription to the dispenser giving him only that portion of the prescription called the lens formula. Just as a physician's prescription which states the appropriate ingredients, but omits the quantity and time intervals at which the drug is to be administered is not a proper prescription, so the mere statement of the lens formula is not a proper ophthalmic prescription. Only the refractionist is aware of the patient's ocular history and problems; only the refractionist knows whether the lenses should be worn constantly or just for distant viewing or just for near viewing; only the refractionist knows whether the lateral and vertical muscle balances are sufficient to handle the prismatic effects induced by the lenses. Consequently, the responsibility for the proper organization in physical form of the refractive correction is definitely that of the refractionist rather than the dispenser. Where both are the same person few problems are encountered, but the records of many practitioners contain numerous histories of patients who were dissatisfied elsewhere because of the liberties that were taken with the lens prescription.

1. There are many factors which add up to a satisfactory and salutary prescription. The lenses should be centered properly before the eyes to avoid unwanted prismatic effects. The segments of multifocal lenses should be located at a height that will eliminate unnecessary and uncomfortable head and eye movements. The lateral location of the segments should be such that they do not induce prismatic effects that may unnecessarily alter the convergence demands placed upon the patient. The distance of the lens before the eye should be specified in order to completely satisfy the power requirements of the eye. The tilt of the lens, especially if the lens power is great and the tilt is unusual, should be recorded. In addition it should be noted that lenses are designed to produce maximum performance along the optical axis and at a specific angular distance away from the axis. If the lenses are improperly positioned in the frame, the optical effect will be less than optimum.

a. Consequently the complete prescription should designate:

(1) The lens formula including:

(a) sphere
(b) cylinder power and axis
(c) prism power and direction of the base
(d) power of the reading addition
(e) size style and placement of multifocal
(f) tint
(g) center thickness and base curve (or brand name of the lens to be used)
(h) heat treatment
(i) special glass or plastic.

(2) The *lateral placement* of the lenses in the frame. This may be recorded in terms of the position of the optical centers from the geometric center of the lens shape. In the usual case where no prism is required the optical center of the lens will be placed at the point where the visual axis of the eye intersects the lens plane. If prism is required, the optical center of the lens will be located some distance from where the visual axis

of the eye intersects the lens plane. A more modern way of designating the centering of the lens is in terms of the *major reference point.* The major reference point is that point on a lens that gives the power including prismatic effect called for in the lens formula. It differs from the optical center in that the major reference point may have prism power associated with it whereas the optical center, by definition, cannot. The major reference point has the advantage that it is not necessary to have prior knowledge of the size of the frame that is to be used in order to specify the precise lateral centering of the lens. Lateral placement is designated in terms of the distance between major reference points.

(a) In either case, whether designating the lateral placement of the lens using optical centers and decentration or the distance between major reference points, it is preferable to specify the placement in monocular terms. This results in separate decentration specifications for each eye if the optical center is used or separate distances from the major reference point of each eye to the center of the bridge of the nose when the major reference point is used.

(3) The *vertical placement* of the lenses in the frame. This is recorded as the vertical component of the distance of the optical center from the geometric center of the lens shape, called the vertical decentration or the distance of the major reference point above the lower boxing line, called the level of the major reference point. The boxing lines are obtained by making horizontal and vertical lines tangent to the four edges of the lens. This is a means of specifying the size of the lens as well as a means of obtaining reference lines for the lens.

(4) The *inward decentration* of the bifocal segment, from the distance optical center or distance major reference point, also known as segment inset, is specified so that the optical center of each segment will coincide with the converged lines of sight. There are two major advantages to this placement. It minimizes the prismatic effects from the segment thus maintaining the same prismatic effect of single vision lenses at the segment center, and allows lateral scanning eye movements of equal extent when doing near work. When single vision lenses are used for near work only, similar benefits are obtained by centering these lenses for the converged lines of sight also.

(5) The *vertical position* of the segment is specified so that the wearer will naturally tend to look through the proper part of the lens, i.e. he will only look through the segment when viewing near objects and vice versa. The position can be specified in terms of the location of the top of the segment below the distant optical center, called the *segment below;* or the distance from the lower boxing line to the top of the segment, called the *segment height.*

(6) The distance of the back pole of the lens from the cornea is called the *vertex distance.* This is especially important when the prescription is very strong, as in the case of corrections for aphakia or severe myopia.

(7) If an unusual amount of tilt is required because of special head and eye posture, perhaps imposed by extraordinary viewing conditions, or because of facial configurations that produce unusual fitting requirements, the amount of tilt should be specified.

b. It is then the task of the dispenser to select an appropriate frame or mounting that will be comfortable, cosmetically attractive, and appropriate for the lenses that have been prescribed. In some instances the refractionist may also specify the frame that is to be used. The *frame specification* is then considered to be a part of the prescription.

II. SPECIFICATION OF LENS POWER

A. The same lens formula may be written in several ways. In the past, when few choices of lens forms were available to the refractionist, the manner of expressing the lens power was based primarily on convenience. Thus, a simple sphero-cylindrical correction might be: +1.00 ⊃ –0.50 axis 90, or +0.50 ⊃ + 0.50 axis 180. Both formulas denote lenses of identical focus and power. However, the formulas do imply that the lenses are constructed differently. As a result these lenses would have certain different optical properties even though the powers would be the same.

1. If the lens formula is written with a minus sign before the power of the cylinder, it is said to be in minus cylinder form. If it is written with a plus sign before the power of the cylinder, it is said to be in plus cylinder form. The procedure used to express the lens formula in an alternate form is called transposition. The transposed formula describes a lens of a different physical form, but with identical power. Since some lenses are made in plus cylinder form and some in minus it is important to be able to express the lens formula properly and appropriately. Lens catalogues list the availability of designs and the cost according to the cylindrical notation that is appropriate to the construction of the lens. Thus, transposition is necessary to locate these listings and to specify the choice of lens properly.

2. For *transposing* one sphero-cylindrical combination into another form:

   a. Algebraically add the power of the sphere to the power of the cylinder. The result is the sign and power of the new sphere expressed in transposed form.

   b. Change the sign of the cylinder. If the sign of the original cylinder is plus, change it to minus. If it is minus, change it to plus. Do not change the power of the original cylinder. The result is the sign and power of the new cylinder expressed in transposed form.

   c. Either add or subtract 90° to the axis of the original cylinder whichever produces a total that is 180° or less. The result is the axis notation of the transposed cylinder.

      (1) Transpose the following from minus cylinder to plus cylinder form: +1.50 ⊃ –0.50 x 180.

         (a) Add the power of the sphere to the power of the cylinder: +1.50 + (–0.50) = +1.00 (sign and power of the new sphere).

         (b) Change the sign of the cylinder and keep the same power of the cylinder: +0.50 (sign and power of the new cylinder).

         (c) Change the axis of the original cylinder by 90°: 180 – 90 = 90 (axis of the transposed cylinder).

            [1] Note that if 90 had been added to 180 the new axis would have been greater than 180. By convention this would not be acceptable.

         (d) +1.00 ⊃ + 0.50 x 90 transposed formula in plus cylinder form

3. For transposing a *simple cylinder* into a *sphero-cylinder* follow the same rules using 0.00 for the power of the sphere.

   a. Transpose + 1.25 x 60 to minus cylinder form:

      (1) 0.00 + (+1.25) = + 1.25 (sign and power of the new sphere)
      (2) –1.25 (sign and power of of the new cylinder)
      (3) 60 + 90 = 150 (axis of the transposed cylinder)
      (4) + 1.25 ⊃ – 1.25 x 150 transposed formula in minus cylinder form.

4. *Two simple cylinders* whose axes are 90° apart may be converted into *a sphero-cylinder* by transposing one cylinder into a sphero-cylinder and adding the second cylinder to it.

a. Express the combination of a + 1.00 x 90 and + 3.00 x 180 in sphero-cylindrical form.

(1) (+ 1.00 ⊃ – 1.00 x 180) + (+3.00 x 180)
(2) + 1.00 ⊃+ 2.00 x 180 transposed form or alternatively
(3) (+ 3.00 ⊃ – 3.00 x 90) + (+ 1.00 x 90)
(4) + 3.00 ⊃– 2.00 x 90 transposed form

5. A *sphero-cylinder* can be considered to be a combination of *two simple cylinders.*

a. Use the sphere as one cylinder with its axis 90° from the axis of the cylindrical component of the sphero-cylinder.

b. Algebraically add the power of the sphere and the cylinder of the sphero-cylinder for the sign and power of the second cylinder.

c. The axis of the second cylinder is the same as the axis of the original cylinder of the sphero-cylinder.

(1) Express the following sphero-cylinder as a combination of two simple cylinders: –3.00 ⊃ + 2.00 x 45.

(a) –3.00 x 135 ⊃–1.00 x 45

6. *A sphere* can be considered to be a *combination of two simple cylinders.*

a. Use the power of the sphere for the power of each cylinder and assign axes 90° apart to each of them.

(1) Express a + 2.00 diopter sphere as a combination of two simple cylinders.

(a) + 2.00 x 90 ⊃ + 2.00 x 180

B. The power diagram or optical cross is a method of recording the power of a lens formula.

1. *The meridians of maximum and minimum power of a lens are called the principal meridians.* In a power diagram two lines intersecting at right angles are drawn to conform with the orientation of the principal meridians of the lens formula. Each line is labeled at one end with the degree notation of a principal meridian. The power of the lens in each principal meridian is written at the opposite end of the appropriate line.

a. Spherical power is always written at the ends of both lines of the power diagram since every meridian of a sphere has equal power.

b. Cylindrical power is recorded as zero on the line representing the axis meridian and the full power of the cylinder on the line that is 90° away (the power meridian). For example, if a + 1.00 x 180 were to be recorded on a power diagram, the + 1.00 would be located on the line corresponding to the 90th meridian and zero power would be located on the line corresponding to the 180th meridian.

c. Sphero-cylindrical lenses can be recorded as the algebraic sum of the powers of the sphere and the cylinder. The sums represent the actual refractive powers of the lens formula in the two principal meridians.

d. Two or more simple cylinders can be recorded directly on a power diagram if the principal meridians are coincident. The algebraic sum of powers in each principal meridian represent the actual refractive power of the lens formula in each of the corresponding principal meridians.

2. It is possible to express the powers of the power diagram as a lens formula.

a. Designate the power in one meridian as the power of the sphere.

b. Subtract the power of the sphere from the power of the second meridian of the power diagram. The result is the power of the cylinder.

c. The axis of the cylinder is at right angles to the second meridian.

(1) Express the powers of the following power diagram (Figure XXVI-1) as a lens formula:

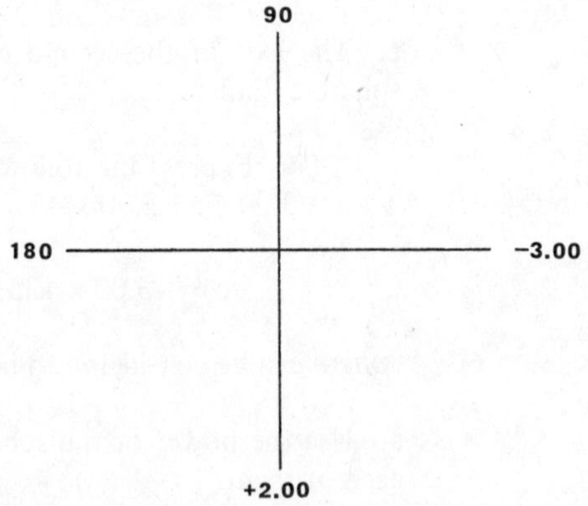

Figure XXVI-1 – Power Diagram

(a) Designate the +2.00 meridian as the sphere.

(b) Subtract the power of the sphere from the power of the second meridian −3.00 − (+2.00) = −5.00. This is the power of the cylinder.

(c) The axis is at right angles to the second meridian.

(d) + 2.00 ⊃ − 5.00 x 90 lens formula

(e) If the − 3.00 meridian had been chosen as the sphere, the result would have been − 3.00 ⊃ + 5.00 x 180.

[1] This is the plus cylinder form of the previous lens formula.

(2) The power diagram could be considered to be composed of two component diagrams, one for a sphere and another for a cylinder. The sum of these components must total the power in each of the principal meridians of the power diagram.

(3) The power diagram (A) is broken into two components. Component (B) is a + 1.00 sphere, component (C) is a simple plus cylinder +1.50 x 90 (Figure XXVI-2). If component (B) had been considered to be a +2.50 sphere, component (C) would be a −1.50 x 180 (Figure XXVI-3).

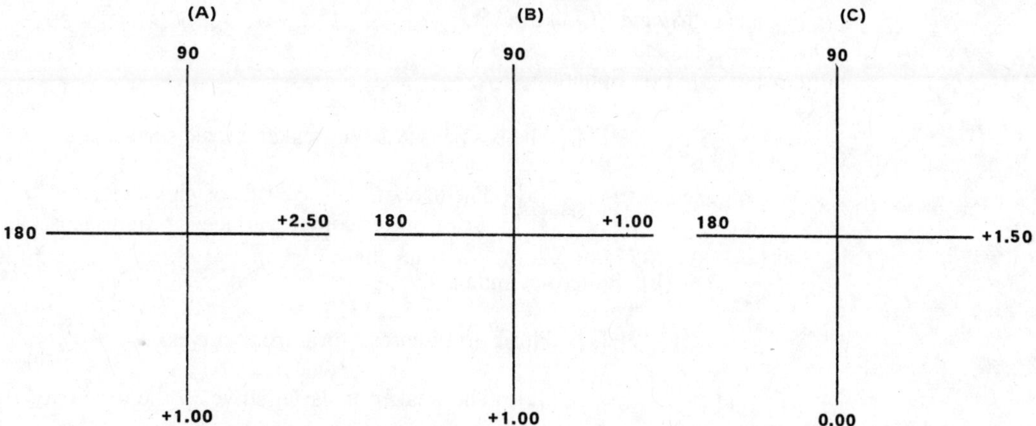

Figure XXVI-2 – Power diagram as two components, plus cylinder.

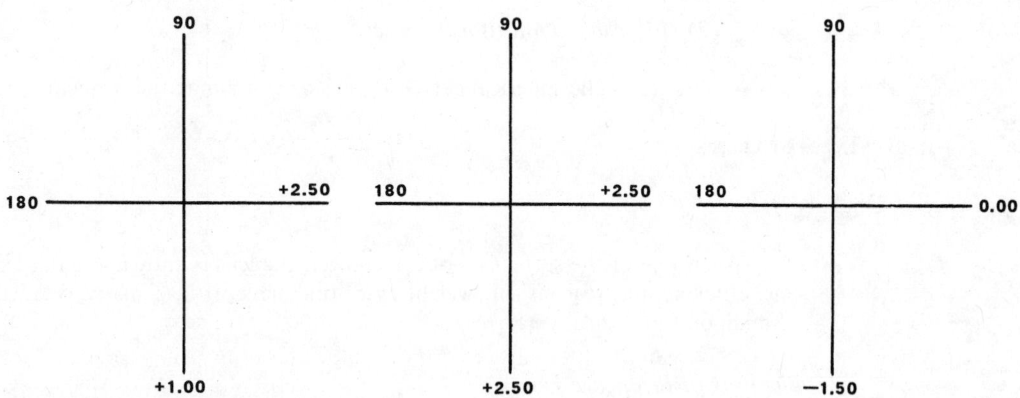

Figure XXVI-3 – Power diagram as two components, minus cylinder.

III. PHYSICAL FORMS OF LENSES

A. **Physical form** is determined by the center thickness of the lens and the curvatures of its surfaces. It is possible to make lenses of the same power in different physical forms. These variations in form constitute the "bending" of the lens. If lenses are made with the proper bending, they will produce better images since certain aberrations will be minimized or eliminated.

1. It is a common manufacturing practice to group lenses into ranges of powers and to make all lenses within the group with the same curvature on one surface. The power differences of the lenses in the group are obtained by selection of different curves for the other surface. Theoretically this is not an ideal situation because each power requires a different bending for optimum performance. However, by judicious choice of curves the performance differences between the ideal and the compromise design can be made very minor. The economies of manufacture are allowed to outweigh the theoretical advantages of design. The fixed curve that is found on lenses over a range of powers is called the base curve and is ordinarily ground at the factory.

a. The base curve is used to designate the lens form and varies not only for different ranges of powers but also for the same ranges of powers among different manufacturers. Exceptions to the following can be found, but the definitions given below are essentially standard.

(1) *Single Vision Lenses*

(a) Spheres

[1] The base curve is the weaker curved surface, i.e.:

[a] The back or concave side of plus lenses,
[b] The front or convex surface for minus lenses.

(b) Sphero-cylinders

[1] Plus Form Lenses, (toric front curves)

[a] The weaker or flatter curve on the toric (front) side

[2] Minus Form Lenses (toric back curve)

[a] The spherical front surface curve

(2) *Bifocal and Multifocal Lenses*

(a) The spherical curve on the side containing the segment

B. Types of Lenses

1. *Flat Lenses*

a. When one of the surfaces is of zero power, the lens is known as a flat lens. While this lens is efficient for reasons of weight and thickness, it has many disadvantages from the standpoint of optical performance.

2. *Biconvex or Biconcave Lenses*

a. Lenses which have both surface powers of the same sign are known as biconvex or biconcave lenses. They provide a means for securing high powers in a single lens, but exaggerate the defects of the fat lens. Except for trial case lenses they are seldom used for refraction.

3. *Periscopic Lenses*

a. To overcome the aberrations of flat lenses, lenses were constructed with a fixed curve on one surface of 1.25 D. Such lenses are called periscopic. Periscopic plus lenses are made with a base curve of – 1.25 D. on the back surface, while minus periscopic lenses are made with a + 1.25 D. curve on the front surface. It can be seen that in either case, the lens will appear slightly bent or curved. The summation of the powers of the two surfaces provides the resultant power of the lens, so that a lens with a base curve of –1.25 and a front curve of +2.75 results in a +1.50 lens.

b. Except in limited powers, these lenses did not minimize the defects of flat lenses sufficiently, so lenses with deeper base curves were developed to supersede them.

4. *Meniscus Lenses*

a. Originally meniscus lenses were manufactured with a single base curve of 6.00 D. Convex meniscus lenses were made with a – 6.00 D. on the back surface. Concave meniscus lenses were made with a + 6.00 D. on the front surface. Variations of the above generalizations are common. Bausch and Lomb uses a + 6.00 curve on the front surface, but the American Optical Co. uses curves from – 6.00 D. to – 14.00 D. curves on the back surface to cover the range of lens powers.

b. By general usage the term meniscus has been applied to lenses which have a base curve greater than 3.00 D. Actually the term meniscus, when not qualified by other specifications, signifies a 6.00 D. base curve. It is acceptable terminology to specify a 4.00, 7.00 or 10.00 D. meniscus lens if the lens is a sphere with that particular base curve. Lenses of 3.00 D. base curve or less are commonly called "flat," whether actually flat, biconvex, biconcave or periscopic.

5. *Sphero-cylinders and Toric Lenses*

a. There are two common forms of sphero-cylindrical lenses. One form is made with the sphere on one surface and the cylinder on the other surface. It is essentially a flat lens with a cylinder in place of the surface of zero power. This construction was popular at one time, but is less common now. The second form is made with the cylinder added to the curve of the convex side. The curves on the convex surface are the base curve and a curve equal in power to the sum of the base curve and the plus cylinder. The concave side is made equal to the difference between the sphere of the lens formula and the base curve. Since the convex surface is toric, these lenses are called toric lenses. Ordinary toric lenses are made with a +6.00 D. base curve, but could be made with any other base curve.

b. If a lens formula calls for + 1.75 ⊃ 0.75 x 180, the curves on a toric lens would be determined by first transposing the lens to + 1.00 ⊃ + 0.75 x 90. The weakest curve on the toric front surface is the base curve. This is usually + 6.00 D. The strongest curve on the toric surface is the sum of the base curve and the cylinder (+6.00) + (+0.75) or + 6.75 D. The concave surface is the difference between the sphere of the prescription and the base curve (+ 1.00) – (+ 6.00) = –5.00 D. The curves can be shown in terms of power diagrams (Figure XXVI-4).

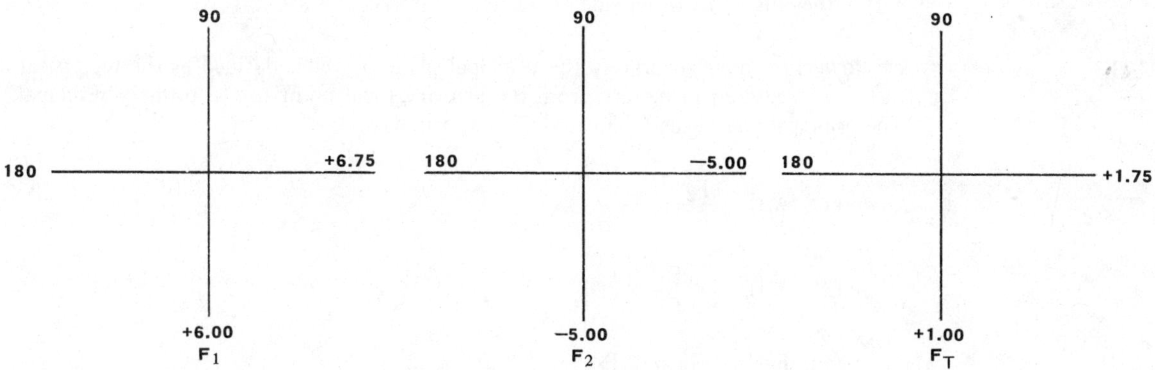

Figure XXVI-4 – Toric Lens Variations.

6. *Corrected Curve Lenses*

a. In general, the form of corrected curve lenses resembles that of toric lenses. This is not surprising since one surface is toric and the other surface is spherical. They could be classified as toric lenses, but since they are more carefully designed and manufactured than the common toric lens they are referred to by the name of corrected curve lenses. These lenses are specifically designed to reduce aberrations. They may be made in either plus cylinder (front surface toric) or minus cylinder form (back surface toric) and are distinguished by their large range of base curves. A further description of corrected curve lenses will follow the section on lens aberrations.

IV. POWER OF OPHTHALMIC LENSES

A. There are very few difficulties in specifying power as long as considerations are restricted to paraxial ray optics and thin lenses. However, the eye moves behind the ophthalmic lens so that the situation is not paraxial. Lenses do have finite thicknesses, especially in the case of plus lenses. Theoretically this would dictate the use of the principal planes in the specification of power.

1. *In thin lens* paraxial ray optics power is measured as the reciprocal of the distance, measured in meters, from the primary focal point to the vertex of the lens. The primary focal point is that object point to the vertex of the lens. The primary focal point is that object point that gives rise to an image at infinity, i.e., produces rays parallel to the optic axis after refraction. The unit of lens power is the diopter.

a. For a single refracting surface the refracting power can be computed from the formula $F = \frac{n' - n}{r}$ in which n' is the index of the medium, n is the index of the air, and r is the radius of curvature of the surface. If thickness is neglected, the power of a thin lens can be considered to be the sum of the powers of the two surfaces, or $F = F_1 + F_2$.

b. This can be expressed in terms of the radii of curvature $F = \left(\frac{n' - n}{n}\right)\left(\frac{1}{r_1} - \frac{1}{r_2}\right)$

2. *For thick lenses* and rays that are not close to the optical axis (the line connecting the centers of curvature of the two surfaces) it is often desirable to use the principal planes when specifying power.

a. These are the object and image positions at which an object gives rise to an erect image of the same size as the object. The points at which the principal planes cross the optical axis are called the principal points.

b. The locations of the principal planes depend on the form of the lens. They may be within the lens or on either side of the lens.

c. Power, or more accurately the principal plane power is defined as the reciprocal of the distance, measured in meters, from the primary focal point to the primary principal plane. The principal planes can be located by the formulas:

(1) $A_1H = \frac{cF_2}{F}$

(2) $A_2H' = -\frac{cF_1}{F}$, where

(3) $F = F_1 + F_2 - cF_1 F_2$.

(a) The symbols used are: A_1 is the front vertex of the lens; A_2 is the back vertex of the lens; H is the primary principal plane; H' is the secondary principal plane; c is the thickness of the lens measured in meters divided by the index of the lens material; F_1 is the power of the front surface; F_2 is the power of the back surface; F is the total power of the lens.

d. Illustration

(1) Locate the primary and secondary principal planes for a lens made of glass of index 1.5, whose front surface is + 8.00 D., whose base surface is – 3.00 D., and whose thickness is 5.0 mm.

(a) $F = +8.00 + (-3.00) - (\frac{.005}{1.5})(+8.00)(-3.00) = +5.08$ D.

(b) $A_1H = \frac{\left(\frac{.005}{1.5}\right)(-3.00)}{+5.08} = -1.97$ mm.

(c) $A_2H' = \frac{-\left(\frac{.005}{1.5}\right)(+8.00)}{+5.08} = -5.23$ mm.

(2) The location of the primary principal plane H is 1.97 mm. in front of the first surface (minus direction means a measurement from the front vertex A_1 to the left). The secondary principal plane is 5.23 mm. in front of the back vertex A_2. Since the lens is 5.0 mm. thick the secondary principal plane is 0.23 mm. in front of the front vertex. The principal planes are separated by 0.74 mm.

e. The value of the principal planes is that they provide a basis for equivalence independent of the form of the lens. Thus, even though the principal planes vary in position with lenses of different form, the power of the lens can be specified easily and lenses can be compared. Lenses having equal principal plane power will have equal distances between the primary focal point and the primary principal plane regardless of the forms of the lenses. Since the location of the principal planes vary with the different lens forms and since the focal lengths will be equal for lenses of the same principal plane power, it can be seen that the distance of the focal points from the vertex of the lens will not be the same. Thus, the form of the lens could influence the power of the lens to be prescribed if the measurement of focal length were to be made from the vertex of the lens.

3. *Thickness* can influence the power of the lens. The effect can be large as illustrated in the accompanying diagram by Pascal (1947) (Figure XXVI-5).

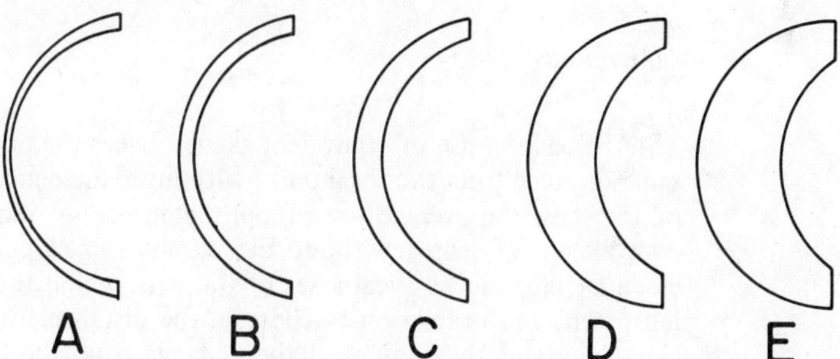

Figure XXVI-5 – Two surfaces of constant difference in radius and varying distances between. (A) *t* less than *d*, concave in form and concave in effect. (B) *t* equals *d*. plano in form and concave in effect. (C) *t* greater than *d*, convex in form and plano in effect. (D) *t* three times *d*, convex in form and plano in effect. (E) *t* more than three times *d*, convex in form and convex in effect. *d* difference in radius of two surfaces: *t* thickness of lens.

4. It will be noted that two surfaces of constant values will produce lenses of different dioptric signs depending upon the distance between the surfaces. While this effect is of primary importance in lenses of high surface curvatures such as contact lenses, it serves to graphically illustrate the influence of thickness upon the refractive value.

B. Designations of the powers of lenses.

1. *Approximate power*

a. The approximate power of a lens can be determined by the simple formula, $F = F_1 + F_2$, or the total power is the sum of the power of each surface. This method ignores the form and thickness of the lens.

b. The approximate method is, however, the method commonly used when a lens measure is employed to determine the power of a lens.

(1) If a lens consists of two surfaces, one of + 2.00 power and one of +3.00 power, the approximate method would result in a total power of +5.00 D. The thickness factor can be also explained upon the basis of the power of the light wave reaching each surface. It would be assumed that parallel rays of light would have a vergence of +5 upon emerging from the lens. If the vergence of the wave is determined by each surface independently, it is assumed that the plano wave takes the power of +2 upon emerging from the first surface and that the +2 wave assumes the added 3 from the second surface. However, the vergence of a non-parallel wave front varies with the distance which the wave travels. As the wave emerges from the first surface, its vergence is +2, but as it travels toward the second surface, its vergence is no longer +2. The thicker the lens or the greater the distance from the first to the second surface, the stronger the wave becomes, if convergent, before it reaches the second surface. The approximate formula can only be correct or accurate if the lens is infinitely thin, which would mean that the two surfaces actually occupied the same spatial position.

2. *Equivalent power*

a. Another method of designating the power of the lens is by means of equivalent power, which has been briefly discussed earlier. The power of the lens in such a case is expressed in terms of the distance of the focal length as measured from the principal plane. It can be computed by the formula: $F = F_1 + F_2 - c(F_1)(F_2)$. (Symbols explained earlier)

3. *Vertex power*

a. Whereas the use of equivalent power places the principal planes of different lenses at the same distance from the focal point without coincidence of the position of the actual surfaces of the lens, the average use of ophthalmic lenses requires some means of determining the equivalency of lenses without the cumbersome operation of the formulas required. The essential tangible physical asset of the lens, which the refractionist can readily note, is the lens itself, and in relation to the eye, the distance from the back surface of the lens to the eye. Consequently, the use of the distance from the back surface to the focal point of the lens as a determinant of the power of the lens has become practically universal in ophthalmic optics. This distance is known as the vertex focal length, to distinguish it from the diopter determined by the equivalent method, and the power is known as the vertex power or vertex diopter, or D_V. The symbol F_V is used to designate it in formulas. The lenses of equal vertex power, in contrast to lenses of equal equivalent power, have the back surfaces of the lenses equidistant from the focal points, although the principal planes are not equidistant from them. Figure XXVI-6 shows the contrasts between vertex and dioptric power.

b. Vertex power can safely ignore the matter of thickness and form. Modern lenses and trial sets are constructed on this basis.

c. The vertex power of a lens can be determined by the following formula:

$$F_V = \frac{F_1}{1 - c(F_1)} + F_2$$

which, when expanded by an infinite series reduces to $F_V = F_1 + F_2 + cF_1^{\ 2} +$ . . . . when the higher order terms are dropped.

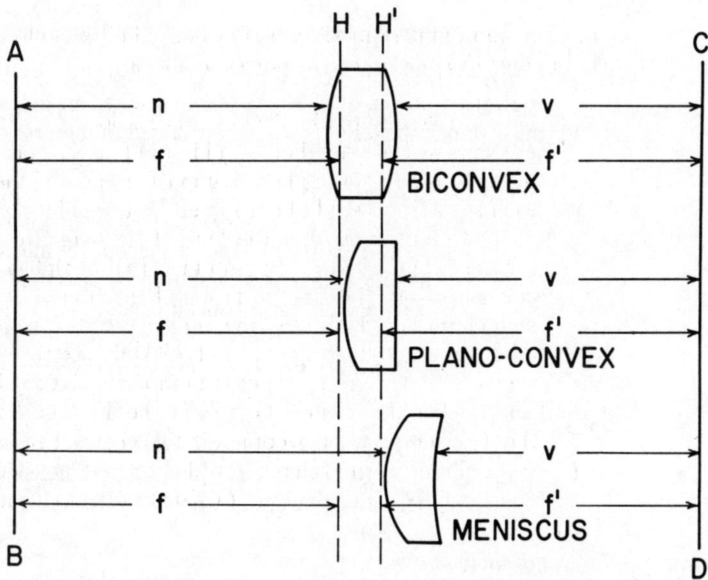

Figure XXVI-6 – Illustrating the relationship between equivalent vertex and neutralizing power. AB primary focal plane; CD secondary focal plane; *n* neutralizing focal length; *f* and *f'* primary and secondary equivalent focal lengths; *v* back vertex focal length; H principal plane; H' secondary principal plane.

4. *Effective power*

a. If a focus is required at some point, there are an infinite number of lenses that could produce a focus at that point provided there are no restrictions placed on the location of the lens. Lenses that focus in the same place are said to have the same effective power, even though they have different equivalent or vertex powers. This is shown in the accompanying diagram (Figure XXVI-7).

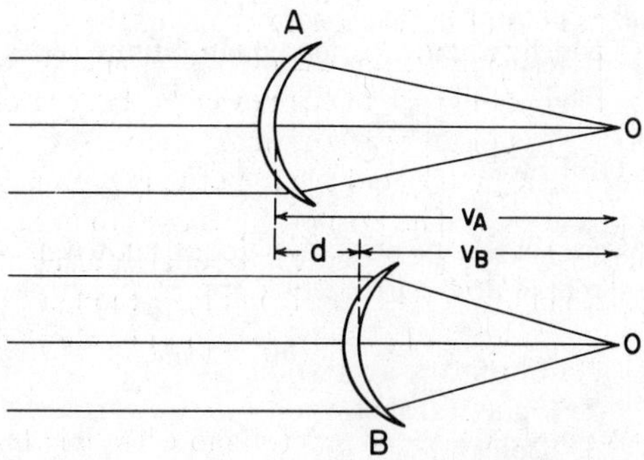

Figure XXVI-7 – Illustrating effective power. Two lenses, A and B of different focal lengths f_1 and f_2 with the same effective power at eye, O, due to difference in position, *d*.

b. Alternatively, the same lens when moved farther or closer to the eye alters its effective power without altering the vertex power. This is important if the refraction of the eye is performed with lenses placed at one distance from the eye and the correcting lens is fitted at a different distance. If the power of the lens is high a significant difference in effective power may result. Examples of this are cataract corrections and high minus corrections. If the fitting distance is greatly different from the refracting distance, as it would be when contact lenses are prescribed, significant changes in effective power can be expected.

c. To determine the equivalent lens with the same effective power as a known lens in a new position from the eye, the following formula is used: $Fe = \frac{F}{1 - dF}$, in which Fe is the equivalent power of the new lens measured in diopters F the known lens in diopters and d the distance the lens is moved, expressed in meters.

(1) Illustration:

(a) A + 10.00 D.S. is placed 15 mm. from the eye to give a patient his best acuity. What power should be specified in the lens formula if the frame locates the lens 20 mm. from the eye?

$$[1] \quad Fe = \frac{+10.00}{1 - (-0.005)(+10.00)} = +9.55 \text{ D.S.}$$

(b) A plus lens gains effective power as it is moved away from the eye, therefore the lens should be reduced in vertex power to maintain the same effective power. The reverse is true for minus lenses.

5. *Neutralizing power*

a. The power of a lens can be neutralized by placing another lens of equal, but opposite power in a position with it. Ideally zero refraction should result from the combination, but this rarely happens since the thicknesses of the lenses produce a thick lens combination, and because the surfaces of the two lenses, since they are not usually matched very closely produce air gaps. This is especially true for lenses of high power. It is preferable to place the neutralizing lens against the front surface of the lens being neutralized. This results in the determination of the power as measured from the front vertex to the primary focal point. This is called the front vertex power or, because it is the power measured by neutralization, the neutralizing power. It can be determined by a formula similar to that used for back vertex power, but with the surfaces reversed:

$$F_N = \frac{F_2}{1 - cF_2} + F_1$$

which, when expanded in an infinite series reduces to $F_N = F_1 + F_2 + cF_2{}^2 + \ldots$ when the higher order terms are dropped.

V. ABERRATIONS OF LENS

A. Lenses are subject to defects of focus known as aberrations. The principal types of aberrations that are encountered in ophthalmic lenses are:

1. Chromatic aberration
2. Spherical aberration
3. Coma
4. Radial or marginal astigmatism
5. Curvature of field
6. Distortion

B. Chromatic aberration

1. Since the velocity of light is dependent on the wavelength and the medium through which it is passing, each wavelength is focused at a different point. The linear spread of these foci along the optical axis is called longitudinal or axial chromatic aberration (Figure XXVI-8). For an object point that is off the optical axis there will be an image that is also off axis. If a screen is placed in the place of the violet focus the spread of the red and violet foci is a measure of the lateral or transverse chromatic aberration (Figure XXVI-9).

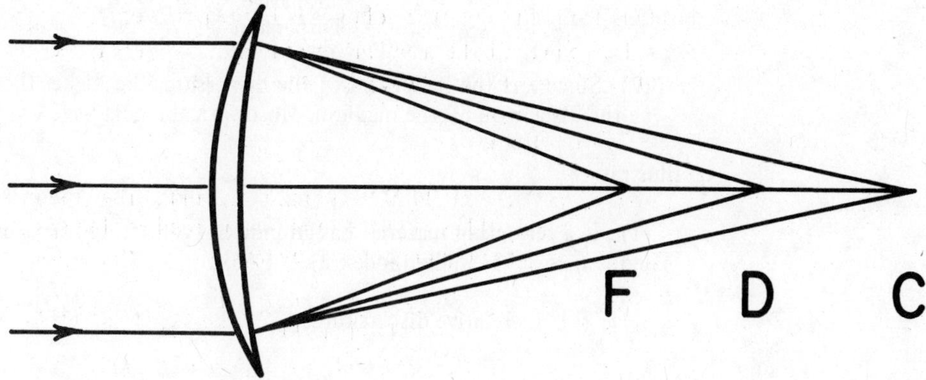

Figure XXVI-8 – Chromatic aberration. Longitudinal chromatic aberration is the difference in focal length for the C and F rays.

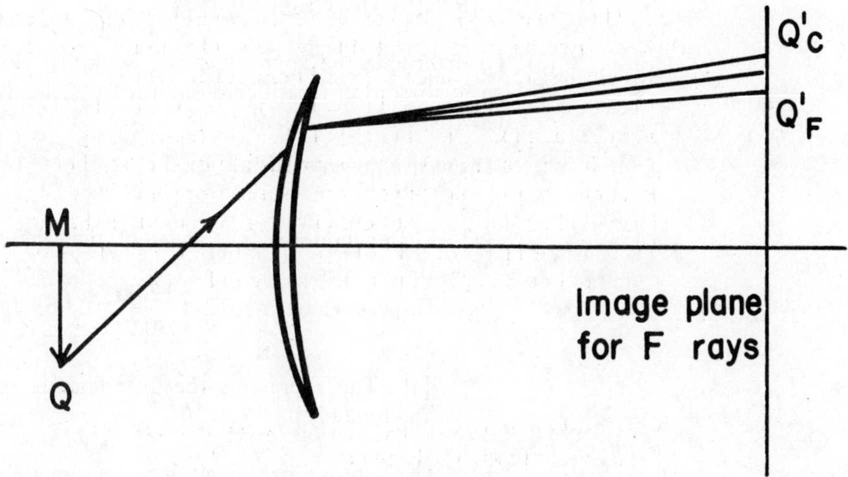

Figure XXVI-9 – Chromatic Aberration. Lateral chromatic aberration is the distance between the C and F chief rays measured in the plane of the F focus.

2. The chromatic aberration is measured in terms of the dispersive characteristics of the optical system.

a. One method used to quantify the amount of dispersion is by the formula:

(1) Relative Dispersion $= \frac{n_F - n_c}{n_D - 1}$

where n_F is the index for the F line (light blue) of the Fraunhofer hydrogen spectrum (λ_F = 486.1 nm.), n_c is the index for the C line (red) of the hydrogen spectrum (λ_C = 656.3 nm.), n_D is the mean value of the D doublet (yellow) of the sodium spectrum (λ_D =589.3 nm.).

b. Frequently, the dispersive power is specified instead of the dispersion. This is known as the nu value (ν value).

(1) Dispersive power (ν) = $\dfrac{1}{\text{Relative Dispersion}} = \dfrac{n_D - 1}{n_F - n_C}$

(2) Since ν is the reciprocal of the dispersion, the higher the ν value, the smaller will be the dispersion by the medium. Most optical media have ν values between 30 and 60.

c. Illustration

(1) If a refracting material has an index of refraction for sodium light n_D = 1.556; an index n_c = 1.541 and an index n_F = 1.559;

(a) its relative dispersion is:

$$\text{Relative dispersion} = \frac{n_F - n_C}{n_D - 1} = .0324$$

(b) and its nu value is:

$$\nu = \frac{1}{\text{Relative Dispersion}} = \frac{1}{0.0324} = 30.9$$

(c) To determine the approximate longitudinal chromatic aberration, i.e., the chromatic aberration measured along the optical axis, the dispersive power may be calculated with the formula:

$$\text{Dispersive power} = \Delta F = \frac{F}{\nu}$$

[1] For example, if the power of the lens is +2.00 D. and nu value is 30.9; the

$$\text{Dispersive power } (\Delta F) = \frac{+2.00}{30.9} = 0.065 \text{ diopter}$$

[a] This represents the difference in refracting power for the red and blue rays.

[2] The approximate longitudinal chromatic aberration can be expressed in linear units by the formula:

$$\text{Dispersion} = \frac{f}{\nu}$$

[a] The distance between the red focus and the blue focus is approximately:

$$\text{Dispersion} = \frac{f}{\nu} = \frac{+0.50\text{cm.}}{30.9} = 1.62 \text{ cm.}$$

(2) The approximate lateral or transverse chromatic aberration can be determined for

a prism or an extra-axial point in a lens according to the formula:

$$\text{Dispersion} = \frac{\text{Deviation}}{\nu}$$

(a) Since the prismatic deviation can be determined by using Prentice's Rule, the dispersion can be calculated using the following variation of the above formula.

[1] Dispersion $= \frac{Fd}{\nu}$, where F is measured in diopters and d is in centimeters from the optical axis.

[a] The dispersion of the above lens at a point 12 mm. from the optical axis is: Dispersion $= \frac{(+2.00\text{ D.})\,(1.2\text{ cm.})}{30.9} = \frac{2.4\,\Delta}{30.9} = 0.078\Delta$, where Δ stands for prism diopters.

[2] Therefore, the blue and red rays would be deviated differently. The amount of difference in this case is about 2.6 minutes of arc.

3. Chromatic aberration cannot be corrected in a single lens. It would be possible to make an achromatic lens, i.e. the foci for C, D, and F lines coincide, using a doublet lens made up of two lenses of the same dispersive power but of different refractive indices. The dispersions could neutralize one another while the refractive power did not. However, even this would be color corrected for only one viewing distance. In addition, the eye is not an achromatic system having about one diopter of chromatic aberration. Plus, ophthalmic lenses tend to increase the total chromatic aberration of the lens eye system and negative lenses tend to correct the chromatic aberration of the eye.

C. Spherical Aberration

1. Rays that strike the periphery of a lens will ordinarily by brought to a focus some distance from the paraxial focus and the focus of the peripheral rays, measured along the optical axis, is called the longitudinal spherical aberration. It may also be expressed in terms of diopters. Alternatively the spread of rays from the periphery of the lens measured on a screen that is placed at the paraxial focus is a measure of the lateral spherical aberration (Figure XXVI-10).

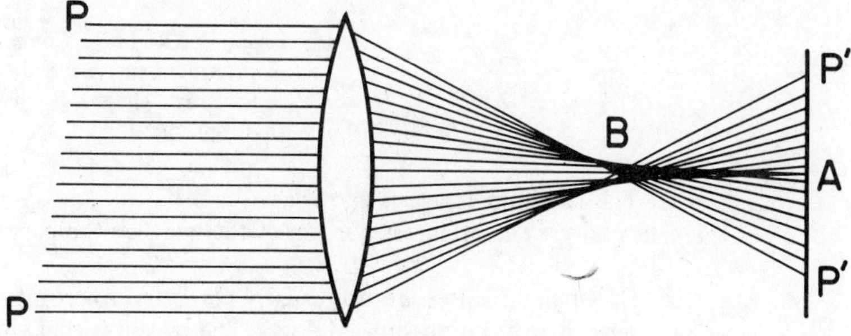

Figure XXVI-10 – Spherical aberration. Pheripheral rays (P) displaced from paraxial focus A along axis from A to B (longitudinal spherical aberration); Peripheral rays (P') displaced in paraxial focal plane from paraxial focus A (lateral spherical aberration).

2. The amount of spherical aberration varies with the bending of the lens, but the size of the aperture stop plays a major role in the control of this aberration. The iris of the eye serves to

admit only a small bundle of rays from a limited surface area of the lens. For normal pupil sizes the amount of spherical aberration in ophthalmic lenses is not very important.

3. For distant objects when using ophthalmic crown glass of index n = 1.523, minimum spherical aberration occurs when the total power of the lens is eight times the power of the back surface of the lens: $F = 8\,F_2$.

a. Since this requires both front and back surfaces to be of the same sign, it is evident that modern ophthalmic lenses of meniscus shape are not designed to minimize spherical aberration.

D. Coma

1. Coma is an aberration associated with the image of an object point that lies off the axis of the lens. There is a difference in magnification for rays that pass through different zones of the lens. The focus of the rays through the marginal zone of the lens is at a different place than the focus through the central portion of the lens (Figure XXVI-11).

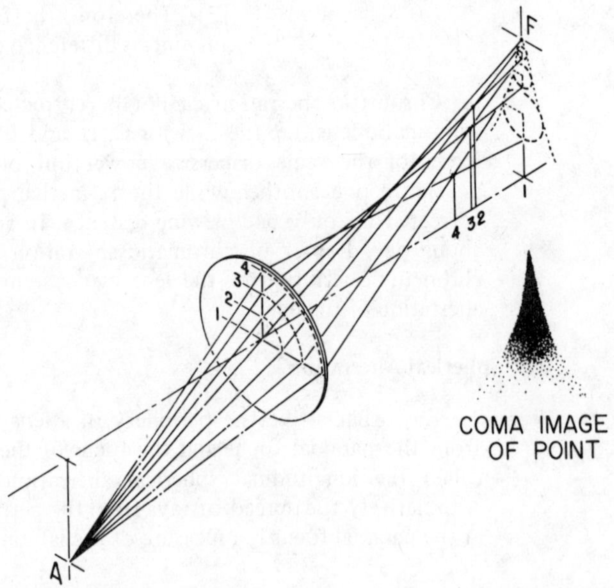

Figure XXVI-11 – Coma. AF chief ray. Note the longitudinal displacement of focal points of peripheral rays as compared to the central ray. The image on the screen shows the comet-like image that is produced.

2. The resultant image is extra-axial, fan-shaped, and spreads out from the focus produced by the central rays. The brightest portion of the image is the part formed by the central rays.

3. Ophthalmic lenses are not usually corrected for coma even though, with the proper bending of the lens, it may be possible to do so. The reason is that the pupil of the eye is the aperture stop of the system. It is small enough to limit the bundle of rays from the lens to a very small diameter which in turn limits the coma. Consequently coma is considered to be of little significance in ophthalmic lenses. The form of lens that minimizes coma is similar to the form that minimizes spherical aberration.

E. Radial or Marginal Astigmatism

1. The aberration known as astigmatism is usually referred to as radial astigmatism or marginal

astigmatism or astigmatism of oblique incidence in order to distinguish it from the refractive error and the cylindrical correction of the astigmatic refractive error.

2. A small bundle of rays from a point source that strike a lens surface obliquely will form an ellipse on the surface of the lens. The major axis of this ellipse is called the meridian section or tangential plane. The minor axis of the ellipse is the sagittal section or plane. The rays that pass through these planes form images that are known as the tangential focus and sagittal focus respectively. The foci that are produced are lines that are perpendicular to their respective planes. The distance between the tangential and sagittal foci is called the astigmatic difference. If the tangential focus lies closer to the lens than does the sagittal focus, it is said to be a positive astigmatism; if the reverse, it is called negative astigmatism. In general, increased obliquity of the rays results in increased astigmatism and greater departure of these foci from the axial image plane (Figure XXVI-12).

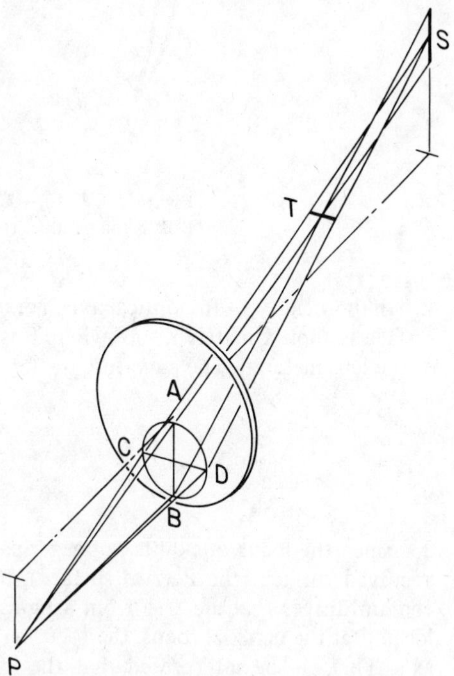

Figure XXVI-12 – Radial or marginal astigmatism. ABCD is an ellipse formed by the oblique bundle of rays from P. AB is the tangential plane; CD is the sagittal plane; the line T is the tangentail focus; S is the sagittal focus; and the distance TS is the astigmatic interval.

3. Astigmatism will occur for small bundles, hence the size of the pupil cannot eliminate it. The result is that points are imaged as lines in the astigmatic focal planes and as conic sections in between. That conic section which has the smallest area is called the circle of least confusion.

4. Marginal astigmatism (or radial astigmatism) is one of the principal aberrations of ophthalmic lenses. It can be sufficient to cause a decrease in vision when the eye is looking through the peripheral part of the lens. The reduction of marginal astigmatism is a major objective of the designer of ophthalmic lenses. The choice of the proper bending of the lens can reduce or eliminate this aberration.

F. Curvature of Field

1. When marginal astigmatism is eliminated, the sagittal and tangential foci coincide to form a surface containing point image. The shape of this surface, called the *Petzval surface,* is paraboloidal. The Petzval surface coincides with the paraxial focal plane along the optical axis. The

distance between the focal plane and the Petzval surface increases with the distance away from the optical axis (Figure XXVI-13).

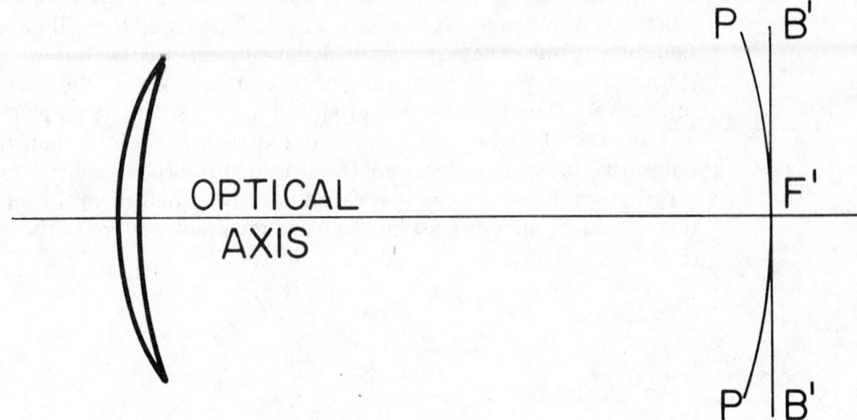

Figure XXVI-13 – Curvature of field. F′ is the secondary focal point; B′B′ is the paraxial focal plane; PP is the Petzval surface.

2. In the vicinity of the optical axis, i.e., the extended paraxial region, the radius (r) of the Petzval surface is approximately r = nf′ where f′ is the secondary focal length of the lens and n is the index of the lens material. The curvature of the field is:

$$c = \frac{1}{r} = \frac{F'}{n}$$

3. Since the locus of points in image space that have no astigmatism (locus of stigmatic points) is a curved surface (the Petzval surface), it is impossible to have a plane image surface that will contain images that are free from astigmatism. If, for example, the desired image surface is a plane located at the paraxial focus, the focusing error will be greater at greater distances from the optical axis. This can be interpreted that the lens is the wrong power for off-axial points. The power difference between the desired power and the obtained power is called the power error. Power error, therefore, varies with obliquity.

E. Distortion

1. A lens may produce an angular magnification in the periphery that is different from the paraxial magnification. The image of an extended object either will be compressed more in its periphery because of a diminishing magnification, thereby producing barrel distortion or expanded in the periphery because of an increasing magnification thereby producing pincushion distortion (Figure XXVI-14).

2. All positive spectacle lenses produce an apparent pin-cushion distortion, all negative lenses produce a barrel distortion. The amount of distortion is specified as the percent difference in magnification between a peripheral point and the axial point on the lens.

3. Distortion can be diminished by the proper bending of the spectacle lens, but it is rarely possible to eliminate it. Those lens forms having minimum distortion are much more highly curved than those normally used in ophthalmic optics.

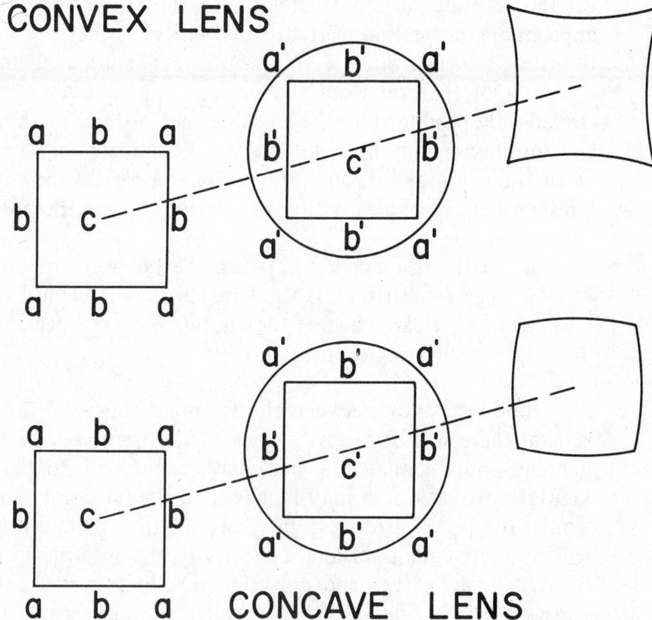

Figure XXVI-14 – Distortion. Image of a square represented as it strikes a lens indicating image produced. Points *a* strike the lens farther from the center than points *b* as indicated by *a'* and *b'*. In a convex lens, the points falling farthest from *c* provide a larger object, *ca*, than the object size *cb*. The farther from the center, the greater the magnification and *ca* appears more greatly magnified than *cb*, producing a distorted pin-cushion effect. In the concave lens, the larger object is minified more by falling farther from the center, producing a barrel effect.

VI. ABERRATIONS AND THE EYE

A. Of the various aberrations, coma and spherical aberration are not important in ophthalmic lenses because the pupil of the eye acts as a stop to regulate the area of the lens through which light enters the eye. This limits the magnitude of these aberrations to relatively small amounts. Although distortion is affected by the bending of the lens, lenses are not commonly corrected for distortion because of the extreme curves that are required. Chromatic aberration can be corrected only with combinations of lenses, therefore it must be ignored in ordinary ophthalmic lenses. Radial astigmatism and curvature of the field, however, are of prime importance since they alter the focus of light passing through peripheral portions of the lens, and affect the dimensions of the total visual field throughout which clear vision can be secured.

B. The Far Point Sphere

1. The far point of the eye is that point in space for which the eye is correctly focused when accommodation is totally relaxed. As the eye rotates about a point (very nearly) called the center of rotation of the eye, the far point or punctum remotum traces out a spherical surface. This surface is known as the far point sphere. The radius of the far point sphere is different for different refractive conditions. The ametropia or refractive error is measured as the reciprocal of the distance from the cornea to the far point sphere (the ocular refraction) or from the spectacle to the far point sphere (the spectacle refraction). An object or an image of an object that is located on the far point sphere will be seen clearly without the use of any accommodation.

2. In adapting an ophthalmic lens for the correction of the eye for distant viewing, the appropriate correction is that lens which forms a point image on the far point sphere for all positions of gaze. Such a lens would create a visual image that would be equally clear for any direction of fixation from the optical axis to the extreme periphery of the lens. However, the curved field produced by the lens does not ordinarily coincide with the far point sphere of the eye, and the discrepancy between the two constitutes one measure of how much the vision is blurred when the eye looks through the peripheral part of the lens. In strong powers, this has the effect of limiting the area of clear vision to a region around the pole of the lens.

a. If the discrepancy between the far point sphere of the eye and the focal field of the lens is negative, that is, if the lens focus falls behind the far point sphere, accommodation can restore a clear image. If the discrepancy is positive, with the focus falling before the far point sphere, blurring occurs.

3. The discrepancy between the far point sphere of the eye and the Petzval surface means that in general there will be a power error in the periphery of the lens. If a lens is made with a different bending and thickness the peripheral focus will no longer be stigmatic, but the tangential and sagittal astigmatic foci may be closer to the far point sphere than was the stigmatic focus. In other words, the power error may be reduced with a different lens binding, but the marginal astigmatism will be increased. Decisions concerning the interplay between these two variables of the focus (marginal astigmatism and power error) constitutes one of the major activities of the lens designer. Lenses which are designed to minimize the deleterious effects of one or more of these aberrations through the proper choice of bending and thickness are designated *Corrected Curve Lenses.*

VII. CORRECTED CURVE LENSES

A. Wollaston first showed that by altering the form of a lens the radial astigmatism could be reduced or eliminated. Ostwalt later demonstrated a second solution to the same problem. It was Tscherning who showed that both were solutions to a mathematical equation that related lens power, form, viewing distance, stop distance, peripheral angle and index of refraction of the lens material to produce a lens with zero marginal astigmatism. The plot of the equation is an ellipse, hence, it is now known as the Tscherning Ellipse (Figure XXVI-15).

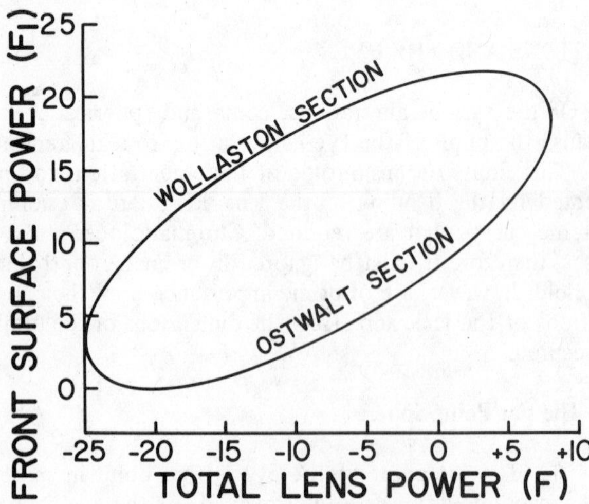

Figure XXVI-15 – The Tscherning Ellipse.

1. The upper half of the curve, describing lenses of rather steep curvature, is called the Wollaston Section. The lower half, describing lenses of more conventional ophthalmic form, is called the

Ostwalt Section. Both designs eliminate marginal astigmatism, but since each will, in general, produce a different curvature of the field, the designs are not necessarily equivalent.

a. As shown in Figure XXVI-15, the abscissa gives the power of the lens (F) and the ordinate, the power of the front surface (F_1). It can be seen that +6.00 lens can be constructed in two ways, with a front curve of +14.73 D. or with a front curve of +21.04 D. Similarly a minus six diopter lens can be constructed with a front curve of either +5.05 or +18.73 D.

2. A plus 2.00 D. lens based on the Ostwalt curve has a radial astigmatism of .00 D. and a curvature of the field of –.14 D., while one based on the Wollaston curve has a radial astigmatism of –.02 D. and a curvature of the field of +.14 D.

a. In this case, both designs result in power errors which would create a blur of the image, but the patient could accommodate to clear up the blur caused by the minus power error. Of course, nothing could be done physiologically to overcome the plus power error of the latter design. Therefore, the Ostwalt solution is preferred in this case.

(1) In determining the power error the circle of least confusion is usually considered to be the reference standard. The location of this circle is compared to the far point sphere of the eye. For example, a –10.00 D. meniscus lens has a sagittal power of –9.43 D. and a tangential power of –8.87 D. The radial astigmatism is 0.56 D. and the circle of least confusion lies at –9.15 D. The power error is therefore +0.85 D. The lens design that places the midpoint of the astigmatic interval on the Petzval surface is sometimes referred to as the no-curvature form of the lens.

(2) Henker and others have computed the curvature of the field on the basis of the discrepancy between the far point sphere and the sagittal focus. According to these standards, the curvature of the field of the –10.00 D. meniscus would be +0.57 D.

3. Similar solutions exist for other viewing conditions. Lenses designed to eliminate radial astigmatism for objects located at the reading point will be flatter by approximately 2.50 diopters than a similarly powered lens used for viewing distant objects.

B. Punktal Lenses

1. Punktal lenses, designed by von Rohr and manufactured by Zeiss in 1911, were the first commercial attempts to correct radial astigmatism. These lenses eliminated radial astigmatism for powers from +7.78 to –24.68 D., but ignored the curvature of the field. Power error exceeded 0.10 D. for all powers except those in the range of –2.00 to –4.00 and –20.00 D.

a. These Punktal lenses were based on a peripheral angle of vision of 35° for plus lenses, 30° for minus lenses, and on a distance of 25 mm. from back surface of the lens to the center of rotation of the eye, and for objects located at infinity.

2. Above the ranges included in the Punktal lenses, radial astigmatism cannot be corrected with spherical surfaces. Therefore, an aspheric surface must be used. Such lenses of silicate glass were made under the name of *Katral lenses.* These lenses were expensive and were manufactured only by Zeiss.

3. Each lens of the Punktal series was ground on a different curve, and some 15,000 lens blanks were required to encompass the usual range of prescriptions. This made the lens practically a factory order lens in every case, and the delay involved and the cost prevented widespread use of the lens in this country. However, since it was the usual situation in Europe to have the manufacturer fill the ophthalmic prescriptions, it constituted no special problem for the European

practitioners. Punktal lenses have enjoyed a widespread popularity throughout Europe almost from the time of their introduction.

4. The Punktal series was redesigned in 1946-47 by Roos. In its new form the lenses are corrected to reduce the radial astigmatism for objects at infinity and 25 cm. to: a) less than 0.10 D. for a distance of 15° in all directions from the optical axis, b) less than 0.20 D. for most powers, and less than 0.25 D. for high minus lenses for a distance between 15° and 30° in all directions from the optical axis. Beyond 30° the emphasis is on the correction of oblique astigmatism for infinitely distant objects. In all cases the astigmatism never exceeds 0.20 D. This amount of astigmatism is allowed in order to permit a favorable choice of curves for the reduction of astigmatism for near objects.

5. Zeiss Punktal lenses use front surface toric design for plus lenses and the weaker minus lenses. Inner toric design is used for high minus lenses.

C. Orthogon Lenses

1. The Orthogon lens was produced by Bausch and Lomb in 1928. The lenses are based on the Punktal calculations but were modified by W. B. Rayton. The different powers were grouped together so that all lenses were manufactured on some fifteen base curves. The radial astigmatism was allowed to increase as high as 0.25 D. in some cases. However, in most cases, the astigmia is within 0.05 D.

2. As with the Punktal, no attempt is made to correct for curvature of the field. Also, as with the Punktal, the distance from lens surface to center of rotation of the eye is 25 mm. Calculations are based on points on the lens surface that are located 30° from the optical axis.

3. Orthogon lenses which are factory finished as stock uncut lenses are made with the toric surface on the front. The base curve is usually the weakest curve on the front surface, but it is the spherical curve on the back surface for some plus lenses.

D. Tillyer Lenses

1. Edgar Tillyer, whose series was introduced commercially by the American Optical Company in 1926, compromised the full correction of astigmatism in order to partially correct for curvature of the field. He allowed the marginal astigmatism to become as great as 0.12 D. for weak prescriptions and 0.25 D. for strong prescriptions, if this permitted better control of the power error.

a. The Tillyer series of lenses were computed for a 27 mm. distance from the back surface of the lens to the center of rotation of the eye and for an angular distance of 30° from the optical axis.

b. The power range covered by the Tillyer design is calculated on the basis of 19 base curves. In all cases the base curve is the weakest curve on the front surface. Usually the front surface is the toric surface. However, for some of the higher minus lens powers the back surface is the toric surface.

2. In 1964 the American Optical Company introduced the Tillyer Masterpiece lens series. This lens is selected on the basis of considerations involving: 1) viewing distances of infinity, 30 inches, 16 inches and 13 inches; 2) viewing angles of 20°, 30° and 40° from the optical axis; 3) distances from the back surface of the lens to the center of rotation of the eye that are claimed to include 90% of the population having amounts of refractive error covered by the lens series. Calculations are based on the power meridian, the axis meridian and for the meridians 45° from these meridians. The designers are John K. Davis, Henry H. Fernald and Arline W. Rayner.

E. Widesite

1. The Widesite lens, by Shuron, is a front surface toric lens series. The base curves are from –5.00 to –12.00 diopters in 0.25 diopters jumps and from +5.50 to +9.00 diopters.

F. Kurova

1. The Kurova lens series of the Continental Optical Co., originally introduced in 1920, was redesigned in 1925 by F. E. Duckwell. The parameters of the design were: 1) an infinitely distant object; 2) a 30° viewing angle; and 3) a 25 mm. center of rotation distance. It gives first priority to the correction of marginal astigmatism, but also attempts to correct plus power errors and minus power errors as second and third priorities respectively. It is a front surface toric design with the base curve on the front surface. There are 37 plus base curves ranging from 4.50 to 12.50 in 0.12 and 0.25 diopter steps.

G. Kurova Shursite

1. With the merger of Shuron and Continental into the Shuron-Continental Division of Textron, Inc. a new lens series was introduced in 1966. This design, known as the Kurova Shursite, is corrected for: 1) object distances of infinity and 14 inches using 2) viewing angles 20°, 30° and 40° and 3) center of rotation distances of 26.5 mm. to 31.0 mm. depending on the lens power. The longer distances are used for the minus lenses. It is a minus toric design with each of the 20 base curves located on the spherical front surface. The performance characteristics are based on a compromise correction of marginal astigmatism, power error and lateral chromatic aberration.

H. Normalsite

1. The Titmus Optical Company produces a corrected curve lens series known as Normalsite. The designer was F. E. Klingaman who decided to use a viewing distance of 13 feet in computing the design. The viewing angle is 30° and the center of rotation distance is 27 mm. The lens became available in 1950 as a front surface toric with front surface base curves. It was redesigned in 1962 for a 60 mm. lens blank size. For lens powers above –13.00 Diopters the front surface is a concave toric, but for weaker minus powers and all plus powers the surface is a convex toric. First priority was given to the correction of marginal astigmatism, but power error was also corrected as a second priority.

I. Best-Form (Uniform)

1. In 1963 Univis Inc. marketed their first single vision lens design under the name Best-Form. It has been up-dated and renamed the Uni-Form lens. The designer is E. Bechtold. The viewing distance used in computing the design is infinity. The viewing angle is 30° and the center of rotation distance is 27 mm. It is a rear surface toric with a front surface spherical base curve. The performance was evaluated using the modulation transfer function. This is a mathematical criterion based upon a spatial frequency resolution analysis that is often used for complex optical components.

J. Most cylindrical and toric corrected curve lenses are corrected either for the spherical component of the lens formula or for a power between the powers of the principal meridians since it is not possible to correct both meridians simultaneously with one spherical and one cylindrically curved surface. A lens designed by B. Maitenaz of the Société de Lunetiers (ESSEL), which is named Atoral, is now being marketed. This makes use of aspheric curves on the back surface of the lens to correct for marginal astigmatism in both principal meridians. The lens is a molded plastic (CR-39). The Atoral lens is being made only for prescriptions of +5.50 D. S. to +15.50 D. S. and will be covered more fully in the section on aspheric lenses.

K. The other advantages of corrected curve lenses are that they are polished to a finer degree, the tools are kept within a tolerance of .03 diopters, and the axial thickness of lenses of a given power are uniform.

VIII. DETERMINING THE POWER OF A LENS

A. There are many different methods of determining the power of a lens, but the clinician usually confines himself to three: the lens gauge or lens measure; neutralization; and a focusing device such as a lensometer, vertometer, or focimeter.

B. The Lens Measure

1. Since the power of a lens is related to the curvature of its surfaces, it is possible to measure the depth of the curve and specify this sagittal depth in terms of diopters of power (Figure XXVI-16).

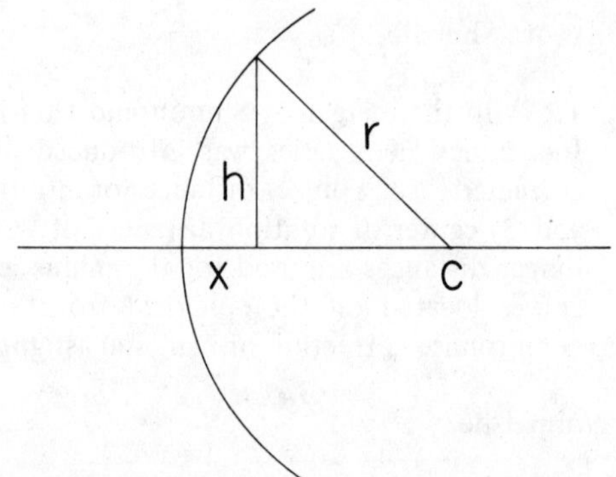

Figure XXVI-16 – Construction of arc indicating principle of lens measure. *r* radius; *h* the half chord of the arc; *x* depth of arc; *c* center of curvature.

a. The sagittal depth (x) is related to the radius of curvature (r) and the half chord (h) as follows:

(1) $r^2 = h^2 + (r - x)^2$ which can be rewritten as

(2) $$x = \frac{h^2 + x^2}{2r}$$

(a) However, the power of the surface (F) is related to the radius and the difference between the indices of refraction n and n′

(3) $$F = \frac{n' - n}{r}$$

(a) So that the final formula becomes:

(4) $$F = \frac{2x\,(n' - n)}{h^2 + x^2}$$

(a) Frequently an approximation is made to simplify the calculation. Since x is usually small when compared to h, a small error is introduced if the x^2 term is dropped. The approximate sagittal equation becomes:

(5) $$F = \frac{2x\,(n' - n)}{h^2}$$

2. *The lens gauge* is an instrument in which h is expressed as the distance from the center movable pin to the outer fixed pin. The center pin is movable and is geared to a pointer which indicates on a scale the depth of the curve, x. Assuming a constant for n' of 1.53, the scale can be calibrated directly in diopters (F), since h and n' are constants and x is the only variable.

a. The pins of the gauge are placed normal to the surface and the gauge is rotated about the axis of the movable pin. If the reading remains constant, the surface is spherical. If the reading varies, the points of maximum and minimum readings represent the powers of the principal meridians of a cylindrical surface.

(1) The power of the cylinder is the difference between the two readings.
(2) The powers of both surfaces are determined and added algebraically.
(3) The axis must be marked and determined from a protractor.

3. Lens gauges are manufactured with the calibrations determined for glass of an index of 1.53. Most optical glass today has an index of 1.523. To allow for this discrepancy, the readings of the gauge must be modified by the following formula:

a. F_t (true power) = Fm (measured power) x (0.987).

b. If glass of another index is used, the formula reads,

$$F_t = \frac{Fm\ (n' - 1)}{.530}$$

C. Neutralization

1. The elementary method of determining the power of a lens is by the procedure termed neutralization. This is based upon the concept that thin lenses, when placed in contact with one another can be considered to be a single lens whose total power F is the sum of the powers of the individual lenses $F_1 + F_2$. $F = F_1 + F_2$

a. Therefore, if a lens of known power, say F_1, when added to the lens F_2 whose power is unknown, results in zero power for F, $F_1 + F_2 = 0$ then the power of $F_2 = F_1$.

2. In practice a large supply of lenses of known powers are made available. Then by a trial and error procedure the proper combination of known and unknown lenses is found to give zero power.

3. This procedure works reasonably well with lenses of low power and slight axial thickness. When high powered lenses are neutralized, the process leads to error, both because of the thickness of one lens and the technique itself.

4. When flat lenses were commonly used, Prentice disclosed that lenses of high powers did not neutralize accurately and special neutralizing sets were developed in which the minus lenses were taken as standards and the plus lenses designed to neutralize these. Figure XXVI-17 illustrates that two lenses of equal curvatures will not neutralize each other since both are part of a single convex sphere. When toric and corrected curve lenses were introduced, the problem became more complex since an air space between the lenses actually imposed a combination of three lenses into the problem. To avoid this complication, toric and curved lenses are neutralized by holding the neutralizing minus lens against the front surface of the plus lens. But, as discussed previously, this is in effect a measure of the *front vertex power or the neutralizing power.* If all lenses were infinitely thin, as has already been noted, neutralizing power would represent the effective power. However, it is possible to measure most lenses with a reasonable degree of accuracy, or to compensate mathematically for the discrepancy once the neutralizing power is known.

5. *Principles*

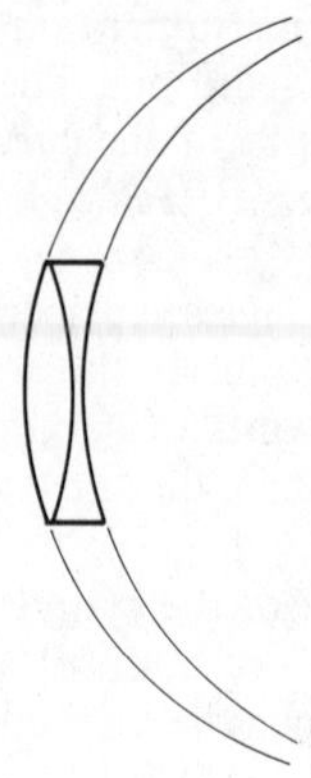

Figure XXVI-17 – Prentice's illustration of two lenses of equal curvature placed in neutralizing position.

a. A plus lens may be considered a series of prisms with their bases coming together at the optical center of the lens and their apices at the margins. A minus lens may be considered a series of prisms with the apices at the center and the bases at the periphery. As the incident ray strikes a lens away from the optical center, the deviation of the emergent ray will be increased as a result of the combination of the power of the lens times the distance from the center. As is apparent, the image of an object viewed through the lens will be displaced towards the apex of the theoretical component prism. Thus, as a plus lens is moved so that the incident ray strikes it above the optical center, the image will be displaced upwards. If the lens is slowly moved downwards, the incident ray will strike the lens farther and farther from the center, and the image of the object viewed through that point of the lens will appear displaced farther and farther upwards. If the lens is now moved in an upwards direction, the ray will be bent less as the optical center is approached, the displacement will diminish, and in contrast to its former position the image will move downwards. When the optical center is passed, the prismatic effect will now be base up, and the image will appear displaced farther downwards. A minus lens will produce the opposite effects due to the inverted prismatic positions.

(1) If the plus lens is now moved more rapidly throughout a range equal to its entire diameter, it can be seen that an object viewed through it will always appear to move opposite to the direction towards which the lens is being moved (Figure XXVI-18).

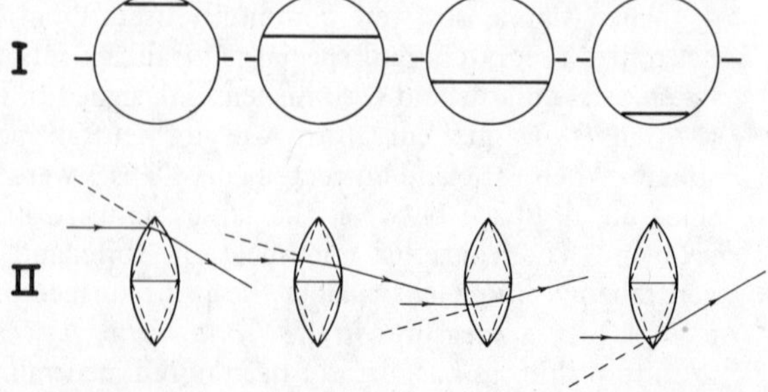

Figure XXVI-18 – Prismatic effect of plus lens in neutralization. Series I, showing how horizontal arm of cross appears to move down as lens is moved up. Series II, lenses considered as prisms, showing action of displacement of incident ray.

b. A cylindrical lens can be considered to represent a series of prisms lying with their base-apex lines at right angles to the axis. If the lens is moved in the axis, no motion, or motion due to the spherical component only, if any, is revealed. If the lens is moved in the meridian of power, the cylinder displaces the image just as the sphere did, in plus lenses away from the center, and in minus lenses towards the center of the lens. But if the cylinder is moved obliquely so that the incident rays travel along a meridian between the axis and power meridians, then the prismatic effect of the cylinder is exerted in an oblique manner. As the lens is being moved, the incident ray will be farther from the axis at the periphery than at the center and the oblique prismatic effect will be more marked at the periphery. A straight line viewed through a cylindrical lens held with its axis oriented obliquely to the line is farther displaced at the periphery than at the center, and the line appears to lean or tilt.

(1) If a cylindrical lens is rotated so that its axis moves clockwise and then counterclockwise, a line viewed through the lens will also appear to rotate or tilt. Since any cylindrical lens formula can be expressed with the sign of the cylinder either plus or minus, i.e. +1.00 D.C. x 60 can be written as +1.00 D.S.⊂−1.00 D.C. x 150, any cylindrical lens can be considered as having both a plus cylinder axis and a minus cylinder axis. If the image of the line, which is colinear with the object line appears to rotate in the opposite direction to the direction of lens rotation, the axis is the plus axis. If the image rotates in the same direction, the axis is the minus axis (Figure XXVI-19).

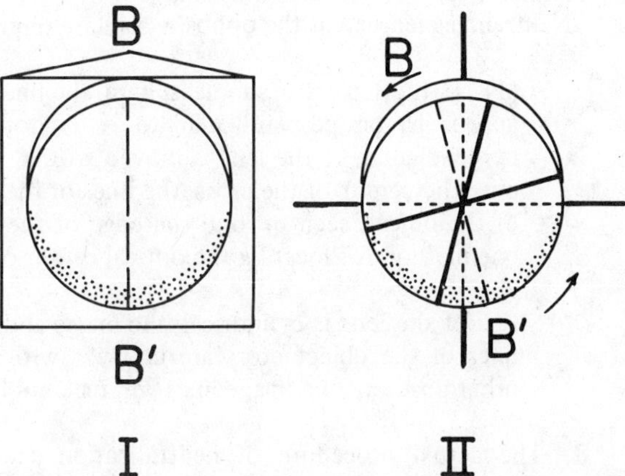

Figure XXVI-19 – Cylindrical lens viewed from its prismatic components and illustrating apparent displacement of arms of cross when cylinder axis is not coincident. (I) Dotted outlines represent theoretical prismatic alignment of cylinder. (II) Dotted lines indicate points on lens struck by corresponding points of the arms of the cross. Peripheral points fall farther from base-line BB′, than central points and are displaced farther towards the apices. BB′ base line of component prisms and meridian of axis of the cylinder.

c. When a sphero-cylindrical lens is moved, the resultant movement of the images of the lines will be a combination of the effects produced by the spherical and cylindrical components. This motion of the image will depend on the power of these components and whether the lens is given a translational or rotational movement. Since it is necessary to move the lens in neutralization the technique is sometimes referred to as "shaking out" a lens.

6. *Technique*

a. There are three major aspects of neutralization.

(1) Determination of the type of lens, such as sphere, cylinder, sphero-cylinder, prism and the like.

(2) Determination of the power of each of these components.

(3) Determination of the principal meridians of the lens.

b. In the first step there is no need to use neutralizing lenses since the determination of the type of lens can be made simply by observing image motion relative to lens motion.

c. In the second step the spectacle lens is held before the eye, and a lens of opposite power is held against the front surface. Usually, a cross is used as a target since this provides a line target for either meridian. The periphery of the lens may produce disturbing motion, and a mask limiting the observation to a central portion of the lens may be placed against the lens. The farther the lens is held from the eye, the greater the span of the deviated ray when the lens is moved, and slight motions will be noted which might escape observation if the lens is held too close to the observer. The unknown lens is moved along the direction of each arm of the cross, that is, vertically and horizontally. If no motion is observed, the lens contains neither cylindrical nor spherical power. If the lines move against the lens motion, the unknown lens is plus; if they move with the lens motion, the unknown lens is minus. "Neutralizing lenses" of the opposite sign are required to eliminate the motion.

(1) If the lens is a simple sphere, the images of the lines seen through the lens will appear to be perpendicular to one another, just as the lines of the object are perpendicular. If the lens is moved so that the optical center of the lens falls directly over the center of the cross, the lines of the image, seen through the lens, and the lines of the object, seen beyond the edge of the lens, will appear to be continuous. This is one method for locating the optical center of a lens.

(2) If the lens is cylindrical, the image and object lines will only be continuous if the lines of the object cross are colinear with the principal meridians of the lens. In all other positions the image lines will make oblique angles with one another.

d. The actual procedure of neutralization can be done by following this step-by-step procedure.

(1) The lens is held before the cross and centered so that both the horizontal and vertical lines are continuous. Then the lens is rotated and the continuity of the lines observed.

(a) If they remain continuous in all meridians, the lens is a sphere.

(b) If rotation breaks the continuity, a cylinder is included, and the lens is now rotated back to a position where continuity is restored.

(c) If in the first attempt to center the lens, the lines appear oblique, so that continuity of all four ends cannot be achieved, the lens contains cylindrical power, and must be rotated to a position in which continuity is gained.

(2) Once all four ends are continuous, the lens is moved rapidly along the directions of the arms of the cross, usually the horizontal and vertical meridians.

(a) If image motion is against the direction of the lens movement, the lens is plus and minus lens power is needed to neutralize it; if with the lens movement, the lens is minus and plus lens power is needed to neutralize it.

(3) A lens of opposite power is held against the front surface of the unknown lens and the motion again noted. The power of the neutralizing lens is increased until the motion in one meridian, at least, disappears.

(a) If too strong a neutralizing lens is selected, the motion will be reversed from its original direction.

(4) If the same lens neutralizes both meridians, the unknown lens is a sphere, and the power of the neutralizing lens indicates its power. The sign is opposite to the sign of the neutralizing lens.

(5) If only one meridian is neutralized, mark the meridian which still has motion with a wax pencil by two marks which agree with the arm of the cross at right angles to the direction the lens is moved when it still shows motion. That is, if the lens shows motion when moved up and down, the position of the arm which lies horizontal on the lens is marked, when the center of the lens is aligned with the center of the cross.

(a) This marking indicates the axis of the cylinder.

(6) A cylindrical neutralizing lens is placed over the neutralizing sphere so that its axis coincides with the lines marked on the lens.

(a) The power of the cylinder is increased until a point is reached at which no motion is detected when the lens is moved in either principal meridian.

(b) In stong combinations, it is well to check the spherical meridian after the cylindrical one appears to be neutralized.

(7) The sphere and cylinder before the unknown lens when all motion is halted, measures the power of the unknown lens. The sign of the unknown lens is opposite to that of the neutralizing lens.

(a) If the lens is a sphero-cylinder combination in which one meridian is minus and one is plus, the same technique applies.

(8) A sphero-cylinder may also be neutralized by using two spheres. One sphere is used to neutralize the motion in one meridian and the other sphere is used to neutralize the motion in the second meridian. These powers represent the powers in the principal meridians of the unknown lens. It is then necessary to interpret these powers in terms of the spherical and cylindrical powers of the usual lens formula.

(a) If a −3.00 D.S. neutralizes one principal meridian and a −1.25 D.S. neutralizes the other principal meridian of the unknown lens, the power of the unknown lens is equal, but opposite in sign.

+3.00

+1.25

(b) This can be written as +1.25 D.S.⊃+1.75 D.C. x 180 or +3.00 D.S.⊃−1.75 D.C. x 90 or +3.00 D.C. x 180⊃ +1.25 D. C. x 90.

(c) Care must be taken with this method to avoid confusing the meridians and lenses which apply to these meridians.

(9) The lens is placed upon a protractor to determine the axis, by means of the wax markings made during the neutralization.

(a) If only a fragment of the lens is available, the exact axis cannot be determined unless some clue in the shape or drilling indicates the horizontal mounting lino denoting the position the fragment occupied before the eye.

(10) *Prism*

(a) Prism effect may be secured by either grinding a prism into the lens or by decentering the lens. In decentering the lens, the optical center (or front pole) is moved away from the geometrical center of the finished lens, by cutting the pattern of the lens a given number of millimeters to either side, above or below the centered position. This produces prismatic effect by permitting the lines of sight to pass through the lens at a point other than the optical center.

(b) If the lens has been decentered, it will be noted that the center of the cross viewed through the lens does not lie at the center of the lens when the arms are continuous.

(c) If the prism has been ground into the lens, the center of the cross may lie outside of the lens itself no matter how the lens is placed.

(d) To neutralize the prism, a known prism is placed against the front surface of the lens with its base opposite to the base in the lens. Since a prism displaces towards its apex, the base of the neutralizing prism need only be placed in the direction towards which the center of the cross appears moved when seen through the lens. The amount of prism which restores the cross to a central position measures the prismatic effect.

D. The Lensometer, Vertometer or Focimeter

1. The lensometer or vertometer consists of a movable luminous target, a fixed standard lens, a lens holder so designed that the back surface of any unknown lens can be positioned in the optical system at a constant distance from the standard lens, and a fixed telescope focused for infinity.

2. The general principle is that light entering the telescope must be parallel in order to make the luminous target appear clear without accommodative effort. This can be done by moving the target so that the standard lens forms an image of the target in the secondary focal plane of the unknown lens. The amount that the target must be moved to produce the desired focus can be calibrated in diopters. This is a function of the power of the standard lens used in the instrument, but it is always a constant amount of movement of the target throughout the dioptric scale for each diopter of power of the unknown lens.

3. When there is no unknown lens in the instrument the target must be placed in the primary focal plane of the standard lens. However, when an unknown lens is in place between the standard lens and the telescope the light will be refracted and will no longer be parallel as it enters the telescope. It is necessary to move the target away from the primary focal plane of the standard lens so that the light will be non-parallel as it emerges from the standard lens. When these non-parallel rays focus in the secondary focal plane of the unknown lens the image, seen through the telescope, will be clearly in focus.

4. The usual way of expressing the power of an ophthalmic lens is in terms of the *back vertex power.* This can be determined by placing the ocular surface of the unknown lens against the lens stop of the instrument. The target is designed so that the lines comprising it, can be focused and aligned only when the principal meridians of the lens coincide with those lines. To achieve this the

target itself can be rotated to any position. The principal meridians of the unknown lens are indicated by a protractor scale on the instrument.

5. It is also possible to measure the *front vertex or neutralizing power* using a lensometer or vertometer by placing the front surface of the lens against the lens stop.

E. Comparisons

1. The vertometer or lensometer gives the vertex power of the lens independent of its form or construction. The lens gauge yields the approximate power. Neutralization provides the neutralizing power. In the discussion of the power of a lens, the formulas for the various types of power were given. From these, it is possible to determine the true powers of lenses measured by either neutralization or the lens gauge.

a. To determine the vertex power from the neutralizing power, the equations may be combined by indicating the error as $F_N + x = F_V$. Substituting from F_N and F_V, the formula may be simplified to $x = c(F_1 + F_2)(F_1 - F_2)$.

b. To determine the vertex power from the lens gauge, the true power of the gauge method is first determined by the formula allowing for the difference in index noted in that section. The error is $F - F_V = x$. By substituting, it will be found that $x = cF_1{}^2$.

(1) F_1 is the power of the first surface, F_2 is the power of the back surface, and c is the fraction, thickness divided by the index.

c. It will be found that the variations are far greater in plus lenses than in minus lenses, and if .10 D. is assumed as a tolerance, a lens of only 1 mm. thickness has no practical discrepancy, a lens of 2 mm. thickness has approximate power reasonably close until +9.00 D. is reached, a lens of 3 mm. thickness varies significantly at +7.00, of 4 mm. at +6.00, and 5 mm. at +5.50.

2. Gamble (1949) describes a simple method of converting the neutralized power of a lens to the vertex power.

a. The thickness of the lens at the center is stated in meters. A lens 3 mm. thick at the center would be .003 meters thick.

b. The thickness is multiplied by .66. (In the above example, .003 x .66 = .00198.)

c. Square the dioptric power of each surface and multiply each value by the result found in step (b) above.

d. Subtract the answer for one surface from that for the other to find the difference between the vertex and neutralized power.

e. Example: Given a lens of +16.00 D., 8 mm. thick at center, and the back curve measured to be −4.00 D.

(1) Front curve measures +20.00 D.
(2) Thickness is .008 M. x .66 = .00528.
(3) $(20)^2 = 400$; $(4)^2 = 16$.
(4) (400 x .00528) − (16 x .00528) = +2.03 D. difference.

f. This is a means of calculating the value of F_v from the derived expression that relates $F_v = F_N + c(F_1{}^2 + F_2{}^2)$

IX. PRISMS AND PRISMATIC EFFECT

A. A prism is an optical component whose two plane surfaces are not parallel and which would meet only in one direction, even if the surfaces were extended indefinitely in all directions. The intersection of the surfaces is a straight line called the apex of the prism. The angle between the surfaces is the refracting angle (β) of the prism. The side opposite the apex of the prism is called the base. A line perpendicular to the apex along a surface is called the base-apex line. A plane through a base apex line perpendicular to the surface is a principal section of the prism.

B. Power of a Prism

1. A thin prism produces a deviation of a ray of light. This amount of deviation ($\in$) is a measure of the power of the prism.

2. The deviation ($\in$) is related to the refracting angle (β) and the index (n) in a thin prism by the approximate formula:' $\in = (n - 1)\beta$ (Figure XXVI-20).

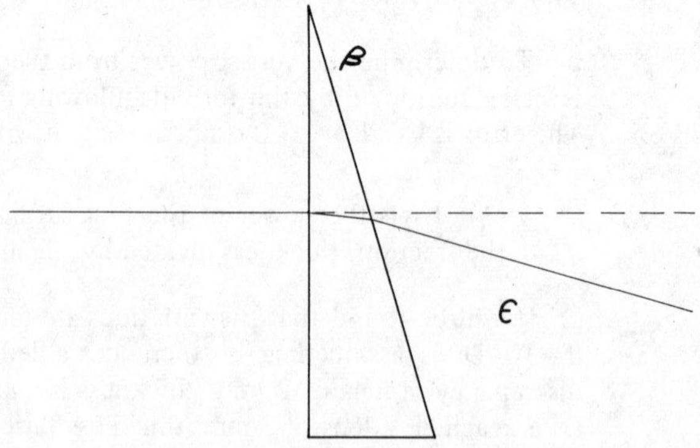

Figure XXVI-20

3. The units of the deviation are dependent upon the units used to measure the refracting angle of the prism. If β is measured in *radians,* the deviation will also be measured in radians. If β is measured in degrees, the deviation likewise will be in degrees. Formerly it was the custom to express the power of a prism indirectly, that is in terms of its refracting angle rather than its deviation. As a result some confusion may occur because the deviation is approximately half the angle since the index of ophthalmic crown glass is 1.523.

a. Occasionally the power of an ophthalmic prism will be expressed in terms of *centrads* (v). A centrad is 1/100 of a radian.

$\in^{\triangledown} = 100\,(n - 1)\,\beta$ where β is measured in radians.

(1) It is an angular measure and can be related to degrees and radians.

$1^{\triangledown} = 0.01 \text{ radian} = 0.573°$

b. It is much more convenient to measure the linear deviation of a ray on a flat surface than on the curved surface that all of the above angular units require. A deviation of one centimeter measured on a flat surface one meter away is produced by a prism of one *prism diopter* (Δ) power. (Figure XXVI-21)

(1) If the refracting angle β is measured in radians the power of the prism measured in prism diopters is

$\in^{\Delta} = 100\,(n-1) \tan \beta$

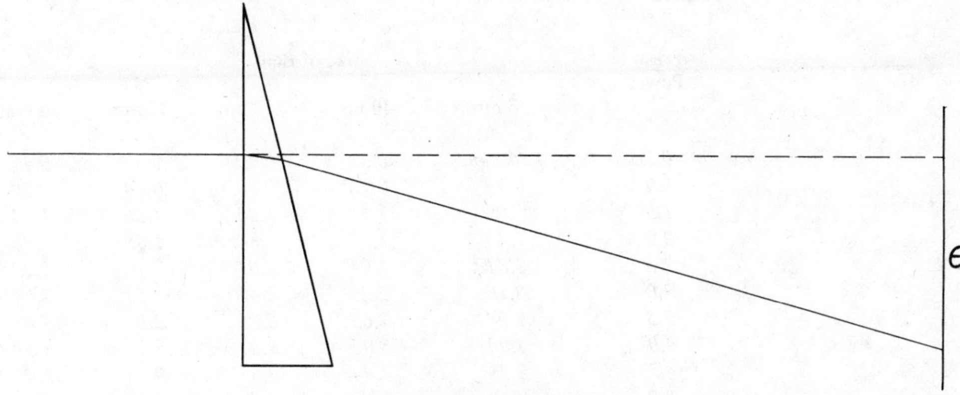

Figure XXVI-21

(2) The relationship for small angles makes it possible to substitute β measured in radians in place of tan β. There is little error introduced for the useful range of ophthalmic prisms using the approximate formula.

$$\epsilon^{\Delta} = 100\,(n-1)\,\beta$$

(3) It should be noted that centrads are essentially numerically equal to prism diopters $1^{\nabla} = 1^{\Delta} = 0.573^{\circ}$

4. The power of a prism varies according to the angle between the base apex line and the meridian in which the power is measured.

$$\epsilon^{\Delta}_{\circ} = \epsilon^{\Delta} \cos \Theta$$

a. Where $\epsilon^{\Delta}_{\circ}$ is the power in the meridian oblique to the base apex line; ϵ^{Δ} is the power of the prism measured along the base apex line; and Θ is the angle between the two meridians.

5. The thickness difference at any two points of a simple ophthalmic prism can be calculated using the following formula:

$$\Delta t = \frac{x\epsilon^{\Delta} \cos \Theta}{100\,(n-1)}$$

where Δ t is the difference in thickness; x is the distance between points; Θ is the angle that the line that includes the two points makes with the base apex line of the prism; and n is the index.

a. A reference chart for the differences in thickness of the base and apex for a prism of given power and size of the lens blank can be developed as in Table XXVI-1 for the formula T = .0191 x prism power x diameter of lens, for glass of index 1.523.

(1) It can be shown that the difference in thickness between the apex and base of a 1 prism diopter prism is the same number of points as one-tenth of the diameter in mms. That is, if the diameter is 50 mm., the difference in thickness will be 5 points; if the lens is 45 mm. in diameter, the difference in thickness will be 4.5 points, and so on. If a 2 prism diopter prism is desired, the number of points is multiplied by the desired power so that the latter lens would have a difference of 9 points, and so on. A point is a measure of thickness. In this case it is equal to one-fifth of a millimeter.

(a) However, a point is also defined as one-sixth or one-tenth of a millimeter besides the one-fifth millimeter just referred to above.

(2) **Table XXVI-1 – Difference in apex-base thickness for varying lens sizes.**

Prism Power	Size of Lens 38 mm.	40 mm.	42 mm.	44mm.	46 mm.	48 mm.
0.5Δ	*0.36 mm.*	*0.38*	*0.40*	*0.42*	*0.44*	*0.46*
1.0	*0.73*	*0.76*	*0.80*	*0.84*	*0.88*	*0.92*
1.5	*1.09*	*1.15*	*1.20*	*1.26*	*1.32*	*1.38*
2.0	*1.45*	*1.53*	*1.60*	*1.68*	*1.76*	*1.83*
2.5	*1.81*	*1.91*	*2.01*	*2.10*	*2.20*	*2.29*
3.0	*2.18*	*2.29*	*2.41*	*2.52*	*2.64*	*2.75*
3.5	*2.54*	*2.67*	*2.81*	*2.94*	*3.08*	*3.21*
4.0	*2.90*	*3.06*	*3.21*	*3.36*	*3.51*	*3.67*
4.5	*3.28*	*3.44*	*3.61*	*3.78*	*3.96*	*4.13*
5.0	*3.63*	*3.82*	*4.01*	*4.20*	*4.39*	*4.58*
6.0	*4.35*	*4.58*	*4.81*	*5.04*	*5.27*	*5.50*
7.0	*5.08*	*5.35*	*5.62*	*5.88*	*6.15*	*6.42*
8.0	*5.81*	*6.11*	*6.42*	*6.72*	*7.03*	*7.33*
9.0	*6.53*	*6.88*	*7.22*	*7.56*	*7.91*	*8.25*
10.0	*7.26*	*7.64*	*8.02*	*8.40*	*8.79*	*9.17*

6. Clear, flexible sheets of modified polyvinyl chloride plastic have been fabricated to produce prismatic effects. Utilizing an adaptation of the Fresnel lens principle, these molded sheets can be considered to be composed of a series of small prisms, all aligned with their base-apex lines parallel, and lying adjacent to one another on a thin platform of plastic. The plastic is cut to the desired shape with scissors and pressed onto the surface of a conventional ophthalmic lens (Figures XXVI-22a and b).

a. The thickness of the bases of these Fresnel Press-On Prisms is markedly less than the base of a conventional prism i.e. length of the base-apex line, since the groove width is usually 1.5 mm. instead of the customary conventional ophthalmic lens blank size of 50 to 60 mm.

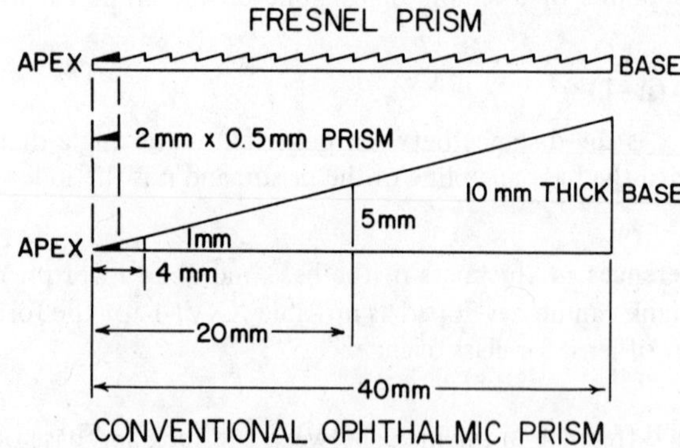

Figure XXVI-22A – The Fresnel Prism Principle. A Fresnel prism, much thinner than a conventional ophthalmic prism of the same power, can be imagined to be a series of small plastic prisms (see shaded prisms) lying adjacent to each other on a thin platform of plastic.

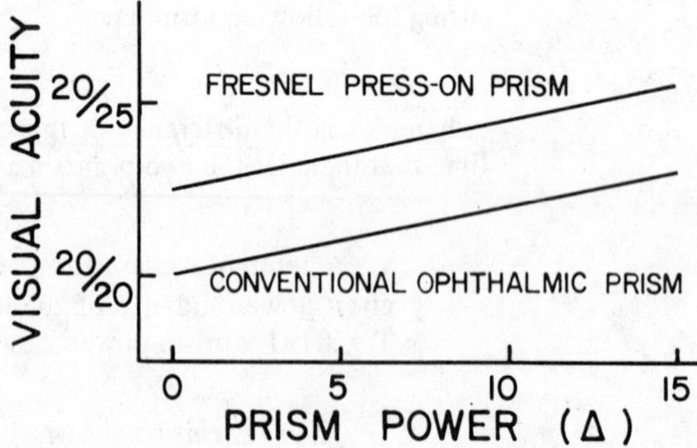

Figure XXVI-22B – Acuity Performance of Prisms. Both OSG Press-On and conventional prisms demonstrate clinically insignificant acuity decrement even for high powers. Conventional glass prisms had a 3.0 D. ocular curve and 2.1 mm. apex thickness. Fresnel prisms were pressed onto plano lenses with the same ocular curve and thickness. Visual acuity was measured psychometrically with Landolt Cs after a method described by Flom, Weymouth & Kahneman, J. Optical Soc. Am. 53 (9): 1026, 1963.

b. Since the Fresnel Press-On Prism is made of a number of equal prisms there will be no large variation in edge thickness of the lens even for prisms of high power.

c. These membrane prisms are light in weight because of the low specific gravity of the plastic and the thinness of the prism.

d. The Fresnel Press-On Prism is currently available in powers of 0.5Δ to 20Δ.

e. The prism is generally applied to the ocular surface of the lens. Both the lens and the prism are cleaned with soap and water. The membrane prism is applied to the lens with both components under running water to eliminate entrapment of dust and air. The prism is patted dry, reorienting it if necessary during the process, and allowed to dry for about five minutes. It is simple to remove one prism and replace it with another.

C. Prismatic Lenses

1. A prism may be incorporated into an ophthalmic lens. In this case the surfaces of the lens may be curved, but one edge, the base, will be thicker than the opposite edge, the apex. The prism may still be considered to be distinct from the rest of the lens.

a. Ogle (1952) has described the non-uniform magnification (distortion) that is produced by a prism. In general for ophthalmic prisms the distortion decreases with steeper base curves. For a fitting distance of 23 mm., measured from the rear surface of the lens to the entrance pupil of the eye, the distortion becomes zero for all of the common powers of ophthalmic prisms when the base curve is about +9.00 diopters. It should be noted that the base curve that minimizes this unsymmetric magnification is not usually the same that minimizes the other common optical aberrations.

2. Prisms are prescribed according to the direction of the base, and if placed obliquely, both the meridian of the base-apex line and the position of the base are given.

a. Example: O.D. 3^{Δ} base-up and base-out at 45 is often shortened to O.D. 3^{Δ} BU @ 45.

D. Decentration

1. A *displacement of the optical center* from the line of sight is called decentration. The result of decentration is a deviation of the image. Consequently decentration may be used in place of prism.

a. While reference has been made to the optical center, this actually may lie anywhere within the lens, between the surfaces or outside the surfaces. Actually, what is commonly termed the optical center is the pole of the principal axis at one surface.

2. The *amount of prism in prism diopters* can be calculated for a spherical lens by formula $\&^{\Delta} = dF$ where d is the decentration in centimeters and F is the dioptric power of the lens. If the sign is positive, the direction of the prism base is in the direction of decentration; if negative, the base is opposite to the decentration. Decentration is always considered to be positive.

3. It is also possible to calculate the prism due to decentering a cylinder or sphero-cylinder by considering the decentration to be the composite of decentrations in each of the two principal meridians. Each of these decentrations will produce prism except in the case when the power in one of the principal meridians is zero.

a. Example: A +2.00 D.S. ⊂ −2.00 D. C. x 45 is decentered in 5 mm. along the 180th meridian before the right eye. What is the prismatic effect that is produced (Figure XXVI-23)?

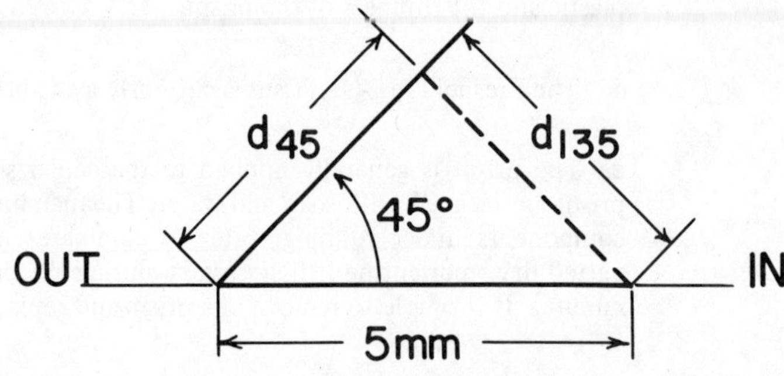

Figure XXVI-23

(1) sin 45° = cos 45°
(2) d_{45} = (5mm.) (cos 45°) = 3.5 mm.
(3) d_{135} = (5mm.) (sin 45°) = 3.5 mm.
(4) ∈45^Δ = (0.35 cm.) (+2.00) = 0.7 base-up and in at 45
(5) ∈135^Δ = (0.35 cm.) (0) = 0 no prism
(6) The net prismatic effect is 0.7^Δ base-up and in at 45.

4. Since the actual prismatic power depends upon the portion of the lens through which the eye will look, the decentration is often in reference to the interpupillary distance. In such instances, decentration may be employed to avoid prismatic effect as well as to provide it.

a. For example, if the interpupillary distance were 66 mm. and 46 mm. lenses (horizontal dimension) were to be prescribed with a distance between the lenses (DBL) of 24 mm., the total distance from geometric center to geometric center of the lenses would be 70 mm. This would exceed the interpupillary distance by 4 mm.

(1) If the poles of the lenses were permitted to remain at the geometrical centers, the lines of sight would pass a total of 4 mm. nasal to the poles; if the lenses were 3.00 D. in power, 3 x .4 would equal 1.2 prism diopters of prismatic effect.

(2) To avoid this, the lenses could be ordered decentered in, 2 mm. each, making the distance from pole to pole 66 mm. without affecting the sizes of the lenses.

b. The decentration would be accomplished by moving the lenses in that distance from the center of the pattern. Since most lens blanks are about 58 mm. round and 1 mm. is required for edging, the practical limitations of decentration in the above case, unless oversize blanks were used, would be 5½ mm. for each lens.

5. A plus lens, as noted, exerts prismatic effect with the base towards the pole of the lens, while a minus lens exerts prismatic effect with the apex towards the pole. If in the above case the lenses were not decentered, 1.2Δ would have been the effect; base-out if the lenses were plus, and base-in if the lenses were minus. If the lenses were plus and base-in effect had been desired, it can be seen that the physical limitations of decentration would not have permitted sufficient base-in to be provided by that means to be significant. In such a case, a prism would have had to be ground on the lens.

a. There is no difference in prismatic effect or in the form of the lens between a decentered lens and a lens which has prism ground in it. The advantages of a lens which has prism ground in it are:

(1) Larger amounts of prism may be incorporated

(2) The base curve may be selected according to any criterion of lens design that one wishes to follow.

6. *Obliquely combined prisms*

a. Occasionally, it is desired to combine prisms having their bases in opposite directions or at oblique angles into one resultant prism. When the base-apex lines are parallel, the powers need merely be added if the bases lie in the same position, or subtracted if they lie in opposite positions. If the base-apex lines are not parallel, the resultant may be found by calculation.

(1) To determine the resultant power, use the formula: $R^2 = A^2 + B^2 + 2AB \cos a$.

(a) R = resultant; A = power of one prism; B = power other prism; a = angle between the base-apex lines of the two prisms.

(2) To determine the position of the resultant base-apex line, the following formula is used: $\sin b = \frac{B}{R} \sin a$.

(a) A simpler method consists of drawing vectors (Figure XXVI-24).

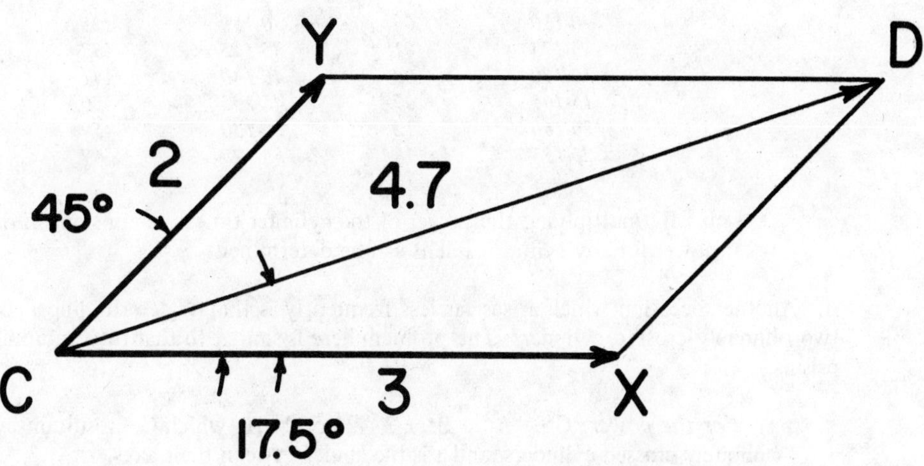

Figure XXVI-24 – Combining oblique prisms by Vector method (1 cm. per prism diopter). Combining 3Δ base-in in 180th meridian with a 2Δ base-in and down in the 45th meridian, to secure 4.7Δ, base-down and in, in the 17½ meridian.

[1] Lay off as a vector in a positive direction a straight line of length equal to the power of the prism with its base-apex line located in the meridian nearest zero.

[2] At an angle equal to the angle between the two base-apex lines, lay off the second prism power as a vector in a positive direction.

[3] Complete the parallelogram and draw a diagonal from the origin of the vectors, C.

[4] The length of the diagonal CD represents the resultant prismatic power.

[5] The angle XCD between the first vector and the diagonal is the angle between the first prism's position and that of the resultant prism.

X. CYLINDERS

A. Occasions may arise in which it is desirable to know the power of a sphero-cylinder in a meridian other than the axis or power meridian in order to compute the prismatic effect. This is particularly true when the cylinder has an oblique axis and decentration horizontally or vertically is desired.

1. The formula for this is: $Fe = Fs + Fx \sin^2 a$, in which Fe is the effective power; Fs, the power of the sphere; Fc, the power of the cylinder; a, the angle between the axis and the meridian under consideration. If a simple cylinder is used, the formula becomes, $Fe = Fc \sin^2 a$.

2. Morgan (1940) has presented a table of constants for a 1.00 D. cylinder (Table XXVI-2):

a. Power of +1.00 D. cylinder at five degree intervals with angle measured from axis of cylinder.

(1) **Table XXVI-2**

Angle	Power	Angle	Power	Angle	Power
0-180	*00*	*30-150*	*.25*	*60-120*	*.75*
5-175	*.01*	*35-145*	*.33*	*65-115*	*.82*
10-170	*.03*	*40-140*	*.41*	*70-110*	*.88*
15-165	*.07*	*45-135*	*.50*	*75-105*	*.93*
20-160	*.12*	*50-130*	*.59*	*80-100*	*.97*
25-155	*.18*	*55-125*	*.67*	*85-95*	*.99*

b. By multiplying the power of the cylinder times the constant in the above table, the total power for any cylindrical lens can be determined.

B. Another occasion which arises far less frequently is that of determining a compound lens to replace two obliquely crossed cylinders. The problem here is similar to that of combining two obliquely crossed prisms.

1. *For the power:* $C^2 = A^2 + B^2 + 2\,AB \cos 2\,a$; in which C = resultant cylinder, A and B are the obliquely crossed cylinders, and a is the angle between their axes.

2. *For the axis of the resultant cylinder:* $\sin 2\phi = \frac{B}{C} \sin 2\,a$. ϕ is the angle between the first cylinder axis and the resultant cylinder axis.

3. *For the resultant sphere:* $S = \dfrac{A + B - C}{2}$

4. The vector method can also be applied to the solution of obliquely crossed cylinders (Figure XXVI-25).

a. Transpose the combination so that the signs of the cylinders are both alike.

b. Represent the power of the cylinder whose axis location is nearer zero as a vector in a positive direction in the direction of the cylinder axis.

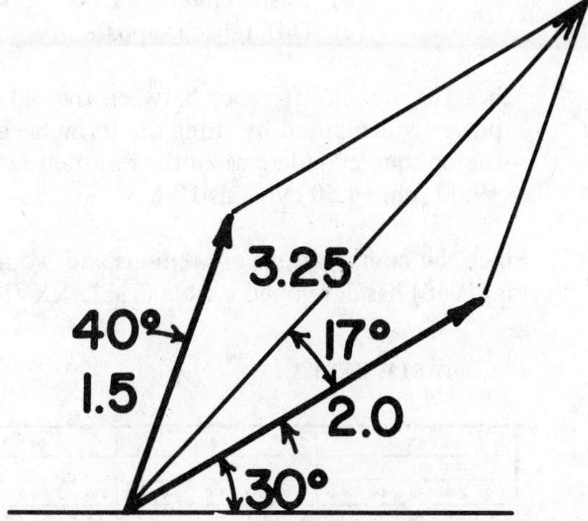

Figure XXVI-25 – Combining two oblique cylinders by vectors (1½ in. per diopter). +2.00 D. cyl. axis 30 and +1.50 cylinder axis 50 combined to produce a resultant cylinder of +3.25 axis 38½.

c. Represent the power of the second cylinder as a positive vector at an angle from the first equal to twice the angle between the cylinder axes.

d. Complete the parallelogram and draw the diagonal. The length of the diagonal indicates the power of the resultant cylinder.

e. The angle between the first vector and the diagonal is twice the angle between the axis of the first cylinder and the axis of the resultant cylinder.

f. The sphere is determined by the formula, $S = \frac{A + B - C}{2}$

It should be noted that the result of adding two simple cylinders will be a sphero-cylinder.

5. If sphero-cylinders are being added, it is necessary to add the power of both the spheres to the sphere (s) determined in f.

C. Comparison of Old and New Sphero-cylinder Rxs.

1. A common problem involving the concept of obliquely crossed cylinders is that raised by comparison of a patient's entering spectacle prescription with that found by the refractionist during the examination when the axes of the cylinders are at variance. If the axes are fairly close, or the powers are quite close, the spherical equivalent is occasionally employed to estimate the difference between the older correction and that revealed during examination and under contemplation for the new prescription. However, if the powers are markedly different and the axes not too similar, an error of large amount may be compounded, as the following example reveals:

a. Given a precataract correction of +2.00 sph ≏ +1.50 cyl. axis 130, and a post surgical correction of +12.00 sph ≏ +4.00 cyl. axis 180

(1) Spherical equivalents would show a difference of:

(a) Precataract; +2.00 + .75 = +2.75
(b) Postcataract: +12.00 + 2.00 = +14.00
(c) Difference is apparently, +11.25 D.

b. The actual difference between the old and new corrections, if spherical and cylindrical power is computed by using the formulae discussed and working backwards to derive one of the oblique cylinders when the resultant cylinder and the other oblique cylinder is known, is +9.00 sph. +4.50 cyl. axis 10.

2. Since the computations are tedious and would have to be freshly performed for each patient, Naylor (1968) has developed a table (Table XXVI-3) which helps simplify the process.

a. **TABLE XXVI-3**

a°	Cr = 1 D					Cr = 2 D					Cr = 3 D					Cr = 4 D					Cr = 5 D				
	C_1					C_1					C_1					C_1					C_1				
	1·0	2·0	3·0	4·0	5·0	1·0	2·0	3·0	4·0	5·0	1·0	2·0	3·0	4·0	5·0	1·0	2·0	3·0	4·0	5·0	1·0	2·0	3·0	4·0	5·0
10 170	0·4 51 129	1·1 81 99	2·1 85 95	3·1 87 93	4·1 88 92	1·1 20 160	0·7 50 130	1·3 75 105	2·2 81 99	3·2 84 96	2·1 14 165	1·3 26 154	1·0 50 130	1·6 70 110	2·4 77 103	3·1 13 167	2·2 19 161	1·6 30 150	1·4 50 130	1·9 66 114	4·1 12 168	3·2 16 164	2·4 23 157	1·9 34 146	1·7 50 130
20 160	0·7 54 126	1·4 76 104	2·3 82 98	3·3 84 96	4·3 86 94	1·4 34 146	1·4 55 125	2·0 69 111	2·8 76 104	3·7 80 100	2·3 28 158	2·0 41 139	2·0 54 126	2·6 65 115	3·3 72 108	3·3 26 154	2·8 34 146	2·6 45 135	2·7 55 125	3·2 63 117	4·3 24 156	3·7 30 150	3·3 38 142	3·2 44 136	3·4 55 125
30 150	1·0 60 120	1·7 75 105	2·7 80 100	3·6 83 97	4·6 85 95	1·7 45 135	2·0 60 120	2·7 70 110	3·5 75 105	4·4 79 101	2·7 40 140	2·7 51 129	3·0 60 120	3·6 67 113	4·4 71 109	3·6 37 143	3·5 45 135	3·6 53 127	4·0 60 120	4·6 66 114	4·6 35 145	4·4 42 138	4·4 48 132	4·6 54 126	5·0 60 120
40 140	1·3 65 115	2·1 76 104	3·0 80 100	4·0 83 97	4·9 84 96	2·1 54 126	2·6 65 115	3·3 72 108	4·2 78 104	5·1 78 102	3·0 41 131	3·3 58 122	3·9 65 115	4·6 70 110	5·4 73 107	4·0 43 137	4·2 55 125	4·6 60 120	5·1 65 115	5·8 69 111	4·9 43 137	5·1 52 128	5·4 57 123	5·8 62 118	6·4 65 115
45 135	1·4 67 113	2·2 77 103	3·2 81 99	4·1 83 97	5·1 84 96	2·2 58 122	2·8 68 112	3·6 72 108	4·5 77 103	5·4 79 101	3·2 54 126	3·6 62 118	4·2 67 113	5·0 72 108	5·8 74 106	4·1 52 128	4·5 58 122	5·0 63 117	5·7 67 112	6·4 70 110	5·1 51 129	5·4 56 124	5·8 60 120	6·4 65 115	7·1 67 113
50 130	1·5 70 110	2·4 79 101	3·3 81 99	4·3 83 97	5·3 85 95	2·4 62 118	3·1 70 110	3·9 75 105	4·8 78 102	5·7 80 100	3·3 59 121	3·9 65 115	4·6 70 110	5·4 74 106	6·3 76 104	4·3 57 123	4·8 62 118	5·4 66 114	6·1 70 110	6·9 72 108	5·3 55 125	5·7 60 120	6·3 64 116	6·9 67 113	7·7 70 110
60 120	1·7 75 105	2·7 80 100	3·6 83 97	4·6 84 96	5·6 86 94	2·7 70 110	3·5 75 105	4·4 78 102	5·3 80 100	6·2 82 98	3·6 68 112	4·4 72 108	5·2 75 105	6·1 78 102	7·0 79 101	4·6 65 115	5·3 70 110	6·1 72 108	6·9 75 105	7·8 77 103	5·6 64 116	6·3 68 112	7·0 71 109	7·8 73 107	8·7 75 105
70 110	1·9 80 100	2·8 83 97	3·8 85 95	4·8 86 94	5·8 87 93	2·8 77 103	3·8 80 100	4·7 82 98	5·7 83 97	6·7 85 95	3·8 75 105	4·7 78 102	5·7 80 100	6·6 82 98	7·6 82 98	4·8 74 106	5·7 76 104	6·6 78 102	7·5 80 100	8·5 81 99	5·8 73 107	6·7 75 105	7·6 77 103	8·5 79 101	9·4 80 100
80 100	2·0 85 95	3·0 87 93	4·0 87 93	5·0 88 92	6·0 88 92	3·0 84 96	3·9 85 95	4·9 86 94	5·9 86 94	6·9 87 93	4·0 82 98	4·9 84 96	5·9 85 95	6·9 85 95	7·9 86 94	5·0 82 98	5·9 83 97	6·9 85 95	7·9 85 95	8·9 86 94	6·0 82 98	6·9 83 97	7·9 83 97	8·9 84 96	9·9 85 95
90	2·0 90	3·0 90	4·0 90	5·0 90	6·0 90	3·0 90	4·0 90	5·0 90	6·0 90	7·0 90	4·0 90	5·0 90	6·0 90	7·0 90	8·0 90	5·0 90	6·0 90	7·0 90	8·0 90	9·0 90	6·0 90	7·0 90	8·0 90	9·0 90	10·0 90

3. *To find the difference of cylinder power and axis:*

a. Transpose all sphero-cylinder combinations to plus cylinder form.
b. Measure all angles anti-clockwise, as is commonly done for lenses.

(1) If the angle is greater than 180°, convert to the conventional form.

c. C1 – cylinder power of first or old RX; Cr – cylinder power of new Rx; C2 – cylinder power of difference between old and new Rx.

d. A – value in degrees of angle between the axis of the two cylinders, C1 and Cr.

4. *To use the table for the cylinder power and axis:*

a. Find the heading in the top row which corresponds to the cylinder power, Cr, of the new Rx.

(1) From the example given earlier: +4.00 D.

b. Find the figure in the 3rd row, under the power of Cr, which corresponds to the cylinder power, C1, of the old Rx.

(1) From example given earlier, C1 (+1.50) lies between columns headed 1.0 and 2.0, under Cr = 4.00 D.

c. Find the value of α, the difference between the axes of Cr and C1 along the left-hand vertical column of the table.

(1) In the example given, Cr plus axis is 180, C1 plus axis is 130, difference is 50.

d. Follow the row alongside 50 until it meets the columns under Cr = 4.00, 1.0 and 2.0.

(1) The uppermost figure at the junction is the power of the cylinder, C2.

(a) Since it lies between rows under 1.0 and 2.0, which show powers of 4.3 and 4.8 respectively, the power is 4.5 D.

(2) The figures under that indicate the degrees which the axis of C2 is from the axis of C1.

(a) Since it lies between rows under 1.0 and 2.0 which show 57 and 62 respectively, the degrees are 60.

(b) The resultant axis of C2 is therefore 130 (the axis of C1) plus 60 (the difference in axis), or 190, which is converted to 10°.

e. The cylinder portion of the difference between the old and new Rx, (Cr – C1), or C2 = +4.50 axis 10.

5. *To find the spherical power, two simple additions are used:*

a. The spherical power resulting from the combination of oblique cylinders, Q, is found by:

(1) $Q = \frac{1}{2}(C1 + C2 - Cr)$

(a) In the example given: $Q = \frac{1}{2}(1.50 + 4.50 - 4.00) = \frac{1}{2}(2.00) = 1.00$

b. The final spherical power, S2, of the differences between the Rxs is found by,

(1) $S2 = Sr - S1 - Q$

(a) In the example given: $S2 = +12.00 - 2.00 - 1.00 = 9.00$ D.

6. The precise difference between the entering Rx: +2.00 ⊃ +1.50 axis 130, and the new Rx: +12.00 ⊃ +4.00 axis 180, is +9.00 ⊃ +4.50 axis 10.

7. The importance of the exact difference becomes even more evident as the effects of magnification on perspective and prismatic effects in different positions of the field, discussed in the following sections and in Chapter VIII, are considered.

XI. MAGNIFICATION

A. Magnification, while not usually the characteristic that is of primary importance, is always present in ophthalmic lenses. Angular magnification can be readily appreciated by the eye.

B. Paraxial angular magnification for distance prescriptions can be calculated with the formula:

1. $$\alpha/\beta = \left(\frac{1}{1 - \frac{t}{n} F_1}\right)\left(\frac{1}{1 - hF_v}\right),$$

where α/β = angular magnification; t is the thickness of the lens measured in meters, n is the index, F_1 is the dioptric power of the front surface of the lens, h is the fitting distance measured from the back surface of the lens to the entrance pupil of the eye in meters, and F_V is the back vertex power of the lens measured in diopters. Since the term in the first bracket includes the parameters of the thickness and power of the front surface, and therefore indirectly also specifies the power of the second surface, it is sometimes referred to as the shape factor in the magnification formula. The second bracket includes the back vertex power as one of its parameters and is called the power factor.

2. Paraxial angular magnification for near prescriptions can be calculated with the formula

a. $$a_1 \ \alpha/\beta = \left(-\frac{p}{\mu}\right)\left(\frac{1}{1 - \frac{t}{n}\left[F_1 + \frac{1}{\mu}\right]}\right)\left(\frac{1}{1 - h\left[\frac{1}{\frac{1}{F_1 + \frac{1}{\mu}} - \frac{t}{n}} \pm F_2\right]}\right)$$

where p is the distance in meters from the near object to thee entrance pupil of the eye, μ is the distance from the spectacle lens to the near object (a negative distance also measured in meters), and all other terms having the same interpretation as in 2 above.

3. It is possible to determine the variation in magnification for any change in the variables of base curve, center thickness, fitting distance and vertex power by differentiating the appropriate equation. However, simplified forms of these differentiated equations for distance objects, neglecting the higher order terms, are:

a. Shape Factor Contributions

(1) $$\Delta(\alpha/\beta)\% = \frac{100\, t\, \Delta F_1}{n}$$

(2) $$\Delta(\alpha/\beta)\% = \frac{100\, F_1\, \Delta t}{n}$$

b. Power Factor Contributions

(1) $\Delta(\alpha/\beta)\% = 100\, F_v\, \Delta h$

(2) $\Delta(\alpha/\beta)\% = 100\, h\, \Delta F_v$

c. In all cases thickness (t), fitting distance (h), and changes in thickness (Δ t) and fitting distance (Δ h) are measured in meters; while front surface power (F_1), back vertex power (F_v) and changes in these powers (ΔF_1) and (ΔF_v) are measured in diopters. The resultant answers are in terms of the percent change in magnification $\Delta(\alpha/\beta)\%$. In order to determine the approximate net change in magnification it is necessary to multiply the above contribution by the appropriate factor i.e.: ex: Multiply the Shape Factor Contribution by the total Power Factor.

d. It should be noted that a decrease in the power of F_1 i.e., A negative ΔF_1, results in a decrease in magnification in equation a(1); that a decrease in the center thickness t, i.e., a negative Δ, results in a decrease in magnification in equation a(2); that a decrease in the fitting distance h, i.e., a negative value for Δh, results in a decrease in magnification for plus lenses and an increase in magnification for minus lenses in equation b(1); that a decrease in the value of F_v, less plus or more minus, i.e., a negative value for ΔF_v, results in a decrease in magnification in equation b(2).

4. Graphs showing these approximate relationships between variables for both the shape factor and the power factor have been published. In Figure XXVI-26 the contour lines represent combinations of F_1 and t that will produce various amounts of magnification.

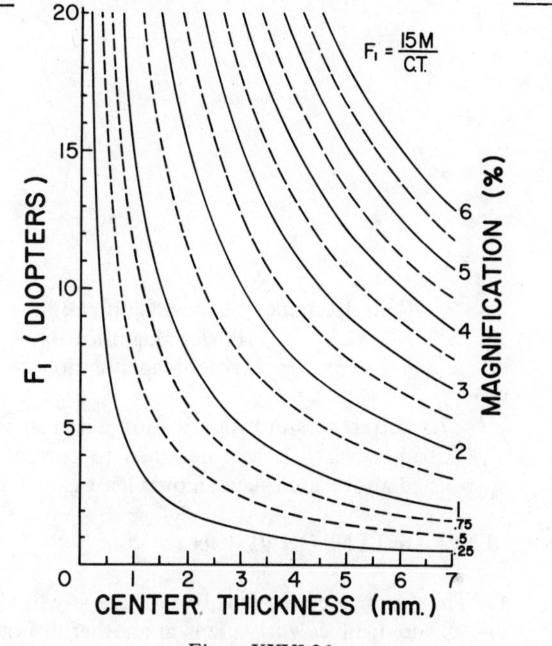

Figure XXVI-26.

a. As an example, a lens having a front surface power of +15.00 diopters and a center thickness of 2.0 mm. will have a shape magnification factor of 2%.

(1) Similarly, a lens with a front surface power of +5.00 diopters and a center thickness of 6.0 mm. will also have a shape magnification factor of 2%.

5. In Figure XXVI-27 the contour lines represent combinations of h and F_v that will produce various amounts of magnification.

a. As an example: a lens of back vertex power of +2.00 diopters having a fitting distance of 1.0 cm. will have a power magnification factor of 2%.

(1) Similarly, a lens of back vertex power of +1.00 diopter having a fitting distance of 2.0 cm. will also have a power magnification factor of 2%.

b. Negative values of F_v (minus lenses) will have similar interrelationships, but will produce negative magnification (minification).

6. A lens having a 2% shape magnification and a 2% power magnification will have a 4% total magnification since the total magnification is the product of the shape and power magnifications.

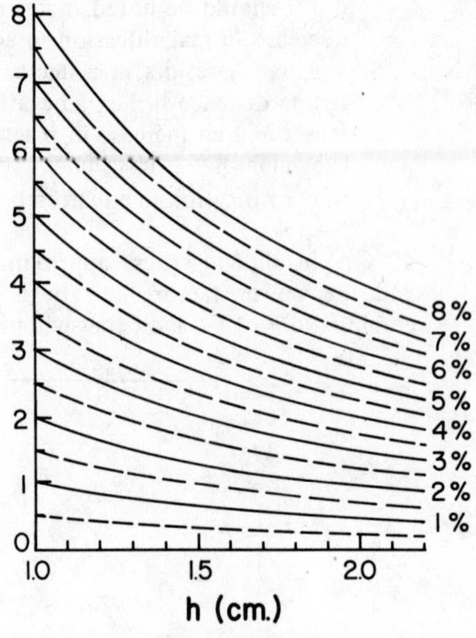

Figure XXVI-27.

a. Example: Shape Magnification = 1.02
Power Magnification = 1.02
Total Magnification = (1.02) (1.02) = 1.04 or 4% magnification

7. Differences in magnification between the two eyes produce the condition of aniseikonia (see Chapter VIII). Lenses designed to correct this condition, based upon the magnification criteria listed above, are called eikonic lenses.

XII. INFLUENCE OF LENS ON VISION

A. The distance of the lens from the eye will alter its effective power as has been shown. To replace a lens at one distance with a lens at another distance with equal effectivity, the variation in distance must be compensated by the formula given earlier in this chapter under effective power.

1. A significant implication of the effectivity of a lens in relation to its position before the eye is noted when it is remembered that common practice designates the extent of refractive error by the lens which apparently corrects it. Since the correction lens is always placed at a finite distance

a. **Table XXVI-4**

Plus Correct. Lens	Error at P'P' of Eye	Minus Correct. Lens	Plus Correct. Lens	Error at P'P' of Eye	Minus Correct. Lens
.986	*1.00*	*1.01*	*10.30*	*12.00*	*14.45*
1.95	*2.00*	*2.03*	*10.90*	*13.00*	*15.78*
2.88	*3.00*	*3.14*	*11.70*	*14.00*	*17.40*
3.79	*4.00*	*4.25*	*12.40*	*15.00*	*19.00*
4.67	*5.00*	*5.38*	*13.10*	*16.00*	*20.30*
5.53	*6.00*	*6.54*	*13.70*	*17.00*	*22.20*
6.36	*7.00*	*7.75*	*14.40*	*18.00*	*24.10*
7.20	*8.00*	*9.00*	*14.80*	*19.00*	*25.90*
8.00	*9.00*	*10.30*	*15.63*	*20.00*	*27.80*
8.94	*10.00*	*11.60*	*16.25*	*21.00*	*29.80*
9.55	*11.00*	*13.00*	*16.80*	*22.00*	*31.80*
			17.40	*23.00*	*33.90*

before the eye, and since this distance actually alters the effectivity of the lens, Neumueller (1948) and Curcio (1950) have pointed out that the true refractive error may vary materially from that designated by the lens. While this difference is mainly significant in errors of high amount, it should be noted that hyperopes are almost always undercorrected in relation to the real state of refraction, while myopes are almost always overcorrected, by comparisons of the power of lens used and the error 'at the eye'. This discrepancy is indicated in Table XXVI-4 by Curcio (1950), for a spectacle plane 14 mm. in front of the eye.

b. It is significant that the actual *amount of accommodation* required by an uncorrected hyperope for clear distance vision is in excess of the amount indicated by a correction lens. If the near point is considered, it is found that the effectivity of the correction lens varies even more markedly, and that a corrected ametrope is not an emmetrope. Pascal (1952a) has, as described in Chapter VI, developed the concept of the accommodative unit to indicate the actual discrepancy involved. Curcio (1950) further elaborates this by the following graph, Figure XXVI-28 which, allowing for the effectivity of the lens at a near point of 13 inches, and for the difference in the true ametropia and that indicated by the lens at 14 mm. from the eye, shows the actual accommodative discrepancy for the hyperope and myope of a given amount of refractive error. In prescribing lenses for presbyopes, if of reasonably high refractive error, these considerations become pertinent. Sinn (1949) points out that the thinner or flatter a lens is, the closer its effective value at near approximates its known vertex power, and that in thick lenses, the actual position of the bifocal segment, whether on the front or back surface, may vary the effectivity appreciably. This is especially pertinent when the same prescription is to be used for both regular and safety glasses, particularly if the type is one in which the segment is on the back surface.

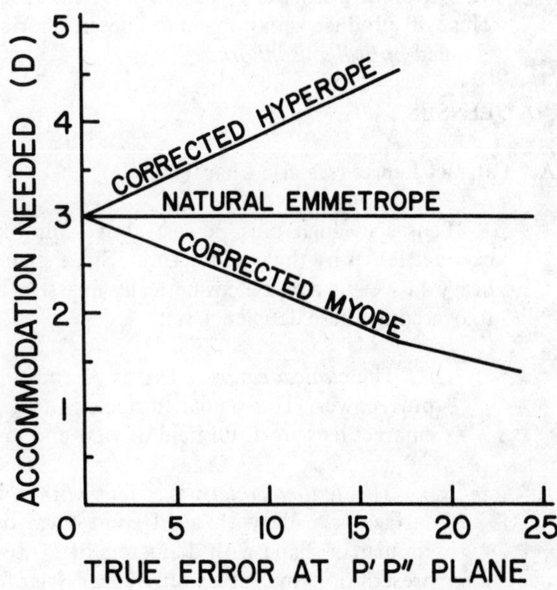

Figure XXVI-28 – Graph of effectivity of lens at 14 mm. in relation to accommodative effort and true error for fixation at 33 cms. (after Curcio).

B. The lens will usually produce a subjective variation in the *size* of perceived objects. The size of the retinal image of a corrected myope will be decreased and that of a corrected hyperope will be increased over that of the uncorrected state when no accommodation is used. However, the uncorrected hyperope, who has, in addition, decreased the image size by accommodating, will see objects as larger when he no longer has to accommodate. The myope, who does not use accommodation when viewing distance objects, will not have this as a complicating factor in the perception of the size of distant objects. The astigmat may note a change in shape of the image when he is corrected. This is due to the different magnification that accompanies the different powers of a cylindrical lens. The patient may notice this as a form of distortion. These effects may be calculated using the equations of Section XI of this chapter.

1. *Perspective,* especially at nearer points, will be influenced since the angle of the rays into the eye is altered. The hyperope will assume objects to be closer, while the myope will assume them to be farther away.

2. *The fixed field* of vision for a hyperope will be limited in relation to his uncorrected vision since the rays are converged by the lens. The reverse holds true for the myope since objects that are ordinarily beyond his view will be brought into his field by the diverging power of his correcting lens. In both instances the size of the lens and the frame tend to limit the field. In the case of the myope the thick edges of the lens also tend to obscure peripheral objects and thereby limit the field.

3. *Eye movements* will also tend to be quite different because of the prismatic effects that are produced in the periphery of the lens. The hyperope will have to increase the extent of his eye movements and the myope will have to decrease his when corrected. In cases of anisometropia different convergence and divergence demands will be incurred as a result of the prismatic effects that are induced by the lenses.

4. Different *prismatic effects* will be induced through different regions of the correcting lens. This will produce variations in the heterophoria with different directions of gaze. Such a condition is called *optical anisophoria.*

XIII. SPECIAL LENSES

A. **Cataract Lenses** (see also Chapter XXII)

1. Lenses of high plus power, above approximately +7.00 diopters, are often designated as cataract lenses by the manufacturer. Since strong plus lenses have large amounts of aberrations, are heavy in weight and are cosmetically unattractive, some lenses have been designed in special forms to overcome these deficiencies.

a. The *clinical cataract lens* is of conventional design. The front surface is a sphere of high plus power. The ocular surface is toric and shallow. The major advantages of a clinical cataract lens are a full field of view and low cost.

b. The *lenticular lens* is a lens with a restricted visual area. The periphery of the front surface is made with a different form or curve, so that the useful portion is central, and circular in shape with diameters of 20 to 40 mm. The peripheral region does not carry the prescription and serves only as a carrier for the central region so that it may be inserted into a conventional spectacle frame. Since aberrations tend to restrict vision to the central paraxial region of a conventional lens, the severe reduction of lens area does not result in a comparable reduction of the field of view. The major advantage of the lenticular design is weight reduction.

(1) The *Ultex cataract* lens is made of one piece of glass; a central area 27 mm. in diameter is ground biconvex. The periphery of the back surface is almost flat. This form reduces thickness and weight and is better appearing. Vision is confined to an area in which aberrations are not too prominent despite its form.

(2) Similar to the above is the *fused cataract lens* which consists of a barium crown central section fused to ordinary crown. The dispersive values of the two are nearly the same. As barium crown has a high index, the lens need not have extremely strong curves. The diameter of the barium disc varies from 26 to 30 mm. The back surface is almost flat.

(3) The *fused Nokrome* lenticular cataract lens is similar in construction to the Univis lens, but uses a non-tarnishing barium glass. It is obtainable on Tillyer or Orthogon curves.

(4) The *Orthogon* one piece lens is made with the lenticular portion ground on the front surface and upon the Orthogon series of curves. The lenticular portion is 30 mm. round.

(5) The *Tillyer "E"* is made like the Orthogon, but on the Tillyer series of curves.

c. Various lenticular designs are also available in plastic. The lightness in weight of a plastic lens combined with the lenticular design offer distinct advantages where weight must be kept to a minimum.

2. Bifocal cataract lenses are also made and will be considered in that chapter.

B. High Minus Lenses

1. Since strong minus lenses are heavy and unattractive, lenticular lenses, similar in principle to the lenticular cataract lenses have been made. The correction is in a central, circular area while the periphery has little or no correction and serves as a carrier. This design reduces the weight by reducing the edge thickness. Although the central region does not contribute to the appeal many people prefer the appearance of these lenses to the more conventional design. The smaller edge thickness offers advantages in mounting that the thicker lenses do not have.

a. The minus lenticular was originally made by cutting off the peripheral curve with a flat tool so that the peripheral curve of the front surface was plane. A variation was to substitute a convex tool for the flat tool. Neither procedure of manufacture is now in common use.

b. *The myo-disc lens* is made by grinding a smaller concave section into a flat disc. The disc is thin and the usable areas vary with the power of the lens.

(1) For powers of –6.25 to –9.00, the corrective field is 30 mm.; from –8.00 to –16.00, 25 mm.; from –14.00 to –20.00, 22 mm., and from –18.00 to –30.00, 20 mm. Cylindrical corrections are ground on the outer surface.

c. Minus lenticular lenses are also manufactured in plastic. Although the size of the corrective field may vary from manufacturer to manufacturer these plastic lenses have approximately the same dimensions as myo-disc glass lenses.

2. *Thin-lite lenses* are conventional lenses made from flint glass of index from 1.61 to 1.70 depending on the prescription and the manufacturer. This higher index reduced the thickness and curves but not the weight. Thin-lite lenses are provided in both white and tinted glass.

C. Microscopic Lenses

1. Lenses of very high power are sometimes prescribed for people with low visual acuity to enable them to read printed material. These microscopic lenses are available in either single vision (lenticular design) or bifocal form in powers from +8.00 diopters (2X) to +48.00 diopters (12X). Higher powers can be obtained on special order. The corrective portion of the lens can be from 25

to 40 mm. in diameter. These lenses may be of glass or plastic in one-piece construction. Usually the higher powers are made in plastic with aspheric curves.

2. Microscopic lenses require very short viewing distances. They have a very limited depth of field for high powers.

D. Safety Lenses

1. Lenses having special physical properties to offer protection against flying objects, glare and/or radiation, and which may incorporate an ophthalmic correction are called safety lenses.

2. A glass lens having a minimum thickness of at least 2.0 mm. can be *tempered* by a heat treatment process. Such lenses, although they do not meet safety specifications, do offer added protection from flying objects. In circumstances where weight and extra thickness are undesirable, these dress-safety thickness lenses are often prescribed.

3. *Industrial safety lenses* are designed to meet the specifications of the U.S.A. Standards Association for Eye and Face Protection (USAS Z87.1 – 1968).

a. These lenses must be at least 3.0 mm., except high plus lenses may be as thin as 2.5 mm. if they can withstand the force of a 1 inch diameter steel ball that weighs 2.4 ounces falling from a height of 50 inches onto the front surface of the lens without breaking the glass.

b. These lenses are generally heat treated to obtain added strength and can be identified by the distinctive polarization pattern that this treatment provides as light is transmitted through the finished lens.

4. Surface irregularities in hardened lenses may precipitate lens fractures when struck by a flying object. Peters (1962) reports that light scratches reduce the impact resistance by 12% and deep scratches cause a reduction by 44%. Such scratches can occur through normal use and ordinary cleaning.

5. *Plastic lenses may also be used as safety lenses.*

a. These lenses must withstand penetration by a number 25 solid needle fastened to a holder weighing 1.56 ounces which is dropped from a height of 50 inches onto the front surface of the lens.

b. Plastic lenses require no special treatment in order to make them resistant to penetration. The plastic is sufficiently elastic to give with the blow, thereby absorbing much of the force.

6. Safety lenses made of a *laminate* of a sheet of plastic between two crown glass components are available from several manufacturers. The glass which may be broken by a flying object is prevented from flying into the wearer's eye by the plastic sheet. These lenses are known as I-Safe lenses (American Optical) or Motex.

E. Aspheric Lenses (See also Chap. XXII)

1. When the power of a lens exceeds –21.00 diopters or +8.00 diopters, it is no longer possible to obtain correction of marginal astigmatism using spherical surfaces. It is then necessary to use aspheric surfaces.

a. Aspheric curves have constantly changing radii of curvature from the center to the outer edges. It is possible to select aspheric curves so that spherical aberration, marginal astigmatism, power error, or distortion may be minimized, but it is not possible to simultaneously correct all of the aberrations. Usually the decision is made to correct for marginal astigmatism or power error or to partially correct for both aberrations. The lens is most frequently made with an ellipsoidal front surface and a toric or spherical rear surface. Some designs use other conic sections such as paraboloids or hyperboloids for the aspheric surface.

2. The principle of the design usually is based on an infinitely distant object, a 30° viewing angle, and a stop distance of about 25 mm.

a. *The Volk Catraconoid* lens is a glass aspheric bifocal lens with the aspheric surface, an ellipsoid of revolution, on the front. For noncylindrical prescriptions the rear surface is a −3.00 diopter sphere. For cylindrical prescriptions the toric surface is on the rear and the cylinder is divided equally on each side of the −3.00 diopter base curve.

b. *The American Optical Aolite Aspheric* cataract lenses are cast in lenticular form of CR-39 plastic. There are 29 base curves based upon a front surface which is an ellipsoid of revolution. It corrects partially for marginal astigmatism and power error. Major attention is given to the correction of the tangential meridian when it is not possible to correct for marginal astigmatism completely.

c. *The Bausch and Lomb Pan-Aspheric Cataract* Lenses are cast in both full field and lenticular forms of CR-39 plastic. There are 8 base curves based upon a front surface which is an ellipsoid of revolution. It corrects mainly for marginal astigmatism.

d. *Armorlite,* a pioneer in the field of plastic lenses, uses a higher order conic shape as the front surface aspheric. The back surface is either spherical or toric, depending on the prescription requirements.

e. Other aspherics are available from Zeiss as the *Katral;* from Univis as the *Uni-Form Aspheric Uni-Lite;* from Titmus as the *Cristyl full field* or lenticular aspheric. The Zeiss Katral is a glass lens, the others are plastic.

f. *The Essel Atoral* lens is a CR-39 plastic lens made with a rear surface aspheric. This surface is basically elliptical, but also incorporates a correction for astigmatism, i.e., the surface is both aspheric and toric, hence the name Atoral. The design of this surface is unique because this aspheric surface is not a surface of revolution. It is possible to correct for the marginal astigmatism in all meridians instead of just one meridian. The front surface is spherical regardless of the prescription. The field that is free from marginal astigmatism is greatly enlarged by this design.

XIV. PLASTIC LENSES

A. Another relatively recent innovation is the manufacture of spectacle lenses utilizing plastic materials rather than glass. While this development had been in progress for some time, it was not until molded long-chain and cross-linked resins became available that quality plastic lenses were marketed. Today lenses are made of either thermoplastic (plastic at temperatures varying from 122 to 254°F., but solid below that temperature) or thermosetting (not affected by heat after once set) plastics. The methyl methacrylates seem to be the best of the former, while the allyl diglycol carbonates, CR-39, are the more popular examples of the latter.

1. Comparison of glass with plastic lenses involves comparison of a number of properties. Among these are optical clarity, water absorption, light stability (resistance to hazing), rate of thermal expansion, thermoplasticity, shrinkage, warping, abrasion resistance, impact resistance, and weight.

2. Generally, modern plastic lenses provide properties equal to or superior to those of glass, for all practical purposes, with the exception of abrasion resistance. Another feature of plastic lenses is that the curvatures may be molded on the lens and that aspherical surfaces can thereby be

provided when needed. Graham (1949) gives the following comparison of glass, methyl acrylates and allyl diglycol carbonates:

a. **Table XXVI-5**

	Glass	Methacrylate	Resin (ADC)
Specific Gravity	*2.5*	*1.2*	*1.25*
Refract. Index	*1.52*	*1.49*	*1.5*
Resist. to Fogging	*1*	*5*	*4.5*
Light Transmission	*88%*	*90-92%*	*90-92%*
Resist. to Abrasion	*No. 5*		*No. 3*

b. The resistance to abrasion test is based upon the Mohs scale, which merely lists ten minerals in order of ascending hardness, each of which will scratch the one below it but not the one above it. There is no definite mathematical relationship between the various minerals so that a substance scratched by mineral 4 as compared to one scratched by mineral 8 is not half as hard but may be much more than half, or more likely, much less than half as hard. Other tests are available, but while physicists describe hardness in terms of scratch resistance, abrasion resistance, impact resistance, cutting resistance, and resiliency, no correlation precisely exists between these factors. Consequently, claims of manufacturers may vary according to the type of hardness and the method of testing employed.

3. Keeney and Duerson (1953) performed some tests comparing various types of commercially available plastic and glass lenses. Their results are listed below:

a. Armorlite and Plastolite lenses were found to be much harder than Plexiglas, with standard I-Gard lenses softest. The special I-Gard lenses, Transpex, were apparently not tested, and these are definitely much harder than the standard I-Gard lenses.

b. Armorlite, Plastolite and Plexiglas are not distorted apparently by even boiling temperatures. I-Gard softens at 80°, and Transpex at 105° according to the manufacturer.

c. Armorlite, Plastolite and case-hardened crown did not shatter under impacts which did ordinary crown, Plexiglas and I-Gard lenses. The manufacturer of I-Gard lenses reports tests which show that the I-Gard lens is superior to hardened crown, however.

d. Almost all plastic lenses show a good resistance to chemical and electrical spattering but Plastolite and Armorlite were hardly affected by even acetone.

4. CR-39, a material made and patented by the Pittsburgh Plate Glass Company, is an allyl diglycol carbonate. The basic material is a monomer, which is a liquid. When a catalyst is added, the material polymerizes into a clear, hard solid. The liquid material is put into glass molds. Careful temperature control during the polymerization procedure is necessary during the 16 hr. curing period to maintain the desirable optical and physical characteristics. All that is necessary to produce a finished lens or a semi-finished lens is to remove the plastic from the molds. When finishing of the second surface is required, grinding and polishing may be done using comparable techniques to those used in finishing glass lenses. Longer periods for generating, fining and polishing are necessary.

B. Comparative advantages and disadvantages of plastic as compared to glass lenses include:

1. *Disadvantages*

a. Plastic lenses are more readily scratched unless particular care is employed in cleaning them.
b. Thermoplastic forms may distort by sudden heat exposure, although usually most will stand any heat that the body will.

c. Chemicals affect plastic lenses much more than they do glass.
d. The index of refraction is less than that of glass. This variation must be noted if lens measures are used.
e. Ordinary edgers are not efficient on the softer types.
f. Plastic lenses are flammable. However, they are difficult to ignite and burn rather slowly.
g. The cost of plastic lenses is slightly more than of glass lenses in general. The difference in cost is becoming negligible since more plastic lenses are now being prescribed.
h. Drilling weakens the lenses.

2. *Advantages*

a. Impact resistance is greater than for glass, even exceeding case-hardened glass in some types.
b. Fragmentation, when it does occur, yields larger pieces with less jagged edges than does glass.
c. The weight is only from 40-50% that of glass.
d. Light transmission is from 5-8% better.
e. Fogging tendency is reduced from 60-75%.
f. High velocity particles and welder's spatter affect plastics less than they do glass.
g. Fewer internal reflections are apparent, especially in strong prescriptions.
h. Molding eliminates some surfacing procedures and permits aspherical curves.
i. A tinted lens, since it is a coated lens, has uniform transmission despite having variations in thickness.

C. Plastic lenses are now available in most single vision combinations, in lenticular forms, and in bifocals.

XV. LENS REFLECTIONS AND COATINGS

A. Reflections occur frequently and unintentionally in ophthalmic work. For the most part these reflections are not bothersome, but occasionally and especially under certain viewing conditions they may be very noticeable and extremely annoying. The factors that contribute to awareness of reflections are:

1. intensity
2. clarity
3. location
4. contrast

B. Figure XXVI-29 indicates the surface at which reflection occurs and the percent of light reflected into the eye for each of the five reflections that are most intense and bothersome.

1. For light striking the lens surface normally the intensity of the reflected ray is given by

$$I_r = \left(\frac{n-1}{n+1}\right)^2 I_o$$

Where I_r is the intensity of the reflected ray, I_o is the intensity of the incident ray, and n is the index of the reflecting material.

2. Certain substances may be coated onto the surface of the material to reduce the intensity of the reflection.

a. These coatings, called anti-reflection coatings must bear certain relationships of index and thickness to the substrate onto which they are deposited.

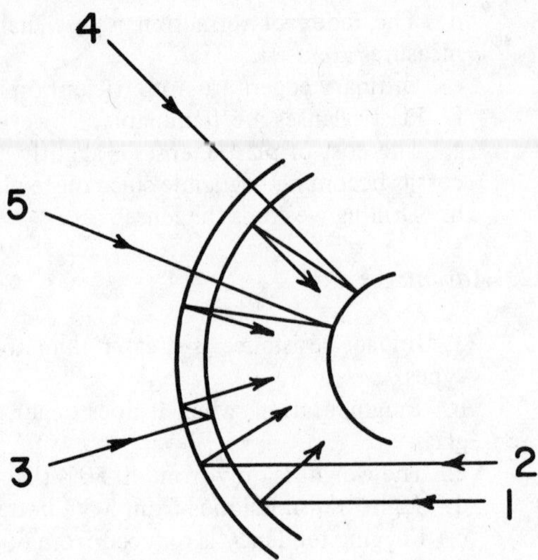

Figure XXVI-29 – Schematic Representation of Single and Double Reflections of an Ophthalmic Lens (after Jones, 1948).

	% of Stray Light	
	Before Coating	After Coating
1. From rear surface into eye	*4.26*	*1.42*
2. From front surface into eye	*3.90*	*1.30*
3. From double reflection within lens	*0.17*	*0.057*
4. From cornea to rear surface and back	*0.09*	*0.03*
5. From cornea to front surface and back	*0.08*	*0.027*

(1) The index of the coating must be equal to the square root of the index of the substrate to be maximally effective.

(2) The optical thickness must be ¼ wavelength of the light.

b. This means that for ophthalmic crown glass of index 1.523 the coating should have an index of 1.23. No durable coating has been found which has so low an index. Instead, magnesium fluoride of index 1.38 is used. This means that even though some light is reflected at the surface, the coating will be hard and durable and therefore more permanent.

(1) Since white light is light of all wavelengths, it is impossible to have a single coat whose optical thickness will be a quarter of a wavelength.

(a) Consequently all wavelengths will not be equally attenuated and therefore the intensity of the reflected light will not go to zero.

(b) However, it is possible to adjust the thickness of the coating so that it is maximally effective for wavelengths at the peak of photopic sensitivity of the eye, i.e., around 555 nanometers, in the green region of the spectrum. Therefore light from the red and blue ends of the spectrum will predominate in the reflection and will give the lens a purplish cast known as the residual purple.

(2) The table accompanying Figure XXVI-30 indicates the intensity of these five reflections, A through E, after coating. Since the optical thickness varies with the path that the light takes through the coating the wavelength of minimum reflectivity will

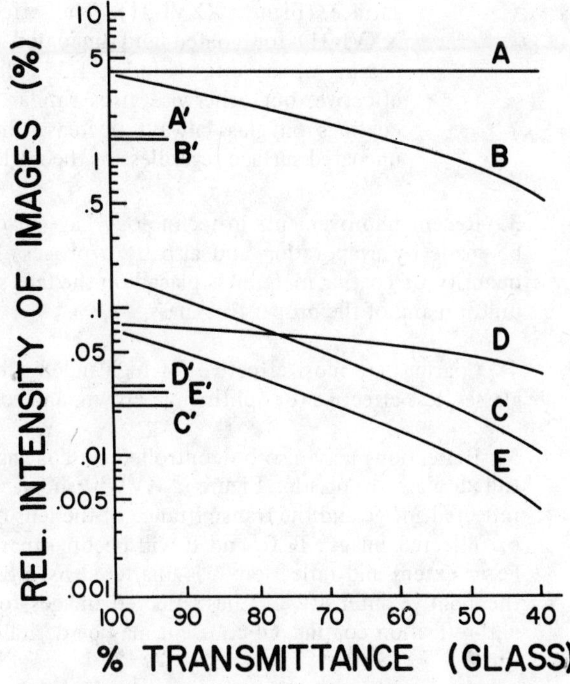

Figure XXVI-30 – Percent relative intensity of reflections A through E as a function of lens transmittance.

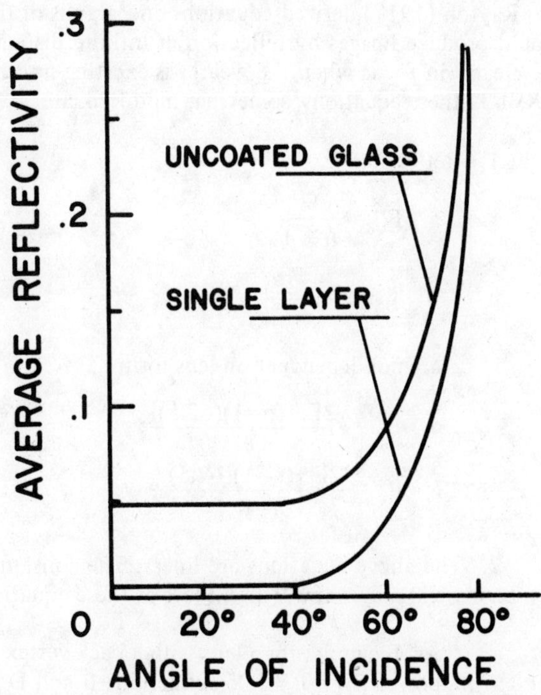

Figure XXVI-31 – Angle of incidence ϕ versus R_{av} of uncoated glass and the minimum R_{av} of the same glass coated with a single layer.

shift toward the blue end of the spectrum when light is incident obliquely onto the surface (Figure XXVI-31). The effectiveness of the coating is shown in (Figure XXVI-31) for coated and uncoated glass lenses for glass of index 1.52 and for a coating of cryolite of index 1.35. Magnesium fluoride of index 1.38 is not quite so effective, but otherwise gives similar results. It should be noted that anti-reflection coatings on glass always decrease the average reflectivity to lower values than the uncoated surface regardless of the angle of incidence.

3. Recent improvements in technology have made it possible to coat plastic lenses. Deposits can be made by evaporation and also by a process known as spin coating. In this process a small quantity of coating material is placed on the lens surface and the lens is rotated until the coating is uniform and of the proper thickness.

4. Coatings are most effective for high index substrates such as flint glass and the dense barium glasses, less effective for ophthalmic crown, and somewhat less effective still for plastic lenses.

5. Reflections may also be controlled by coating the lens with an absorbing material, or by using tinted glass or plastic. Figure XXVI-30 shows the relationship between the intensity of the reflected image and the transmittance of the lens material. If the lens is lightly tinted, the intensity of reflected images B, C, and E will become markedly less. Reflection D is diminished, but to a lesser extent and reflection A is unaltered by a tint. The points marked A′, B′, C′, D′ and E′ show the relative intensity of the reflected images for white, ophthalmic crown glass which has an anti-reflection coating. Of course it may be desirable to both coat the lens and to use an absorptive tint.

a. It should be noticed that those rays that pass through the lens most often, i.e., C and E, are those reflections that can be most effectively controlled by an absorptive tint.

C. Rayton (1917) derived equations and graphs of the relations between lens form and lens power that would produce images by reflection at infinite distances from the lens for distant objects. These images are clearly in focus when the wearer is exerting no accommodation. For the reflections shown in Figure XXVI-32 these equations, somewhat modified, are:

1. Reflection:

a. $F_v = \frac{2F}{n+1}$

b. $F_v = -\frac{2F_1}{n-1}$

c. not dependent on lens form

d. $F_v = \frac{2F - (n-1)(62.5)}{n+1}$

e. $F_v = \frac{2F + (n-1)(62.5)}{n-1}$

2. The above equations are linear. The constants are based upon a fitting distance of 16 mm. and a corneal radius of 8.0 mm. Plots of these equations are shown in Figure XXVI-32.

a. Example: for a lens with a back vertex power (F_1) of –8.75 diopters and a front surface power (F_1) of +2.25 reflections B and D would be clearly in focus when the wearer looked at distant objects, but reflections A and E would be out of focus and therefore would be lacking in clarity. It may be possible to choose different curves for the lens to throw these images out of focus, thereby making them less obvious. In this example a lens whose front surface power(F_1) is +6.00 diopters would throw reflection B approximately 14.00 diopters

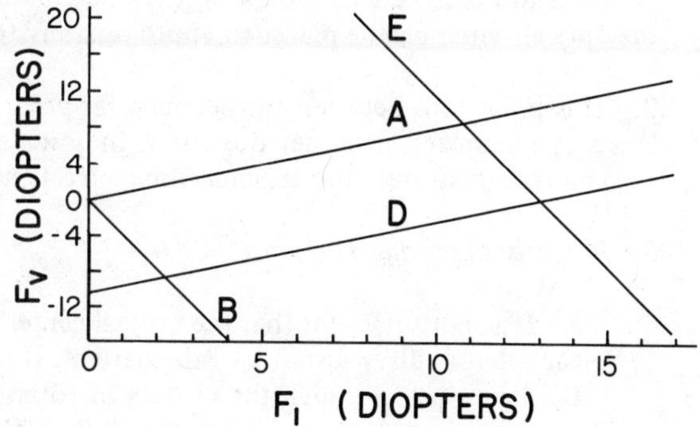

Figure XXVI-32 – Locus of reflected images in focus without accommodation–16.0 mm fitting distance, 8.0 mm corneal radius.

and reflection D about 0.50 diopter out of focus. It would probably be necessary to resort to changing the fitting distance slightly to make reflection D even more blurred. It is unlikely that reflection B would be bothersome after the base curve were changed.

3. The location of reflected images can often be changed by tilting the lens. This is usually most effective for reflections A, B, and C. These reflections are ordinarily rather large, in contrast to reflections D and E which tend to be quite small. These small reflected images, in part the result of reflection off the cornea, move very little with a tilt in the lens. They are most effectively controlled by changing the fitting distance and by using absorptive materials.

4. Occasionally, the environment offers conditions of high contrast so that dim reflections, not customarily noticed, will become visible. It may be possible to alter the surround to diminish the contrast sufficiently to render the reflections unnoticeable. Obviously, this solution is sometimes impossible to carry out.

D. Among the advantages ascribed to coated lenses are:

1. Magnesium fluoride actually provides a more resistant surface than either plastic or glass. Despite its extreme thinness it offers some advantages in durability over the usual lens surface.

2. Surface reflections are decreased.

3. Transmission is increased.

4. Internal reflections and the resultant ring images that are apparent in high minus lenses and some high plus lenses are diminished, resulting in an improved cosmetic appearance.

XVI. PLACING THE LENS BEFORE THE EYE

A. Fry and Ellerbrock (1941), in discussing the position of lenses before the eye, indicate that two main schools of thought exist. Some recommended that the optical centers be placed so that the lines of sight pass through them when directed straight ahead; while others maintain that the line of sight should pass three mm. above the optical centers.

1. The position of the optical center will vary with the tilt of the lens before the eyes. Based on conditions assumed by manufacturers of optical frames and mountings, the ideal tilt of the standard lens appears to be 8°. Such a tilt places the optical center 4 mm. below the center of the

pupil when the line of sight passes normally through the lens surface. As the guards arms are designed to hold the lens mounting the line closer to the pupil center than 3 mm., the position of the optical center can be placed at approximately that distance below the pupil centers.

2. This point falls between the near and far point directions of gaze so the prismatic effect of the lenses is minimized in either direction. In some cases it might be desirable to lower the centers even more to distribute the anisometropic effects more evenly for both directions of regard.

3. *Properly Centering The Lens*

a. It is not sufficient that the optical center of the lenses be spaced only in accordance with the interpupillary distance of the patient. It is also necessary to be sure that the optic axes of the lenses pass through the centers of rotation of the eyes. Since the exact location of the centers of rotation is not known, it is sufficiently accurate to assume that they lie on the lines of the sight (the line connecting the center of the entrance pupil and the point of fixation). All lenses perform best when the center of rotation is on the optical axis of the lens, giving thereby the widest field and suffering the least aberrations.

(1) If a lens is decentered to match the interpupillary distance of the eyes, but the plane of the lens is such that the optic axis does not traverse the centers of rotation of the eyes, the benefit of the decentration is markedly affected, particularly when the powers are strong. Allen (1962) illustrates several situations involving misalignment of the optic axis both vertically and horizontally (Figure XXVI-33).

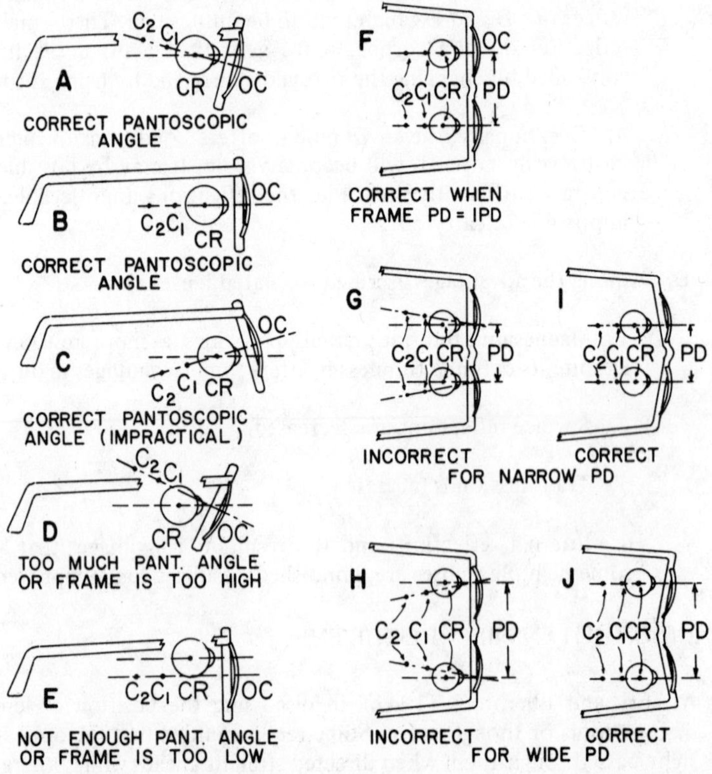

Figure XXVI-33 – Illustration *n* of various correct lens placements in both vertical and horizontal alignment. A, B, C = correct vertical alignment; D, E = incorrect vertical alignment; = F, I, J = correct horizontal alignment; G, H = incorrect horizontal alignment. C_1, C_2 = optic axis; CR = Center of Rotation, OC = Optical Center.

(2) To insure the placement of both the optical centers and optic axis as desired, Allen (1962) proposes the following technique:

(a) The patient fixates either a retinoscope or ophthalmoscope light source while his pupil is observed through the peephole of the instrument by the observer. The latter moves the source until the reflections on both the front and back surface of the lens coincide and appear centered in the patient's pupil.

(b) Raising, or lowering; movement to either side; or tilting of the eyewear may be necessary to produce such alignment of the two images and the center of the pupil, and the position at which this is attained indicates the correct placement and angle of the lens planes and centers.

B. Cylindrical Effect of Obliquity

1. The position of the lenses before the eyes in relation to the direction of sight becomes important when the effects of tilting are considered. When a lens is tilted, the incident light strikes the lens obliquely, introducing marginal or radial astigmatism, even though the light passes through the center of the lens.

a. The change in the power of the sphere through tilting is determined by the formula: $F(1 + 1/3 \sin^2 a)$. The created cylinder power is disclosed by $F \tan^2 a$.

b. A 3.00 D. sphere tilted 20° will result in a compound effect of +2.12⊂+0.40 cyl.

c. A 1.00 D. sphere tilted as much as 45° will result in a compound effect of +1.16⊂+1.00 cyl.

d. An aphakic +12.00 lens tilted the usual angle of 10° will provide a resultant of +12.12⊂ +0.37 cyl.

2. A small angle of tilt is not important in small powers, but where bifocals or aphakic lenses are concerned, the angle of the lenses before the eyes may explain undesirable results (see Chapter XXII – Aphakia).

3. Pascal (1950) offers several simplifications of the formula for determining the effect of tilt upon a correction. The percentage of power added to the original sphere is determined by the square of one tenth the degrees of tilt. For example, if a lens is tilted 20°, the percentage of power added is $\left(\frac{20}{10}\right)^2$, or 4%; if tilted 30°, $\left(\frac{30}{10}\right)^2$, or 9%.

a. For a lens of 8.00 D., tilted 30°, we find the new spherical power to be determined by adding the original sphere, S, to the % of added power of the tilt, S X 9%, to find the new sphere S'; or, S' = 8.00 + 8.00 X .09 = 8.72.

b. The cylinder is found by the formula C = S' X $\tan^2$ angle of tilt.

(1) In the above example, C = 8.72 X $\tan^2 30°$ = 2.91.

c. The total cylindrical power may be found by the formula:

$$\frac{S'}{\cos^2 \text{angle}}, \quad \text{or,} \quad \frac{8.72}{\cos^2 30°} = 11.63 = (8.72 + 2.91).$$

d. If a cylindrical lens is tilted, the tilt is significant only if the lens is tilted on its axis. In that case, no actual spherical power is induced, but S′ is found from the cylinder power, as described above in section a, and the new total cylinder power is found by the formula in section c.

e. In compound lenses, both methods are used and the results combined.

4. The following charts are also utilized by Gamble (1949) and Duke-Elder (after Percival, 1928):

a. Gamble's Chart for effect of a lens tilted in vertical meridian for each diopter:

(1) **Table XXVI-6**

Degrees of tilt	Horiz.	Vertical	Degrees of tilt	Horiz.	Vertical
0	*1.000*	*1.000*	*20*	*1.175*	*1.041*
5	*1.010*	*1.002*	*25*	*1.297*	*1.166*
10	*1.042*	*1.010*	*45*	*2.464*	*1.232*
15	*1.097*	*1.023*			

b. Percival's (1928) chart for resultant spherical and cylindrical power for a lens tilted in vertical meridian, per diopter:

(1) **Table XXVI-7**

Degrees of tilt	Sphere	Cylinder	Degrees of tilt	Sphere	Cylinder
0	*1.0101*	*.0314*	*25*	*1.0648*	*.2315*
15	*1.0228*	*.0734*	*30*	*1.0948*	*.3349*
20	*1.0409*	*.1379*	*35*	*1.1314*	*.5547*

XVII. PRESCRIPTION STANDARDS

A. The Committee on Standards of the American Optometric Association (Morgan, et al., 1952) has reported the following series of standards for prescription lenses. These are summarized in tabular form:

1. **Lenses**	**Tolerance**	**Provision**
a. Type	As specified on Rx.	
b. Color	As specified on Rx.	
c. Surface Defects	No waves, pits, scratches, watermarks, grayness, etc., visible to naked eye.	Inspected by grazing incidence of beam of light from R40 type bulb.
d. Imperfections	No bubbles, striae, etc.	
e. Edge thickness	+ or – .2 mm.	Standard edge thickness of 1.8 mm. at nasal strap unless lens power necessitates variance or Rx requests it.
f. Segment size, inset and height	+ or – .25 mm. and symmetrical upon inspection.	
g. Lens size		
rimless	+ or – .25 mm.	Measured along horizontal and vertical meridians through major reference point.
bevel for zyl	+ or – .25 mm.	
bevel for metal	Fit standard lens size for specified size.	

h. Bevel		
rimless	Edges flat and smooth	
insert	Bevel smooth and straight.	
i. Power		
0 - 5.75	+ or – .06D.	Each meridian of a toric lens is considered separately. The total power through the segment for a bifocal is considered.
6.00 - 12.75	+ or – .12	
13.00 - 16.75	+ or – .18	
17.00 - 20.00	+ or – .25	
j. Cylinder Axis		
0 – .87 D.	+ or – 2½°	
1.00 D. and up	+ or – 1°	
k. Prism Power		Direction of power as specified, and measured at major reference point. A lens with no prism power called for is a 0 lens.
vertical	+ or – .25	
horizontal	+ or – .5	
l. Eye size	+ or – .25 mm.	The horizontal dimension of a rectangle whose sides touch the edge of the lens.

2. In referring to the thickness of the lens, it must be remembered that the thickness will be influenced by the magnification required, by the cosmetic appearance and weight of the lens, the problem of supporting the lens before the eyes, and the factors inherent in the power of the lens. The thickness of the lens can be determined from the formula for magnification given earlier in this chapter, and the effect of the power on the thickness from the formula,

$$\text{Vertex thickness} = \frac{F\,h^2}{2a},$$

in which F is the power of the lens, h is one-half the diameter of the lens, and a is the amount of difference between the indices of the lens and air.

B. The United States of America Standards Association, formerly the American Standards Association, a voluntary organization devoted to the establishment of standards for numerous industries has devised a code, USASA Z80.1-1964, for first quality ophthalmic lenses. This incorporates the features of prescription standards of the American Optometric Association listed under A and adds some criteria for the design of corrected curve lenses.

1. Surface defects in otherwise acceptable prescriptions have been reported to produce impaired acuity and/or annoyance in patient. No relationship was established between sensitiveness to such lenses and prescription, nor to age, sex or race of person.

2. The use of small, intense light sources such as the Sylvania c-100w lamp or the Modernarc is valuable in the detection of surface waves, striae, cracks, pits, veins, bubbles, grayness and orange peel, which are difficult to detect by other methods.

3. Long filament lamps in clear glass envelopes, such as those used in certain showcase displays, can be used to detect surface defects. The reflection of the filament by the irregular lens surface will reproduce breaks or curves in the image whereas smooth surfaces will reproduce continuous, regular images.

REFERENCES AND BIBLIOGRAPHY

Allen, M.J. (1962): How Do You Fit Spectacles? Indiana J. Opt., 32: 5.

**Bailey, N.J. & Hofstetter, H.W. (1959): Effect of Ophthalmic Lens Fluorescence on Visual Acuity. A.A.A.O., 36: 643.*

**Balding, G. & Balding, W. (1954): Clinical Experience With Hard Resin Lenses, E.E.N.T., 33: 677.*

**Bechtold, E.W. (1958): The Aberrations of Ophthalmic Lenses, A.A.A.O., 35: 10.*

**Bechtold, E.W. & Langsen, A.L. (1965): The Effect of Pantoscopic Tilt in Ophthalmic Lens Performance. A.A.A.O., 42: 515.*

**Bender, A. (1955): Prismatic Effect in Single Vision Lenses, O.J.R.O., 92 (24): 44.*

**Bennett, A.G. (1950): Prismatic Effects of Sphero=Cylinders: A New Graphical Construction. Opt., June 30.*

**Bryant, R.J. (1969): Ballistic Testing of Spectacle Lenses, A.A.A.O., 46: 84.*

**Curcio, M.: Lens Effectivity in Relation to True Ametropia. Penn St. Coll. Alum. Bull. 3: 11.*

Davis, J.K. (1957): The Optics of Plano Lenses. A.A.A.O., 34: 540.

**Davis, J.K. (1959): Problems and Compromises in the Design of Aspheric Cataract Lenses. A.A.A.O., 36: 279.*

**Davis, J.K. (1962): Corrected Curve Lenses and Lens Quality. A.A.A.O., 39: 135.*

**Davis, J.K. (1967): Stock Lenses and Custom Design. A.A.A.O., 44: 776.*

**Davis, J.K. & Clotar, G. (1956): An Approach to the Problem of a Corrected Curve Achromatic Cataract Lens. A.A.A.O., 33: 643.*

**Davis, J.K.; Fernald, H.G. & Rayner, A.W. (1964): An Analysis of Ophthalmic Lens Design. A.A.A.O., 41: 400.*

**Davis, J.K.; Fernald, H.G. & Rayner, A.W. (1965): The Design of a General Purpose Single Vision Lens Series. A.A.A.O., 42: 203.*

**Davis, J.K. & Rich, J.B. (1967): Spectacle Lenses for the Myopic Patient. A.A.A.O., 44: 424.*

**Emsley, H.H. (1946): Visual Optics, 4th ed., Hatton Press, London.*

**Fry, G.A. (1950): American Standards for Ophthalmic Lenses. Opt. Weekly, 41: 1469.*

**Fry, G.A. (1960): Lens Prescription and Orders for Eyewear. A.A.A.O., 37: 138.*

Fry, G.A. & Ellerbrock, V. (1941): Placement of Optical Centers in Single Vision Lenses. Opt. Weekly. 32: 933.

Gamble, J.D. (1949): Points in Practical Optics, O.J.R.O., 86 (5): 46; (6): 32.

**Gartner, W.F. (1965): Astigmatism and Optometric Vectors. A.A.A.O., 42: 459.*

**Glancy, A.E.: The Focal Power of Ophthalmic Lenses. Am. Opt. Co. reprint.*

**Goldstein, D. (1964): A Critique of the Sine-Squared Law. A.A.A.O., 41: 549.*

**Graham, R.C. (1946): Reduction of Reflections. A.A.A.O., 23: 145.*

**Graham, R.C. (1949): Plastic Lenses Made of Thermosetting Resins. A.A.A.O., 26: 358.*

**Grolman, B. (1966): New Single Vision General Purpose Lens. J.A.O.A., 37: 553.*

**Gunning, J.N. (1950): Coated Lenses. Opt. Weekly, 41: 201, 239.*

**Hirsch, M.J. (1965): New Ophthalmic Lens Series and Base Curves. A.A.A.O., 42: 370.*

Jones, R.S. (1948): Lens Coatings – Value and Practical Use. O.J.R.O., 85 (11): 36.

**Kaplow, E.L. (1952): Suggestions for Lens Improvement. O.J.R.O., 89 (19): 34.*

Keeney, A.H. & Duerson, H.L. (1953): Evaluation of Plastic Spectacle Lenses. Arch. Oph., 49: 530.

**Knoll, H.A. (1953): The Measurement of Oblique Astigmatism in Ophthalmic Lenses. A.A.A.O., 30: 198.*

**Knoll, H.A. (1962): Ophthalmic Lens Reflections. Opt. Weekly, 53: 1517.*

**Marks, R. (1950): A Progress Report on Plastic Ophthalmic Lenses. A.A.A.O., 27: 242.*

**Mason, W.M. (1948): The Coated Lens. Optics, March.*

**Mattern, R.P. (1948): Reflection Reduction in Spectacle Lenses. Opt. Weekly, 39: 2295.*

**McConnell, J.W. (1965): Minus Cylinders in Single Vision Lenses – An Opposing Position. O.J.R.O., 102 (22): 35.*

**Medoff, H. (1955): The Corrected Curve Story. O.J.R.O., 92 (1): 25.*

**Miles, P.W. (1952): The Importance of Corrected Curve Spectacle Lenses, Am. J. Oph., 35: 1320.*

**Morgan, M.W. (1940): Optometric Optics, U. Calif.*

**Morgan, M.W. (1961): The performance of Ophthalmic Lenses, J.A.O.A., 31: 447.*

**Morgan, M.W. (1963): Distortions of Ophthalmic Prisms. A.A.A.O., 40: 344.*

**Morgan, M.W.; Fry, G.A. & Shepard, C. (1952): Prescription Tolerances and Standards, J.A.O.A., 24: 101.*

Naylor, E.J. (1968): Astigmatic Differentiation in Refraction Errors. Br. J. Oph., 52: 422.

**Neumueller, J. (1948): The Correction Lens. A.A.A.O., 25: 247, 326, 370, 417.*

Ogle, K. (1952): Distortion of the Image by Ophthalmic Prisms. Arch. Oph., 47: 121.

**Pascal, J.I. (1947): Lens Thickness Relative to Form and Power. Opt. World. 35 (1): 15.*

**Pascal, J.I, (1950a): Effects of Tilted Lenses. A.J. Oph. 33: 1599.*

**Pascal, J.I, (1950b): True and Approximate Surface Power. Opt. World. 38 (3): 34.*

**Pascal, J.I. (1952): Selected Studies in Visual Optics. C.V. Mosby & Co., St. Louis.*

**Pascal, J.I. (1952): A Simple Exposition of Image Magnification. Opt. Weekly, 44: 2079.*

Percival, A.S. (1928): The Prescribing of Spectacles. Bristol.

**Peters, H.B. (1962): The Fracture Resistance of Industrially Damaged Safety Glass Lenses. A.A.A.O., 39: 33.*

**Petrie, G.R. (1950): Optical Components in Plastic. Opt., 119: 143.*

Rayton, W.B. (1917): The Reflected Images in Spectacle Lenses. J.O.S.A., 1: 137.

**Sheard, C. (1922): The Effective Power of an Ophthalmic Lens. Am. J. Phys. Opt., 3: 338.*

**Silberstein, I.W. (1964): The Fracture Resistance of Industrially Damaged Safety Glass Lenses. Plano and Prescription – An Expanded Study, A.A.A.O., 41: 199.*

**Sinn, F.W. (1948): An Introduction to the Aberrations in Lenses. Penn. St. Coll. Opt., Alumni Bull., Feb.*

**Sinn, F.W. (1949): Form And Thickness Consideration of Ophthalmic Lenses for Various Near Points. A.A.A.O., 26: 202.*

**Snyder, H.M. (1956): Afocal Lenses in Optometric Practice. Opt. Weekly, 47: 195.*

**Southhall, J.P.C. (1933): Mirrors, Prisms, Lenses, McMillan Co., N.Y.*

**Starkle, D. (1948): Plastics as an Ally of Optical Glass in England. Opt. World, Jan.*

**Volk, D. (1958): Conoid Refracting Surfaces and Conoid Lenses. A.J. Oph., 46: 86.*

**Volk, D. (1965): Aspheric Ophthalmic Lenses in Refraction. I.O.C., Vol. 5, No. 2.*

**Wild, B.W. (1963): Optical and Physical Properties of Safety Glasses. J.A.O.A., 34: 1207.*

Wild, B.W. (1968): A Low Vision Lens For Reading. Opt. Weekly, 59 (15): 36.

**Tehcnical Publications of various manufacturers of lenses and of special optical devices.*

Southhall, J. P. C. (1933): Mirrors, Prisms, Lenses. McMillan Co., N.Y.
Starkle, D. (1948): Plastics as an Ally of Optical Glass in England. Opt. World, Jan.
Volk, D. (1958): Conoid Refracting Surfaces and Conoid Lenses. A. J. Oph., 46.
Wild, B. W. (1963): Optical and Physical Properties of Safety Glasses. J.A.O.A., 34:16.
Technical Publications of various manufacturers of lenses and of special optical devices.

Absorption Lenses 27

I. WAVE LENGTHS

A. Electromagnetic energy includes cosmic rays, x-rays, light, radar, radio waves, etc. The classifications, based upon the wavelengths, are not distinct. These extend from smaller than 0.0001 nanometer (1 nanometer = 10^{-9} meter) to beyond 30,000 meters. The visible spectrum occupies the very narrow range between approximately 390 and 780 nanometers.

1. The sun, usually used as a criterion for light, emits energy to 800,000 nanometers. The short wavelengths are attenuated by the atmosphere. Very little energy below 200 nanometers reaches the earth. Conversely, high energy radiation of short wavelengths presents a danger to life and well being above the earth's atmosphere.

B. The visible spectrum gives rise to the sensation of light.

1. Attributes of light are hue, saturation and luminosity (brightness). (See also Chapter XV.)

a. *Hue* is that characteristic to which we refer when we name a color, i.e., red or green. The correlate of hue is wavelength. For light that is a mixture of a number of wavelengths, the wavelength of the spectrum that most closely matches the mixture color is called the dominant wavelength. Hue can therefore be described by its dominant wavelength. A light of 650 nanometers describes a light having a red hue; 480 nanometers describes a blue light.

b. *Luminosity* refers to the visibility of light. This is a function of the energy of the radiation and the wavelength. Since the eye is the ultimate determinant of visibility, it is customary to establish the energy necessary to just stimulate the eye (the absolute threshold) for each wavelength. The reciprocal of this energy (the sensitivity) plotted against the wavelength specification is called the scotopic spectral luminosity curve (Figure XXVII-1).

2. At absolute threshold the eye does not perceive hue, but merely a gray color. Scotopic vision is, therefore, achromatic. It represents the variation with wavelength of the sensitivity of the rod system of the retina of the eye. The maximum sensitivity is at 510 nanometers.

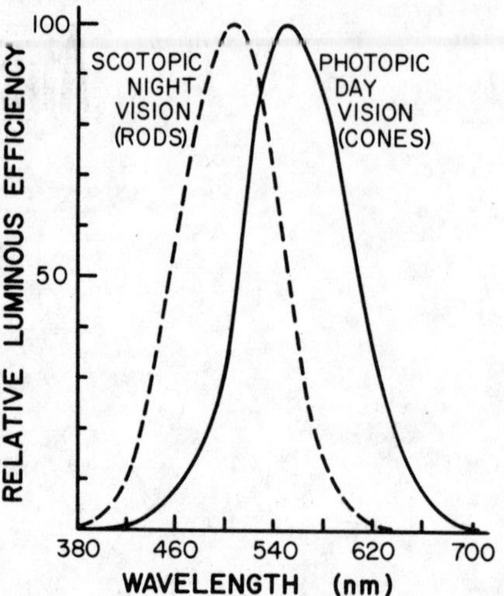

Figure XXVII-1 – Photopic (P) and Scotopic (S) Luminosity Curves.

3. At higher energy levels color begins to be perceived. The photopic spectral luminosity curve is a measure of the sensitivity of the eye for the wavelengths of the visible spectrum based upon a comparison of the luminosity of lights of different colors. In such determinations the observer matches only the luminosity and disregards the differences in hue. The photopic luminosity curve represents the variation with wavelength of the sensitivity of the cone system of the retina. The maximum sensitivity is at 555 nanometers.

C. The portion of the total spectrum which is of primary ophthalmic concern is usually divided into the actinic or ultra-violet, the visible, and the thermal or infra-red.

1. Other radiations such as x-rays, gamma rays and many other forms of nuclear radiations are damaging to the eye, but since they are also damaging to other bodily functions they tend not to be treated as solely an ophthalmic problem. In addition, eye protection from these radiations is not attained by absorptive lenses.

2. In considering the effects of the different portions of the spectrum to the eye, Morgan (1940) divides the spectrum into five sections:

a. Short ultra-violet–13.6 to 310 nanometers
b. Long ultra-violet–310 to 390 nanometers
c. Visible–390 to 780 nanometers
d. Short infra-red–780 to 1,500 nanometers
e. Long infra-red–1,500 to 100,000 nanometers

3. It should be noted that the actinic portion of the spectrum has some thermal effects and the thermal portion has some actinic properties. In addition, absorption of radiation may result in re-emission of the energy in the longer wavelength or thermal portion of the spectrum.

II. ABSORPTION BY THE EYE

A. Absorption follows the Laws of Beer and Bouguer which state that equal thicknesses of liquid or solid absorb equal percentages of the radiation incident upon them. Since each wavelength is treated independently it is possible to have selective absorption and still obey these physical laws.

1. The absorption varies with the individual, age, the specific anatomical region of the eye, and the wavelength. A major factor in absorption, according to Duke-Elder (1938), is the presence of high molecular weight proteins (Figure XXVII-2).

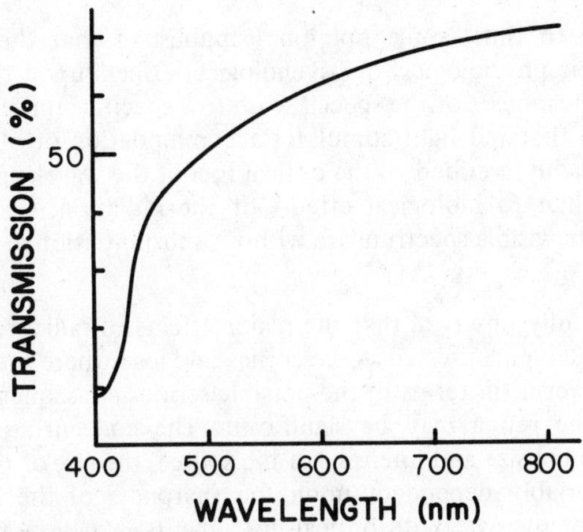

Figure XXVII-2.

B. The absorption of the infra-red varies with the different media of the eye.

1. The *tears* seem to have little absorptive property.

2. The *cornea* absorbs almost all the infra-red above 1500 nanometers and part to the level of 1000 nanometers, but none of the rays below that wavelength.

3. The *aqueous* has the same general absorption as the cornea, but absorbs an additional 20 to 30% of the infra-red which penetrates the cornea.

4. The *lens capsule* exhibits negligible absorption, while, the nucleous exceeds the cortex. Another 30% of the remaining infra-red is absorbed in the lens.

5. Some 60% of the residual of the infra-red is absorbed by the *vitreous.*

6. Approximately 3% of the original infra-red finally reaches the *retina.*

a. Some authorities differ in their interpretations of the effects of infra-red on the eye. Morgan (1940) cites the absorption of the long infra-red by the cornea and the short by the lens. Luckiesh and Moss (1937) report an experiment in which the effects of ordinary sources of infra-red are considered negligible. Others credit infra-red with various effects which will be considered later.

C. The absorption of the ultra-violet seems to take place mainly in the cornea. All ultra-violet, of natural light, below 300 nanometers is completely or markedly absorbed there.

1. The ultra-violet which penetrates the cornea with a wavelength less than 300 nanometers is absorbed almost totally by the lens. As the lens scleroses, the lower level of absorption rises toward 450 nanometers, and in advanced conditions some of the visible violet may also be absorbed.

2. Some ultra-violet may reach the retina.

D. **The effects of radiant energy** are dependent upon the amount of energy absorbed. This means that the inter-relationships of relative absorption and available energy cannot be dissociated. If high energy sources are present, a low absorption by the tissue may still result in a significant alteration of the tissue. Conversely, if there is little energy emanating from the source, it may be immaterial that the tissue absorbs strongly at that wavelength. Ordinarily light is absorbed by the media to so slight a degree that any effects other than those due to photic stimulation of the retinal receptors are too small to matter.

1. From time to time, some opinion is published that the visible portion of the spectrum produces specific physiological or psychological effects upon the visual mechanism which are not the customary responses of the special sense to a specific stimulus. Such claims are highly dubious, and statements that red light stimulates accommodation or blue light inhibits convergence, etc., can be more readily ascribed to the optical foci of the wavelengths in regard to the location of the yellow focus than to biological effects of the radiation. Claims for therapeutic or restorative properties for the visible spectrum are without substantiation at the present time.

2. It can be readily observed that the major effects of radiant energy of the near ultra-violet and near infra-red will be manifested in the cornea and lens where the greater portion of the absorption takes place. However, in terms of the possible serious consequences of damage to the retina, slight absorption at the retina may be significant. The concentration of radiation on the retina is dependent upon the size and intensity of the source, the size of the pupil, and the size of the image. The latter is variably dependent upon the sharpness of the focus which is a function of the refractive state of the eye. With optical instruments it may be possible to concentrate the radiant energy on the cornea, iris, lens or any other site. Such concentrations may prove injurious.

III. EFFECTS ON THE EYE

A. Effects may be either physiological or pathological. Since there is no confirmation of claims that infra-red or ultra-violet is directly beneficial to the eye, only pathological effects may be assumed to result from these radiations.

B. Infra-Red

1. The *long infra-red rays* will produce mild conjunctival irritations. Keratitis is also ascribed to these by some authorities.

2. The *short infra-red rays,* which concentrate mainly in the lens, may produce clouding of the lens, developing into lamellar cataracts. Burn-like lesions of the choroid or retina may also be produced. Others cite clouding of the aqueous and hemorrhagic congestion of the iris as results.

3. Permanent changes are almost exclusively due to local heating of the tissue. When the heat is dissipated slower than the rate of heat inflow, protein coagulation results. Secondary heating can also be produced, such as heating of the lens by heating the iris or electrocautery of the retina through the sclera.

4. Lasers, which are coherent sources of high energy, present unique problems. Some are capable of emitting extremely brief, but strong impulses of light. The heat produced by the laser can be highly concentrated on a small area and can be delivered so quickly that the tissue temperature will be raised above the burn threshold. Burns can be caused by pulsed lasers even after the laser beam is reflected off several surfaces in the room before it enters the eye.

C. Ultra-violet

1. The *short ultra-violet* usually produce inflammation of the conjunctiva and cornea. If the eyes

are exposed for long intervals or for frequent short ones, which have an accumulative effect, abiotic effects such as swelling of the lens capsule, changes in the cell structures of the lens nucleus, and even retinal lesions may result. The latter are thought due to excessive physiological over-stimulation since the affected areas are larger than the areas struck.

a. Experiments by Cogan and Kinsey (1947) upon rabbits have demonstrated the production of ultra-violet keratitis by exposure to wavelengths of 280-295 nanometers.

2. The longer ultra-violet rays produce little damage other than that ascribed by some to fluorescence in the lens. This fluorescence may affect acuity by the haze produced, and it has been observed that cataracts may develop upon exposure to extreme intensities of these rays. Duke-Elder (1938) suggests that the fluorescence serves the purpose of altering harmful short rays to less harmful longer ones.

a. Further experiments, notably by Wolf (1950; also, in Boeder, 1950), have indicated that longer ultra-violet, below approximately 365 nm., definitely affects the dark-adaptation rate and threshold of the rods, and perhaps even the cones to a lesser extent. Direct sunlight may be assumed to include this effect. It should be noted, however, that ordinary sun-glass tints are not sufficiently absorptive to be of great benefit in this regard (Peckham and Harley, 1951).

b. Another interesting report is that of the visibility of certain ultra-violet wavelengths in conditions of aphakia, leading to the apparent conclusion that the upper limitation of the visible spectrum is partially due to absorption of some otherwise visible ultra-violet by the lens and its capsule.

D. Visible Light

1. Although no definite abiotic effects are ascribable to the visible spectrum, excessive light may produce discomfort and asthenopia. This has been related to the motor activity of the iris and ciliary body since the discomfort disappears when drugs are used to paralyze the involved muscles.

2. *Acuity* is affected by the level of illumination. At very low levels of illumination an increase will produce slight improvement in acuity. At levels approaching 5 foot-candles small increases result in marked increases in acuity. Between 5 and 10 foot-candles the acuity continues to improve, but at a distinctly lower rate (Tinker, 1935). Above 10 foot-candles the acuity improves very slightly until finally excessive illumination results in additional scattered light within the eye which in turn produces a veiling glare and lowered acuity. (See also Chap. X, Visual Acuity.)

a. Part of the improvement in acuity is attributed to retinal function and part is due to the smaller pupil size which accompanies high retinal illuminance.

b. Visual performance measured by standards of efficiency or production, and the subjective observations of ease of performance are not wholly in agreement. Since the major task of the refractionist is to provide comfortable as well as efficient vision, the patient's subjective complaint must be given major consideration. Many individuals who exhibit no physical or pathological basis for light sensitivity, do suffer from discomfort when exposed to ordinary levels of illumination, and seem to see better or easier with the slightly reduced illumination. Such cases may be, as is often stated, mainly psychological.

c. Certain cases of ocular pathology may show unusual reversals to lowered acuity at normal levels of illumination. Reduction of the illumination will enhance acuity.

3. Genuinely *excessive illumination* will be painful. Also bothersome and even painful will be glare produced by peripheral light sources, reflections and the uneven illumination of a room or

large area. To most individuals, glare is mostly expressed in terms of excessive lighting, although as seen in Figure XXVII-3, glare may be present under more ordinary amounts of illumination.

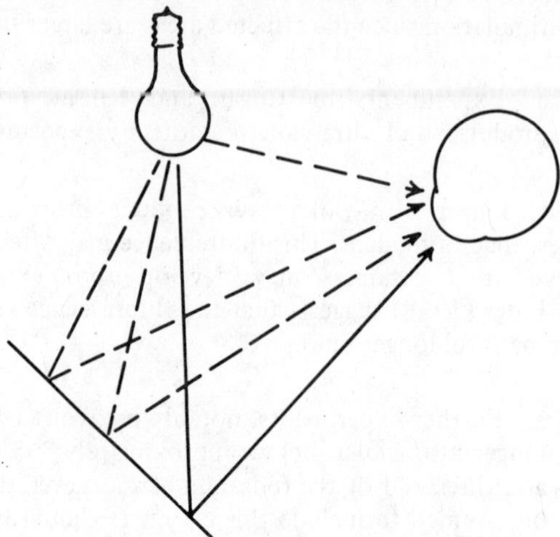

Figure XXVII-3 – Illustrating glare from source of illumination and from surface viewed. Dotted arrows represent light producing glare.

a. It can be observed that a neutral reduction of the light entering the eye will occasionally improve the visual acuity. This is ascribed to several factors–the reduction of the peripheral haze due to glare, the reduction of the slight haze due to reflections between the lens surfaces, and the partial neutralization of the scattered blue rays. In addition, the comfort which tinted lenses seem to provide some individuals is explained not only by the factors affecting acuity, but also by the reduction of the contrasts between surroundings of different illumination levels, or so-called contrast shock. Since absorption lenses reduce illumination upon a percentage basis, a case can be made for the lesser percentage contrast between two levels of illumination with absorption lenses before the eyes.

IV. ABSORPTIVE LENSES

A. Absorptive lenses are frequently called tinted lenses because the glass is not as clear as ordinary crown glass. The tint is not a major factor, but merely a result of the chemicals used to increase the absorption of the glass. The nature of the color or the depth of the color, within limits, is not important, except from a cosmetic standpoint or as a means of identification. The major factor is the absorption curve of the lens. The same color of a lens may be produced by different chemicals, but the absorption properties may not be alike. As Morgan (1940) points out, unscrupulous manufacturers may imitate the appearance of an absorption lens by matching color but without actually matching the absorption curves.

1. Ordinary white crown glass transmits about 92% of the visible wavelengths. Essentially all of the light that is not transmitted is reflected at the surfaces. The amount of visible light that is absorbed for standard lens thicknesses is negligible. Crown glass absorbs almost 100% of the rays above 4,000 nanometers and below approximately 290 nanometers.

2. Absorptive lenses may be classified as either non-selective, uniform absorbers (neutral density filters) or selective (non-uniform) absorbers.

a. Other common terms used for descriptive purposes are *sharp cut-off filters*, implying that the transmission shifts rapidly from a high transmission at one wavelength to a low transmission at a neighboring wavelength; and,

b. *Bandpass filters*, implying a high transmission over a limited range of wavelengths and very low transmission over all other wavelengths.

B. Terms involved in absorption

1. *Transmission (T)* is the amount of light, usually expressed in percent, that passes through the lens compared to the light incident upon it.

2. *Attenuation (A)* is the amount of light, usually expressed in percent, that does not pass through the lens. Attenuation includes the light lost by reflection, scattering and absorption.

a. $T(\%) = 100 - A(\%)$

3. *Transmissivity (t)* is the transmission for a unit of thickness of the material. In ophthalmic work the standard thickness is usually 2.0 mm. although occasionally a 1 mm. standard thickness is employed.

4. *Optical density (D)* is the negative logarithm to base 10 of the transmission.

a. $D = -\log_{10} t$

b. Densities of several components can be added and from the sum the transmission can be calculated.

5. Each of the above terms can be calculated for any wavelength, but custom dictates that, unless otherwise specified, the effects are summed and expressed for the entire visible spectrum.

6. According to Bouguer's Law equal thicknesses of a material transmit equal fractions of the radiation incident upon them. This can be expressed mathematically:

a. $T = t{-}kx$, where T is the transmission, t is the transmissivity, k is the attenuation coefficient and x is the thickness.

b. The graph of transmission versus thickness is an exponentially decreasing function. However, if the percent transmission is plotted on a logarithmic scale and the thickness is plotted on a linear scale, the following is true:

(1) $\log T = -kx, \log t$

(a) For any value of the transmissivity, the graph will be a linear plot.

c. This enables one to use a nomograph to establish the transmission for any thickness.

(1) The maximum transmission for any infinitely thin lens will be the incident light diminished by the light lost by reflection.

(a) For glass of index 1.523 for light that is normally incident upon the surface, this loss will be about 4% per surface or a total of 8%.

(b) If the transmissivity is known, or if the transmission for any thickness is known, a straight line drawn through the points 92% transmission at zero thickness and the second point will establish the straight line graph.

(c) As an example, if in Figure XXVII-4 the transmissivity of Ray-Ban 2 is known as 53% for a 2 mm. thickness, the straight line thereby established will give transmission for any thickness. The transmission for a 1.5 mm. thickness will be 60% and for a 4.5 mm. thickness will be 25%.

7. For industrial work the specification of the transmission is often in terms of Shade Numbers. Shade Number = $\frac{7}{3}$ D + 1

   a. A lens that transmits 10% of the light has a density of 1.0 and a shade number of 3.3.

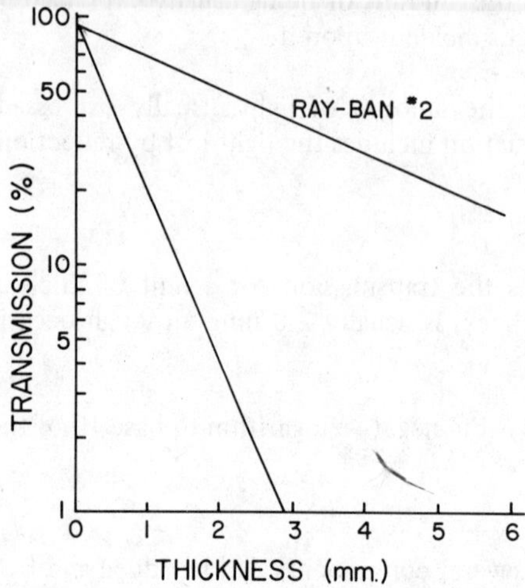

Figure XXVII-4 – Transmissivity per thickness graph.

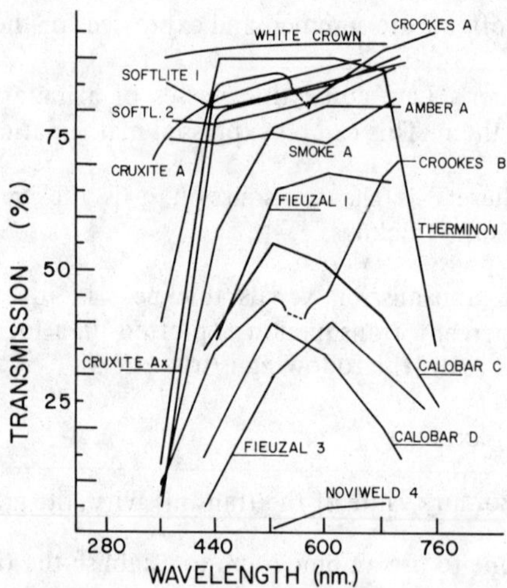

Figure XXVII-5 – Representation of absorption of commonly used tinted lenses.

B. Relation of color to chemical composition

1. As previously stated, the color is due to the nature of the chemical added. Typical colors and chemicals used to secure them are:

   a. Cobalt for blue; chrome and ferrous oxides for green; gold oxide for red; dydinium oxide for salmon; silver and uranium oxides for yellow; manganese oxide for violet; and cerium oxide for brown.

2. Lenses which are identifiable by color and commonly used include (Figure XXVII-5):

   a. Amber–yellow; Amethyst–violet; Blue–blue; Calobar, Rayban, Willsonite–blue-green;

Crookes–brownish-grey; Cruxite–flesh; Soft-Lite–flesh; Fieuzal, Euphos–yellow-green; Noviol–yellow; Viopake–brownish-yellow; Therminon–pale green.

3. If the chemically produced color is uniform throughout the lens, the absorption will only be uniform if the lens is of uniform thickness throughout its area. This is not possible with lenses of refractive power. Convex lenses are usually darker at the centers than at the edge, while concave lenses are usually darker at the edge. By fusing a white refraction lens with a tinted plano lens, uniform absorption can be provided. Similarly, by fusing a tinted section of varying thickness to a white lens, a lens of gradually increasing absorption from one section to the next can be produced.

4. Polarizing lenses are also used as absorption lenses. These lenses absorb about half of ordinary light and almost totally block light polarized by reflection from horizontal surfaces. They are especially effective in reducing glare from water or wet surfaces, or metal surfaces.

5. Absorption is also achieved by partial silvering of a surface of the lens, making the lens into a transparent mirror which reduces the transmission of light by reflecting a portion of it.

V. CLASSIFICATION AND USES OF ABSORPTIVE LENSES

A. Absorptive lenses may be classified in several ways.

1. *Classification by Absorptive Properties* (Obrig, 1935)

a. Neutral density lenses

(1) These lenses are designed to transmit the spectrum in proportion to white crown glass. They are non-selective absorbers and, therefore, reduce the transmission without altering the relative proportions of the various wavelengths. Their benefits result from a reduction in the intensity of the light, a modification of contrast and glare.

b. Ultra-violet absorbers

(1) Almost all glass absorptive lenses absorb strongly in the ultra-violet. Distinction should be made between lenses that absorb strongly only in the ultra-violet and those that absorb strongly throughout the spectrum including the ultra-violet. Cruxite and Viopake are typical of the best known of the former category, but Hallauer, Euphos and Fieuzal also should be included. In the latter category are the neutral greys such as TO-20, True Color, G-15 and the green glasses such as Ray-Ban, Calobar, Contra-Glare and the like.

(2) These are useful for many of the same conditions. In general ultra-violet absorbers transmit large quantities of the visible energy whereas those that absorb throughout the spectrum are of the sunglass category transmitting rather small percentages of the visible.

c. Infra-red absorbers

(1) Relatively few glasses are good absorbers of infra-red radiation. Very few transmit large amounts of the visible and absorb large amounts of the infra-red. It is easier to obtain lenses that absorb large amounts of both visible and infra-red. In the former category are Therminon and Infra-Bar. In the latter category are Ray-Ban, Calobar, Contra-Glare and similar deep tints.

(a) These lenses usually contain some ferrous oxide and, therefore, have a greenish cast of varying intensity depending on the degree of absorption.

(b) The elimination of the infra-red has a cooling effect which is often pleasant to the patient.

(c) Many lenses that absorb strongly in the near infra-red transmit large amounts in the middle and deep infra-red. Where the presence of infra-red radiation is of critical importance the transmission curve of the material in the deep infra-red should be examined carefully.

d. Selective absorbers

(1) Special glasses, often with sharp cut-offs, are used in unusual conditions and for vocational use. Such lenses should be prescribed with care because of their interference with color evaluation. Among these are cobalt glass and the yellow and amber tints.

(a) Didymium, frequently used for laser protection, is a selective absorber with a very irregular transmission curve.

(b) Crookes glass is relatively neutral, but with a decided irregularity in the yellow region. It is said to be habit forming because of this selectivity.

2. *Classification by Color* (Stair, 1948)

a. Colorless lenses include most of the common types which show little or no color unless viewed edgewise, and in which manganese or selenium is included with less iron oxide. These include the common lenses such as Soft-Lite, Cruxite, Velvet-lite, Azurelite, Therminon and Tonetex.

b. Amethyst tinted lenses, including certain shades of Soft-Lite, Velvetlite, Roseite and similar shades.

c. Neutral tints, including Smoke, Polaroid, Crookes, and certain shades of Cruxite, True Color, G-15, G-31, TO-20, and neutral gray.

(1) Cruxite C and B also have cerium oxide added to absorb ultra-violet.

d. Amber shades, which are generally selective and not recommended for color deficients.

e. Yellow tints, which include Noviol, Kalichrome, Nitelite, Willson Gold, and the like, and which are not recommended for color deficients.

f. Yellow-green tints, such as Fieuzal, Hallauer, Euphos.

g. Blue-green tints, such as Calobar, Cool-Ray, Rayban, Willsonite.

h. Blue tints, such as Cobalt and certain shades of Azurelite. These lenses are selective and not recommended for color deficients.

3. *Classification by Purpose* (Joint Committee on Industrial Ophthalmology, 1953)

a. Tinted lenses for general wear. These are most light shades with transmissions of about 80% or more.

b. Sunglasses

(1) Neutral–absorbing the visible spectrum approximately equally.
(2) Colored–exhibiting selective transmission.

(3) Polaroid–transmitting plane polarized light only.

(4) Reflecting–transmitting part of the light and reflecting the rest. It is possible to coat a lens so that it is highly reflecting in one region and gradually less reflecting over neighboring regions. This is known as a gradient density lens. Often such lenses are prescribed so that it is a double gradient density with both the top and bottom parts of the lens gradient coated. The coatings are either nickel, aluminum or an alloy.

c. Tinted lenses for industrial and special uses

d. Variable density or photochromic lenses

(1) Lenses that change their density when energy is applied to them are called photochromic. Although the active materials of these glasses can be either organic or inorganic, they are usually, for ophthalmic purposes, silver halide crystals. In the presence of ultra-violet radiation or deep violet light the silver halide crystal decomposes into free silver and the halogen. In the absence of this radiation a recombination of these components into the silver halide crystals takes place. The essential feature of the glass is that it is nearly transparent when the material is in its chemically combined state and dark when the silver and halogen are uncombined. The process of going from the combined form through the decomposed form of the crystals and back to the combined form constitutes one complete reversible chemical cycle. No significant changes in photochromic behavior have resulted from 30,000 cycles.

(a) The rate of darkening is primarily dependent on the intensity of the light, but would normally range from a fraction of a minute to several minutes to go from maximum transmission to one half its minimum transmission (Figure XXVII-6).

(b) The rate of clearing is primarily determined by the composition of the glass and the heat treatment used in the manufacture of the photochromic glass. Also it usually takes a fraction to several minutes to go from minimum transmission to one-half its maximum transmission (Figure XXVII-6).

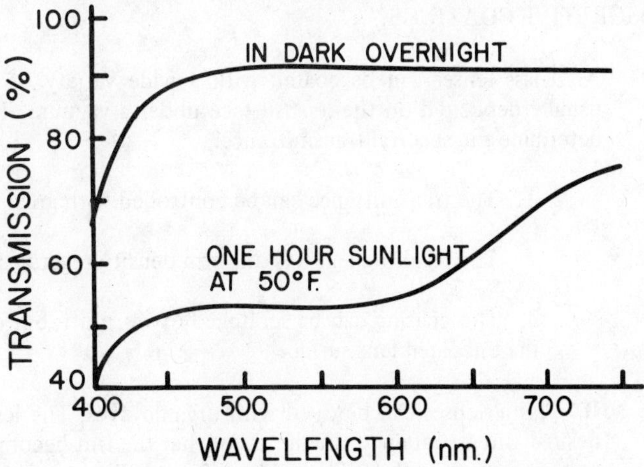

Figure XXVII-6 – Darkening and Fading Curves for Bestlite Photochromic Glass.

(c) Temperature affects both the optical density and the rate of change. Higher temperatures result in higher transmittance for the dark cycle and lower temperatures result in lower transmittance for the dark cycle.

(d) In general, glasses that become the darkest take longer to clear than other glasses that do not become very dark. The clearing can be accelerated by external heating or by exposure to wavelengths longer than those used for darkening.

(2) The transmittance of photochromic glasses is usually low in the ultra-violet and violet and higher in red and in the infra-red (Figure XXVII-7).

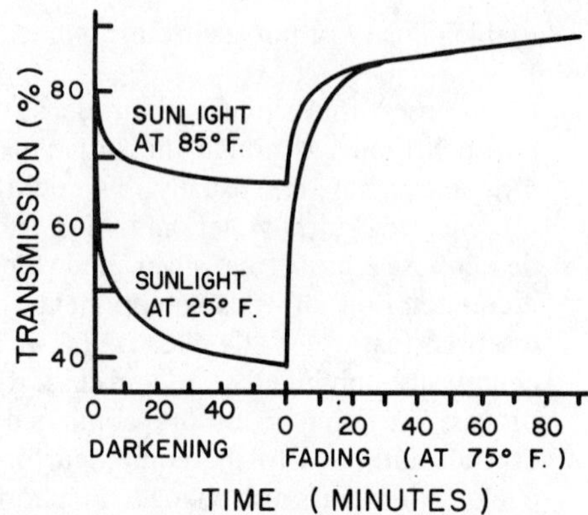

Figure XXVII-7 – Spectral Transmittance Curves for Bestlite Photochromic Glass.

(3) Photochromic glass can be used satisfactorily for single vision or one-piece multifocal lenses because much of the absorption occurs near the surface of the lens and because the optical density of the lens is usually quite low. The lens, especially if of low power, has nearly uniform transmittance over its entire surface.

(4) Photochromic lenses are only marginally useful as sunglasses because of their relatively high transmittance even when they are at their maximum density.

VI. ABSORPTIVE COATINGS

A. Glass lenses can be coated with a wide variety of inorganic absorbing materials. The material is usually deposited on the lens surface under a vacuum. The amount of absorbing material deposited will determine the spectral transmittance.

1. The transmittance can be controlled with great precision to any desired value.

2. The resulting lens has uniform density regardless of the prescription.

3. The coating can be scratched or worn off, but only under conditions that would be harmful to the uncoated lens surface.

B. Plastic lenses can be dyed with organic dyes. The lens is dipped in a warm solution of dye until the desired tint is obtained. In the event that the tint becomes too deep it is possible to remove some of the tint by immersing the lens in a bleaching solution.

1. Several different tints can be applied to obtain the desired tint and transmission.

2. The resulting lens has uniform density regardless of the prescription since the absorption of the dye is essentially a surface effect.

3. The tint is relatively permanent and fades only slightly with age.

C. Purposes and Uses

1. A great deal of propaganda surrounds the entire field of tinted ophthalmic lenses. In an attempt to clarify the atmosphere, a sub-committee of the Joint Committee on Industrial Ophthalmology (1953) derived the following conclusions regarding the subject:

2. *Ordinary Tints*

a. Tinted lenses of the lighter shades, most commonly used, may be useful from a cosmetic standpoint, and where the patient subjectively feels that they are beneficial, but they should not be promoted for relief of photophobia, which is usually pathologic in origin, nor promulgated upon the basis of any physiologic advantages such as reducing difficulty associated with fluorescent lighting, improving the acuity, or similar claims.

b. The primary function of commonly tinted lenses is to reduce the intensity of light. If sunlight produces discomfort, sun-glass shades should help. Where an actual sensitivity to glare from other sources exists, shades dark enough to reduce the glare may be advocated.

(1) Reduction of light to some 60% is required to protect against glare.

c. The denser shades of the milder types of tint may be used for actual photophobia, as ordinarily associated with corneal, conjunctival, or iritic pathology or dysfunction.

3. *Sunglasses*

a. By more or less voluntary standardization, the leading manufacturers of sunglasses have classified the shades of sunglasses into three, or sometimes four, classes. The lightest shades transmit not more than about 60%; the next about 30%, the third about 20%, and where a fourth exists, about 10%. Some distinction of grading by letter or number still exists but generally, a Rayban 1 and Calobar B fall in the first category, while Rayban 3, and Calobar D, as well as Univis Green 3, fall in the third, or most widely used category. The same general groupings apply to most other makes. The transmission curves for the various makes, Calobar, Rayban, Willsonite, etc., are sufficiently similar to be of little importance in prescribing (Stair, 1948).

(1) Of interest in this connection and in regard to the claims previously made about the influence of the ultra-violet upon the threshold adaptation, is the study of Peckham and Harley (1951) in which the conclusion is reached that most sunglass tints are not dark enough to avoid influencing the adaptation rate. Exposure to sunlight at a beach with ordinary sunglass shades provided protection for only one day of exposure. Thereafter the cone sensitivity is affected. Shades as dark as 10 to 12% transmission provided protection for over a week of exposure. The effects are ascribed purely to the excessive light of the visible spectrum, since the ultra-violet and infra-red are eliminated by either type.

4. *Night-Driving Glasses*

a. The use of yellow glasses, under various names, has been advocated for assistance in increasing visibility and guarding against headlight dazzle when driving at night. Broom and Cole (1952) published one study in which the contrast of oncoming headlights was markedly reduced and the general visibility apparently increased. However, as Fry (1952) pointed out in discussing the study, several factors are involved in night driving. These include not merely the dazzle of oncoming headlights, but the ability to see pedestrians and objects on the side of the road, as well as the outlines of the road itself. Any tinted lens can be expected to reduce the total illumination of oncoming lights, but the problem exists of the total reduction of visibility of the road and of objects seen by reflection of the markedly reduced light. Richards (1952) in a report for the Highway Research Board, concludes that yellow glasses do not increase visibility under conditions of night driving levels of illumination, and that they do not compensate for night myopia. The Joint Committee previously mentioned (1953), likewise condemns the advocation of tinted lenses for night driving, as well as heavily tinted windshields, while the National Safety Council (Connolly, 1952) found unanimous opinion among authorities that any advantage gained by reduction of headlight glare is more than overbalanced by extra hazards arising from reduction of visibility of objects at night.

(1) Miles (1954) reports that the use of any tinted lens, particularly the use of green windshields, is dangerous for night driving. He found that acuity, ordinarily reduced to 20/32 under night driving conditions, fell to 20/40 with the second shade of ordinary tinted lenses, and to 20/46 through the green windshield, while the combination of tinted lenses and a green windshield reduced it further to 20/60. Resolution also fell from a threshold of 10 seconds of arc to 42 seconds, which means that two objects discernible as two at 100 feet through the clear windshield would have to approach to 25 feet through the green one to be equally discernible. (See also Chapter X, Visual Acuity, Night Vision.) Other factors, such as stereoscopic acuity, discrimination of angular velocity, contrast, etc., were also adversely affected.

(2) Allen (1965, 1966, 1967, 1968, 1969, 1970) has repeatedly warned of the hazards of tinted windshields. He points out that the greatest hazard is to the older driver whose reduced ocular transmission can ill afford any light loss due to windshield tint or excessive tilt angles. The likelihood of running into a white lighted object at night is not greatly increased by windshield tint, but the likelihood of running into a pedestrian or an animal is. Contrary to popular opinion, the tinted windshield in the daytime is especially hazardous. Because the daytime ambient luminance is often higher than the luminance of the taillight, turn or brake signal, the differentially greater reduction of red by "heat" absorbing (tinted) windshields is not desirable. (In modern automobiles a tinted band at the top of the windshield is always accompanied by a green tint throughout the remainder of the glass).

(3) Allen notes, in addition, that for protanopic and protanomalous color defective drivers, red is almost completely invisible, i.e., a red light may not appear to be lighted. Since tinted windshields absorb red light more than the yellow and green parts of the spectrum, the protanopic and protanomalous color defective driver is even more severely handicapped by windshield tint.

(4) In addition, most yellow absorption lenses almost totally eliminate the blue and violet rays of the spectrum and thus constitute an additional hazard by effectively reducing the total luminance available and by inducing anomalous color vision effects such that blue police lights and other blue warning lights cannot be seen.

5. *Special Purpose Tints*

a. Certain yellow lenses which eliminate the blue end of the spectrum are claimed to be useful for early morning hunting, boating, etc. This claim has not been substantiated despite the fact that there is an apparent increase in brightness when such lenses are worn. It appears that the detectability of threshold objects is impaired. Also there is some fluorescene in most of these lenses which might be a problem. Such lenses include the Noviol, Kalichrome, Rifilite, and Wilson Gold.

b. Polaroid lenses are also advantageous where reflections from the surfaces interfere with visibility into deeper waters. They are especially suitable for automobile driving as they greatly minimize windshield reflections and for certain headings and times of day, they significantly reduce highway, hood, and sky glare.

c. For industrial use in which welding arcs, electric arcs, and other high intensity levels of light are common and must be closely observed, a series of special tints for these industrial purposes have been developed in accordance with federal specifications. These specifications provide that almost all the extra-visual rays of the spectrum be absorbed. To conform with this, most of the red and blue end of the spectrum is markedly reduced or eliminated, with a maximum transmission in the blue-green or yellow-green bands. The following table (U.S.A.S. Z87.1-1968) of standardized shades applies to the commonly used industrial tints such as Noviweld, Arc-Ban, Immunite, Wilson-weld, and so forth.

(1) **TABLE XXVII-1**

Transmittances and Tolerances in Transmittance of Various Shades of Absorptive Lenses, Filter Lenses, and Plate

Shade Number	Optical Density Maximum	Optical Density Standard	Optical Density Minimum	Luminous Transmittance Maximum Percent	Luminous Transmittance Standard Percent	Luminous Transmittance Minimum Percent	Maximum Infrared Transmittance Percent	Maximum Spectral Transmittance in the Ultraviolet and Violet 313mμ Percent	334 mμ Percent	365 mμ Percent	405 mμ Percent
1.5	*0.26*	*0.214*	*0.17*	*67*	*61.5*	*55*	*25*	*0.2*	*0.8*	*25*	*65*
1.7	*0.36*	*0.300*	*0.26*	*55*	*50.1*	*43*	*20*	*0.2*	*0.7*	*20*	*50*
2.0	*0.54*	*0.429*	*0.36*	*43*	*37.3*	*29*	*15*	*0.2*	*0.5*	*14*	*35*
2.5	*0.75*	*0.643*	*0.54*	*29*	*22.8*	*18.0*	*12*	*0.2*	*0.3*	*5*	*15*
3.0	*1.07*	*0.857*	*0.75*	*18.0*	*13.9*	*8.50*	*9.0*	*0.2*	*0.2*	*0.5*	*6*
4.0	*1.50*	*1.286*	*1.07*	*8.50*	*5.18*	*3.16*	*5.0*	*0.2*	*0.2*	*0.5*	*1.0*
5.0	*1.93*	*1.714*	*1.50*	*3.16*	*1.93*	*1.18*	*2.5*	*0.2*	*0.2*	*0.2*	*0.5*
6.0	*2.36*	*2.143*	*1.93*	*1.18*	*0.72*	*0.44*	*1.5*	*0.1*	*0.1*	*0.1*	*0.5*
7.0	*2.79*	*2.571*	*2.36*	*0.44*	*0.27*	*0.164*	*1.3*	*0.1*	*0.1*	*0.1*	*0.5*
8.0	*3.21*	*3.000*	*2.79*	*0.100*	*0.061*	*0.061*	*1.0*	*0.1*	*0.1*	*0.1*	*0.5*
9.0	*3.64*	*3.429*	*3.21*	*0.061*	*0.037*	*0.023*	*0.8*	*0.1*	*0.1*	*0.1*	*0.5*
10.0	*4.07*	*3.857*	*3.64*	*0.023*	*0.0139*	*0.0085*	*0.6*	*0.1*	*0.1*	*0.1*	*0.5*
11.0	*4.50*	*4.286*	*4.07*	*0.0085*	*0.0052*	*0.0032*	*0.5*	*0.05*	*0.05*	*0.05*	*0.1*
12.0	*4.93*	*4.714*	*4.50*	*0.0032*	*0.0019*	*0.0012*	*0.5*	*0.05*	*0.05*	*0.05*	*0.1*
13.0	*5.36*	*5.143*	*4.93*	*0.0012*	*0.00072*	*0.00044*	*0.4*	*0.05*	*0.05*	*0.05*	*0.1*
14.0	*5.79*	*5.571*	*5.36*	*0.00044*	*0.00027*	*0.00016*	*0.3*	*0.05*	*0.05*	*0.05*	*0.1*

(2) The following table lists respective uses for such lenses for welding operations (USAS Z87.1 – 1968):

(a) **TABLE XXVII-2**

Welding Operation	**Suggested Shade Number**
Atomic Hydrogen	*10 - 14*
Shielded Metal Arc, electrode diameter	
5/16, 3/8 in.	*14*
3/16, 7/32, 1/4 in.	*12*
1/16, 3/32, 1/8, 5/32 in.	*10*
Carbon Arc	*14*
Gas shielded Arc (ferrous)	
1/16, 3/32, 1/8, 5/32 in. diam. electrode	*12*
Gas Shielded arc (nonferrous)	
1/16, 3/32, 1/8, 5/32 in. diam. electrode	*11*
Gas welding	
heavy, over 1/2 in.	*6 or 8*
medium, 1/8 to 1/2 in.	*5 or 6*
light, up to 1/8 in.	*4 or 5*
Cutting	
heavy, over 6 inches	*5 or 6*
medium, 1 to 6 inches	*4 or 5*
light, up to 1 inch	*3 or 4*
Torch Brazing	*3 or 4*
Soldering	*2*

C. Summary

1. The employment of the lighter shades is prevalent. While the definite evidence seems to indicate that these shades are of exceedingly doubtful physiologic benefit, many patients prefer them for either cosmetic advantages or because of apparently psychologically induced assumptions of assistance. Whether the cause is purely psychological or not, the tints serve a therapeutic purpose in those cases in which the patient appears to feel an added measure of relief by their inclusion. However, the wearing of tinted lenses seems to have an addictive characteristic so that patients often request increasingly darker shades as time goes on. Likewise, many patients are unhappy if the tint is omitted after one has been worn for some years.

2. The subjective influence is not necessarily one which the refractionist should bow to upon all occasions. Many drivers are personally convinced that night-driving lenses or even sunglasses worn at night are definitely beneficial and that their night vision is improved, despite all measurable evidence to the contrary. However, since decreasing the visibility in this respect carries with it responsibilities and implications of an order entirely different from the mere possible catering to a whim which the ordinary mild tints involve, it may become the definite responsibility of the refractionist to deter the wearing of such darker tints for night driving (Miles, 1954, Richards, 1952).

3. The use of correction sunglasses is increasing. A definite use is served for individuals who are annoyed by bright sunlight. Also, the indication that some adaptation to decreased illumination is affected by sunlight is of concern, particularly, for example, to individuals who spend a day at the seashore and then drive home at twilight (Peckham and Harley, 1951).

4. The use of special purpose tints for vocational and recreational uses is also on the increase, particularly, in the former instance, due to increased government and industrial concern with working standards and safety. The refractionist may only upon occasion be required to consult upon or prescribe such lenses.

REFERENCES AND BIBLIOGRAPHY

**Allen, M.J. (1964): Misuse of Red Light on Automobiles. A.A.A.O., 41: 695.*

Allen, M.J. (1965a): Tinted Windshields Are a Hazard. Opt. Weekly, 56 (18): 76.

Allen, M.J. (1965b): Automobile Visibility Problems. J.A.O.A., 36: 807.

Allen, M.J. (1966): Automobile Windshields: A New Car Study, 1966 Models. Opt. Weekly, 57 (28): 14.

Allen, M.J. (1966): Vision, Vehicles, and Highway Research News (Nat. Acad. Sc.), 25.

Allen, M.J. (1967): The Visual Environment in the Modern Automobile. The Prevention of Highway Injury Symposium, U. Michigan, Highway Research Inst., April.

Allen, M.J. (1967): Tips for Older Drivers. Opt. Weekly, 58 (23): 19.

Allen, M.J. (1968): Report on Windshield Tint and Angles. Physicians for Automobile Safety News Letter, Springfield, N.J., April.

Allen, M.J. (1969): Vision and the Driving Task. Canadian J. Opt., 31 (1): 41.

Allen, M.J. (1970): Vision and Highway Safety. Chilton Books, Phila.

**Allen, M.J. & Crossley, J.K. (1965): Automobile Liquid Glass Tint: A Research Report. A.A.A.O., 42: 344.*

**Bergevin, J. & Millodot, M. (1967): Glare with Ophthalmic and Corneal Lenses. A.A.A.O., 44: 213.*

**Blackwell, H.R. (1953): The Effect of Tinted Optical Media Upon Visual Efficiency at Low Luminance. J.O.S.A., 43: 815.*

Boeder, P. (1950): The Effect of Ultraviolet on the Human Eye. A.A.A.O., 27: 437.

**Bosshard, E. (1957): Vacuum Coated Sun Glass Lenses. A.A.A.O., 34: 394.*

Broom, M.E. & Cole, O.N. (1952): Automobile Headlighting in Night Driving. Opt. Weekly, 43: 409.

**Carter, J.H. (1964): Photopic Ophthalmic Lenses, J.A.O.A., 35: 411.*

**Clark, B.A.J. (1969a): Polarizing Sunglasses and Possible Eye Hazards of Transmitted Radiation. A.A.A.O., 46: 499.*

**Clark, B.A.J. (1969b): Color on Sunglass Lenses. A.A.A.O., 46: 825.*

Cogan & Kinsey, (1947): Ultraviolet Keratitis. Vision, 31 (1).

Connolly, P.L. (1952): Motorist Vision Committee Report on Sunglasses for Night Driving. Mich. Opt., August.

**Davis, J.K. & Fernald, H.G. (1969): Prescription Sungalsses. A.A.A.O., 46: 572.*

Duke-Elder, W.S. (1938): Textbook of Ophthalmology, C.V. Mosby, St. Louis, 1.

**Frajola, W.J. & Ellerbrock, V.J. (1959): Ultraviolet Radiation and the Crystalline Lens. Univis Lens Co.*

Fry, G.A. (1952): Letter to editor: Reference to Broom & Cole, Opt. Weekly, 43: 942.

**Guth, S.K. (1961): Discomfort Glare. A.A.A.O., 38: 247.*

**Henderson, H.L., Kele, T., & Shepperd, H.J. (1968). The Effectiveness of Night Driving Glasses Under Part-Task Stimulation. A.A.A.O., 45: 170.*

**Joint Committee on Industrial Ophthalmology of the Am. Acad. Ophthal. & Otol. (1953): Tinted Optical Media. Reprinted from National Safety News in New Jersey, J. Opt., July.*

**Lauer, A.L. (1951): Further Studies of the Effect of Certain Transmission Filters on Visual Acuity With and Without Glare. Highway Research Board Bull., 43: 44.*

Luckiesh, M. & Moss, F.K. (1937): Infrared Radiation and Visual Function, J.O.S.A., 27: 69.

**McFarland, R.A., et al. (1960): Dark Adaptation as a Function of Age and Tinted Windshield Glass, Highway Research Board Bulletin, 255.*

**Miles, P.W. (1953): Alleged Effects of Tinted Lenses to Aid Vision in Night Driving by Reducing Ultraviolet Light. A.J. Oph., 36: 404.*

Miles, P.W. (1954): Visual Effect of Pink Glasses, Green Windshields, and Glare Under Night Driving Conditions. Arch. Oph., 51: 15.

Morgan, M,W. (1940): Optometric Optics Absorption Lenses, U. Calif.

Obrig, T.E. (1935): Modern Ophthalmic Lenses and Ophthalmic Glass, New York; 3rd ed. (1944) Chilton Press, Phila.

Ogilvie, J.C. (1953): Ultraviolet Radiation and Vision. Arch. Oph., 50: 748.

Peckham, R.H. & Harley, R.D. (1951): The Effect of Sunglasses in Protecting Retinal Sensitivity. A.J. Oph., 34: 1499.

**Publications of various manufacturers of tinted lenses.*

Richards, O.W. (1952): Vision at Levels of Night Road Illumination. Highway Research Board Bulletin, 56.

**Richards, O.W. (1964): Do Yellow Glasses Impair Night Driving Vision? Opt. Weekly, 55 (9): 17.*

**Savell, A.L. (1958): Absorptive Lenses. B.J. Phys. Opt., 15: 236.*

Stair, R. (1948): Spectral Transmission Properties and Use of Eye-Protective Glasses. Nat. Bur. Standards, Circular 471.

Tinker, M.A. (1935): Quoted by Vandergrift and Pascal from A.J. Oph. (1938).

USAS Z 87.1 – 1968 – USA Standard Practice for Occupational and Educational Eye and Face Protection. United States of America Standards Institute.

**Vandergrift, O.W. & Pascal, J.I. (1938): Absorptive Lenses and Their Value. Softlite Lens Co.*

**Van Nus, F. (1967): X-rays and Flint Glass. Opt. Weekly, 58 (16): 21.*

**Wild, B.W. (1961): The Effect of Ultraviolet Light on the Eye. A.A.A.O., 38: 15.*

**Wittekind, J.M. & Hall, R.M. (1952): Compendium on Protective Eye Devices. A.A.A.O., 29: 369, 430.*

Wolf, E. (1950): Night Vision and Ultraviolet. Vision, Am. Opt. Co., 34 (2).

**Wolf, E.; McFarland, R.A. & Zigler, J. (1960): Influence of Tinted Windshield Glass on Five Visual Functions. Highway Research Board Bulletin, 255.*

28 Bifocals, Multifocals, and Progressive Addition Lenses

I. DEVELOPMENT

A. The first lens to have two regions, each of different power, was a composite lens. Benjamin Franklin, bothered by presbyopia and annoyed at having to use two pairs of glasses, had his single vision lenses cut into two pieces. He then had the pieces joined together so that the lens used for seeing distant objects was placed above the lens used for seeing near objects. This design became known as the *Franklin bifocal.* The flat edges of the two portions of the lens made a distinct and sharp line across the width of the lens. The two portions of the lens were held together by the eyewire of the frame. The lens was mechanically weak and tended to come apart, so subsequent innovators tried to cement the two lenses together. When that proved ineffective they resorted to a notch and bevel junction. That was a mechanical improvement, but an optical disadvantage since it broadened the already too obvious dividing line.

1. There were optical advantages to the design. The optical centers were both at the dividing line, so that the wearer experienced no sudden prismatic changes in going from distant to near viewing. No added chromatic aberration resulted. Field of view was excellent.

2. There were also disadvantages. The wide dividing line made the lens cosmetically unattractive, especially after it collected dirt that lodged between the two halves of the lens.

B. The *Solid Upcurve bifocal* was the first commercially successful bifocal that was made from a single piece of glass. This one-piece bifocal was relatively simple to make. The distance prescription was ground on the front surface of the lens and the power of the addition was ground on the rear surface. In order to make this a useful bifocal all that was required was to grind the top portion of the rear surface to make it flat. It was invented in 1837 by Isaac Schnaitmann of Philadelphia.

1. The advantages were numerous. The lens was mechanically strong, provided a wide field of view and was cosmetically attractive. The dividing line was not very obvious.

2. The disadvantages were several. The choice of curves was dependent upon the power of the prescription. This choice rarely coincided with the curves that would have been selected using optical criteria, so aberrations were usually present in significant amounts. Prismatic effects were customarily large since the eye rarely looked along the optical axis.

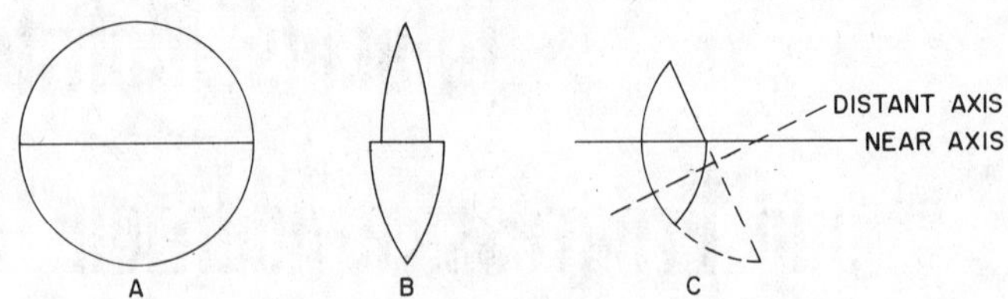

Figure XXVIII-1 – Franklin and solid upcurve bifocals. (A) and (B) front and sideview of Franklin bifocal. (C) Solid upcurve bifocal showing how distant portion is attained by flattening one curve, and how principal axes of distant and near sections are at variance.

C. *The Perfection bifocal*, invented by August Marick in 1888, was similar to the Franklin bifocal. It was made of two different lenses, one having the distance prescription and the other the near prescription. The lenses were cut so that the dividing line was a common arc. The two lenses were then joined. The major advantage to the design was that it was mechanically stronger than the Franklin bifocal. In appearance it resembled the modern Ultex bifocal.

D. *The Cement bifocal* made use of a small lens that was cemented to the distance lens. The distance lens was made with at least one surface spherical. The small lens which provided the additional power for near was made with the radius of one surface, usually the convex surface, equal to the radius of one surface, usually the concave surface, of the distance lens. These matched surfaces were then cemented together using Canada Balsam. The small lens was very thin and was called the wafer. The rear surface of the wafer was chosen to provide the proper amount of additional power for near. The design has been credited to G. W. Wells, G. M. Gould and August Marick. The last named obtained the actual patent in 1888.

1. The advantages were that the lens was mechanically strong and relatively attractive, at least when new. It also offered the possibility of changing the power of the addition quickly and inexpensively without changing the distance lens. It was only necessary to warm the lens to soften the cement, slide one wafer off and replace it with a new wafer. The cement bifocal is still used for temporary prescriptions where frequent changes of bifocal additions are anticipated, such as in post-surgery or in visual training.

2. The disadvantages are that the cement oxidizes as it ages. It becomes discolored and loses its adhesive property. Dirt can collect at the edge of the wafer and, occasionally even under the edge of the wafer. The edges of the wafer may also chip if sufficient care is not used.

E. *The Cemented Kryptok* was the first lens to make use of two different types of glass in the same lens. It was constructed on the same principle as the modern kryptok by grinding a cavity in the front surface of a crown glass lens and filling it with a flint button of matching curves. The button was held in place by a thin crown cover glass. It is credited to John L. Borsch in 1899.

1. The many surfaces which had to be matched made its construction expensive. The fragility of the cover glass made the lens design impractical.

F. *The Monaxial bifocal* is a one-piece bifocal of unique design that was made by grinding the back surface of the reading segment so that its radius of curvature measured from the top of the segment passes through the center of curvature of the back surface of the distance portion.

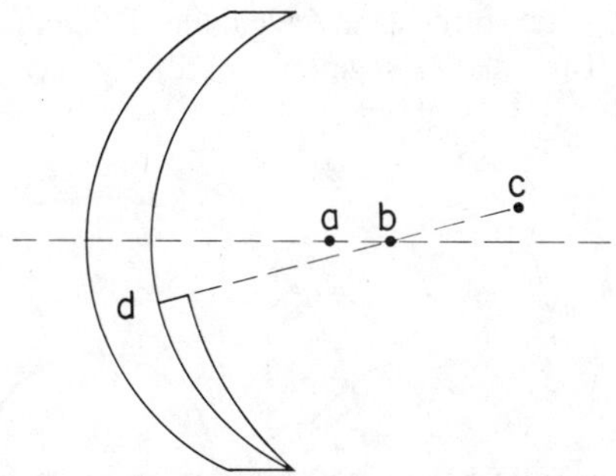

Figure XXVIII-2 – Monaxial bifocal construction, *a* center of curvature of front surface; *b* center of curvature of back surface of distant section; *c* center of curvature of segment placed on radius of curvature joining the point of union of the segment, *d*, with the center of curvature of the back surface, *b*.

II. MODERN BIFOCALS

A. *The Kryptok bifocal* was the first fused bifocal that was commercially available. It is still widely used. The design, as developed by John L. Borsch, Jr. in 1908, made use of a distance lens of crown glass and a segment lens of flint glass. A cavity, the countersink, was ground in the front surface of the lens. The segment glass was made into a small lens called the button which was then fused to the countersink curve. This eliminated the need of the cover glass which was necessary in the Cemented Kryptok.

1. The back surface of the segment button and the surface of the countersink curve into which the button fits are not ground to identical curves. The process depends upon the melting of the flint button so that it fills the countersink concavity. If the heat is not carefully controlled in the fusing operation the countersink curve will warp and will produce an unwanted cylinder or other optical aberrations.

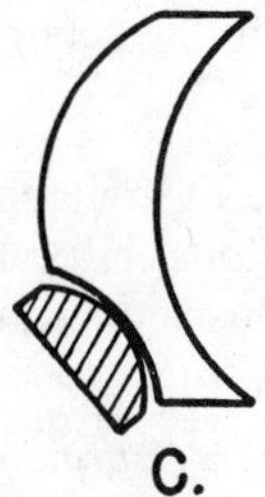

C.

Figure XXVIII-3 – Flint button placed in countersink of major lens for fusing.

B. *The Ultex bifocal* appeared in 1910. It is a one-piece bifocal with the segment ground on the rear surface. It was designed to decrease the amount of chromatic aberration that was found in the fused bifocal designs. The optical center of the segment is usually at a considerable distance from the top of the segment. This results in a large prismatic jump.

1. As seen in Figure XXVIII-4, this type of lens is made by grinding two curves on one surface of a lens blank. After that the blank is divided into two parts, each of which is a semi-finished lens.

2. Various types of Ultex bifocals are available. The major difference between them is the size of the round segment. The smaller segments naturally have a smaller field and smaller amounts of prismatic jump.

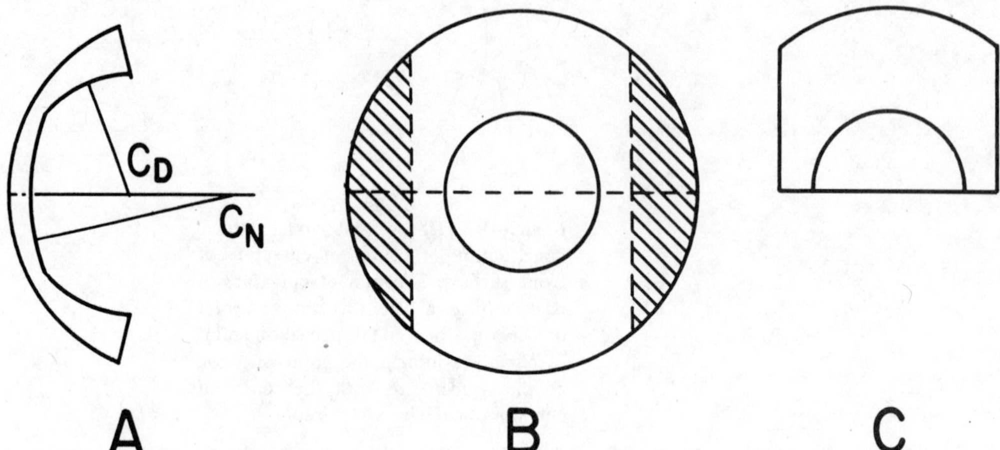

Figure XXVIII-4 – A. Side View of an Ultex A Double Blank. C_d is the center of the curvature of the distance portion of the rear surface. C_n is the center of curvature of the near portion of the rear surface. B. Rear view of the same blank with the segment shape outlined with a solid line and with the two final lens shapes outlined with dashed lines. Cross hatched area is discarded in the final lens blank. C. Finished Ultex A Lens Blank.

C. *The Round Barium (Nokrome) bifocal* differs from the kryptok bifocal in the use of a high index barium crown glass for the segment instead of flint glass and in the close matching of the countersink curve and the rear surface of the button. Close matching of curves cuts down on the heat required for fusing the glasses. This in turn results in more accurate curves and better lenses. The relative dispersion of barium crown glass is almost identical with that of ophthalmic crown glass. Thus, the dispersion produced by the segment of a barium crown bifocal is less than that of a comparably shaped flint segment. However, since it is the dispersion of the whole lens that is important rather than just the segment, the distance lens power is also important in the determination of the total lens performance.

1. Round segment bifocals, especially those of low add power and those having small segments, are among the least conspicuous of conventional bifocals. Only the cosmetic or blended bifocals and the progressive addition lenses are less conspicuous multifocals.

D. *The Tillyer, Sovereign, Panoptik, Univis, Shuron Continental, Kurova, Titmus X-Cel, Kote-line* and other similar lenses are made using comparable techniques. For flat top segments the round button is ground to the desired shape and the portion that was ground away is replaced with ophthalmic crown. (Fig. XXVIII-5) In the next step these two dissimilar glasses are fused to form the segment button. Finally this button is placed in the countersink of the main lens and fused to form the bifocal.

1. For more complex shapes it is necessary to form a button carrier of ophthalmic crown glass into which a hole having the proper segment shape has been milled. In some instances the segment is ground to the same shape and inserted into the carrier hole and fused to form the button. In other instances molten glass is placed in the carrier hole to form the button. In each case the button is fused to the main lens blank which has the receptive countersink already ground in it.

2. Univis and Shuron/Continental employ a barium glass of lower dispersive power to form the button. It is precisely ground to match the countersink curve of the main lens. The congruity of the curves is checked using the Newton Ring Test.

3. The American Optical Company uses a barium glass of 1.66 index for its Fulvue and Sovereign lenses.

4. The Bausch and Lomb Panoptik lenses utilize baryta glass for the segment and Nokrome crown glass for the distance lens.

5. Various other bifocals similar to the above mentioned forms have been described. The names are different, but the principles of construction are similar to those already described.

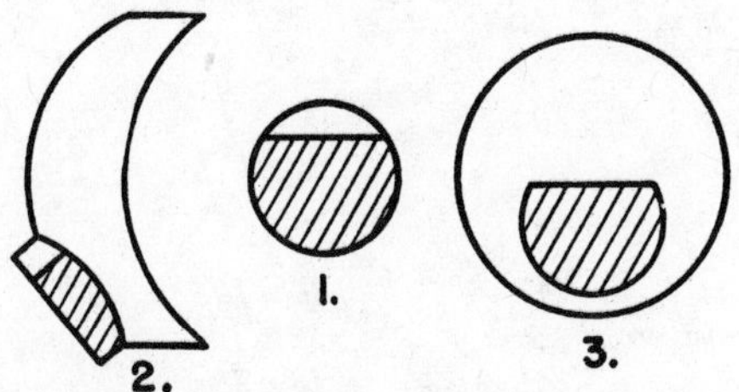

Figure XXVIII-5 – Construction of modern "straight top" type bifocals. 1. Front view of segment button, showing top of flint or barium segment shaped and crown fused to it to complete button. 2. Side view showing exact fit of button to countersink. 3. Front view of finished lens showing blend of crown of button with crown of major lens, leaving modern shaped segment of flint or barium.

E. *The Executive or Dualens* is a one-piece lens bifocal with two different curves ground on the front surface. The dividing line between the distance lens and the segment is a straight line that divides the lens blank in two. The optical centers of both the distance lens and the near lens lie on the dividing line. It is classified as a monocentric bifocal. The difference in curves between the distance and near portions of the lens produces a ledge that is most prominent toward the outer edges of the lens.

III. SPECIFICATIONS OF MODERN FORMS (From data of respective manufacturers)

A. Specifications Of Construction

Table XXVIII-1

Name	Form	Seg glass	Chromatism	Curves	Jump	Usual blank mms.
Kryptok	*fused*	*flint*	*Yes*	*4;6;8;10*	*yes*	*54*
Nokrome	*fused*	*barium*	*no*	*4;6;8;10*	*yes*	*54*
	known as Orthogon, Tillyer, CFR, etc. when on corrected curves					
Sovereign	*fused*	*barium-baryta flint*	*little*	*corrected curves*	*reduced*	*58*
X-Cel	*fused*	*barium type*	*slight*	*corrected curves*	*reduced*	*55x60*
Titmus	*fused*	*barium-baryta*	*little*	*corrected curves*	*reduced*	*54*
Panoptik	*fused*	*baryta*	*little*	*corrected curves*	*reduced*	*54*
Kote-Line	*fused*	*barium type*	*little*	*4.25;6.25;8.25; 10.25 and special*	*reduced*	*58*
Vision-Ease	*fused*	*barium type*	*little*		*reduced*	
Kurova D	*fused*	*barium type*	*slight*	*0;4.25;6.25;7;25;9.25; 10.25;12;13;15;16*	*reduced*	*55x60;60 rd.*
Ultex	*ground*	*crown*	*none*	*−4;−6;−8*	*varies*	*52-55 x 46-62*
Executive	*ground*	*crown*	*none*	*corrected curves*	*none*	*60 x 56*

B. Appearance, Sizes, Etc. (Table XXVIII-2)

Table XXVIII-2

Shape	Name	Style and/or	Size	Seg Pole from seg top	Prism in seg
1. Round segs	*Kryptok*		*22*	*22*	*no*
(fused)	*Nokrome*		*13*	*6½*	*no*
	Orthogon	*C*	*16*	*8*	*no*
	Tillyer	*D*	*20*	*10*	*no*
	Titmus	*F, O, CFR*	*22*	*11*	*no*
	Unachrome				
	Kurova				
	Vision-Ease				
	X-Cel				
(one piece)	*Ultex*	*B*	*11*	*5.5*	*no*
	Kurova	*M*	*22*	*11*	*yes*
2. Hemispheres	*Ultex*	*A*	*38 x 19*	*19*	*yes*
(one piece)	*Kurova, etc.*	*E*	*32 x 16*	*16*	*yes*
		AL	*33 x 38*	*33*	*yes*
		AA	*38 x 30-32*	*19*	*yes*
		L	*32 x 24-26*	*16*	*yes*
3. Arched top	*Sovereign*	*C*	*20, 22, 25 x 14.5, 16, 17.5*	*3.5-4*	*to 4½ vert. & slab off*
Round Bottom	*Panoptik*	*B&L Reg*	*22 x 14.5*	*3.5*	*to 1½ in or out*
(fused)		*LS*	*24 x 16*	*3.5*	
		PR	*21.5 x 14.5*	*3.5*	*to 4 any merid.*
	Titmus	*CT*	*22 x 14.5; 24 x 16*	*3.5*	
	Univis	*F*	*22 x 14.5*	*3.5*	
(one piece)	*X-Cel*	*D*	*20, 22, 25, 28, 35 wide*		
4. Straight Top	*Univis*	*D*	*20, 22, 25 x 15, 16*	*5*	*slab-off*
(fused)	*Tillyer*	*S*	*20, 22, 25, 28 x 15, 16, 17.5, 20*	*4-5*	*slab-off*
	Titmus	*ST*	*22, 25, 28, 45 x 14, 15*	*5*	*slab-off*
	Kurova	*D*	*22-28 x 16-19*	*5*	*slab-off*
	Vision-Ease	*D*	*20, 22 x 15, 16*	*5*	*slab-off*
	Kote-Line	*D*	*22½, 25, 28, 35 wide*	*4-5*	*slab-off*
	Univis	*B*	*22 x 9*	*4.5*	*slab-off*
	Vision-Ease	*B*	*20, 22 x 9*	*4.5*	*slab-off*
	Kote-Line	*R*	*22 x 9*	*4-5*	*slab-off*
	Univis	*R*	*28 x 14*	*7*	*slab-off*
	Vision-Ease	*R*	*22, 26 x 14*	*7*	*slab-off*
	Kote-Line	*R*	*22 x 14*	*7*	*slab-off*
	Univis	*R Comp*	*20 x 14*	*4-10*	*to 1½ vert.*
	Vision-Ease	*R Comp*	*22, 26 x 14*	*0-10*	*by varying pole*
	Univis	*Prism D*	*20 x 14*	*7*	*to 2 base-in*
	Univis	*D 28, 35*	*28 x 19; 35 x 22.5*	*5*	*to 1½ base-in*
	Vision-Ease	*Cen-Cor D*	*28 x 19*	*5*	*by decentration*
	Univis	*IS 22*	*22 x 15*	*4*	
(one piece)	*Executive*	*one piece*	*60 x 25*	*0*	*no*

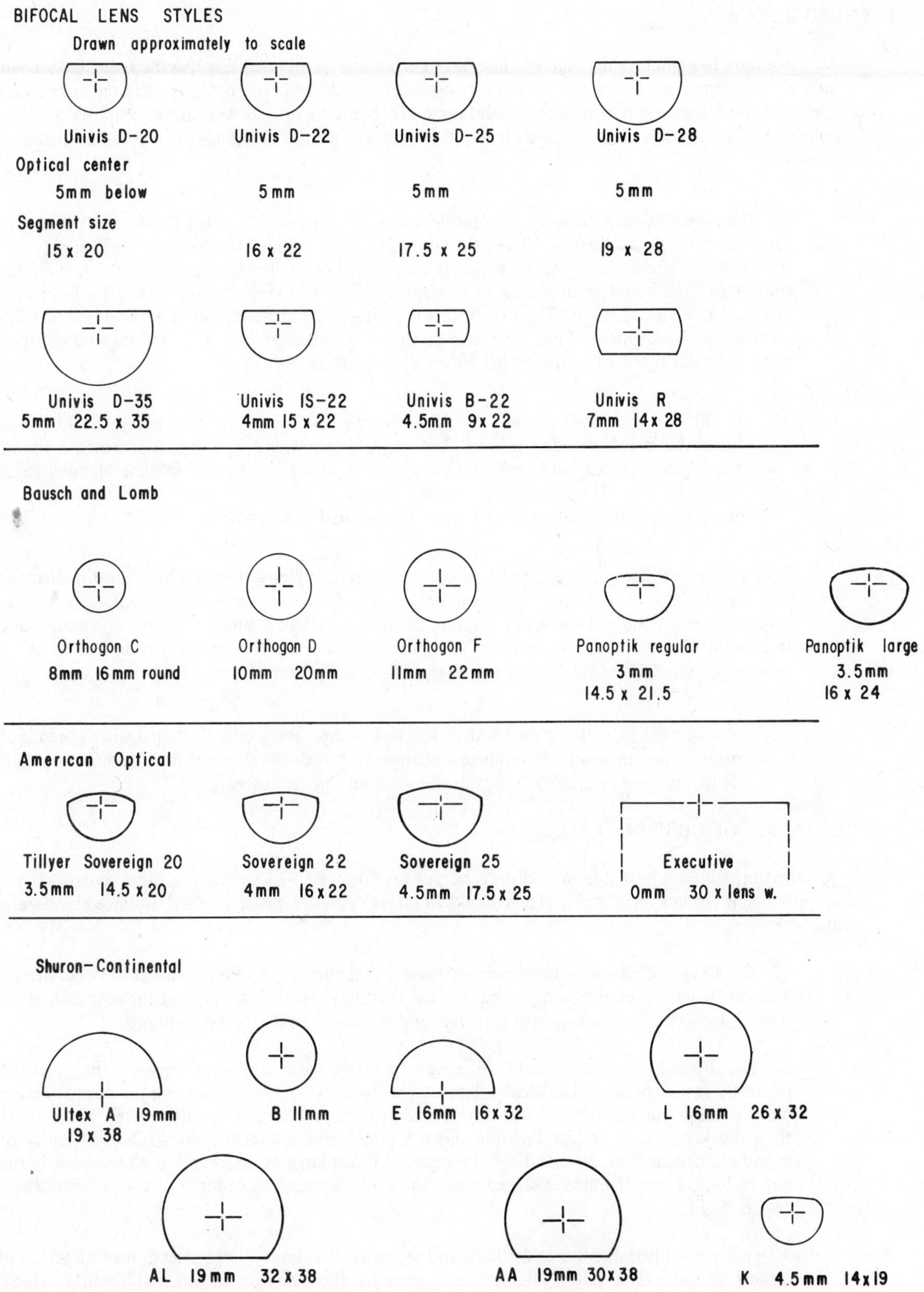

BIFOCAL LENS STYLES
Drawn approximately to scale

Univis D-20 | Univis D-22 | Univis D-25 | Univis D-28

Optical center
5mm below | 5mm | 5mm | 5mm

Segment size
15 x 20 | 16 x 22 | 17.5 x 25 | 19 x 28

Univis D-35
5mm 22.5 x 35

Univis IS-22
4mm 15 x 22

Univis B-22
4.5mm 9 x 22

Univis R
7mm 14 x 28

Bausch and Lomb

Orthogon C
8mm 16mm round

Orthogon D
10mm 20mm

Orthogon F
11mm 22mm

Panoptik regular
3mm
14.5 x 21.5

Panoptik large
3.5mm
16 x 24

American Optical

Tillyer Sovereign 20
3.5mm 14.5 x 20

Sovereign 22
4mm 16 x 22

Sovereign 25
4.5mm 17.5 x 25

Executive
0mm 30 x lens w.

Shuron-Continental

Ultex A 19mm
19 x 38

B 11mm

E 16mm 16 x 32

L 16mm 26 x 32

AL 19mm 32 x 38

AA 19mm 30 x 38

K 4.5mm 14 x 19

Figure XXVIII-6 – Specifications of Some Modern Bifocals.

IV. BLENDED BIFOCALS

A. Attempts to eliminate the segment line have been made in order to disguise the fact that the lens is a bifocal. The lenses currently available are one-piece bifocals with the obvious differences between the curves of the distance and near portions eliminated by blending one curve into the other by grinding and polishing. The only advantage to such lenses is cosmetic since the blending introduces unwanted optical effects.

1. The *Beach Blended Bifocal* was developed in 1946 by Mr. Howard D. Beach. The segment is located on the front surface. The optical correction is contained in a circular area roughly 10 mm. in diameter. The blended region which is an annulus encircling the segment is approximately 18 mm. wide. The blending produces an unwanted cylindrical effect whose power is about equal to the power of the addition. The axis of this unwanted cylinder is oriented parallel to a line tangent to the circular segment. Thus, the axis of this unwanted cylinder will vary depending upon the portion of the annular blend through which the patient is looking.

a. In a second study made by Knoll in 1962 an analysis was made on the so-called Improved Beach Blended Bifocal. The major differences noted were a decrease in the size of the segment to about 8 mm. and a decrease in the width of the annular blended region to about 12 mm. The more rapid change that results from the narrower blended area causes more unwanted cylindrical power than the original Beach bifocal.

2. The *Younger Seamless Bifocal* is also a bifocal with a blended region between the distance and segment regions of the lens. The segment is on the front surface. The optical correction is contained in a circular area about 16 mm. in diameter. The blended region is an annulus about 7 mm. wide. The blending produces an unwanted cylindrical effect of considerable magnitude. The unwanted cylinder is several magnitudes larger than the power of the addition.

a. According to the manufacturer the lens is now being manufactured with a blended zone of 11.75 mm. in width. With abrupt changes of power the segment line becomes more visible. Thus, for lenses of high add power the segment line is noticeable.

V. CONSIDERATION OF DIFFERENT FORMS

A. Most bifocals are available in additions of powers from +0.50 to +4.50 diopters, but other powers are obtainable upon special order. Lens blanks of larger diameter, usually called oversize blanks, are also available.

1. The Kryptok bifocal is not made with corrected curves. The flint segment has high dispersion. The construction requires a high heat to fuse that may result in warping of the segment. However, it is relatively inexpensive, almost invisible, and popular despite its shortcomings.

2. The Round Barium segment bifocals are made with corrected curves. The segment has relatively low dispersion. The close tolerances of the curve of the button and the countersink curve make possible the use of low heat during the fusing operation. It is only slightly more expensive than the kryptok, is almost invisible and is a popular high quality bifocal. One difficulty of the round segment is that the width of the segment is not large at the very top. Consequently, the eye has to look a considerable distance down into the segment in order to get a satisfactorily wide reading field.

3. One piece bifocals offer wide fields and segments that have a large selection of locations of the optical centers. The latter characteristic governs the amount of prismatic jump. One piece segments have relatively small amounts of dispersion. Ultex style bifocals are not very visible because the ledge formed by the segment is small. The Executive style bifocal is quite conspicuous

because of the large differences in curves of the distance and near portions of the lens. The wide field of the Executive bifocal has made this design very popular.

4. The modern fused bifocal types, including the flat top and the arched top segments, are more noticeable than the round segments, at least insofar as the top of the segment is concerned. This is especially true of the 35 mm. and 45 mm. diameter flat top segments. The conspicuousness of the top of the segment is often lessened by the application of a coating. The bifocals of this type offer greater reading field upon crossing the segment line. They may, depending on the type and size of segment, offer a large distant field around the segment.

B. The modern high quality bifocals generally use three different types of glass: flint, barium, and baryta, which is a barium and flint mixture. If the mixture contains, for example, 30% of barium oxide, 40% silica, and less than 10% each of other components, it is known as barium crown glass; but if it contains 25% barium oxide, 35% silica, and 20% lead oxide with other minor elements, it is known as baryta or barium flint. Most companies use some baryta in higher adds in order to obtain the necessary refractive power.

1. Sinn (1948) made a study of the dispersion of different types of segments in prescriptions of varying distance power. His results show that the dispersive value of barium crown and of one piece bifocals is practically equal at all points, while that of barium crown as compared to flint itself varied in accordance with the add called for and the distance prescription.

a. Thus for the following range of adds, the comparative dispersion was found to be:

(1) Adds of 1.00 D:

(a) Flint has a higher dispersion from +5.00 to –2.00 D. distance power of the lens, but less dispersion from –3.00 up to –20.00 D. distance power.

(2) Adds of 2.00 D:

(a) Flint has a higher dispersion from +5.00 to –5.00, but less from –6.00 to –20.00.

(3) Adds of 3.00 D:

(a) Flint has a higher dispersion from +5.00 to –8.00, but less from –9.00 to –20.00.

C. Morgan (1963) analyzed the optical performance of eight common bifocal designs for distance prescriptions of +4.00, +2.00, –2.00 and –4.00 diopters for an addition of +2.00 diopters. He concluded that the image seen through the bifocal segments, although blurred by oblique astigmatism, longitudinal chromatic aberration and chromatic dispersion, was dependent upon the interrelationships of the aberrations. The aberrations interact and the errors may tend to cancel. Image quality was best for different bifocal designs depending upon the distance prescription. With a +2.00 add, the best image qualities were produced by the Nokrome for the +4.00 distance power, the Univis D-22 for the +2.00 distance power, and the Executive for the –2.00 and –4.00 distance power.

1. Thus, it may be seen that no one best type of glass for bifocals exists. The choice of the required bifocal must be made in accordance with the distance power, the power of the add, the size and position of the segment, the need of the patient, the characteristics in other regards such as the location of the poles of the segments, etc.

VI. TRIFOCALS AND MULTIFOCALS

A. Lenses which contain powers prescribed for visual functions at more than two distances or through more than two different areas of the lens are usually called trifocals. Customarily, trifocals are adapted for distant vision, for near vision and for a plane between the two. While originally recommended for vocational purposes, their prescription for ordinary wear for individuals requiring bifocal additions of 1.75 D. and upwards is becoming more and more prevalent. They provide the most flexible visual range when presbyopia is quite advanced, although they must be carefully placed and adjusted and require a period of adaptation. Most trifocals have the intermediate addition in fixed proportion to the reading addition. Also, most trifocals are confined to either one piece construction or to the fused forms of so-called modern design having either straight or curved tops. Trifocals are made with an intermediate section placed between the distance and reading segments, or with two separated segments in the distance lens.

1. The increased employment of trifocals has been due to a variety of factors. These include a more general awareness of the advantages of trifocals, a policy by some manufacturers of guaranteed replacement of trifocals with bifocals in an attempt to reassure hesitant practitioners to use trifocals, the introduction of trial lenses to facilitate demonstrating the advantages of trifocal lenses, and the design and manufacture of new and varied types of trifocals. In addition, are the increasing number of older persons in a steadily increasing population, the employment of older people at tasks and duties involving a greater range of vision, and the increased availability of recreational time for a wider range of avocations and hobbies. From a purely physiologic standpoint, the optical necessity of the intermediate power can be readily demonstrated by a consideration of the far and near limitations of the distance and near corrections of the usual range of bifocal powers. The following charts indicate the variations in the range of the usual bifocal powers as compared to various trifocals. (Borish, 1947)

a. Table XXVIII-3

Using a 13-inch Near Working Distance

		Bifocal			**Trifocal**								
					Ultex-Univis-Kurova Modern-Fulvue			**Orthogon ST Panoptik**			**Orthogon A**		
Add	**Amp**	*PP***	*P*	*PR***	*PP*	*P*	*PR*	*PP*	*P*	*PR*	*PP*	*P*	*PR*
1.5	*3*	*9*	*13*	*26*	*11*	*18*	*53*	*11½*	*20*	*80*	*9-10*	*14-16½*	*29-45*
1.75	*2.5*	*9½*	*13*	*23*	*12*	*19*	*45*	*12½*	*21½*	*64*	*10-11*	*15-17*	*29-35*
2.	*2*	*10*	*13*	*20*	*13*	*20*	*40*	*12½*	*14*	*36*	*12-13*	*17-19*	*29-35*
2.25	*1.5*	*11*	*13*	*18*	*15*	*22*	*35*	*14*	*16*	*32*	*14-15*	*19-22*	*29-35*
2.5	*1*	*11½*	*13*	*16*	*18*	*23*	*32*	*17*	*21*	*28½*	*17*	*22*	*29*
2.75	*.5*	*12*	*13*	*14½*	*22*	*25*	*29*	*20*	*23*	*26*	*22*	*25*	*29*
3.	*0*	*13*	*13*	*13*	*26*	*26*	*26*	*20*	*20*	*20*	*29*	*29*	*29*

Using a 16-inch Near Working Distance

		Bifocal			**Trifocal**								
					Ultex-Univis-Kurova Modern-Fulvue			**Orthogon ST Panoptik**			**Orthogon A**		
Add	**Amp**	*PP*	*P*	*PR*	*PP*	*P*	*PR*	*PP*	*P*	*PR*	*PP*	*P*	*PR*
1.5	*2.0*	*11½*	*16*	*26*	*14½*	*23*	*53*	*16*	*18*	*80*	*12*	*17*	*29*
1.75	*1.5*	*12*	*16*	*23*	*17*	*25*	*45*	*11½*	*29*	*64*	*14*	*19*	*29*
2.	*1.0*	*13*	*16*	*20*	*20*	*26*	*40*	*14*	*25*	*36*	*17*	*22*	*29*
2.25	*.5*	*14½*	*16*	*18*	*25*	*29*	*35*	*22*	*26*	*32*	*22*	*25*	*29*
2.5	*.0*	*16*	*16*	*16*	*32*	*32*	*32*	*28½*	*28½*	*28½*	*29*	*29*	*29*
2.75	*.0*	*14½*	*14½*	*14½*	*29*	*29*	*29*	*26*	*26*	*26*	*29*	*29*	*29*
3.	*.0*	*13*	*13*	*13*	*26*	*26*	*26*	*20*	*20*	*20*	*29*	*29*	*29*

*Bausch and Lomb manufacture an Ultex trifocal with a fixed intermediate add of 1.37 regardless of the reading addition; American Optical Co. varies their Tillyer one piece intermediate as prescribed.

**PP designates the near point of the range, PR the far point.

2. However, many other considerations besides the purely focal features of the lens powers are involved. Ellerbrock and Zinnecker (1950), studying the ranges of the various lenses and powers as compared to the amplitudes of accommodation, similar to the charts used, call attention to the fact that different authorities vary in their interpretation of the relative amount of accommodation which should be held in reserve for comfort. While the customary amount is considered to be one-half the amplitude, some authorities recommend that at least two-thirds the amplitude be reserved, while some even establish a fixed amount, 2.50 D., to be held in reserve at any age, or all of it if the total is below that quantity. They establish four factors which would call for the use of an intermediate segment.

a. A consideration of the range of available vision through the different powers of the lens.

b. The distance of the far-points of the near, intermediate and far sectors.

c. Elimination and reduction of the "uncomfortable distance" where more than a given percentage of the amplitude must be used for prolonged and critical vision.

d. Elimination or reduction of the "blurred distance" when attempts are made to employ more than the total amplitude or less than zero accommodation through the far or near portion respectively.

(1) Of the factors, the ranges developed by consideration of the optical factors determine all of them except c., which depends upon the theory of accommodative reserve employed. Upon the basis of all theories, Ellerbrock and Zinnecker believe that a trifocal is helpful in all conditions in which an add of 1.25 D. or over is needed.

(2) Yeates (1949), in a study of a number of cases personally fitted, recommends the following indications for their employ. In all cases in which the amplitude is over 2.00 D., trifocals will give a good range; where the amplitude is over 1.00 but less than 2.00, they give a complete range; where it is less than 1.00 D., they improve the range but do not give a complete one. Hence, the judgment of their utility is not only dependent upon the range but upon the utility of the respective lenses in the individual case. He finds that more women than men may need the lenses due to the consistent employment of the intermediate field in housework, and that tall persons find them more useful than short ones. Bannon (1951), analyzing the reports of a number of refractionists totalling 22,640 trifocal prescriptions, also finds that the major criterion for their successful employ is the need of the patient for the respective working distance. Other features such as age, amplitude, and range based on the amplitude were chiefly significant only in relation to the above. The value of trial lenses for demonstration and the utilization of a careful history which not only determined the need but also indicated the neurotic tendency, if any, of the patient towards multifocals, assisted materially in establishing a high rate of success: 92% being totally satisfied, and 7% partially satisfied. Bannon found that trifocals seemed more suitable for patients with an accustomed nearpoint of 13 inches rather than the customarily used 16 inches.

(3) Miles (1953), reporting on a number of personally fitted bifocals, recommends that they be used early, and suggests that first adds of .75 be changed to trifocals with 1.50 near powers and 50% intermediates. He comments on the use of small additions to help students doing nearwork even when the amplitude is sufficient, and suggests that this assistance is ignored in principal when the intermediate assistance is omitted in moderate bifocal powers. Miles believes that difficulties in accommodative-convergence relationships at near are helped by using trifocals and moderating the transition to near, but Tait (cited by Miles) disagrees with this, finding no alleviation

of such problems by mere lens changes, and recommending that such problems be aided by convergence training or prism base-in.

3. Among the major problems involved in fitting trifocal lenses is that concerned with the placement of the segments in relation to the pupil. As Shepard (1951a) comments, the area between two locations of clear vision is that area which avoids interruption of the pencil of light entering the pupil. Consequently, the dividing lines are actually equal in width to the size of the pupil. In moving from one section of the lens to the next, a movement sufficient to place the entire pupil in a homogeneous lens area is required. Also, since a segment in the lens plane of approximately 19-20 mm. in width is needed to encompass a page width, the actual dividing line of any bifocal or trifocal is the distance from the lowest part of the distance portion which encloses the entire pupil to that portion of the segment which has this width. The total determination is then based not only upon this factor which is actually itself determined by the width of the segment and its shape, but also upon such factors as the habitual posture of the patient, the accustomed head-tilt, the pupil size, the relative width and heights of the segments. and whether the patient is more habitually a head mover or eye mover. (Shepard, 1951b)

a. To encompass these varied influences, the manufacturers of bifocals and trifocals offer a large diversity of shapes, sizes and positions of multifocal lenses. It is thus possible to prescribe intermediate segments of varying widths, and even in varying positions, or totally encircling the near field.

b. Likewise, certain standardizations of prescription positions of trifocals have become evident. Almost all reviews indicate that the chief cause of failure is the setting of the segments too low, so that the reading field itself is out of ready reach. The use of a frame with adjustable pads is recommended so that the positioning of the trifocal can be altered if need be. Some recommend that the top of the intermediate be placed at the geometrical center of the lens, or not more than 1 mm. below (Goldberg, 1948; Yeates, 1949). Others recommend that the reading segment itself be placed exactly as if the lens were a bifocal or at least not more than 2 mm. below that position. Simecik (1952) summarizes his experience as follows:

(1) In 86% of male patients, the top of the intermediate was successfully worn at the lower pupil edge; in another 13% of male patients, a fraction lower in the upper half of the iris beneath the pupil. This latter position also satisfied most women.

(2) The summarization of Bannon indicates the following three fitting positions:

(a) For most men, the top edge of the trifocal is satisfactory at the upper edge of the iris beneath the pupil.

(b) For most women, the top edge of the trifocal is satisfactory midway in the upper half of the iris below the pupil.

(c) For people rarely requiring close vision, or with neurotic tendencies in regard to the dividing lines, or who carry the head well back, the top of the trifocal should be placed in the middle of the lower part of the iris beneath the pupil.

4. Bannon also reports that 50% of patients reported that trifocals were as easy to adapt to as were bifocals, 36% found them easier to adapt to, and only 14% more difficult. Yeates and Miles both point out that trifocals are of little value in anisometropic cases, and are little appreciated where the overall acuity is poor. Monocular cases seem to adapt to them readily. Miles also recommends that a 7 or 8 mm. intermediate segment be used unless the lens plane is very close to the eye or the pupil quite small. Finally, since various trifocals have varying intermediate

proportions of the near power, it is well to consider the range provided by the different forms for given purposes as well as the shape and size of the trifocal applicable to a given case.

B. Types of trifocals – standard

1. *Univis, Kurova, Titmus, Vision-Ease, Orthogon ST., X-Cel, Kote-Line*

a. The Univis CV lens consists of a D shaped segment with the intermediate varying from the standard Nu-line of 7 mm. in height, to a vocational model of 8 mm. in height, with a 6 mm. height also available. The width in the usual forms varies from 20 to 28 mm. The reading segment is from 1 to 2 mm. less in height than the D bifocal.

(1) The power of the intermediate is usually 50% of the near add, although it can be supplied in powers of 40%, 60% and 70%. The B and R forms of the reading segment can also be supplied.

b. The Kurova MC 3-way is available in the D shaped form with an intermediate of 6.5 mm. in height and 23 and 25 mm. in width. The power of the intermediate is 50% in standard form, but is also available in 60% and 70% powers.

(1) A 3-way round top form is also available with a 7.5 mm. high intermediate.

c. The Titmus trifocals are also D shaped segments presenting 6 or 7 mm. intermediate segments. The lens otherwise resembles the Univis CV and Kurova form and characteristics, with widths of 22, 23, 25, and 28 mms.

(1) Titmus also supplies a 6.8 x 25 Panoptik, and a 7 mm. intermediate straightline, one-piece trifocal.

d. Vision-Ease makes a similar trifocal with 6, 7, 8 or 10 mm. intermediates and in 22, 23, 25, 28 or 35 widths.

e. Bausch and Lomb make the Orthogon ST which is a straight-top trifocal with a 7 mm. high intermediate and an overall width of 23. It observes the same range of powers as does the Panoptik trifocal.

f. Lantz Kote-Lines are made in widths of 22, 23, 25, or 28 mms. The 22 wide seg has an intermediate of 6 mm. in height, while the others have intermediate seg heights of 7.

g. The Tillyer S trifocal is available in a 7 mm. intermediate with a 24 mm. wide segment. The power of the intermediate is 50% of the power of the addition.

2. *Panoptik*

a. The Panoptik trifocal supplies an overall segment of 25 x 19 mm. in the typical Panoptik shape, of which the intermediate occupies 7 mm. in height. The intermediate is provided in powers of 55% of the add.

3. *Sovereign*

a. The Sovereign trifocal follows the Sovereign shape, with the intermediate an arched segment following the standard Fulvue C bifocal top. The entire section is 24 x 19 mm. of which the intermediate occupies 6.5–7 mm. in height. The power is standardized at 50% of the reading.

4. *Ultex and Kurova*

a. The Ultex X is a one-piece trifocal similar in appearance to the Ultex A bifocal, with the intermediate comprising a band completely around the reading field. The total seg size is 48 x 32 maximum of which the intermediate comprises 7½ to 8½ mm. in height.

(1) Shuron/Continental has standardized the ratio of intermediate to near dioptric power in the Ultex series which it manufactures at 50%.

b. Upon request, any of the three sections of the Ultex trifocals can be ground for far, near, or intermediate power.

(1) A so-called bifocal, known as See-Step, is actually a trifocal in which the near power is ground into the intermediate band, which is 9-10 mm. in height. The lower portion, which exhibits the same power as the distance correction, is 28 mm. wide by 14 mm. high, with the top of the intermediate (near power) set at a maximum of 23-24 mm. This lens is useful to individuals working upon scaffolds, in dangerous footing, etc.

5. *AO Tillyer Executive Trifocal and Titmus Horizon*

a. This is a one-piece trifocal with straight tops in which the field is as wide as the Rx frame. The trifocal segment is 7 mm. wide, the reading segment can be prescribed as high as 18 mm. The trifocal power is 50% of the power of the reading addition.

C. Double Seg Trifocals

1. *Univis, Titmus, Kurova, Vision-Ease, X-Cel, and Kote-Line*

a. The lower segment is either D, B, or R in shape and size with an inverted D segment at the top of the lens. The distance between the two may be independent in power.

(1) A standard Univis D-D segment is now available consisting of two 22 or 25 mm. wide segments separated by a standard 13 mm. Each segment is decentered in 2 mm. and provided in a regular series of related powers.

(2) The Shuron/Continental, Vision-Ease, Kote-Line, and Titmus lenses consist of similar constructions to the Univis D-D, with the characteristic sizes of each manufacturer. The Titmus Occupational ST has a standard 13.5 mm. separation between segments.

(3) All the above manufacturers also supply a 4-way, in which a trifocal constitutes the lower segment.

2. *Panoptik*

a. The lower segment is a standard Panoptik segment measuring 23 x 16 mm. in the usual position, with a circular upper segment, inverted at the top of the lens, measuring 19.5 x a maximum of 13.5 mm. The distance between may be varied from 9 to 12 mm.

(1) The lens is available with:

(a) Lower seg for near, major lens for far, and upper for either near or intermediate.

(b) Lower seg for near, major lens for intermediate, upper seg for far.

3. *Sovereign*

a. The Sovereign, Tillyer D lens resembles the Panoptik in having an inverted upper segment. The relationship of far, near and intermediate may be varied, as with the Panoptik. The Sovereign seg is 20 x 14 mm., while the upper seg is 20 mm. wide by any designated height.

(1) A similar lens, known as the Univis F; is made by Univis.

b. The Sovereign C-C lens is similar in characteristics to the Sovereign, Tillyer D except that the upper segment has the Sovereign form.

4. *Double Round Segs*

a. The Tillyer D-D consists of two round nokrome segments of 20 mm. width spaced at any designated distance from each other and at variable heights.

b. The Titmus Occupational Kryptoks consist of two kryptok segments spaced at a standard separation of 13.5 mm. although special separations can be supplied.

c. The Kurova 0 0 is a similar lens consisting of two round barium segments.

5. *Ultex-Nokrome*

a. The Ultex-Nokrome consists of a fused lower segment of 20 mm. diameter with an inverted ground Ultex A form for the upper segment. The height and separation is variable according to specifications.

(1) The lens is also available in a form in which the lower segment is a Kryptok.

6. *Double Executive*

a. The AO Tillyer Executive Double segment consists of a large reading field, a 12.5 to 13 mm. distance portion and an upper segment extending across the lens. A variety of combinations of upper and lower additions are possible providing great versatility.

b. The Horizon lens made by Titmus is similar.

7. *Tillyer A-A*

a. This lens consists of two ground Ultex A segments, with the upper inverted. The distances and powers are variable.

D. Comparative Chart of Trifocals

Table XXVIII-4

Type	Name	Seg Shape	Size of Near	Size of Intermediate	Power % of Add
Standard (fused)	*Univis CV*	*flat-top*	*20→28 x 11-12*	*6 & 7*	*40, 50, 60, 70*
	Kurova 3 way	*flat-top*	*22→28 x 13-15*	*6.5 - 7*	*50, 60, 70*
	Titmus	*flat-top*	*22→28 x 11-16*	*6, 7*	*50*
	X-Cel	*flat-top*	*23→35 x 11-16*	*7*	*50*
	Kote-Line	*flat-top*	*22→28 x 12-14½*	*6, 7*	*50*
	Vision - Ease	*flat-top*	*22→28 x 11½-16½*	*6, 7, 8, 10*	*40, 50, 60, 70*
	Tillyer S	*flat-top*	*24 x 11-12*	*6.5 - 7*	*50*
	Orthogon ST	*flat-top*	*23 x 13*	*7*	*55*

Table XXVIII-4 continued.

Type	Name	Seg Shape	Size of Near	Size of Intermediate	Power % of Add
standard (fused)	*Monocentric (Kurova)*	*flat-top*	*25 → 25 x 14½*	*6.5*	*50, 60, 70*
	Panoptik (B&L)	*arched top*	*25 x 12*	*7*	*55*
	Panoptik (Titmus)	*arched top*	*25 x 12*	*6.5 - 7*	*50*
	Tillyer Sovereign	*arched top*	*24 x 12*	*6.8*	*50*
(one piece)	*Executive*	*straight-top*	*60 x 21*	*7*	*50 & variable*
	Horizon	*straight-top*	*60 x 21*	*7*	*50 & variable*
	Ultex X	*round-top*	*32 → 33 x 16*	*7½-8½*	*50*
Double-Seg (fused)	*Univis*	*upper-inverted D lower-D, B, R, CV*	*variable*	*variable*	*variable*
	Kurova	*upper-inverted D lower-B, D, R, 3 way*	*variable*	*variable*	*variable*
	Titmus	*upper-inverted D lower-inverted D*	*variable*	*13.5 mm.*	*variable*
	Vision - Ease	*upper-inverted D lower-D, B, R, D trifocal*	*variable*	*variable*	*variable*
	Kote-Line	*upper-inverted D lower-D, trifocal*	*variable*	*variable*	*variable*
	Panoptik	*upper-inverted circle lower-Panoptik*	*19½ x 13½*	*variable*	*variable*
	Tillyer D-D & Kryptok	*upper-inverted circle lower-circle*	*20 x variable*	*20 x variable*	*variable*
(fused & one piece)					
	Kryptok or Nokrome Ultex	*upper-inverted hemisphere lower-inverted circle*	*20 x variable*	*38 x variable*	*variable*
(one piece)	*Tillyer Executive*	*upper-straight lower-straight*	*variable x 13*	*variable*	*variable*
	Kurova M	*upper-straight lower-straight*	*each 20.5*	*14 mm.*	*variable*

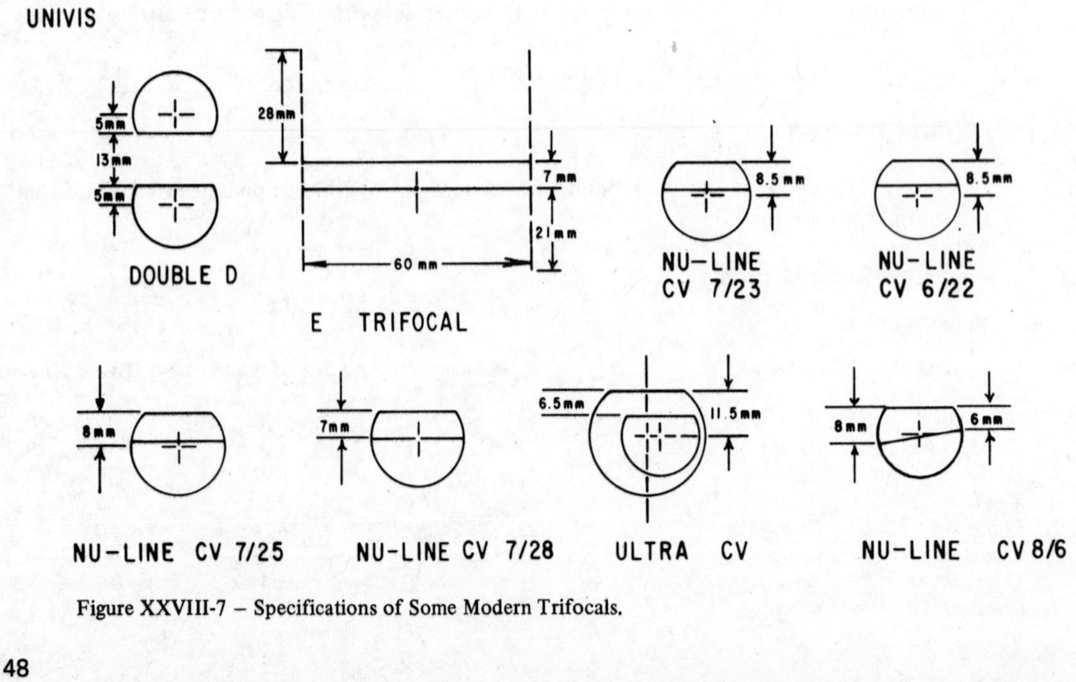

Figure XXVIII-7 – Specifications of Some Modern Trifocals.

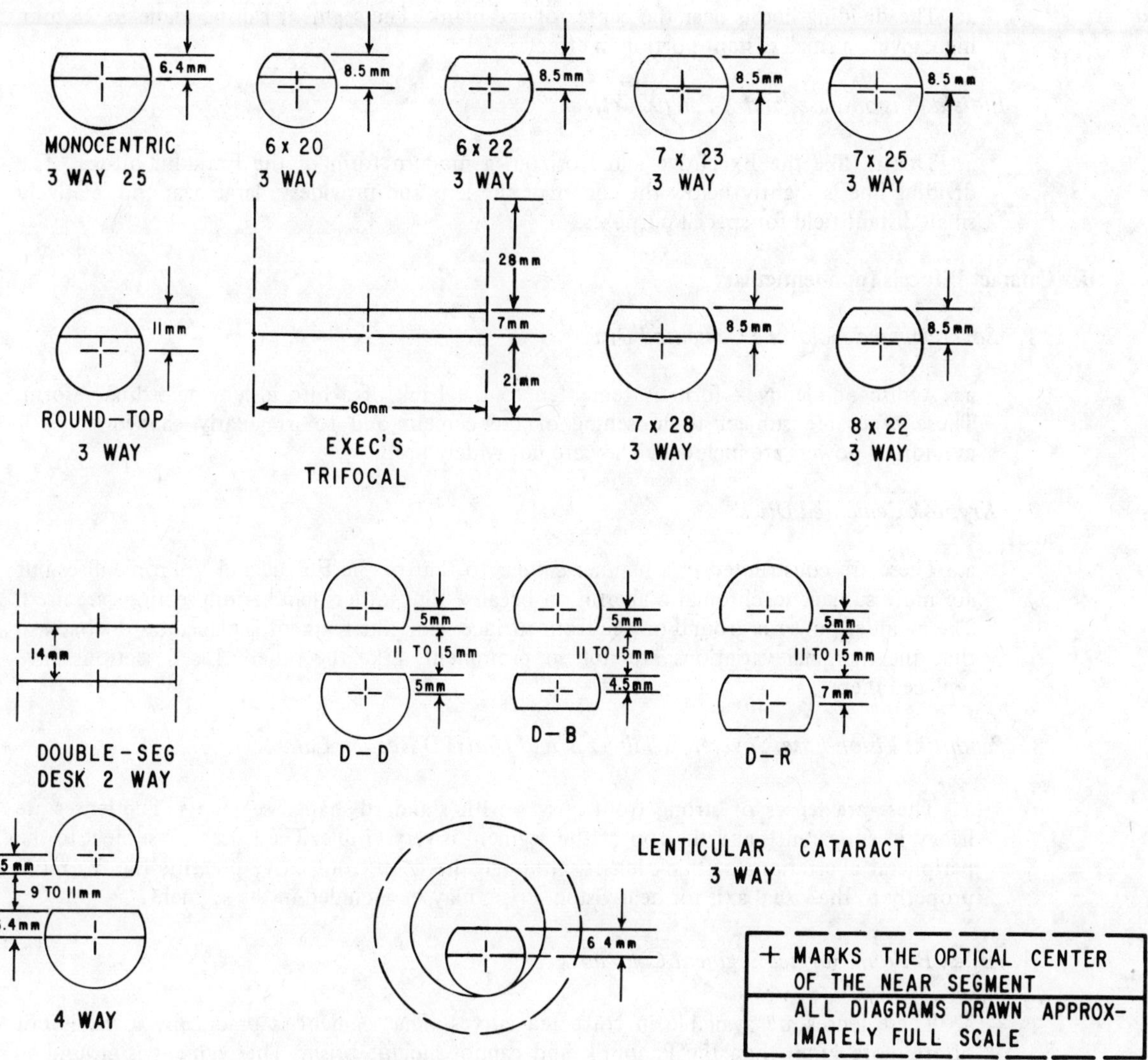

VII. SPECIAL TYPES OF MULTIFOCALS

A. Minus ADD forms

1. *Rede-Rite or Minus Segment Ultex*

a. The Rede-rite bifocal is a near point lens with a segment ground in the top which provides the distant power. This enables the wearer to gain a large near field and still have a "window" for distant vision. The size of the seg is the same as that of the A type Ultex. This lens should never be used when the distant correction is over 1.00 D. or the add over 3.00 D. as it has the pronounced jump of all one piece bifocals of the hemispheric seg type.

2. *Fulvue Minus Seg*

a. This lens is similar but is a fused bifocal with a Sovereign shaped and sized distant window.

3. *A. O. Tillyer Executive and Horizon (Titmus)*

a. The dividing line is near the center of the blank. The segment can be made to 25 mm. high, giving a small distant portion in effect.

4. *Di-field (Vision-Ease) and X-Pan (X-Cel)*

a. This is, like the Executive and Horizon, a modern form of the Franklin bifocal. The dividing line is slightly below the center of the lens and provides a large near and relatively small distant field for special purposes.

B. Cataract Bifocals (non-lenticular)

1. *Sovereign and Nokrome Cemented Disc*

a. A disc of biconvex form is cemented to the back of a bifocal lens of ordinary form. These types are subject to loosening of the cement and to irregularly shaped edges if cylindrical powers are included. They are not widely used.

2. *Kryptok Cemented Discs*

a. These are constructed in a manner similar to that of the Fulvue and Nokrome discs but are more subject to chromatic aberration because flint rather than barium sections are used. The cylinder power is ground on the front surface while the segment is placed on the back so that the marginal variations are not so prominent. Like the others, fused sections have replaced them.

3. *Panoptik, Vision-Ease, Sovereign, Tillyer S, and Univis D Regular Cataract*

a. These are lenses of strong front curves with standard shaped segments. The lenses are heavy in appearance and the top of the segment is very visible. The lenses are subject to the peripheral aberrations of thick lenses, although the deep front curve presents the seg more properly to the visual axis for near vision. Prism may be included in the segment.

4. *Ultex B Front Surface Segment Cataract*

a. These lenses are available in corrected curves. The segment is practically invisible but offers more jump than the Panoptik and cannot include prism. The segment is ground so that it offers proper incidence to lowered lines of sight for near.

5. *Titmus Fused Regular Cataract*

a. The straight top and curved top segments are available in standard 22 mm. widths. The round barium segment in 22 mm. size and a standard kryptok in 22 mm. size (clinical cataract) are also available from Titmus.

6. *Univis Bifocal*

a. This lens consists of a fused lenticular section of 25 mm. above a fused reading segment of 18 mm. The segment has a slightly curved top rather than the characteristic Univis straight top. Baryta flint or barium is used to minimize chromatic aberration. The lens is the lightest in weight and the thinnest of these types, and the segment and distance portion are independent except when a high cylindrical correction is involved.

7. *Univis Trifocal*

a. A trifocal lens of similar construction to the standard Univis Cataract D is also made. The straight-top intermediate section is supplied.

8. *A.O. Clinical Cataract*

a. A full field bifocal 22 mm. round segment on Tillyer curves for post operative use is also made by American Optical Co.

C. Lenticular Cataract Bifocals

1. *Panoptik Lenticular Cataract*

a. A distance lenticular section contains a standard Panoptik shaped lenticular segment placed within the distance field as in a normal lens. The segment is 19.5 x 13.5 within a customary 32 mm. lenticular section. It is usually placed 3 mm. below the center of the distance portion. It has the same features of construction that the standard Panoptik has.

2. *A.O. Lenticular F Style*

a. This lens is an adaptation of the Sovereign shape of bifocal to the lenticular style. The segment is placed within the distance field, which is 34 mm. in diameter. The segment is slightly smaller than the Panoptik segment in the same type of lens, being 18 mm. wide. The series is built on Tillyer curves and is supplied regularly in Cruxite A shades. The top of the seg is placed 2 mm. below center.

3. *Univis Lenticulars*

a. *Lenticular D*

(1) The lenticular section of this bifocal is 34 mm. in diameter. The D shaped segment is 22 mm. wide, giving one of the largest reading fields in this form.

b. *Lenticular T (trifocal)*

(1) The lenticular section is also 34 mm. in width. The segment is 22 mm. in width and contains an intermediate section of 6.5 in height.

4. *Titmus Lenticulars*

a. The lenticular bowl is 34 mm. in width. Segment types available include the Straight Top and Curved Top in 22 mm. widths, as well as Straight Top 7 x 22 mm. lenticular trifocal.

5. *Aolite Aspheric-Lenticular Bifocal*

a. This lens is made in 29 aspherized base curves. The segment is a 22 mm. round segment to counteract the prismatic effect of the strong distance lens. Size of the distance field is 40 mm. round.

6. *Shuron/Continental Lenticulars*

a. *Lenticular D*

(1) The lenticular section for distance is 31 and 36 mm. in diameter. The segment is 19 mm. wide by 13.5 mm. high. The pole of the segment is 4 mm. below the top line.

b. *Lenticular 3-Way*

(1) The distance section is 31 and 36 mm. in diameter. The segment width is 19.5 mm., with the near height being 12 mm. high, and the intermediate 6 mm. high. The reading pole is 1 mm. below the top line.

c. *Ultex High-Power Adds*

(1) The lens consists of a distant portion upon which is ground a segment of either 22 or 36 mms. upon a blank of 80 mm. The segment is ground in the precise center of the lens so that the near field occupies the entire central portion while distant vision can only be secured at the periphery. This is definitely a vocational lens of specialized purposes, but can be used similar to regular bifocals.

7. *Vision-Ease Catarex Lenticular*

a. *Bifocals*

(1) The lenticular section of the bifocal is 34 mm. in diameter. The segment is 18 mm. wide and 14 mm. high and is decentered in 1.5 mm. and down 2 mm. The lens is designed to be ground on a plano minus cylinder ocular curve.

b. *Trifocals*

(1) The lenticular section of the trifocal is 34 mm. in size and the segment is an R style trifocal 20 mm. wide with the reading or bifocal part 8 mm. in height and the intermediate 6 mm. in height. The segment is decentered in 1.5 mm. and down 1 mm. The lens is designed to be ground on a plano minus cylinder ocular curve.

8. Most cataract bifocals used today are of the lenticular type. These are decentered for each eye, usually 1½ mm. in, and placed at a fixed distance below the distance center. They offer a lighter, more attractive, and optically advantageous lens in comparison to older forms. The peripheral portion usually is of little service even if not ground away because of the excessive aberrations of such high powers.

D. Lenticular Minus Bifocals

1. *Myodisc*

a. The myodisc bifocal is a standard myodisc distance lens with an additional, independent section ground for the near correction. The segment is placed lower than normal segments, but no obvious chromatic aberration or lack of definition is noticed. Jump is present. The dividing line between distant and near sections is not too noticeable. The lens is constructed as a one piece bifocal and cylinder is included on the front surface.

2. *Panoptic Minus Lenticular*

a. This bifocal has the appearance of the standard Panoptik with the segment located as in a non-lenticular lens. The segment is of standard Panoptik shape and is 21.5 mm. x 14.5. The pole is 3 mm. below the top edge. The lenticular portion is normally about 30 mm. round.

3. *Ultex Minus Lenticular*

a. This lens consists of a standard Ultex form bifocal containing the reading segment on the back surface. The front surface is ground to a concave curve of lesser radius than the back curve, forming a biconcave lens. The usable area is determined by the individual specifications and powers ordered.

4. *Kryptok Minus Lenticular*

a. This lens is constructed in a similar manner to the Ultex Minus lenticular but with a fused flint round segment on the back surface.

VIII. PROGRESSIVE ADDITION LENSES

A. In the 1950s a new type of lens was made commercially available. It was designed to provide a range of clear vision between the far point and the reading distance that was continuous and uninterrupted. These lenses have been given the generic name of progressive addition lenses. Progressive addition lenses differ from bifocals and trifocals in that there is no segment and hence no dividing lines between distance and near viewing. In addition there are no sharp discontinuities of power in a progressive addition lens. Progressive addition lenses differ from blended bifocals in that the blended region of a blended bifocal is not optically useful whereas the transition zone of a progressive addition lens contains powers that can be used for viewing at distances that are intermediate between distance and near.

1. All progressive addition lenses have certain common characteristics.

a. *A distance center.* This is the point on the lens that provides the power called for in the distance prescription.

b. *A near center.* This is the point on the lens that provides the power called for in the near prescription.

c. *A transition zone.* This is the region on the lens that has continually varying power. In some progressive addition lenses the transition zone is found only between the distance and near centers. In other progressive addition lenses the transition zone may extend above the distance center and below the near center. In these cases the distance and near centers would be points within the transition zone.

B. Omnifocal

1. The progressive addition lens that was first available in the United States was the Omnifocal. This lens, developed by Joseph Weinberg and David Volk in 1962, is characterized by a transition zone that extends from the top of the lens to the very bottom. The rate of increase of power is non-linear with distance, i.e., the increase of power is slower at the top of the lens than at the bottom.

2. The 57 mm. round glass lens is of one piece construction.

a. The *front surface* has the progressive addition curves and, in addition, the base curve and a front surface plus cylinder axis 90°. The magnitude of the cylinder is 0.75 diopter greater than the power of the addition. For example, if the prescribed add is +1.25 diopters the cylinder on the front surface would be +2.00 diopters.

b. There are three base curves available +4.25, +6.25, and +8.25 diopters. The selection of the base curve is dependent upon the power of the distance prescription and, in some cases, the axis of the cylinder that is prescribed to correct the patient's astigmatism.

(1) An example of this is a pair of prescriptions, identical in power, but differing in axis which would be made on different base curves as follows:

(a) +3.50 −0.50x10 +6.25 diopter base curve

(b) +3.50 −0.50x45 +8.25 diopter base curve

3. The *distance* and *near* centers are separated by 25 mm. There is no inset of the near center.

4. The *back surface* of the Omnifocal is finished by the laboratory to produce the desired prescription. Ordinarily the back surface will be toric since it will be necessary to compensate for the front surface cylinder. It is also usually necessary to place the axis of the cylinder at an oblique angle to the front surface cylinder in order to produce the desired amount and axis in the resultant cylinder in the finished lens. Thus, it is to be expected that the Omnifocal lens will have bitoric construction with the back surface cylinder axis at an oblique angle to the front surface cylinder.

5. *Additions* are available in powers of 0.75 to 1.75 diopters.

6. The line between the distance and near centers represents a *line of symmetry* in the finished Omnifocal. It is along this line that the best imagery is produced. Aberrations are encountered laterally from this line.

a. The major aberration is astigmatism The magnitude of the astigmatism increases with increasing distance from the line. The largest amounts of this aberration are encountered in the lower lateral regions of this spectacle lens. The axis of the astigmatic error of the Omnifocal varies from location to location on the lens.

7. The *field of clear vision* is sometimes considered to be that field that has no more than 1.00 diopter of astigmatic aberration associated with it. Using this arbitrary definition it is possible to describe the field in terms of the lens. The width of the field is greater at the top of the lens than at the bottom. The shape of the field is triangular. This means that the width of the reading field is limited. (Figures XXVIII-8 and -9.)

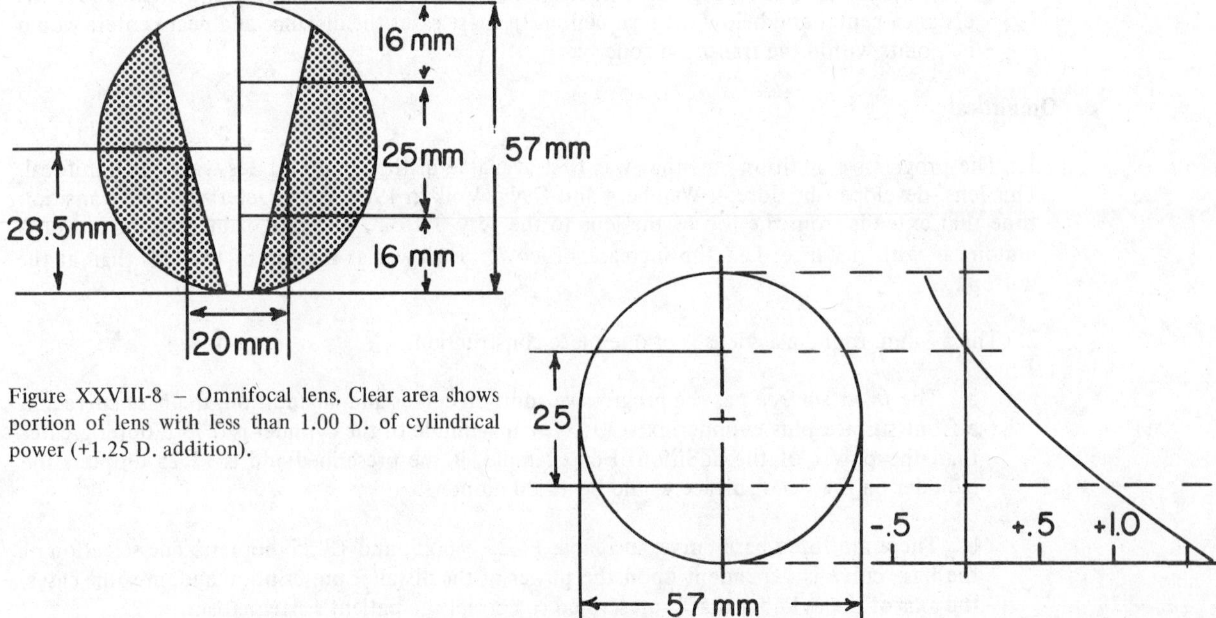

Figure XXVIII-8 – Omnifocal lens. Clear area shows portion of lens with less than 1.00 D. of cylindrical power (+1.25 D. addition).

Figure XXVIII-9 – Omnifocal design showing nonlinear progression of power from the top of the lens to the bottom (+1.00 diopter addition).

a. The amount of the addition determines the width of this field. The higher additions have narrower reading fields.

C. Varilux

1. The second progressive addition lens available in the United States was the Varilux. It was developed in France in 1951 by Bernard Maitenaz and improved in several stages throughout that decade. The current Varilux is characterized by an upper half that contains the distance prescription, a 12 mm. transition zone that contains the progressive addition, and a bottom portion that contains the near prescription power. The rate of increase of power is linear, i.e., equal fractions of the addition are found with equal distances in the transition zone.

2. The 60 mm. round glass lens is of one-piece construction.

a. The *front surface* has the progressive addition curves and the base curve. There are two base curves available, +6.50 and +9.50 diopters.

3. The *distance* and *near* centers are separated by a vertical distance of 12 mm. The near center is inset 2.5 mm.

4. The *back surface* of the Varilux is finished by the laboratory to produce the desired prescription in the way a conventional Executive bifocal would be finished. The curve on the rear surface would be a sphere for spherical prescriptions and toric for cylindrical prescriptions.

5. *Additions* are available in powers of 0.5 to 3.50 diopters.

6. The upper half of the lens is similar in optical characteristics to the top of a bifocal lens. The line between the distance center and the near center is a *line of symmetry* for the transition zone in the finished Varilux. It is along this line that the best imagery is produced in the transition zone. Aberrations are encountered laterally from this line.

a. The major aberration is astigmatism. The largest amounts of this aberration in the Varilux are in the lateral portions of the transition zone. The axis of the astigmatic error of the Varilux varies from location to location on the lens.

b. The *useful reading area* is roughly circular in shape.

7. The *field of clear vision*, using 1.00 diopter of astigmatic aberration or less as the criterion for clear vision as described previously, is the entire upper half of the lens for distance vision; an area that is roughly circular for near vision; and a narrower channel for the transition zone. The width of this channel is wider for lower power additions. (Figures XXVIII-10 and 11)

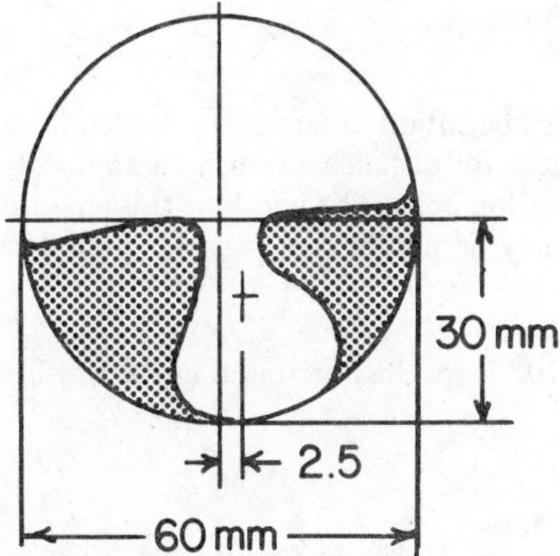

Figure XXVIII-10 – Varliux lens. Clear area shows portion of lens with less than 1.00 D. of cylindrical power (+1.25 D. addition).

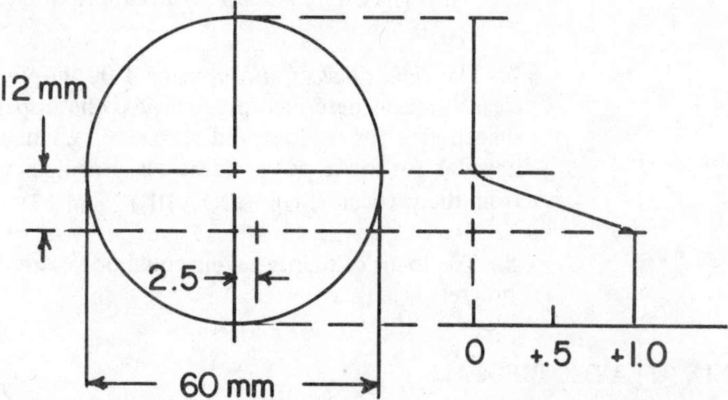

Figure XXVIII-11 – Varliux design of 1966 showing stabilized power at the top and bottom of the lens and progressive increase between (+1.00 diopter addition).

8. The locus of points having equal power are horizontal in the finished lens even though the near center is inset 2.5 mm.

D. Progressor

1. The third progressive addition lens available in the United States was the progressor. It is manufactured in France under the name Zoom BB by the firm of Benoist-Berthiot. There are three areas on the lens. The distance prescription is found in the upper half of the lens. The progressive addition is found in the next 14 mm. in the transition zone. The near prescription power is found in the bottom portion of the lens. The rate of increase of power in the transition zone is non-linear, i.e., the power increases more rapidly in the lower portion of the transition zone than in the upper portion.

2. The 60 mm. round glass lens is of one-piece construction.

   a. The *front surface* has the progressive addition curves and the base curve. Two base curves, +6.00 and +8.00 diopters, are available.

3. The *distance* and *near* centers are separated by approximately 14 mm. The semi-finished lens is rotated approximately 10° in order to produce an inset of 2.5 mm.

4. The *back surface* of the progressor is finished by the laboratory to produce the desired prescription. The curve on the rear surface would be a sphere for spherical prescriptions and toric for cylindrical prescriptions.

5. *Additions* are available in powers from 0.50 to 3.00 diopters.

6. The upper half of the lens is similar in optical characteristics to the top of a bifocal lens. The line between the distance center and the near center is a *line of symmetry* for both the transition zone and the reading area in the finished progressor. Although it is along this line that the best imagery for the progressive addition and near powers are found, there are aberrations in the transition zone and in the upper and lower portions of the reading area. More aberrations are encountered laterally from the line.

   a. The major aberration is astigmatism. The largest amounts of this aberration in the progressor are in the lateral portions of the transition zone. The axis of the astigmatic error of the progressor varies from location to location on the lens.

   b. The *useful reading area* is approximately parabolic in shape.

7. The *field of clear vision*, using 1.00 diopter of astigmatic aberration or less as the criterion for clear vision as described previously is the upper half of the lens for distance vision, a parabolically shaped area for reading, and a narrower channel for the transition zone. The width of this channel is wider for lower power additions. For higher adds there may be no channel. All are tilted 10° from the vertical. (Figures XXVIII-12 and 13)

8. The locus of points having equal power are tilted about 10° from the horizontal in the finished progressor lens.

IX. PLASTIC BIFOCALS

A. As with single vision lenses, plastics have become increasingly useful in the field of bifocal design, particularly because of their advantageous application to strong, heavy lenses such as those required to correct aphakia. The forms of plastic lens bifocals follow those of glass lens bifocals fairly closely, the major difference being that the plastic lenses are molded of the same plastic for both the distance and the addition. Plastic also has a lower refractive index and thereby a lower reflectance factor.

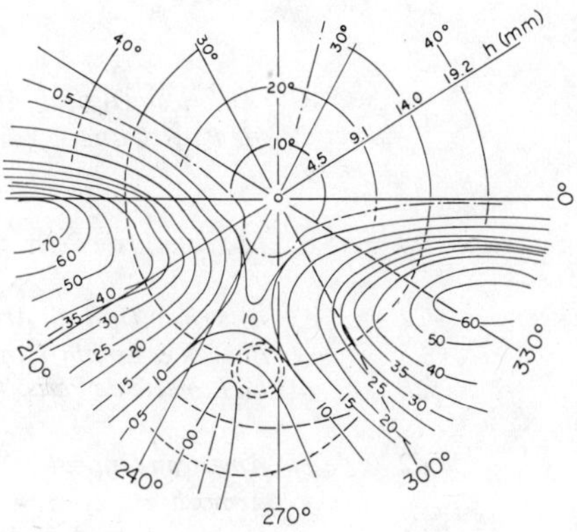

Figure XXVIII-12 – Progressor lens. Clear area shows portion of lens with less than 1.00 D. of cylindrical power (+2.00 D. addition).

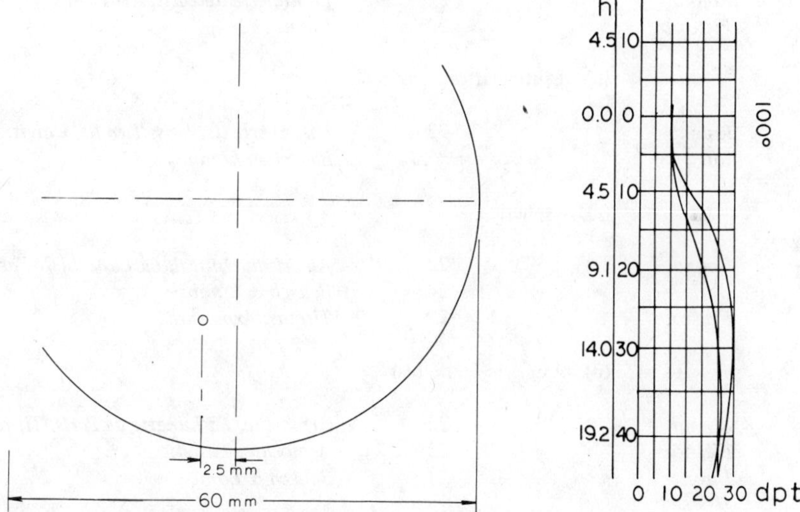

Figure XXVIII-13 – Progressor design showing non linear progression of power from the distance center to the bottom (+2.00 D. addition).

1. *Plastic Trifocals*

a. Table XXVIII-6

Form	Size	Manufacturer
Flat-top	*24 near; 28 x 7 inter*	*Univis*
Round	*22 x 7*	*Armorlite, La Lunette de Paris*
Flat-top	*25 x 7*	*Armorlite*

The major *plastic bifocals* manufactured in this country are tabulated below:

a. **Table XXVIII-5**

Form	Size	Manufacturer
(1) Regular		
Round	*22*	*American Optical; Armorlite; Bausch & Lomb; La Lunette de Paris; Titmus; Younger*
	--	
	28	*La Lunette de Paris*
Flat-top	*22*	*American Optical; Armorlite; Bausch & Lomb Titmus; Univis*
	25	*Bausch & Lomb; Titmus; Univis; Armorlite (in process)*
	28	*La Lunette de Paris; Titmus*
Executive	*62*	*American Optical*
Fulseg		*Armorlite*
Orma-Arc (Ultex)	*26*	*La Lunette de Paris*
(2) Cataract Forms		
(a) Regular		
Round	*22*	*La Lunette de Paris; Armorlite*
Flat-top	*22*	*Univis*
(b) Lenticular		
Round	*22*	*La Lunette de Paris; Titmus; Univis; Armorlite*
Ultex	*30.5*	*Bausch & Lomb*
(c) Aspheric		
Round	*22*	*American Optical; La Lunette de Paris; Titmus Armorlite*
Oval	*24*	*Bausch & Lomb*
Flat-top	*22*	*Titmus; Armorlite*
(d) Aspheric Lenticular		
Round	*22*	*Armorlite; La Lunette de Paris; Titmus*
Flat-top	*22*	*Armorlite; Titmus*
Ultex	*24*	*Bausch & Lomb*

X. JUMP

A. In the course of describing the characteristics of various bifocals, the term "jump" is noted as a negative quality of certain types of construction. Usually, jump is interpreted as that factor of the bifocal whereby the position of an object viewed through the segment is altered as the line of sight passes from the distant portion into the bifocal portion. Almost all bifocals constitute decentered optical systems. As discussed under decentration, a ray of light which does not pass through the poles is bent. Since the poles of the distant and near portions are not coincident, except in the few forms purposely built to gain that objective, it is impossible to avoid some prismatic effect when using the segments of all modern bifocals. The combination of the base-up prismatic effect of a plus lens, with the additional base-down effect of the add at the dividing line, alters the habitual displacement of the object as viewed through the same point of a single vision lens of the same power. If the add is stronger than the distant portion, the prismatic effect will be reversed; if it is weaker, it will be lessened; while if the distant portion is minus, base down effect from the distance will be increased by base down from the seg. Consequently, the jump is affected by:

1. The distance between the pole and the top of the segment.

2. The signs of the lens powers of the two.

3. The strengths of the powers of the two.

B. This jump is manifested at the dividing lines of the distant and added powers, where a ray passing through the lens will be deviated to unequal extents by the two different curvatures. Fry and Ellerbrock (1941) have called this phenomenon *"differential displacement"* rather than jump, and go on to say that this also obviously occurs at other points than the top of the segment. If a horizontal line is viewed through a bifocal lens, it will be noted that the line appears to be displaced in the following manner. The portion of the line seen through the distant portion of the lens, surrounding the bifocal, is not continuous with the part seen outside the lens. The portion seen through the bifocal is also not continuous with that seen through the distant portion. The actual differential displacement is the difference between the lines seen through the distant portion and those seen through the segment, since the displacement of the line seen through the distant portion would be true of the lens even if it were not a bifocal.

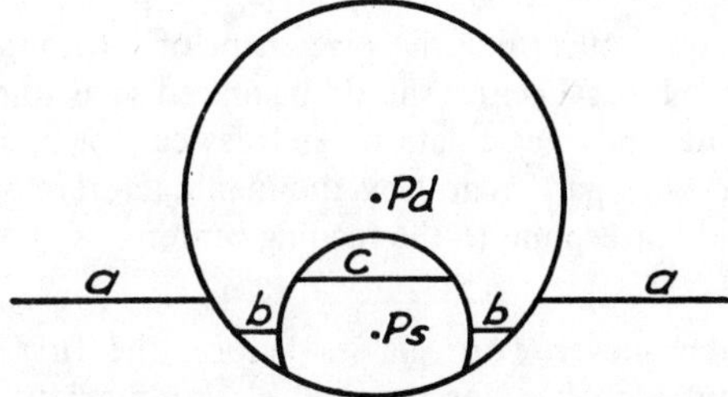

Figure XXVIII-14 – Displacement differential displacement, or jump. *a* position of lines seen outside of lens; *b* position of lines as seen through distant portion of lens, constituting total displacement of distant power; *c* position of line as seen through the seg. Difference inposition of *b* and *c* constitutes differential displacement or jump. If line, *a*, were viewed through pole of segment, *Ps*, only the displacement of the distant portion, *b*, would be evident, eliminating the segment as a factor in "jump."

1. The prismatic effect of the distance portion, therefore, does not actually involve the matter of jump, which is merely an expression of the prismatic effect of the segment or as expressed by Fry and Ellerbrock.

   a. Differential displacement at top of segment = power of add x distance of seg pole to seg top in cms.

2. The differential displacement of the segment can be substantially reduced by placing the seg pole near the top, as is done in the so-called monocentric bifocal. Occasionally, the displacement factor is used to demonstrate that a blind area exists at the top edge. This is only evident if the bifocal is held at some distance from the observer and at normal distances would require an extremely small pupil to be of importance.

3. Since the differences between the distance and the seg also include, as well as the displacement, a *difference in focus and size of the object,* it is of questionable value as to whether elimination of the differential displacement is of much practical importance. Even if it were eliminated by placing the pole at the top of the segment, the other differences would still prevent single vision when looking through the edge.

C. In contrast to the differential displacement due to the prismatic effect of the segment when looking away from the pole of the segment is the Total Displacement at the reading center. This is actually what is understood by jump by many, and merely constitutes the combined prismatic effects of the distant and reading portions. If the pole of the segment is placed at the actual reading center, so that the line of sight passes through it, the total displacement must be due to the distant portion alone.

1. As the authors (Fry and Ellerbrock, 1941) state, an investigation by Ellerbrock places the average reading center at a point 11 mm. below the point in front of the pupil or 5 mm. below the top of the segment.

2. If the wearer were to first look through the distant pole of the lens and then through the reading center, an object would appear displaced due to prismatic effect of the distance portion whether a bifocal were present or not. Usually, the wearer becomes accustomed to this displacement, which is unavoidable ordinarily, within a few days. The wearer of bifocals should also become accustomed to this effect and the undue emphasis placed upon it seems to be unnecessary.

D. Two contrasting theories concerning the placement of bifocal segment poles seem to be prevalent. One seems to hold that the bifocal center should be placed so as to neutralize the prismatic effect of the distance portion. Many ingenuous calculations and devices for choosing the appropriate bifocal under this theory have been devised, particularly by the manufacturers of bifocals. The other holds that the pole of the segment should correspond to the reading center.

1. If the patient has never worn glasses before, the first theory would be more applicable. However, the patient who has not required glasses previous to reaching the bifocal age cannot ordinarily require a distance correction of any noticeable strength. The amount of prismatic effect manifested by the distance portion at the reading center would probably be very slight, and the add would not have to be placed with its pole very far from the actual reading center to neutralize the effect.

2. If the patient has actually required a strong distance correction, he most likely would have been wearing glasses before reaching the age of bifocals. Under such circumstances he would have become accustomed to the displacement of the distance portion. To place the pole of the bifocal in accordance with the first theory, that of eliminating the displacement entirely, would present him with as strange a circumstance as if he first wore glasses.

3. The desired effect is not to eliminate the displacement, but to *avoid changing the conditions* to which he has already been accustomed. Since the previous wearer is already accustomed to jump or displacement, due to the distant correction, the placement of the segment pole at the reading center would best preserve the accustomed conditions.

a. As Fry and Ellerbrock (1941) point out, the exception to this rule is in cases of anisometropia inducing pronounced vertical discrepancies, in which the poles might be manipulated to reduce the vertically induced imbalances.

4. By the simple rules of decentration to compute prismatic effect and using the figure of 5 mm. below the seg top, which is in turn placed 6 mm. below the pupil center, as a standard for the reading center, it is possible to determine just how much change in the accustomed displacement a given type of bifocal of given power will produce if the position of the pole of the bifocal below its top is known.

5. The following table, revised by the author after Morgan, (1940) gives the distances for common bifocals of the pole of the bifocal from the segment top:

a. Table XXVIII-7

Distance From Pole To Top Of Seg	Type
0	*Tillyer Executive, Horizon, Bi-Field, X-Pan*
3	*Panoptik*
3.5	*Panoptik LS & PR; Sovereign*
4	*Sovereign, Titmus CT, Univis & Kurova D, Lenticular Cataract; Kurova CT*
4.5	*Univis B; Kurova B; Vision-Ease B*
5	*Univis D; Titmus ST; Titmus C & N; Tillyer S; all makes, D 28; Orthogon ST; Vision-Ease D; Kote-Line; Kurova D.*
6	*Univis; Titmus CT*
6.5	*Kryptok, type 13*
7	*Univis, Kurova, Vision-Ease R segs;*
8	*Kryptok, type 16; Univis R*
9	*Univis R*
10	*Kryptok, type 20; Univis R; Cen-Cor; Kurova O*
11	*Kryptok, type 22; Ultex B; Fused L; Kurova O*
13	*Ultex Lenticular Cataract*
14	*Ultex Lenticular Cataract*
16	*Ultex E & L; Ultex High Power Add*
19	*Ultex A, AA, AL, Rede-rite*

XI. ANISOMETROPIA

A. If anisometropia is found, and the patient has not previously worn any correction, the possibility of both vertically and laterally induced prism of different amounts for each eye may make a bifocal intolerable. However, if the correction has been worn as a single vision lens with satisfaction by the patient previous to the necessity for bifocals, it is likely that the patient has adapted himself to the imbalance as noted in Chapters VII and VIII and placement of the bifocal so that the habitual total displacement is not altered markedly should eliminate prospective difficulties.

1. The actual position of the reading center must be carefully noted. A single vision lens may be used by a patient with marked anisometropia so that a minimum amount of prismatic effect at the nearpoint is induced by virtue of tilting the head so that the reading center falls very close to the pole of the lens. A bifocal cannot be used in this manner, since its physical construction requires that the reading center be a certain distance from the pole of the distance lens. Therefore, the mere fact that the anisometropic correction has been worn successfully in single vision form does not imply that the bifocal will also be worn without difficulty until it has been determined that the reading center through the single vision lens is at a comparable distance from the distance lens pole to its position as required in the bifocal.

2. If no previous experience had been had with the anisometropic lenses or if the patient had learned to adjust his head through single vision lenses so that the lines of sight passed close to the poles even for close work, it is likely that a bifocal would prove to be difficult to wear without compensation for the anisometropic effect.

a. Ellerbrock (1948) reports, however, that the data do not indicate that patients with anisometropia avoid the prismatic influences at the periphery in the reading position by movements of the head. He finds no correlation between any type of vertical anisometropia and maximum or minimum tilting of the face plane.

B. The determination of the respective vertical prismatic effects is a simple one in spherical lenses or in sphero-cylinders in which the axis position is either 90 or 180. The simple method of computing the prismatic effect due to decentration is used.

1. If the reading center lies 11 mm. below the distant pole, the prismatic effect of the distant lens

is readily determined. From the previous table, the distance of the pole of the seg from its top is known; the distance of the top from the distance lens pole is known and this permits the determination of the distance of the reading center from the seg pole.

a. The distance lens and the seg addition are considered as two separate lenses and the prismatic effect of each is determined individually and then combined.

2. For example, given a distance lens of +1.00 and an add of +2.00, a Kryptok 22 mm. bifocal placed with its top 3 mm. below the distance pole is to be used and the reading center is 11 mm. below the distance pole (Figure XXVIII-15).

a. Prismatic effect of distant lens: 1.00x1.1. cm.=1.1. Δ base-up.

b. Prismatic effect of near add: Top of seg 3 below distance pole; pole of seg 11 below top; therefore, pole of seg is 14 below the distance pole. Reading level is 11 below distance pole; therefore, reading level is 3 above the seg pole: 2.00x3= .6 Δ base-down.

c. Total prismatic effect=1.1 Δ base-up and .6 Δ base-down, or .5 Δ base-up at reading level.

3. Referring to Figure XXVIII-15, it is possible to derive a formula for determining the prismatic effect of a bifocal at the reading distance, which would read as follows: Prismatic effect = $F_a\,(r+a) - h\,(F_a + F_d)$.

a. F_a = power of add; F_d = power of distance; r = distance of pole of seg from top of seg; a = distance of top of seg from pole of far lens; h = distance of reading level from pole of distance lens.

b. Lens powers are given plus or minus dioptric signs; distances are stated in centimeters; and a minus answer indicates prism base-up, while a plus one indicates prism base-down.

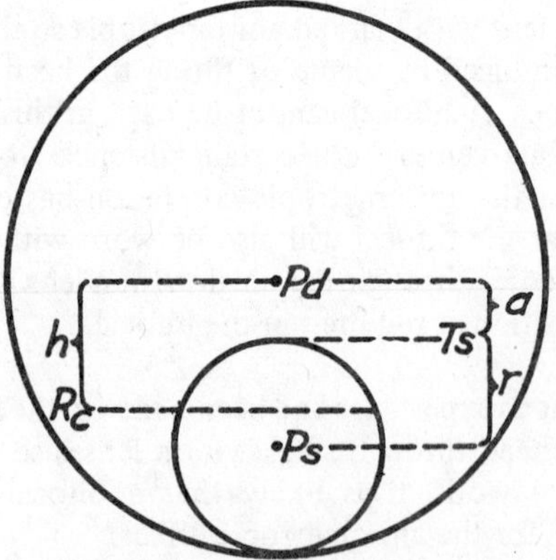

Figure XXVIII-15 – Illustrating important points of reference in determining prismatic effect of a bifocal. *Pd* pole of distant portion; *Ps* pole of reading addition; *Ts* top of segment; *Rc* reading center or level; *a*, position of seg top from distance pole, or "below center"; *r*, distance of pole seg from top of seg; *h*, distance of reading center below pole of distant lens.

C. The above calculations are most simply effective with distant corrections which are simple spheres. When a sphero-cylindrical correction is involved, it is necessary to determine the total power of the distance correction in the vertical meridian. If the cylinder is at axis 90, producing 0 power vertically; or at axis 180, producing its total power in the vertical meridian; or at axis 45 or 135, producing a vertical effect of exactly one-half its total power, the calculation is simple, since the power of the sphere and cylinder in the vertical meridian need merely be combined.

1. If the cylinder is in an oblique meridian other than 45 or 135, it is necessary to first compute the power of the cylinder in the vertical meridian and then combine that with the spherical power.

a. This can be computed by the formula, $F_e = F_e \sin^2\phi$, or for the entire sphero-cylinder, $F_e = F_s + F_e \sin^2\phi$, in which Fe is the effective power of the combination in the desired meridian; F_s is the power of the sphere; F_e is the power of the cylinder; and ϕ is the angle between the axis of the cylinder and the desired meridian.

(1) Chapter XXVI, Section X, subdivision A,2,a lists a table which indicates the power of a cylinder at various angular distances from its axis.

(a) From this table we find that the power of a 1.00 D. cylinder axis 30 would be .75 in the 90th meridian (60° away). If we wished to find the vertical power of a 3.00 D. cylinder at that axis, we merely multiply the factor .75 by 3.

2. Once the vertical power of the oblique cylinder is known, the total vertical effect can be readily determined by the simple calculations noted earlier in this section.

D. In placing bifocal adds, the pole of the add is not merely below the pole of the distance lens, but is also displaced or decentered inward to compensate for the convergence of the lines of sight at the nearpoint.

1. Morgan (1940) has derived a simple formula for determining the amount of inset for various near-point distances of fixation.

a. The amount of inset $= \dfrac{\text{interpupillary distance}}{34}$

b. For each inch the fixation is closer than 16 inches add .1 mm. to amount of inset; for each inch farther than 16 inches deduct .1 mm from the inset for each segment.

2. Morgan's formula does not allow for the power of the lens. Scott Sterling (1935) has derived a suggested table of insets in which the prismatic effect of the lens power is considered. The table is derived from the following formula (Ellerbrock, 1948):

$$i = \frac{P}{1 + w\left(\frac{1}{s} - \frac{1}{f}\right)}$$

in which P is ½ the interpupillary distance, w is the distance of the lens to the working nearpoint, s is the distance from the lens to the center of rotation of the eye, and f is the focal length of the lens. The derived table results in fractions of tenths of millimeters, but since .5 mm. fractions are as accurate as can customarily be used, the following summary is modified accordingly. (Table XXVIII-8)

3. Since the pole of the segment is displaced not only vertically but laterally from the distance pole, not only the induced vertical but also the induced lateral prismatic power may be significant.

Table XXVIII-8. Insets to make reading fields coincide at 16 inches.

Power of distance lens in 180th	Distance from nose to center of pupil									
	27	28	29	30	31	32	33	34	35	36
+15	*2.5*	*2.5*	*2.5*	*2.5*	*3*	*3*	*3*	*3*	*3*	*3*
+14	*2.5*	*2.5*	*2.5*	*2.5*	*2.5*	*3*	*3*	*3*	*3*	*3*
+12	*2*	*2.5*	*2.5*	*2.5*	*2.5*	*2.5*	*2.5*	*3*	*3*	*3*
+10	*2*	*2*	*2*	*2.5*	*2.5*	*2.5*	*2.5*	*2.5*	*2.5*	*3*
+ 9	*2*	*2*	*2*	*2*	*2.5*	*2.5*	*2.5*	*2.5*	*2.5*	*2.5*
+ 8	*2*	*2*	*2*	*2*	*2*	*2.5*	*2.5*	*2.5*	*2.5*	*2.5*
+ 7	*2*	*2*	*2*	*2*	*2*	*2.5*	*2.5*	*2.5*	*2.5*	*2.5*
+ 6	*2*	*2*	*2*	*2*	*2*	*2*	*2.5*	*2.5*	*2.5*	*2.5*
+ 5	*2*	*2*	*2*	*2*	*2*	*2*	*2*	*2.5*	*2.5*	*2.5*
+ 4	*2*	*2*	*2*	*2*	*2*	*2*	*2*	*2*	*2.5*	*2.5*
+ 3	*1.5*	*2*	*2*	*2*	*2*	*2*	*2*	*2*	*2*	*2.5*
+ 2	*1.5*	*1.5*	*2*	*2*	*2*	*2*	*2*	*2*	*2*	*2*
+ 1	*1.5*	*1.5*	*1.5*	*2*	*2*	*2*	*2*	*2*	*2*	*2*
0	*1.5*	*1.5*	*1.5*	*2*	*2*	*2*	*2*	*2*	*2*	*2*
– 1	*1.5*	*1.5*	*1.5*	*1.5*	*2*	*2*	*2*	*2*	*2*	*2*
– 2	*1.5*	*1.5*	*1.5*	*1.5*	*2*	*2*	*2*	*2*	*2*	*2*
– 3	*1.5*	*1.5*	*1.5*	*1.5*	*1.5*	*2*	*2*	*2*	*2*	*2*
– 4	*1.5*	*1.5*	*1.5*	*1.5*	*1.5*	*1.5*	*2*	*2*	*2*	*2*
– 5	*1.5*	*1.5*	*1.5*	*1.5*	*1.5*	*1.5*	*1.5*	*2*	*2*	*2*
– 6	*1.5*	*1.5*	*1.5*	*1.5*	*1.5*	*1.5*	*1.5*	*2*	*2*	*2*
– 7	*1.5*	*1.5*	*1.5*	*1.5*	*1.5*	*1.5*	*1.5*	*1.5*	*2*	*2*
– 8	*1.5*	*1.5*	*1.5*	*1.5*	*1.5*	*1.5*	*1.5*	*1.5*	*1.5*	*2*
– 9	*1.5*	*1.5*	*1.5*	*1.5*	*1.5*	*1.5*	*1.5*	*1.5*	*1.5*	*1.5*
–10	*1.5*	*1.5*	*1.5*	*1.5*	*1.5*	*1.5*	*1.5*	*1.5*	*1.5*	*1.5*
–12	*1*	*1.5*	*1.5*	*1.5*	*1.5*	*1.5*	*1.5*	*1.5*	*1.5*	*1.5*
–14	*1*	*1*	*1.5*	*1.5*	*1.5*	*1.5*	*1.5*	*1.5*	*1.5*	*1.5*
–16	*1*	*1*	*1*	*1.5*	*1.5*	*1.5*	*1.5*	*1.5*	*1.5*	*1.5*
–18	*1*	*1*	*1*	*1*	*1.5*	*1.5*	*1.5*	*1.5*	*1.5*	*1.5*
–20	*1*	*1*	*1*	*1*	*1*	*1.5*	*1.5*	*1.5*	*1.5*	*1.5*
–22	*1*	*1*	*1*	*1*	*1*	*1*	*1.5*	*1.5*	*1.5*	*1.5*

a. This lateral prismatic power is determined by considering the sphere, the cylinder and the add as three separate lenses.

(1) The lateral and vertical prismatic power of the distance sphere is simply determined by the distance of the reading center from the pole times the dioptric power, first vertically, then laterally.

(a) If the reading center were to be placed 11 mm. below the distance one, and two mm. inwards, the vertical prismatic power would be 1.1 x D. and the lateral power .2 x D.

(2) The *prismatic effect of the cylinder* can be determined by the graphic method. (Figure XXVIII-16)

(a) Draw a lens of the diameter of the dimensions of the lens involved to scale.

(b) Locate the pole of the lens, P, and the reading center C. This is done by measuring the distances PZ, and ZC to agree with the position of the reading center from the distance lens pole. If the reading center were 8 mm. below the pole and 3 mm. in, then PZ would measure 8 and ZC would measure 3.

(c) Use PC as a diameter to draw a circle.

(d) With a protractor, lay off the meridian of power of the cylinder at P.

(e) Draw a line from the intersection of the circle and the meridian of power to C (XC).

(f) Complete the triangle of which XC is the hypotenuse with a right angle at N.

(g) XN gives the dimension of vertical effect of the cylinder and CN the dimension for horizontal effect.

(h) XN x D. of cyl. = vertical prismatic effect; CN x D. of cyl. = horizontal prismatic effect.

(3) Combine the prismatic effects of the sphere and the cylinder for the total prismatic effects of the distance portion of the lens.

(4) Compute the prismatic effect of the add by multiplying the distance from the pole of the add to the reading center times the power of the add, first for the horizontal discrepancy and then the vertical.

(a) If the reading center were 8 below the distance pole and 3 mm. in, and the pole of the reading addition were 11 below the top, which was 3 below the distance pole, or a total of 14, and 2 in, then,

(b) The lateral prismatic effect would be .1 x D. of add; the vertical prismatic effect would be .6 x D. of add.

(5) Total the prismatic effect of the distance and near portions.

(a) It will be found that except in very high powers, the amount of lateral discrepancy is usually so slight that it can be ignored. The major factor in anisometropic corrections involving bifocals is the compensation of the vertical prismatic effect for each lens and the adjustment of discrepancies which may induce discomfort at the reading center.

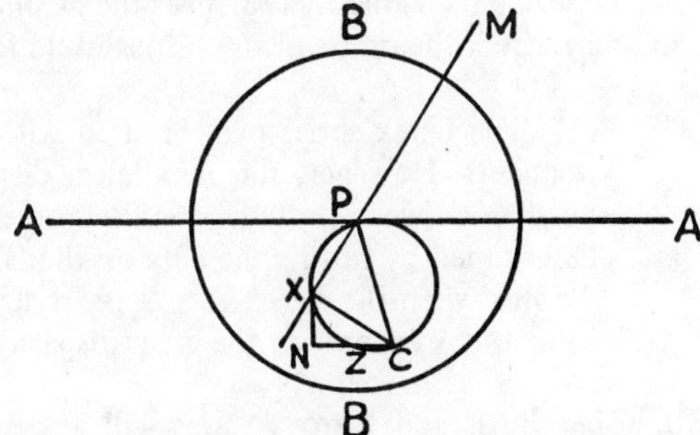

Figure XXVIII-16 – Graphical determination of vertical and lateral prismatic effect of a sphero-cylindrical lens with the cylinder axis in an oblique meridian. *P* pole of distant lens; *C* reading center; *A* horizontal meridian; *B* vertical meridian; *PZ* vertical distance of reading center from pole; *ZC* horizontal distance of reading center from pole; *M* meridian of power of the cylinder (90° from axis); *X* intersection of meridian power and circle of diameter; *PC; XN* dimension of vertical prismatic effect; *NC* dimension of lateral prismatic effect.

4. In those instances in which some lateral prismatic assistance is required to abet a weakened convergence function, particularly when a high ACA ratio exists, so that the added plus power tends to lessen the accommodative-convergence and increase the burden of fusional convergence, some prism base-in power in the near segment is desirable. This may be obtained by either those segments which lend themselves to inclusion of lateral prism in the segment alone, or by decentration of the segment section to move the pole farther nasalward than the interpupillary distance indicates. Several forms of large field segments, such as the straight-top 28 wide segs, or the Ultex segments, lend themselves to such decentration without reducing the size of the nasal reading portion beyond that found in the ordinary sized segments. Up to 1.5 Δ of prism base-in can be achieved with such segments in some powers.

E. Compensation for Anisometropia

1. *Prism in the Segments*

a. The Panoptik, Sovereign, Univis, Kurova, and Ultex bifocals permit the inclusion of prism in the segments with the base in any direction, limited to amounts indicated in the table of bifocals listed previously.

b. The inclusion of prism in a bifocal segment allows for the balancing of prismatic effects at the reading point or for the inclusion of a desired amount of prism to compensate for a muscular imbalance.

c. The R segment, which allows for a selection of the vertical location of the optical center of the segment, can provide prism that is dependent upon the power of the segment and the location of the optical center.

2. *Dissimilar Segments* (Brown, 1942)

a. By using segments for each eye which have their poles at different distances from the distance pole, the amount of prismatic effect can be varied. Each mm. difference in the distance of the poles will vary the prismatic effect .1 for each diopter of add. This can be accomplished by varying the heights of identical segments which is not too practical or desirable except in small amounts. It is also accomplished by using two entirely different shaped segments. While this balances the prismatic effect, it introduces cosmetic disadvantages and may affect the limits of the bifocal field for some purposes.

(1) The Ultex series may be used with reasonable similarity of the appearance of the segments. However, the maximum disparity between various Ultex segments is that possible between those having their poles farthest from each other. This can quickly be determined by noting the data on the Ultex series given earlier. The maximum is .8 per diopter when the Ultex A and B are used (although 1.4 per diopter can be gained by using the A except for the great disparity in appearance).

b. The Univis and Kurova series will also permit the introduction of limited amounts of vertical prism by utilizing different shaped segments. The A introduces base-down; the C, base-up; and combinations of various other shapes can be employed. The R series also permits a choice of segments in which the pole of the add is placeable at various heights. The shape differences in the R series are not so prominent as with others.

3. *Bicentric Grinding*

a. Bicentric grinding or slab-off can be incorporated in a bifocal. The prismatic effect can be located anywhere on the lens, but it is customary to have the dividing line of the slab-off coincide with the top of the segment.

b. The magnitude of the bicentric grinding can be from about 1.5 Δ to 5 Δ depending upon the thickness of the lens blank.

4. Since the introduction of prism is now possible in several varieties of lenses, the use of differently shaped segments is not too common. The introduction of prism does involve a more costly process and usually results in a thicker and heavier lens. The Ultex group may exhibit a shelf around the segment which is hard to keep free of dirt. Where the cost is a greater factor than the appearance, the differently shaped segments may be used. The slaboff has been found to be very popular with many refractionists.

XII. CHOOSING A BIFOCAL

A. Generally, most forms of bifocals are usable by the average patient. While one may have chromatic aberration, and another "jump," these are difficulties which are only a small part of the general adjustment which the bifocal requires in the visual habits of the patient, and are more over-emphasized by the manufacturers of the various forms than by the major run of patients. In using a single vision lens, the patient who wished to see the floor merely dropped his eyes, while when he wished to read, he could hold his print at any point and move his head to sight the matter. With bifocals, the movement of the head is now required to see the floor, while dropping the eyes automatically places them in the bifocal, ready for reading. This reversal of habits, plus the sensation of blur or "dirt" on the lenses which the peripherally seen add presents, constitute the major elements requiring a period of adjustment to the bifocals, assuming that no change in the habitual displacement of the reading point has been affected or that anisometropia is not present at a newly located reading center. Few patients actually complain of either jump or color, but the increased depth of field, the more habitual displacement at the reading point and the ability to enter the reading field close to the margins of the segment, make the better forms of bifocals more desirable and easier for acclimatization when first worn.

B. Besides the question of anisometropia and jump, there are various factors involving the use of the bifocal and the habits of the patient which may influence the choice of a segment or type. The custom of attempting to eliminate displacement altogether instead of merely avoiding a great change in the accustomed displacement, and the application to individuals first requiring lenses at all, still make the choice of the segment by virtue of diminution of differential displacement or total displacement common practice. Part of this is due to the educational endeavors of the manufacturers, who have developed charts and graphs indicating preferable selections based upon purely optical factors of the lenses themselves without too great a regard for the accustomed habits and requirements of the patient.

1. Most single vision lenses, up to recent years, have been made with spherical back curves and cylindrical front curves. Fused bifocals are made with spherical front curves and cylindrical back curves. It has been postulated that this difference in the shape factor in changing from a single vision lens to a bifocal may induce a difference in orientation which the new bifocal wearer may find very disturbing in addition to the other characteristics described earlier. It will be interesting to observe whether the use, advocated by some, of single vision lenses with minus cylinders on the back surface (as is used for many modern bifocals) will show an improvement in patient acceptance.

C. By Optical Performance

1. Morgan (1963), in an experiment involving eight modern bifocal lens designs, demonstrated that aberrations interact and errors tend to cancel. He advocates controlling the astigmatism through the use of appropriate surface curves and controlling the dispersion by selecting the proper position of the segment center with respect to the center of the distance lens and the nu value of the glass.

2. Image quality was found to vary with the power of the distance lens power and the bifocal segment shape. No one bifocal uniformly produced the best image quality. For plus lenses,

segments whose centers were lower tended to produce better image quality. For minus lenses, segments with centers located higher in the lens gave better image quality.

D. By Considerations Involving Displacement, Total and Differential

1. *Where the distance correction is of strong plus power:*

a. The Ultex A, Univis, Vision-Ease, Kurova R or prism segments may be used to present base-down in the segment which will neutralize some of the strong base-up effect of the distance correction.

2. *Where the distance correction is minus in power:*

a. The Univis, Vision-Ease, Kurova, and other prism seg bifocals or any having the pole only a short distance from the top of the seg, such as the Sovereign or Nokrome 16 mm., will either help neutralize some of the base-down induced by the distance portion or will avoid adding to it to any marked extent. Monocentric forms may also be used.

3. *Where the distant correction is plano (in the vertical meridian):*

a. Univis, Kurova, Vision-Ease, Titmus, Sovereign, Executive, Horizon, Panoptik, Ultex B, X-Cel, and most bifocals will induce little prismatic effect if their poles are not too far from the reading center.

4. *Where both the distant correction and add are of strong plus power:*

a. Since the distant correction will induce marked prism base-up, it is desirable to use bifocals which provide stronger base-down effect or do not add to the base-up effect. The Ultex series and the segments with poles practically at the reading center are usable for this purpose. Since certain aberrations are more likely in these powers, the front surface Ultex or Round Barium forms are preferable.

5. *Where the distance correction is weaker than the add:*

a. Since the movement of the visual axis into the segment will produce a sudden reversal of displacement, it is recommended that lenses with a high segment pole such as the Tillyer Executive, Panoptik, Univis, Sovereign, Vision-Ease C, Kurova, Tillyer, Titmus C, X-Cel, etc., or Ultex B or Kryptok type segments be used.

6. *Where prism is desired in the segment only:*

a. Panoptik; Sovereign; Univis & Vision-Ease R prism; Univis & Vision-Ease compensated R; Kurova R; Ultex B & A; or slab-off in the above.

E. Considerations Involving Other Structural Factors

1. *Small Reading Segments:*

a. Kryptok 13 & 16, Univis, Vision-Ease and Kurova B; and others by special construction.

(1) The Univis, Vision-Ease and Kurova B have a segment which is only 9 mm. high. On the average, this permits a vertical field, by projection, of approximately 20-25 cms. at a 40 cm. reading distance.

2. *Segments Permitting Visibility Around The Segment:*

a. Kryptok 13 & 16; Univis, Panoptik, Sovereign, Tillyer S, Titmus, Kurova, Vision-Ease, Kote-Line, X-Cel, etc.

b. Kryptok 20 & 22, Ultex B

3. *Highest Invisibility*

a. Barium type round

b. Kryptok

c. Ultex B

d. Blended and progressive addition forms are totally invisible under usual viewing.

4. *Large Reading Field*

a. Ultex AA or AL

b. Executive, Horizon, Bi-Field, X-Pan, Rede-rite

c. Panoptik, Sovereign, and Univis, Minus-seg and similar types

d. Large sized segs of D/types such as 28, 25 and 45 mm. wide

5. *Intermediate Fields*

a. Small angle – Panoptik, Univis, Sovereign, Kurova, Vision-Ease, Kote-line, Titmus trifocals

b. Large angle – Ultex X, Executive, Horizon

c. Major Intermediate – Univis, Kurova, Vision-Ease, Sovereign, Panoptik, Kote-Line, Tillyer double segs with distance power in major lens and Vision-Ease 10 x 28 trifocal.

6. *Field in Upper Portion*

a. Panoptik, Univis, Sovereign, Kurova, Vision-Ease, Nokrome, Titmus ST, Kote-Line, Tillyer D double segments

b. Standard bifocals in inverted position

F. By Specific Vocations

1. *Customary Use*

a. The usual bifocal is placed from 3 to 4 mm. below the lower pupil margin. The round top types are usually placed in the higher position while the arched or straight tops are placed fractionally lower. This permits the maximum vertical angle of vision at distance without lowering the most usable portion of the segment beyond reasonable range. While the Nokrome and modern types offer a field almost usable to the margins of the segment, the actual dimensions as well as the pole position of the segment do affect the portion of the segment used. Thus, round top bifocals usually require a greater tilt of the head to elevate the wider lower portion to the position of fixation, while the straighter topped types permit a more natural head position for utilization of the major width of the segment. (This permits placement of the latter a bit lower in the lens.)

b. Ellerbrock and Fry (1941) have recommended that the bifocal be set to approximate as closely as possible the position in which the pole of the segment coincides with the reading center. This is impossible in certain types without interference with the distant field.

c. Generally, *stout people* who carry their heads well back will require the top of the segment in a lower position than average, while *stooped individuals* will wear it higher than normal in order to maintain their accustomed posture at near. *Tall persons* will also prefer the segment in a lower position in order to avoid interference with their accustomed inferior range when walking. People doing constant close work will accept a larger or higher bifocal than will those doing only occasional close work.

2. *Large or Highly Positioned Segments*

a. Certain vocations will find highly-positioned or larger segments more useful than the standard types. This group includes architects, barbers, proofreaders, accountants, drafts-men, jewelers, teachers, and others who must have a large near field or who may be required to view the entire top of a desk, drawing board or work bench without too many changes in head position.

b. Such types as the Executive, Ultex series, Cen-Cor, Titmus 28, Univis 28, Kote-Line 28 or 35, Bi-Field, the larger Panoptik, or larger Kryptok types may be used.

c. Occasionally a Kurova, Rede-rite or minus add lens can be used, but such lenses are entirely vocational and best supplied for a specific function only.

3. *Small Segments*

a. Athletes, golfers, builders, mechanics, carpenters, and others who must require a distant field beneath the segment or who may have occasion to use the near field only sporadically, will prefer the small segment for vocational use.

b. The Round Barium type 13 or 16 and Univis, Vision-Ease, and Kurova B lend themselves best for this purpose.

4. *A Large Field Centrally Placed*

a. The surgeon, radiologist, and dentist usually require a full near field which permits a wide angle of vision without too many awkward head positions.

b. The Executive, Ultex AA, AL, L or Target, and the Kurova, Rede-rite or minus add Panoptik, Sovereign or Univis are usable.

5. *A Large Field Above the Center*

a. The ear, nose and throat specialist or others whose field of work may be above the median plane will require a vocational lens which presents the segment in the upper portion.

b. An inverted Ultex, Ultex B, or inverted R or large seg Panoptik can be used.

6. *Specially Placed Segs*

a. The hunter or marksman may require lenses which have the segment placed in a position in which the sighting eye can see both the front and back sights with the gun in firing position (although not necessarily both through the segment). These usually require special placement of the segment.

b. Round Barium type small segments or other types of round segment bifocals can be specially shaped or ground to place the segment in the required position.

c. The AO Executive Segment can be placed at an angle–high, low or even vertically as the occasion requires.

7. *Intermediate Segments*

a. The use of trifocals as a general purpose lens is becoming more popular. It is evident that presbyopia requiring an addition of more than 2.00 D. must leave the patient with an area of indistinct vision between the P.P. of the distance and the P.R. of the add. Besides granting more efficient general visual service, the trifocal often permits continuation at specific vocations which would be otherwise impossible.

b. *Certain vocations may require the trifocal for purely vocational uses.*

(1) The carpenter, laundress, craftsman, chauffeur, and all who work at arm's length may need a trifocal for their vocations. Also the musician, printer and stenographer require vision at distances beyond the range of the bifocal.

(2) Clerks in stores and others who must see at arm's length at a position which makes tilting of the head very awkward, will frequently require an intermediate field. Depending on the vocation of the individual, the size of the intermediate field will vary.

(3) The use of lenses with three distinct focal points may be summarized as follows:

(a) For vocations in which the intermediate field is used for only limited functions, such as the reading of scales, book titles on shelves, etc., the customary small intermediate segments are preferable. These include the Orthogon ST, Univis, Vision-Ease, Kurova, X-Cel, Kote-Line, Titmus, Tillyer S or Executive trifocals with intermediate segments ranging from 6 to 7 mm. in height.

(b) For uses in which the intermediate may be required for a fairly large field and a fairly frequent portion of the time, such as by mechanics, craftsmen, laundresses, and other vocations with similar visual demands, the somewhat larger trifocals found in the Tillyer 724 (C or S), Panoptik, Kurova, Univis, X-Cel, Vision-Ease, Kote-Line, Titmus, Horizon and Executive trifocals in the wider dimensions such as 24 to 28 are available. The Executive and Horizon are available to a width of 60 mms.; the Ultex X has a width of 32 to 33 mms., with an intermediate up to 8½ mm. in height. Vision-Ease makes an intermediate of either 8 or 10 mms. in height and up to 28 mms. wide. X-Cel also makes an intermediate of 8 mms. in height.

(c) For vocations requiring very large intermediate fields such as sculptors, accountants, barbers and similarly employed individuals, the double segment forms with the intermediate as the major lens might be preferable.

(d) For vocations requiring a field above the major lens, inverted bifocals or the double segment trifocals might be used.

(e) Since all trifocals are not a constant fraction of the add in the power of the intermediate, the form alone of the trifocal should not be the final criterion for selection.

(f) Where an intermediate field is required in a special position, as for tailors or stenographers, the Executive, Horizon or Ultex X may provide the largest intermediate field in lateral directions, unless a specially compounded lens is ordered.

REFERENCES

Bannon, R.E. (1951): *Trifocal Lenses – A Clinical Study Based on 22, 640 Trifocal Prescriptions. A.A.A.O., 28: 254.*

*Boeder, P. (1939): *Analysis of Prismatic Effects in Bifocal Lenses. Am. Opt. Co.*

Borish, I.M. (1947): *Trifocals. Indiana Opt., 19 (12): 20.*

*Bronson, L.D. (1952): *A Recent Development in Bifocals. O.J.R.O., 89 (2): 28.*

Brown, J.J. (1942): *Dissimilar Segments Simplified. A.A.A.O., 19: 388.*

*Davis, J.K. & Fernald, H.G. (1969): *The One-Piece (Franklin-Type) Bifocal, A.A.A.O., 46: 163.*

*DuPont, E.C. (1962): *Bifocal Segments, Pt. 1. B.J.P.O. 19: 139.*

*DuPont, E.C. (1963): *Bifocal Segments, Pt. 2. B.J.P.O., 20: 41.*

Ellerbrock, V.J. (1948): *A Clinical Evaluation of Compensation for Vertical Imbalances. A.A.A.O., 25: 309.*

Ellerbrock, V.J. & Zinnecker, K.S. (1950): *Ranges of Clear Vision Through Multifocal Lenses. Opt. Weekly, 41: 1893.*

*Ellerbrock, V.J. & Zinnecker, K.S. (1952): *Effect of Multifocal Lenses on Convergence. A.A.A.O., 29: 82.*

Fry, G.A. & Ellerbrock, V.J. (1941): *Placement of Optical Centers in Bifocal Lenses. Opt. Weekly, 32: 989.*

Goldberg, J.B (1948): *Practical Considerations When Fitting Trifocal Lenses. Opt. Weekly, 39: 2055.*

*Hancock, V. (1938): *An Analysis of Bifocal Prescriptions. Univis Lens Co.*

*Knoll, H.A. (1952): *The Optical Characteristics of Beach Blended Bifocals. A.A.A.O., 29: 150.*

Knoll, H.A. (1962): *The Optical Characteristics of So-Called Invisible Bifocals. A.A.A.O., 39: 538.*

*Lueck, I.B. (1937): *Bifocal Analysis In Anisometropia. Bausch & Lomb, Sci. & Tech., Pub. No. 18.*

*Maitenez, B. (1966): *Four Steps That Led to Varilux. A.A.A.O., 43: 441.*

*Marks, R. (1947): *Trifocals – Their Theory and Application. A.A.A.O., 24: 359.*

*Miles, P.W. (1951): *Experiment in Which Fifty Presbyopes Were Provided With Trifocal Glasses. Arch. Oph., 46: 542.*

Miles, P.W. (1953): *Depth of Focus and Amplitude of Accommodation Through Trifocal Glasses. Arch. Oph., 49: 271.*

Morgan, M.W. (1940): *Optometric Optics. Univ. Calif.*

Morgan, M.W. (1963): *The Optical Performance of Certain Bifocal Lenses. A.A.A.O., 40: 227.*

*Obrig, T. (1935): *Modern Ophthalmic Lenses and Optical Glass. New York. 3rd ed. (1944), Chilton Press, Phila.*

*Pollack, P. (1949): *How to Calculate the Seg Inset in Bifocals. Opt. World, 37 (4): 27.*

*Reed, W.B. (1953): *Why Barium Segments in Bifocal Lenses. Vision, Am. Opt. Co., 37 (1).*

Reiner, J. (1968): *A New Corrective Lens with Progressively Varying Addition. Monthly Clinical Oculists Bulletin, Stuttgart, Germany, 152 (4): 594.*

*Roos, W. (1966): *The Raypath Through the Near Portion of Bifocal Lenses. A.A.A.O., 43: 71, translated by J.W. McConnell.*

*Schwartz, W., Sr. & Schwartz, W., Jr. (1967): *An Evaluation of Our First 100 Varilux Cases. Optical Index, 42 (5): 26.*

Shepard, C.F. (1951): *Locating the Segments. Opt. Weekly, 42: 1371.*

Shepard, C.F. (1951): *The Line of Least Resistance. Opt. Weekly, 42: 1445.*

Simecik, J.F. (1952): *Fitting the Intermediate in Trifocals. O.J.R.O., 89 (11): 34.*

Sinn, F.W. (1948): *Chromatism in Bifocal Segments. A.A.A.O., 25: 211.*

Sterling, S. (1935): *Modern Bifocal Lenses. Ophthalmic Lenses, Bausch & Lomb.*

*Sterling, W. (1952): *The Specifications of Color of Ophthalmic Glasses. A.A.A.O., 30: 335.*

*Swaine, W. (1962): *The Varilux Lens: A Unique Aid for Presbyopia. Opt., 144: 287.*

*Westheimer, G. (1955): *Measuring Bifocal Additions. A.A.A.O., 32 (1): 660.*

*Wild, B.W. (1966): *Progressive Addition Lenses. Opt. Weekly, 57 (28): 18.*

Yeates, F.C.O. (1949): *Prescribing Trifocals. Opt. Weekly, 40: 1269.*

*Zinnecker, K.S. & Ellerbrock, V.J. (1933): *An Investigation of the Factors Affecting the Field of Fixation Through Multifocal Lenses. A.A.A.O., 30: 202.*

*Technical Publications of Manufacturers of Various Bifocals Listed in Chapter.

SECTION V

MONOCULARITY AND STRABISMUS

Strabismus/Definition, Development and Classification 29

I. DEFINITION

A. Morgan (1948) has defined strabismus as "the ocular condition which is characterized by the use of one eye for fixation while the other eye is directed to some other point in the field of vision." Inherent in this definition of strabismus is the concept that strabismus involves at least two factors:

1. *Sensory*
   a. A change in the input of visual information through the two eyes of the visual system.
2. *Motor*
   a. Some kind of mal-alignment of the two visual axes with respect to an object of regard.

B. If throughout his study the student keeps in mind the dualistic problem of the strabismic patient i. e., both sensory and motor factors, he will avoid many of the pitfalls of his predecessors and will be in a position to provide better care by comprehending the totality of the strabismic's problem.

C. Terms used synonymously with strabismus are: squint, manifest ocular deviation, tropia, ophthalmotropia, heterotropia, cross eyes, and wall eyes.

D. The motor anomaly in heterotropia can be caused by a defect in the oculomotor system at any level. For convenience in understanding this system, it can be broken down into subdivisions:

1. The cortical control centers and pathways.
2. The midbrain nuclei, particularly those concerned with accommodative-convergence relationships and convergence itself.
3. The cranial nerves (III, IV, and VI).

4. The origin insertion, integrity or innervation of the extraocular muscles
5. The effects of space-taking lesions in the orbit.

E. The extent and direction of the strabismic deviation manifested depends on the type of deficiency in the visual system and can be reduced to an ocular rotation of the non-fixing eye with respect to the fixing eye about one, two or all of the three axes of rotation (x, y or z.) (Figure XXIX-1).

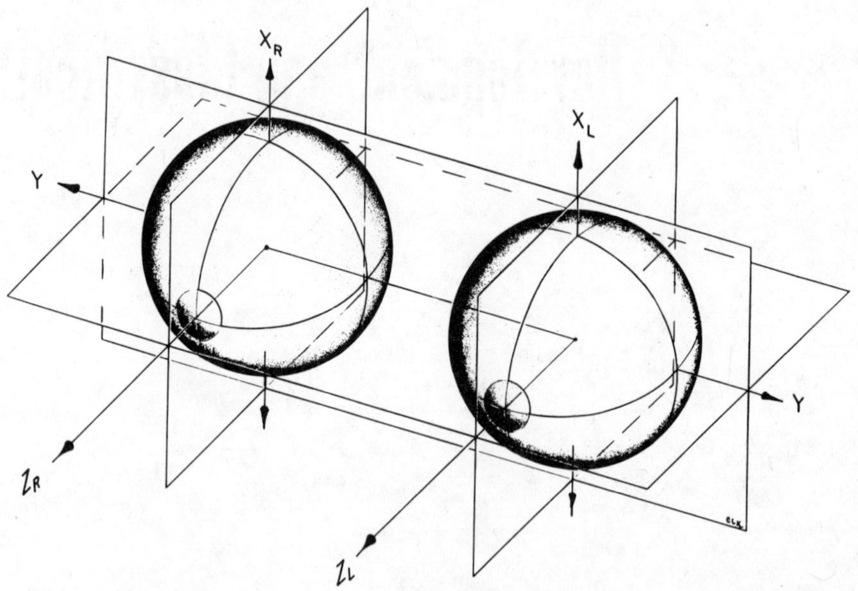

Figure XXIX-1 – Axes about which ocular rotations can be described.

F. The causes and classification will be more completely developed in a later section of this chapter.

II. DEVELOPMENT

A. The presence of two eyes situated on either side of the midline in the head, in addition to providing a safety factor against loss or damage of a single central visual organ, gives additional visual information about the individual's physical surround. Advantages which are well known accrue, such as:

1. The increase of 25% in the size of the field of view;
2. stereopsis gained from comparison of slight disparities in the two retinal images;
3. the improved visual acuity resulting from binocular summation;
4. the kinesthetic cues arising from convergence and accommodation.

B. Derangement of the adventitious, complex, binocular oculomotor apparatus which causes a non-alignment of the two eyes, however, can cause a serious problem for an infant or young child who is learning to unify and integrate his multisensory input with his motor activity in order to explore and manipulate his immediate physical world. It is thus important that the slightly different visual impressions impinged on the retinas of the two eyes be united at some level to form a single visual percept in order to avoid the confusion and contradiction among visual, auditory, tactile and proprioceptive sensations which would result if each eye conveyed a separate sensation of a single object or if two different objects were perceived as lying straight ahead. Such a unified visual impression is known as single binocular perception.

1. The development of single binocular vision in the individual follows an orderly development of specific motor responses of the infant. This development has been cited by some to indicate the empirical or environmental basis of the organization of the entire visual process. It seems more likely, however, that the functional organization follows the physical development of the ocular apparatus, which Chavasse (1939) indicates is far from complete at the time of birth. Thus, certain preliminary eye movements become more complex not solely by virtue of experience or adaptation, but when the anatomy and physiology of the child is sufficiently mature to permit their execution. Ling (1942) notes that a group of children subjected to the same environmental conditions since birth early portray marked differences according to consistent types in regard to the exhibition of certain visual performances.

2. According to Worth (1903) the *pupillary light reflexes* are present at birth. Fixation develops from monocular irregularity to binocularity within 5 to 6 weeks and binocular vision seems to predominate at 6 months. *Fusion* is consistently strengthened up to 6 years of age, at which time it is fully developed. Chavasse maintains that the anatomy of the eye itself is not completed for several months after birth and that the fovea is not fully developed for some time. From these observations he inferred that fusion cannot be perfectly exercised until the anatomical processes are complete.

3. Chavasse postulated that the development of the binocular visual system was based upon orderly sequences in ontological processes. (See also Chapter VII) The first visual reflexes phylogenetically traceable are those known as the *compensatory,* associated with *vestibular stimulation.* These are ascribed to innervation of a neurologically low reflex level.

a. Of a higher order are the reflexes termed *pursuit* (fixation and refixation) or *following reflexes.* These reflexes are not only exhibited in higher orders of life than the previous orders of life, but are attributed to centers lying outside the nucleii, elsewhere in the midbrain or cortex.

b. Of still a more complex order are the *vergence reflexes* associated with single binocular vision and confined mainly to man and the closely related primates.

(a) Ling (1942) found the compensatory reflexes present immediately after birth in humans but not fully efficacious until the age of five or six weeks, at which time the eyes would follow an object while the head was turned.

c. Chavasse (1939) indicated that the culmination of the system of binocular vision was dependent upon the proper anatomical development in sequence of the sensory and motor systems involved, and that an anatomical deficiency affecting one of the more primitive responses depicted above would interfere with the proper development of the response presumed to maturate after it.

(1) Ling listed the order of development of binocular usage of the eyes in the following series of steps: absence of fixation, monocular fixation, monocular dominance, alternation of dominance, binocular fixation. (See also Section 5 below.)

4. *Visual acuity*

a. Chavasse estimated visual acuity to be 10/2000 at birth and 20/166 at the age of one year. Recent results show the acuity to be far in excess of that.

b. Fantz (1961) found the following acuities based upon subjective optokinetic nystagmus and selectivity tests:

(1) **Table XXIX-1**

Age in months	*0.5*	*1.5*	*2.5*	*3.5*	*4.5*	*5.5*
Acuity	*20/400*	*20/400*	*20/400*	*20/200*	*20/200*	*20/100*

c. Dayton, Jansen and Jones (1962) report an accurate acuity determined by optokinetic nystagmus of 20/160 to 20/150 for one month old infants of normal term.

(1) In a later study, the acuity of the newborn was found to be at least 20/150 or better by methods combining electro-oculographic recording with visual confirmation of optokinetic nystagmus (Dayton, et al., 1964a,b).

d. Dayton, et al. (1964a,b), also found the acuity of premature infants to range from 20/800 to 20/1000 while Kiff and Lepard (1966) found it to range from 20/410 to 20/820 for a sample of premature babies.

5. *Fixation*

a. It had been assumed that sustained fixation was absent at birth but appeared in rudimentary form in a few hours and reached a plateau in 4 to 5 weeks (Ling). Chavasse held that binocular fixation seemed to make its first appearance at an average of seven weeks of age, and was then usually accompanied by the appearance of convergence.

b. Dayton and his colleagues, in two separate studies (1964a, 1964b), utilizing electro-oculography, found that 17 of 45 newborn infants seemed able to place and maintain the image of a moving target upon the general macular area, demonstrating an innately more developed fixation reflex than had heretofore been realized. A modicum of binocular vision appeared to be present with what appeared to be conjugate movement in following a target, in a sample of babies from 8 hours to 10 days old.

(1) Wertheimer had earlier demonstrated (1961) in the one infant which he studied, the ability to perform directional oculomotor responses when elicited by an auditory stimulus in 22 out of 45 trials, at an age of 3 to 10 minutes after birth.

6. *Accommodation*

a. Ling (1942) found a different response to stimuli within a foot of the eyes as compared to stimuli presented farther away in infants of 4 to 5 weeks in which the development of sustained visual fixation had been assumed to have reached a plateau. He assumed that this might indicate that while the first signs of visual spatial perception were apparent, accommodation had not been developed.

(1) However, Haynes, White and Held (1965) utilizing dynamic skiametry upon 22 infants ranging in age from 6 days to 4 months, found an inflexible accommodative posture of about 5 diopters which proved invariant for the first month of life but developed into an increasingly flexible skill in accommodative tracking so that by the fourth month, it approximated adult performance.

7. The results of investigations into perceptual developmental aspects of infant's vision by Fantz (1961), Dayton, et. al. (1962, 1964), and Bower (1966) and others have demonstrated responses in form, size and distance which indicate in neonates a far more sophisticated sensorial and perceptual ability in vision than heretofore credited.

a. Bower (1965) from the results of operant conditioning studies of infants concludes: "It has long been assumed that perceptual development is a process of construction – that at birth infants receive through their senses fragmentary information that is elaborated and built on to produce the ordered perceptual world of the adult. The theory emerging from our studies. . . is based on evidence that infants can in fact register most of the information an adult can register but can handle less of the information than adults can. Through maturation they presumably develop the requisite information processing capacity."

b. These more recent studies would thus tend to indicate a radically increased precocity of the visual system in developing infants over that assumed by the more traditional classical view.

C. The individual who cannot develop the ability to "fuse'. the images of both eyes must nevertheless learn to secure, first, a single visual impression, since diplopia would make his surroundings intolerable, and second, a proper localization of the objects seen by him so that he finds agreement between what he sees and what he can touch.

1. The desired single vision is secured by the development of a *monocular* or *uniocular* visual pattern, which may take one of two forms.

a. The eye with poorer vision or with weaker fixation or non-dominancy may have its image suppressed at the higher levels so that only the image of one eye is transmitted and interpreted.

b. If one eye is anatomically deviated so that non-corresponding points are directed at the object of regard and suppression of the image of the eye is impossible or difficult, correspondence between new retinal areas may be developed, a condition known as *anomalous correspondence.*

(1) This adaptation allows a more normal field of view and many of the advantages of binocular vision, such as gross peripheral stereopsis, to the strabismic.

2. Very infrequently a strabismic cannot make a successful adaptation for single vision so that a persistent diplopia is experienced with an inability to fuse termed *horror fusionis.*

a. Cyclotropia has sometimes been found clinically to be responsible for this jump-over at the centration point in strabismus and thus to preclude any bimacular fusion.

D. Whichever course is pursued, *Fusion, Suppression or Anomalous Correspondence,* the individual usually adopts one method of securing single vision. Normal development indicates that fusion is the natural selection, but if for some reason fusion is impossible, the individual will proceed along one of the remaining paths leading to monocularity or ambiocularity rather than binocularity. As Chavasse states:

1. "All varieties of squint appear as perversions or subversions of the normal binocular reflexes by various obstacles operative during the developmental period or afterwards."

E. A major conclusion that can be drawn is that diplopia and confused localization is intolerable and that the development of some perceptual adaptation which permits consistent localization of the images in each eye is an unavoidable consequence of diplopia and confusion.

III. PERCEPTUAL ADAPTATIONS

A. Suppression

1. If the uniocular method of securing single vision is selected, the partial or complete suppression or neutralization of sensory impressions from one eye is usually exhibited. The strabismic may exhibit suppressions of various types:

a. *unilateral,* where parts or all of the visual information coming from one eye are not passed along to the higher cortical centers.

b. *alternating,* where this "blockage" occurs in first one and then the other eye occurring either on a voluntary or involuntary basis.

c. A *combination* of one and two, where one eye is used for fixation at near tasks with the other suppressed, and a switch in the fixating eye occurs for distance vision requirements.

2. *Suppression* is not a pathological function limited to aberrant perception in strabismics. A normal binocular observer does not usually experience diplopia for all objects in his field of view not lying on his instantaneous horopter. That he can be made to do so by calling his attention to this *physiological diplopia* is a readily demonstratable phenomenon. The influence of "attention" in producing even a gross monocular suppression in a normal observer can be demonstrated by the well known "hole in the hand" experiment. If a tube of paper two inches or less in diameter and ten or more in length held close to one eye, is directed at a distant fixation object, and the observer's hand is held up, palm facing the observer at a distance of four to six inches before the other eye, the distant object viewed through the tube is seen framed by the hand as though through an apparent "hole in the hand." (See Figure XXIX-2.) If the observer now switches his attention to the hand rather than the distant object seen through the tube, the hand is seen whole and the suppressed area reappears.

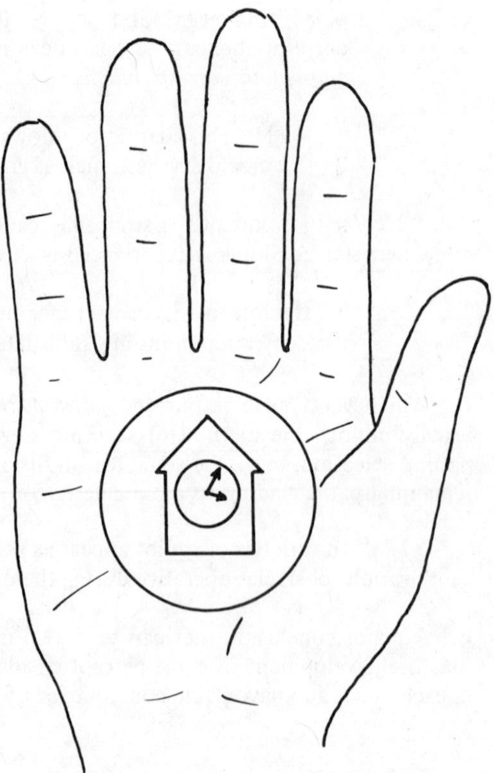

Figure XXIX-2 – Hole in the Hand Experiment.

a. Creating sufficient illumination differences (50 to 1 or less for most observers) between the fields viewed by the two eyes of a normal observer can also cause a complete suppression of the eye confronted by the lower lighting level. Movement of the entire monocular field of view can also cause suppression of part or all of the contralateral immobile field, as is commonly observed in a mirror stereoscope or cheiroscope.

3. The aberrant type of suppression is not confined to cases of strabismus, also being found in cases in which no cosmetic squint is evident, but in which anisometropia, aniseikonia or other interferences with fusional processes exist.

4. It is generally agreed that suppression is a psycho-physiological phenomenon occurring at a high cortical level. A non-objectionable demonstration of electrophysiological changes accompanying suppression is still awaited.

5. *Suppression is classified as:*

a. *Physiological* – during ordinary binocular vision, two identical images, disparately located on the retina, do not result in physiologic diplopia.

b. *Gross* – the image on an extended area of one retina is totally ignored.

(1) Complete or incomplete, or absolute or non-absolute – applying to various distances at which suppression occurs, as at all distances or at near only, etc.

(2) Total or partial – applying to the extent of the field suppressed

(3) Permanent, temporary or intermittent

(4) Suppression is the word usually applied to voluntary neutralization of an image, while suspension is sometimes the term used for involuntary neutralization, but such a differentiation is academic, and hence the term suppression will be used to cover both concepts.

6. Suppression is usually manifested only when both eyes are open, since its main objective is that of securing unconfused single vision. Two principal areas of the retina of the non-fixing eye are involved in conditions of strabismus. The fovea of the non-fixing eye is suppressed so that its percept is not confused with that of the peripheral area of the fixing eye with which it may correspond at the angle of squint, and the peripheral area of the non-fixing eye must also be suppressed to avoid diplopia and confusion. However, the former is usually the area under consideration when suppression is reviewed.

a. This area may expand in size according to the needs of the individual, and may be charted on a tangent screen by appropriate binocular screening methods (Scobee, 1952). An analogy may be drawn between the fusion area of the non-squinter and the suppression area of the strabismus case. Both are similar in shape and location, although not necessarily in size, being generally larger horizontally than vertically and larger temporally than nasally. As stimulation of one fovea and the fusion area results in single vision in one case, stimulation of the fovea and suppression area results in single vision in the other, although the analogy does not predicate a physiological correspondence between the two actions. A stimulation falling outside of the suppression area usually results in diplopia.

7. Jampolsky (1958) in a study of various characteristics of suppression in strabismus, points out that this type of suppression "requires a short latent period to become manifest" and that this phenomenon may be "used to advantage in examination and determination of relative localization" with either similar or dissimilar targets by utilizing instrument flashing or rapid blinking by the patient.

a. Allen (1966) makes use of intermittent stimulation alternating from one eye to the other at a rate of 7 – 15 cycles/sec. as the basis for an entire rationale of strabismus therapy based on the Bartley brightness enhancement phenomenon.

8. Kaufman (1963) has shown that suppression exhibited by normal binocular observers to rivalry phenomena, spreads from the immediate region of the contour overlap as a decreasing monotonic function of angular distance. The occurrence of non-conjugate eye movements increases in this spread. The influence of these movements is attributed to the time lag in recovery from suppression "so that a moving contour can, in effect, leave a wake of suppression in its path in the contralateral field."

9. Electrophysiological evidence on the nature of suppression is reported by Lehmann and Fender (1968).

a. While presenting a steadily illuminated field with varying structure to one eye, and a superimposed light flash of constant parameters to the other eye, of seven normally binocular subjects, they recorded the averaged visual evoked response. It was found that area under the visual evoked response curve decreased monotonically with increased target structure although the peak latencies and relative peak amplitudes do not change. From this they conclude that the reduction of the evoked response was a consequence of "increased informational load" upon the neural populations whose activity is synchronized by the flash.

10. All in all, suppression must be viewed as a useful mechanism for normal binocular observers as well as for those having interferences of the fusional processes.

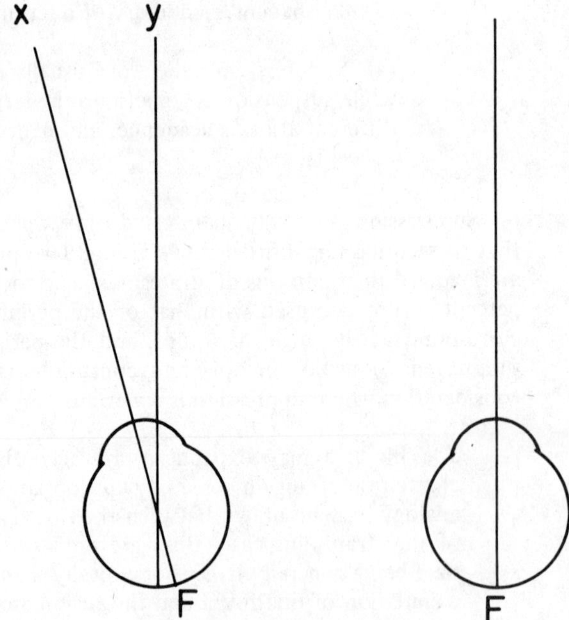

Figure XXIX-3 – Illustrating Suppression.
x – image suppressed to eliminate confusion
y – image suppressed to eliminate diplopia

B. Amblyopia

1. Amblyopia is defined (Schapero, et. al., 1960) as: "reduced visual acuity not correctable by refractive means and not attributable to obvious structural or pathological ocular anomalies." It is classified as:

a. Primary – in which no visible pathological anomaly is found to account for the poor vision.

(1) *Congenital* – reduced vision existing from the time of birth.

(a) It may or may not be accompanied by a total loss of color vision (achromatopsia) and other congenital abiotrophies.

[1] A type formerly called "astigmatic amblyopia" has been found, in some cases, by Ludlam and Wittenberg (1966), to be caused by mal-aligned ocular components which produce optical defects not fully correctible with spectacle lenses. Contact lenses bring about a better alignment and a return to nearly normal visual acuity.

[a] Since this form is attributable to optical anomalies, Schapero (1971) questions its true inclusion among conditions classified as amblyopia.

(2) Acquired or Functional

(a) *Amblyopia exanopsia* or suppression amblyopia

[1] It develops at an early age in the non-fixing eye in monocular strabismus, anisometropia and aniseikonia.

(b) *Psychic* – hysterical or neurasthenic

(c) *Toxic* – due to exogenic poisons

(d) *Nutritional* – usually due to avitaminosis

b. *Secondary* – in which known causes for the lowered acuity are present.

(1) Conditions grouped in this category are usually the results of past pathological conditions and Schapero (1971) considers their inclusion as conditions of amblyopia as stretching a point. However, since the classical differentiations have included such a category, it is given here for the reader's edification.

(a) *Nictalopia* – night blindness, usually due to retinal disease not opthalmoscopically visible or vitamin deficiency.

[1] There is also a type with a genetic transmittance.

(b) *Hemeralopia* – day blindness, usually due to a central scotoma.

(c) *Anesthesia* – insensitivity of the retina, usually due to occipital lesions.

(d) *Hyperesthesia* – excessive sensitivity, usually psychic in origin.

2. The major forms of amblyopia most commonly found are the congenital, toxic and functional types. Differentiation is somewhat difficult since the fundus appearance may be normal or non-indicative.

a. *Toxic amblyopia* usually can be identified more easily than the other two, primarily because a history of either physical impairment or ingestion of a toxic agent can be determined. Also, the visual fields are affected and usually indications are found in both eyes. A final indication is the fact that such patients are usually much older than those in the other categories because, except in severe exposures or to a particularly virulent agent, a long period is required before the poison affects the vision.

(1) Another form of toxic amblyopia has been reported which bears more direct relationship to the confusion about the differing types. Rodger (1953) has reported conditions of nutritional amblyopia in prisoners of war with effects similar to expected endogenic toxicity. Brock (1952) has likewise noted amblyopia with characteristics similar to those reported by Rodger. Such cases may be apparent in children of very low economic levels in which strabismus may also be apparent.

b. Congenital and functional amblyopia, on the other hand, are both customarily monocular (although congenital may be binocular) and exhibit their onset at an early age. The history is frequently inconclusive and testing may leave the diagnosis in doubt. Upon occasion, congenital deformities may be present, or the refraction may reveal an error which favors a judgement of suppression; but frequently, only an attempt to correct the condition may distinguish the two.

(1) In animals Wiesel and Hubel (1963) have demonstrated neurological damage possibly caused by visual deprivation in early life. Kittens deprived of vision monocularly from birth by the suturing together of the lids of one eye exhibited cellular cortical damage. The authors conclude that the physiological defect resulting from the visual deprivation "represents disruption of connections that were present at birth."

3. Recently, Von Noorden (1967) attempted a reclassification of "what in the past has collectively been referred to as *amblyopia exanopsia.*" The five types, not all of which had previously been classified as amblyopia exanopsia , which he now differentiates are:

a. *Strabismic amblyopia*, which he defines as "reduced visual acuity in one eye in patients with strabismus or history of such without ophthalmoscopically demonstratable anomalies of the fundus."

b. *Amblyopia exanopsia* should no longer be applied to describe the functional visual loss that is due to active retinal inhibition in the strabismic or anisometropic patient. It is now used to describe only the substandard acuity resulting from "deprivation of visual stimuli early in life," as for example, from congenital cataracts.

(1) The term "amblyopia exanopsia", however, is still commonly used in connection with conditions separately classified by Von Noorden such as amblyopia associated with strabismus, anisometropia and aniseikonia. The special definition indicated above appears to be used by Von Noorden alone of the authorities noted.

c. *Anisometropic amblyopia* is the deficit of visual acuity in one eye resulting from unequal refractive errors in the two eyes. Anisometropia is frequently accompanied by strabismus and if amblyopia is present in such cases it is difficult to decide how to classify the amblyopia.

d. *Congenital amblyopia,* being a less than normal acuity occurring from the time of birth, is further subdivided into:

(1) Amblyopia secondary to nystagmus
(2) Organic ambylopia
(3) Amblyopia secondary to congenital achomatopsia

e. *Ametropic amblyopia* which occurs "in one or both eyes of children and adults who have significant refractive errors and have not previously worn their glasses."

f. Von Noorden fails to include hysterical, nutritional, or toxic amblyopia in his classification.

4. It must be re-emphasized that, as with suppression, functional amblyopia is not limited to cases exhibiting strabismus or even marked anisometropia. Hallett (1951) reported a number of cases of amblyopia not associated with strabismus, anisometropia or similarly associated conditions. Where the amblyopia was unilateral, the refraction generally showed a high degree of hyperopia in both eyes, and Hallett believed that suppression had been instituted to avoid associated overconvergence; where the amblyopia was bilateral, Hallett believed that definite indications of malingering or psychiatric disturbances existed. Yasuna (1951) also reports a number of hysterical cases of amblyopia. Some 80% of the cases were bilateral, females were twice as prevalent as males, and the age levels extended from 9 to 35. Field charts exhibited typical tubular fields, the edges of the suppressed areas were sharp and steep, and tests for malingering were frequently positive. Brock (1952) reports that amblyopia is almost as frequent without strabismus as with it, although he finds a greater visual impairment when associated with strabismus. In contrast to Hallett, he did find anisometropia in non-strabismus cases, with the amblyopia quite consistently in the eye of greater error.

5. Flom and Neumaier (1966), taking a deeper look at the statistics of incidence of amblyopia in the population, found that the criteria by which it is defined have an important effect on its reported incidence. Using the criterion of monocular ambloypia of 20/40 or worse with a difference between the eyes of *more* than one acuity line, they estimated a prevalence of 1.8% in school children (see also Chapter X, Visual Acuity).

6. Although the factor of reduced acuity defines amblyopia, it is but one feature in a constellation of symptoms and signs which might well constitute a "functional amblyopia syndrome."

a. *Eccentric fixation*

(1) Starting with the clinical observation of Peckham in 1937 that the only improvable amblyopes he found were those with a displaced blind spot in central field testing, it remained for Brock to demonstrate the relationship of the centration of fixation to amblyopia.

(2) Brock (1952) determined by use of his after-image transfer test, that only some 20% of amblyopes retain fixation. This 20% he considered to be truly *exanopsic* i.e., resulting from disuse. The acuity was found to vary with the eccentricity of fixation. He classified amblyopes into four groups: functioning foveas (9.1%); foveas functioning transiently (17.2%); small or relative central scotomas (30.3%); absolute foveal scotomas (43.4%). Amblyopes with foveal fixation respond well to occlusion.

(3) At about the same time, Goldschmidt (1950) utilized the phenomenon of *Haidinger brushes* to subjectively test the effectivity and centration of the macula in direct fixation. He reported "that where the brushes are seen, the acuity is amenable and macular function is not permanently impaired. The brushes are visible independent of the actual visual acuity. Where they are seen, amblyopic vision shows improvement by simple occlusion within two months; where not seen, there is no improvement of vision no matter how long treated." Gording (1951) used Goldschmidt's technique with identical results.

(a) The Haidinger brush phenomenon can only be perceived in the macula area of an eye with intact foveal and macular pathways. A rotating polaroid is thought to act in concert with the 'natural' polarizing effect occurring in Henle's fiber layer in the retina. The effect is eliminated by the layers of the retina present outside the macula. The percept of the rotating propeller is enhanced when a deep blue-violet filter is placed somewhere along the visual path between the eye and the rotating polaroid. The interposition of a sheet of cellophane causes a reversal of the direction of rotation and is useful in checking on the variety of the responses especially when testing young children. Since the Haidinger brush effect is an entoptic phenomenon it is not influenced by ametropia and can actually be enhanced by the interposition of a strong convex lens which will blur the background, thus improving contrast.

(b), A second entoptic phenomenon centered in the macula is *Maxwell's Spot* which appears as a dark red spot when the eye is confronted by a bluish-purple field. It rapidly fades unless this field is alternated at intervals of two to four seconds with a gray filter of similar density.

[1] A review of the literature on the subject and a theoretical basis for the phenomenon may be found in Spencer (1967).

(c) Flom and Weymouth (1961), utilizing the phenomenon of displacement of Maxwell's Spot from the fixation mark to indicate eccentric fixation in strabismus, found a linear correlation of +0.94 between visual acuity and the amount of displacement of Maxwell's Spot from the nominal fixation point. Thus, 86 of 93 non-amblyopes saw Maxwell's Spot concentric with a macularly viewed fixation mark, while all 11 amblyopes demonstrated a Maxwell Spot displaced by at least 15 minutes of arc. They conclude, "The low acuity of the amblyopes here studied can be explained adequately and simply on the basis of the normally low acuity in the parafoveal regions that these subjects use for fixation. It is not justified to propose that all amblyopia is covered by the explanation but it is legitimate to ask what proportion of amblyopes have eccentric fixation capable of explaining the low acuity without recourse to the hypothesis of 'reduction from disuse'." Spencer (1967), citing this work of Flom and Weymouth, offers "two alternative explanations" for their finding that the Maxwell Spot showed a "high incidence of displacement in association with amblyopia and anomalous correspondence."

[1] The first of these is that ". . . the fovea and structure responsible for generating Maxwell's Spot are concentric while the fixation point is displaced."

[2] The alternative is that ". . . the Maxwell's Spot generating structure is not concentric with the fovea."

[3] She concludes: "While bearing in mind that the latter possibility may be true in certain instances, they found little evidence to support this, but ample confirmation in their results for the first possibility."

(4) The introduction of specialized diagnostic and therapeutic equipment by Cüppers (1956) and Bangerter (1955) served to place the testing and treatment of functional amblyopia caused by eccentric fixation on a practical clinical basis, although much of the rationale had been presented earlier by Smith (1935, 1947) and Brock (1941), and was summarized by Smith in 1961.

(a) Cüppers had placed a variety of grids in a modified ophthalmoscope called a Visuskop which can be projected on the patient's fundus. The fixation pattern of a given eye can thus be evaluated directly by the examiner viewing the fundus through the instrument. The patient is asked to view a central fixation target (dot, star, square). The examiner then locates the projected fixation object on the fundus with relation to the macula and observes the pattern of fixation utilized by the patient in that eye.

(b) The *varieties of fixation* to be found can be classified as:

[1] steady central
[2] wavering central
[3] steady eccentric
[4] wavering eccentric

(c) They are also classified by:

[1] the size of the angle of eccentric fixation
[2] the consistency of the response

(5) Von Noorden and Mackensen (1962) have studied the behavior of eyes with eccentric fixation by serial photography. They differentiate between "eccentric fixation" and "eccentric viewing." Eccentric fixation applies only when "eccentric retinal elements have become associated with the principal visual direction." Eccentric viewing, on the other hand, occurs when the principal visual direction." Eccentric viewing, on the other hand, occurs when the principal visual direction still is associated with the fovea but a "parascotomatous retinal area . . . creates the experience of looking above, below or to either side of the objects." Their study of the fixation pattern of 40 amblyopic esotropes showed that the majority fixated with a retinal area nasal to and slightly above the fovea, thus supporting the similar finding of Flom and Weymouth (1961). Von Noorden and Mackensen also found that visual acuity is generally lower, the more peripheral the fixation area. There were, however, significant exceptions which led them to suggest that "inhibition in amblyopia is not limited to the macula alone."

(6) Alpern, et. al. (1967),while measuring a small amount of eccentric fixation in all of the subjects in their sample of amblyopes,found that the amount of acuity loss in these eyes was much greater than that predicted from the amount of eccentric fixation found. From this they concluded that "there is some physiological or pathological process superimposed upon this eccentric fixation which causes a reduction in the acuity over what normally would be expected with the eccentrically fixated area."

(7) Burian (1966) found that in a limited number of young amblyopes with severe loss of acuity, occlusion of the non-amblyopic eye induces eccentric fixation and amblyopia in the previously normal eye in the unexpectedly short time of six weeks.

(8) Enoch (1957, 1959a, 1959b, 1965) has presented some clinical evidence based on Stiles-Crawford Effect measurements and a theoretical case for the concept of "receptor amblyopia." This condition consists of a tilt or shift in orientation or a malorientation of the photoreceptor fiber elements in the fovea which, because of the directional sensitivity of these fibers, is responsible for a generalized lowering of photopic sensitivity and resolution thereshold in central vision. How prevalent this postulated mechanism is in the amblyopic population has been difficult to show because of the cumbersome and arduous evaluation heretofore necessary to make its diagnosis.

(a) Alpern, et al. (1967), after stating that, "The likelihood that such a mechanism accounts for the loss of visual acuity in any appreciable percentage of cases of strabismus amblyopia has been made very small by the theoretical and experimental findings of Dunnewold (1967)," proposes a simpler idea based on measurements of Stiles-Crawford Effect II. In this phenomenon it has been observed that, "The light entering through the edge of the pupil not only is reduced in brightness compared to that entering through the center, but it gives a different color match as well."

(b) In an initial test of three amblyopes using Nagel Anomaloscope color matches, Alpern, et. al., were able to rule out receptor amblyopia "as an important etiological factor in the acuity loss in these (three) subjects."

(c) Marshall and Flom (1969) likewise indicated that the premise of "receptor amblyopia" was probably invalid by indicating that tilted receptor elements do not thereby reduce visual acuity, and that the abnormal Stiles-Crawford response found by Enoch could itself be explained upon the basis of eccentricity of the fixation.

(d) Further investigation on a large number of amblyopes utilizing this simplified approach would be necessary to establish a firmer association of the role played by "receptor amblyopia" with amblyopia as a whole.

b. *Crowding phenomenon or separation difficulty*

(1) Many functional amblyopes exhibit the ability to read small letters in isolation but are not able to discriminate the same or much larger sized letters when an entire line is displayed. This has caused clinicians working with amblyopes to measure and record acuity in the amblyopic eye as 'whole line acuity' and 'single letter acuity' in order to identify those amblyopes who possessed this characteristic to a marked degree.

(2) Flom, Weymouth and Kahneman (1963) found that separation difficulty occurred in normal observers as well as in amblyopes and "that although the extent of the zone of interaction was *angularly* larger for most amblyopic eyes, it was *not* greatly different in normal and amblyopic eyes when expressed in multiples of the interaction free minimum angle of resolution." Compared to the angle of resolution (or visual acuity) the amblyopic eye exhibits relatively the same effect from interaction in that the distance between two letters (or contours) which produces the effect for either depends upon the size of letter (or angle of resolution) describing the acuity. Thus a normal eye with a 1′ angle of resolution would abide contours proportionately closer together without interaction compared to an amblyopic eye exhibiting an angle of resolution of 5′. The zone of interaction of the amblyopic eye would be apparently larger because of the difference of the angles of resolution.

(3) Stuart and Burian (1962) also noted that the crowding phenomenon was universal and dependent upon the level of visual acuity. They found it was not restricted to the horizontal meridian and exaggerated in amount in strabismic amblyopia.

(4) Flom, Weymouth and Kahneman observed that "while the degree to which eye movements affected interaction in normal eyes was unknown, it seemed to contribute to further impairment of resolution in at least some forms of amblyopia."

(5) Von Noorden and Leffler (1966), investigating binocular interaction in amblyopia, compared the measured visual acuity in 42 amblyopic eyes measured both monocularly and when the sound eye was open but was prevented from seeing the letters. They concluded that measured visual acuity of the amblyopic eye is reduced in direct proportion to the intensity of stimulation received by the sound eye. From this they reinforced the previous observation by Murroughs (1957) that prolonged

constant occlusion which completely eliminates light from the non-amblyopic eye is most effective in restoring vision to eyes suffering from functional amblyopia.

(6) Weymouth (1963) points out that visual acuity testing is more complex in measurement of amblyopes than in normals. In normal vision "there exists a size of letter below which the letters are never identified and one above which the letters are always identified. Between these angular sizes is embraced the *region of uncertainty* within which letters are sometimes correctly named and sometimes not." For normal non-amblyopic observers this region of uncertainty is small compared with the angular size difference of succeeding lines and thus a single reading suffices for a clinical measurement. In amblyopia, however, this "region of uncertainty" is much larger and a single, or even a few trials will yield results difficult to interpret. Weymouth points out that the amblyope "reads and sometimes fails 20/40 for example, but instead of reading all of 20/60 he makes several mistakes and even misses a couple in 20/70. In the opposite direction he reads most of 20/30 and even gets one in 20/20." Thus, "his region of uncertainty is very large and order only appears when the proportion of correct answers is plotted and is seen to increase through the entire range tested."

(a) Consequently, to avoid the often erratic and unrepeatable acuity results with amblyopes, Weymouth warns, "it is necessary to make" many trials and plot some sort of a psychometric function. A hasty test will often wildly overrate or underrate the acuity in an amblyopic eye, leading to a wrong diagnosis or a fictitious "cure."

(7) From the foregoing it is obvious that visual acuity testing in amblyopes should be approached carefully and with patience, the conditions of testing should be recorded, and kept uniform throughout the period of treatment.

c. *Poor performance in aiming, pointing and pursuit movements*

(1) Irregular, unsteady, wavering movements of amblyopic eyes on attempts to fixate have been observed by clinicians for many years and recently have been classified and categorized by Kavner and Suchoff (1966) using the Visuskop (the ophthalmoscopic testing devices developed by Cuppers previously described), and by Von Noorden and Mackensen (1962a, 1962b) using electro-ophthalmography techniques.

(a) The movements are characterized by a slow wandering of the amblyopic fovea away from the target followed by a rapid recovery of the fovea to, or near to, the image of the target which the subject is attempting to fixate. The patterns of these movements are very similar to those observed in optokinetic nystagmus.

(2) Von Noorden and Mackensen (1962b) have also examined closely the quality of motor function in attempted pursuit movements of amblyopic eyes and find a greater impairment evident than in the fixation of a steady target by the same eye.

(a) In measuring 30 eyes with varying degrees of amblyopia for horizontal pursuit movements they found especially at slow velocities, a "saccadation" of the pursuit movement so that there was a deterioration in the quality of the pursuit movement and a "superimposition by coarse jerky deviations."

(b) They were not able to establish a direct correlation between pursuit performance and depth of amblyopia, but successive fixation photographs demonstrated a high relationship between the anomalies of fixation behavior and the quality of the pursuit movement.

(3) Lawwill (1966) investigating the fixation pattern in 20 amblyopic patients with eccentric fixation using an infrared measuring device, noted "no change in the area or steadiness of the fixation pattern" for the light or dark adapted state. He did note, however, that, "the oscillatory movements of attempted fixation were noticeably greater in frequency amplitude and randomness" when fixation was tested with a very bright ophthalmoscope fixation device than when observed with the infrared device in a lighted room.

(a) These findings do not seem to compare well with those of Von Noorden and Burian (1958) who found the fixation of the amblyopic eye to be less steady in the light-adapted than the dark-adapted state, and when viewing through neutral density filters.

d. *Relatively good acuity at low levels of luminance*

(1) In a 1921 study, Ammann reported that the introduction of filters which reduced visual acuity by several lines on an eye chart for normal eyes did not similarly reduce vision in amblyopic eyes. This phenomenon was more recently supported by Von Noorden and Burian (1959) who found that "while the normal group showed a constant reduction of visual acuity, vision was only slightly reduced, remained the same or even improved in the group of patients with squint amblyopia." An additional group with organic amblyopia showed a marked reduction in measured acuity.

(a) They conclude that from a practical standpoint, utilization of a neutral filter test can by helpful in deciding if an amblyopia has a functional or pathological etiology.

(2) In a classic paper in 1944, Wald and Burian reported that the absolute threshold of vision in normal and amblyopic eyes was essentially the same. Grovesnor (1957) and Miller (1954) each later found the differential luminance threshold (Δ I/I) to be reduced in eyes with functional amblyopia when compared to their non-amblyopic fellows; for this effect to be more marked for the higher photopic levels than for the mesopic; and, confirming Wald and Burian, to be essentially equal for scotopic luminances.

(a) Continuing this work, Lawwill and Burian (1966) varied the background luminance of acuity symbols over a 4 log unit range for 16 normal, and 21 ambloypic, eyes. They found that normal eyes required a higher contrast when background luminance was low, and that the amount of contrast could be reduced up to a specific minimal level as luminance was increased. Further increase in luminance was not accompanied by a further decrease in contrast when such a level was reached. Eyes with functional amblyopia, on the other hand, approximated the pattern for normal eyes at low background luminances, but needed greater contrast than normals when the background luminance was high.

(3) However, Caloroso and Flom (1969) re-examined the Von Noorden and Burian data and reported that an analysis of the data does not confirm the conclusion that the vision of the amblyopic eye and its function improves in dim light to a point equal to, or better than, the vision of the non-amblyopic eye. In going from photopia to mesopia, the amblyopic eye did not improve in visual acuity but showed a continuing decline in acuity as did the normal eye with reduced luminance. The visual acuity of the amblyopic eye was poorer than that of the non-amblyopic eye at virtually all luminance levels, except at the lowest level where the acuity of both eyes was approximately equal.

(a) Changes in acuity occurring with changes in luminosity might be explained similarly to the reduction in acuity in amblyopia due to use of the parafoveal areas for fixation, rather than to "selective inhibition of form vision" as offered by Von Noorden and Burian.

(4) Alpern, Flitman and Joseph (1960) found that centrally fixated CFF thresholds in amblyopic eyes, which were markedly reduced compared to normal eyes at high intensities, were essentially the same at reduced levels of retinal luminance. Thus, these findings for CFF roughly paralleled those stated for acuity in the earlier studies just enumerated.

7. Several electrophysiological investigations of the nature and site of the neurological defects responsible for the lowered acuity and other altered functions of the amblyopic eye have only recently been completed.

a. Lombroso, Duffy, and Robb (1969), making use of computer-derived, visual, evoked response to high light and patterned targets, demonstrate a difference in response to pattern between amblyopic and non-amblyopic eyes while noting essentially no difference in response to a pure photic stimulus. They postulate a specific inhibition of pattern vision with the site of the defect located in the cortex.

b. Shipley (1969), in further work utilizing the averaged, visual, evoked response in amblyopia in conjunction with direct view ophthalmoscopy, cites evidence to claim:

(1) Responses from normal eyes are markedly affected by contrast in the target structure whereas those from the amblyopic eye are not.

(2) Latency differences between the normal and amblyopic eye are generally not found.

(3) Responses from the normal eye may be made to approximate those of the amblyopic eye by moving the stimulus off fovea often by as much as 2-3°.

(4) Response amplitudes in some amblyopes can be made to approach normal by carefully placing the flash image on the true fovea.

c. Perry and Childers (1969), measuring averaged evoked responses in amblyopic and normal subjects using light flash stimuli, found that the amblyopic eye gives a significantly smaller VER than the normal eye with monocular foveal stimulation. Stimulation of the two eyes simultaneously with unequal intensities yields a binocular VER which approximates the average response for the two intensities in both amblyopic and normal subjects.

8. There is, at present, conflicting evidence and uncertainty in a number of areas in our understanding of functional amblyopia. Some of these clouded areas are:

a. The concepts of amblyopia of "arrest" and "extinction." These are concepts introduced by Chavasse (1939) to serve as models of what might possibly be happening. Schapero (1971) notes that much evidence has been presented to document such phenomena as arrest or extinction of visual acuity in strabismus amblyopia.

b. Brock (1952) has reported the relatively frequent occurrence of small foveal scotomas in strabismus amblyopes. Others have reported an occasional non-functional fovea or foveal area but the high proportion found by Brock has yet to be confirmed by other investigators.

c. The concept of "exanopsia" or loss of vision from disuse has still to be validated. It, presumably, like the terms "arrest" and "extinction," is an attempt at a possible explanation of the improvement in visual acuity following occlusion of the non-amblyopic eye.

d. The idea that a "critical age" exists after which the improvement of the acuity in functional amblyopia cannot occur was apparently introduced by Worth (1903) along with the rule of thumb known as "Worth's fraction" as guides to practitioners. Neither Worth's own data nor anyone else's have ever demonstrated the actual existence of a critical age or the validity of Worth's fraction in determining the extent of possible recorvery of visual acuity.

9. Functional amblyopia is thus a clinical entity, defined by subnormal visual acuity not fully correctable with lenses with no macro-ocular pathology present. It often accompanies the conditions of constant unilateral strabismus and marked anisometropia although functional amblyopia does not necessarily only occur in conjunction with these conditions. In addition to the subnormal acuity evidenced by the amblyopic eye, there is also frequently present eccentric fixation, wavering or unsteady fixation, the inability to perform adequate pursuit or following movements, poor hand-eye coordination with that eye, and a pronounced separation difficulty or crowding phenomenon in which other adjacent contours appear to interact and to reduce measured whole line acuity.

10. For an in-depth coverage of the causes, diagnosis, and treatment of functional amblyopia, see Schapero (1971).

Anomalous Correspondence

1. Instead of suppressing the foveal image of one eye, the squinter may elect to use both foveal images and to develop an artificial correspondence between each *fovea* and a *peripheral point* of the other retina. Such individuals do not perceive diplopia when presented with a single target, but locate both images of the target in the same spatial position. However, as Chodroff (1947) notes, they are frequently conscious of the fact that they are seeing two separate objects in the same place, whereas the normal observer would fuse the two and would be unable to make such a statement. If the stimulus in the deviated eye is moved to the fovea of that eye, the two images will appear a distance apart equal to the angle of anomaly (Figure XXIX-4).

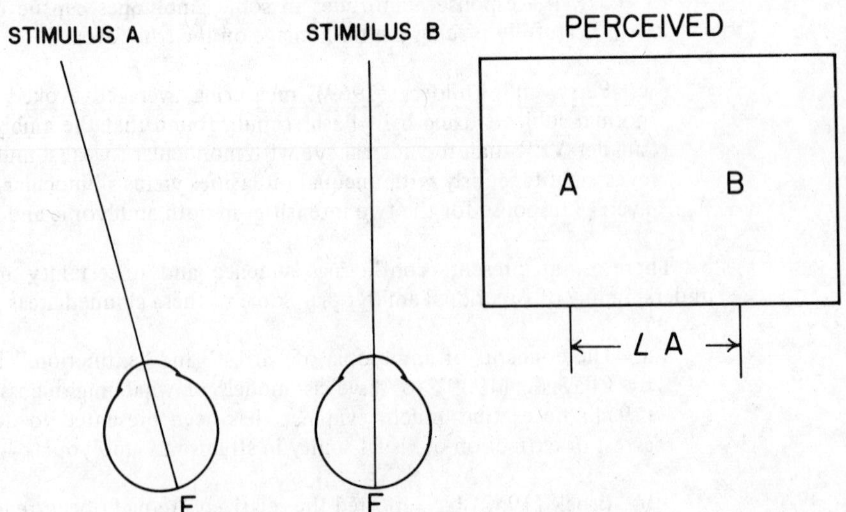

Figure XXIX-4 – Diagrammatic representation of angle of anomaly.
A = Angle of anomaly represented by projection of perceived images from both foveas.

a. Where the objective angle of the strabismus and the subjective angle of directionalization agree, the condition is known as *harmonious.* Where the two differ, the condition is known as *unharmonious.*

(1) Duke-Elder (1949) calls the fraction angle of anomaly over the angle of the squint, the *perversion quotient.*

b. A condition in which faulty projection results in reversal of projection, due to surgical correction of the squint, is known as *paradoxical correspondence.*

2. Almost all investigators maintain that the original innately anatomical correspondence between fovea and fovea, and so forth, still exists, even in these cases, but in a dormant state. Nor is it conceded that a learned association of retinal areas is introduced. Verhoeff (1938) believed that the associated area of the non-fixing eye could lie anywhere between the true fovea and the so-called *false macula,* including the latter, and that what was established was a different method of spatial localization. Brock agrees essentially with Verhoeff in concluding that the actual retinal correspondence is innate, and that anomalous cases develop the ability to identify spatial localization separately with each eye. He ascribes the ability to a learned sense of muscle position for each eye which indicates the localization of the position of the object of regard. He therefore prefers the more precise nomenclature of *anomalous projection* rather than anomalous correspondence.

a. Walls (1951) objects to the entire concept of projection being related to learned or re-learned muscle sense. He believes that anomalous correspondence, just as normal correspondence, is explained in sensory-cortical terms and not motor ones. The projection frame of reference for each eye is expressed in terms of the isomorph of the retina located in layer IV of the cortex in Brodmann's Area 17. Each Area 17 consists of one half of one retina and the half of the other retina viewing the same field. The direction of objects for the eye concerned is dependent upon the particular cell in Area 17 stimulated. This direction is innate and totally determined by the cell involved. Thus, Walls considers that projection is properly cortical rather than retinal. The directions of images in both eyes are determined by a correspondency of the two Areas 17 in the perceptual center, Area 19. Anomalous correspondence can then be considered .a slippage in Area 19 resulting in a new correspondency of Areas 17. This slippage can be considered alterable to some degree.

b. Bielschowsky (1940) confirms the existence of the original anatomical correspondence by Hering after-image test in a dark room, in which no other spatial clues are apparent, and in which both foveas can be brought to project to the same point.

(1) However, other investigators find eccentric projection even with such a test, Burian (1945) using it to determine the extent of deep-seatedness of the condition. Where the projection can be shown to be normal by after-images, Burian holds that the condition is not too firmly established.

(2) Flom and Kerr (1967), utilizing multiple test results in strabismus, obtained results which cause them to question the entire concept of "depth of anomaly."

c. Recently, Boucher (1967), has reported on his measurements of "common visual direction horopters" in exotropes exhibiting anomalous correspondence. He concludes from his measurements of 2 subjects that horopters can be repeatably obtained with alternating exotropes with anomalous correspondence. These horopters were similar in position and shape to those of normal binocular subjects exhibiting fixation disparity except that the horopters measured on the anomalously corresponding exotropes were found to be "considerably more concave towards the subject beyond 10° to 15° from the midline." One of the subjects could exhibit both normal binocular vision with eyes aligned and anomalous correspondence when the eyes were in the divergent state. He showed two distinctly different horopter shapes for the aligned and strabismic positions.

(1) Boucher concludes that, "alternating exotropes with anomalous correspondence used in this investigation have some form of binocular vision and have some form of common visual direction while in this strabismic position."

3. The prevalence of anomalous correspondence appears to be high, although figures vary from one report to the next. Duke-Elder (1949) reports that the condition is common to over half the concomitant squinters, particularly alternating ones. Brock (1939), likewise, found it almost universal among alternators. Duke-Elder also reports it universal among congenital squints.

a. Enos (1950) reports the average incidence at 47.5%.

b. A sample of strabismic patients reported by Jaffee (1953) was found to have the following breakdown for anomalous correspondence:

(1) Monocular esotropia – 31 of 86
(2) Alternating esotropia – 28 of 32
(3) Monocular exotropia – 3 of 12
(4) Alternating exotropia – 8 of 16

c. Adler (1953) reported that 5% of such correspondence was harmonious, 15% was unharmonious, and the balance exhibited a large suppression area which had no relation to the fixating eye.

d. Morgan (1948) finds that these ratios were 15%, 50%, and 35%.

e. The condition appears most likely if the onset of the squint is at an early age before binocular reflexes are established, and generally where the angle of deviation is considerable, being rarely seen in deviations of less than 20° and almost never in those of less than 10° (Duke-Elder, 1949).

(1) It is difficult to correct in small deviations (Scobee, 1952), but otherwise is easiest corrected in deviations of recent origin and short duration.

(2) Like amblyopia, it appears to have no familial or hereditary connotation, (Schlossman and Priestley, 1952).

4. The significant aspect of Brock's (1955) experiments is the definition of the projection habits of the anomalous correspondence as other than those conceived upon a cyclopean eye basis. In normal projection, if a target is placed at the point of intersection of the lines of sight of the two eyes, a single target is projected to a common or unified position. In cases of anomalous projection, a target placed at the crossing point of the lines of sight is seen as two targets, the image of the deviating eye assuming its spatial position in accordance with the position of the fovea in relation to the peripheral area that corresponds with the fovea of the fixing eye. Figure XXIX-5 illustrates this.

a. Brock postulates that the squinter does not develop from suppression to amblyopia but from suppression to a condition which he terms "ambiocular" vision. In this state, the individual utilizes the total stimuli to both eyes even though not consciously aware of the parts of the image seen by each eye to attain an almost normal percept of the object. This phenomenon he terms an *adjustment shift*.

5. Boeder (1964) in attempting to refute the concept of anomalous retinal correspondence in strabismus, reasons as does Brock, that the squinter with single binocular vision makes use of a

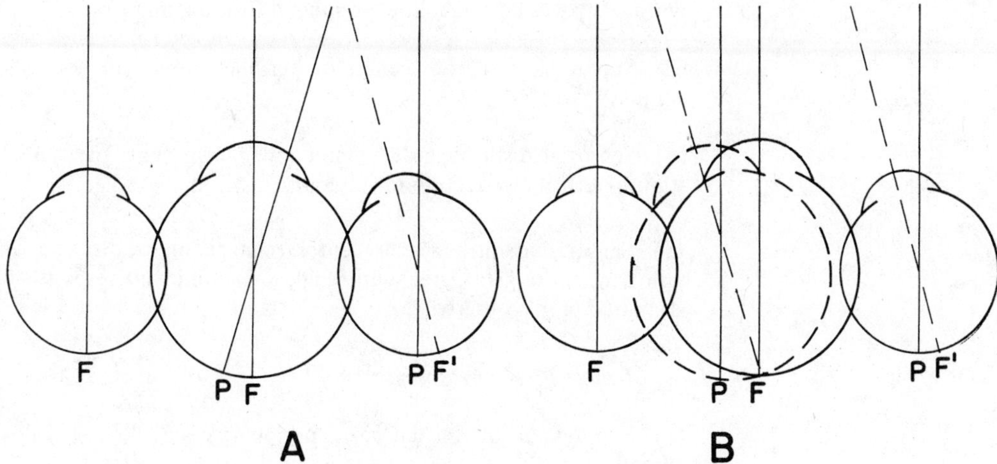

Figure XXIX-5 – Diagrammatic representation of cyclopean eye in normal and ambiocular projection. (A) Normal projection. (B) Ambiocular projection. F fovea of good eye and cyclopean eye; F′ fovea of deviated eye; P peripheral point of deviated eye in correspondence in ambiocular eye.

"*response shift.*" This is a "conditioned reflex," in which stimulation of a retinal receptor elicits a directional response associated with a receptor which is separated from the stimulated one by a shift angle." He feels that strabismic amblyopia in the deviating eye, past pointing, monocular diplopia, and other visual attributes observed of the strabismic, provide strong confirmatory evidence for this "response shift" hypothesis.

a. In a second paper Boeder (1966), analyzing the single binocular vision in concomitant strabismus, found that the absence of physiological diplopia, "the regularly occurring suppression areas and the resulting division of the binocular field between the fixating eye and the deviating eye" were immediate consequences of this hypothesized "response shift."

b. Some of the experiments Brock (1952) describes parallel the percepts of normal binocular vision. However, he notes that the phenomenon is only elicited when the original angle of deviation is maintained and that it may vary with the same patient for different conditions being mainfested under one set of test conditions and being replaced by normal binocular performance in other circumstances.

(1) Some alternating patients accomplish much the same effect by rapid alternation of the eyes. The difference between the condition which Brock describes and that orginarily expected from the concept of cyclopean projection is that two axes of reference seem to be continuously employed by the ambiocular patient, one from the fixating eye serving as the fixation axis, while another from the deviated eye serves as a reference or attention axis. The patient is thereby able to discern foveal detail in two distinct portions of the field without nullifying either impression and without diplopia.

6. Burian (1941) in investigating the fusion movements of strabismus cases, summarized the types of responses as follows:

a. *Cases of normal retinal correspondence*

(1) Single vision when the targets agree with the angle of squint; diplopia otherwise; eyes do not follow peripheral fusion stimuli.

(2) Single vision when the targets agree with the angle of squint; suppression at periphery; eyes do not follow peripheral fusion stimuli.

(3) Suppression at both center or periphery; eyes do not follow peripheral fusion stimuli.

(4) Sensorial disturbance at center (change in angle of squint); peripheral fusional stimuli not followed; constant diplopia.

(5) Sensorial disturbance at center (change in localization or suppression); single vision when targets agree with angle of squint and response to peripheral fusional stimuli; diplopia otherwise.

b. *Cases of anomalous correspondence*

(1) Suppression of one image at periphery; eyes do not follow peripheral fusional stimuli.

(2) Suppression of central and peripheral retinal impressions; eyes do not follow peripheral fusional stimuli.

(3) Eyes follow peripheral fusional stimuli when targets are within range of anomalous correspondence. Otherwise there is suppression or diplopia.

(4) Sensorial disturbance at center (change in localization or suppression); eyes follow peripheral fusional stimuli when targets agree with anomalous correspondence or are displaced according to angle of anomaly; otherwise suppression or diplopia.

c. Burian further notes that patients respond to peripheral fusional movement only if there is a central retinal disturbance such as suppression except in the rare instances in which total suppression of one eye occurs or anomalous correspondence is so highly developed that all aspects of binocularity except stereopsis are present. The lack of stereopsis he found implicit in every case of monocular single vision. If the patient does not exhibit a central retinal disturbance, fusion movements do not occur, the peripheral stimulation being suppressed. The implied rivalry between central and peripheral areas may bear importance for treatment by orthoptics.

(1) Studying the relative effect of foveal and parafoveal stimuli on adductive fusion movements, Ludvigh, et al. (1962) found, in their carefully measured sample of three subjects, that non-foveal stimulation was relatively ineffective in producing adduction when adequate central stimuli were presented to the two foveas under conditions of light adaptation.

(2) In another study Lyle and Foley (1955) found that where similar stimuli were presented to central and peripheral vision, foveal diplopia could only be demonstrated in 20% of their 50 patients.

(3) Goldstein, et. al.(1966), examining the role of the periphery in binocular vision found that the peripheral field contributes significantly to the binocular relationship, and that loss of this peripheral field through retinitis pigmentosa, for example, caused a serious impairment to the quality of binocular vision.

(4) It would seem, then, that depending on the state of binocular vision, the level of light adaptation, the instructions, and the size, location and complexity of the stimuli presented, either central or peripheral predominance can be demonstrated.

d. Among the central retinal disturbances other than suppression is the condition known as *horror fusionis*, in which the patient can be made to see two images, and these can be brought together up to the point of fusion, at which point the patient shifts one eye or the other and places one stimulus away from the corresponding point. Such cases have been considered as evidence of a lack of fusion faculty, but as Bielschowsky (1935) points out, may be due to other impairments such as aniseikonia which interfere with fusion. He believes that horror fusionis is not necessarily a congenital defect but may be due to a neurotic tendency or to factors of image differences such as size disparities which can be corrected by proper lenses and training.

(1) This pioneering effort in 1935 has been followed by at least five reports in the literature reporting successful elimination of horror fusionis by the application of size lenses. The most recent, by Fisher and Ludlam (1963), describes a new approach to aniseikonia measurement in non-fusing squint, utilizing after-images (see Chapter VIII).

7. Duke-Elder (1949) is frequently quoted as commenting that in anomalous correspondence, much of the confusion rests in the fact that different tests seem to test different things.

a. Pascal (1953) attempted to clarify this by indicating that several different correspondences may be involved. He designated them as:

(1) *Normal*

(a) Binocular superposition, in which both maculae project to the same area, fusing like images and interposing compatible ones.

(b) Macula-paramacula separation, in which one macula and one peripheral area project to different spatial positions.

(2) *Anomalous*

(a) Bimacular separation, in which both maculae project to different spatial positions.

(b) Macula-perimacular superposition, in which one macula and a paramacular area of the other eye project to the same area, fusing or superimposing.

(3) Anomalous projection may consist of (1), (a) and (2), (b); of (1), (b) and (2), (a); or of (2), (a) and (2), (b). Each type might respond in various ways to differing tests.

b. Burian (1947) had postulated that the greater the number of different tests which indicated anomalous correspondence, the more difficult the condition was to restore to normal correspondence.

c. Flom and Kerr (1967) questioned the premise stated by Burian that anomalous correspondence was more deeply rooted according to the number of tests which verified it. They felt that measurement errors, unsteady eccentric fixation, changes in the relative position of the eyes (from one angle of deviation to another or from binocularity to strabismus) influenced the results. A small range of measurement error ($\pm 3\ \Delta$) must be exceeded in order to indicate a true anomalous correspondence. A probability of agreement between different methods statistically was reduced as the number of tests were increased.

8. Morgan (1961) presents an analysis of anomalous correspondence viewed as motor phenomenon. He presents a theory which relates many of the clinical observations of the anomalous corresponder to the "type of innervational pattern associated with the strabismus."

a. He makes a differentiation between innervational patterns which are *"registered"* to indicate a change in egocentric direction of a perceived object while others are *"non-registered"* and thus indicate no change in egocentric localization.

(1) Thus, if we deal with a "registered" innervational pattern, "the altered position of each eye with respect to the other is also 'registered' and consequently the 'turned eye' reports that what it sees is displaced with respect to the 'other eye.' This results in anomalous correspondence."

(2) On the other hand, however, "if the innervational pattern associated with the squint is 'non-registered,' the altered position of each eye with respect to the other is not 'registered' and consequently the 'turned eye' does not report that what it sees is displaced with respect to the 'other eye'. This results in normal correspondence."

b. Thus, it may be this motor signal from kinesthetic or other sources which Morgan calls attention to, that triggers the "response shift" or "adjustment shift" which Voerhoef (1938), Brock (1955), and Boeder (1964) have postulated as the actual cortical mechanism acting in anomalous correspondence.

9. In summary, anomalous correspondence is a more common means of securing single vision and proper localization than is ordinarily supposed and is particularly likely in cases of alternating strabismus. There is still serious doubt as to the actual mechanisms at work in this curious perceptual adaptation in strabismus.

a. It is also unknown whether there is an evolution in its development in an individual. A question still remains as to the relative importance of the participation of motor and sensory systems. The proper projection can often be restored by training, the ignored macular area being stimulated in excess of the anomalous area and the patient instructed as to the proper position of an object of interest in space.

(1) The methods in use by which this can be accomplished and the results obtained by these methods will be briefly described in Chapter XXXII.

IV. STRABISMUS

A. Causes of the Deviation

1. Historically, strabismus was first assumed to be due to an abnormal placement of the macula of one eye which necessitated the deviation of the eye in order to secure single vision. This seemed to be corroborated by the paradoxical diplopia which followed surgical correction of the squint, although that is today assumed to be due to anomalous correspondence. Following concepts held that the strabismus resulted from the need to avoid corresponding stimulation when the images of each eye were too different, and also that mal-insertion or unequality of the strength of the respective ocular muscles produced the squint.

a. The Sherrington demonstration of the reciprocal behavior of the ocular muscles invalidated the latter concept. The actual motility of each muscle cannot be determined by the ability to move the eye to the limits of the orbit. This, as Bielschowsky (1940) points out, would only be true if the full contraction of the muscles were required to reach the limits. The fuller implications of this fact will be considered in paralytic strabismus. (See Chapter XXXI.)

2. *Donders'* disclosure of the association of the accommodation and convergence relationship postulated that strabismus was due to excessive convergence innervation aroused by hyperopia. Since he recognized that only a small number of hyperopes exhibited strabismus he also postulated that the probability of strabismus increased with the extent of difference in the acuity of the two

eyes, either due to anisometropia or other interferences with vision. Donders also believed that an absence of accommodation in myopia developed a near-point relationship of accommodation and convergence which resulted in divergency at far.

a. Donders' concept does seem to apply to some squints, but is not totally substantiated by the fact that most refractive patients do not squint; that many squinters exhibit very low refractive errors or errors of opposite sign to that postulated; and that the angle of squint rarely agrees with the extent of excess of deficiency of accommodative effort.

b. Brown (1950) compared cross-sectional studies of strabismus cases with non-squinters at various age levels. From birth to the age of 6, squinters revealed an 80% higher incidence of hyperopia; at seven, 48% more; while from 8 to 11, non-squinters showed a major decrease in the incidence of hyperopia but squinters showed only a 10% lower incidence. The incidence among squinters in the ages from 12 to 15 was some 75% lower than that found in the previous age group. He concluded that:

(1) Strabismic eyes show much more hyperopia on the average and the rate of decrease of the hyperopia is much lower.

(2) While the hyperopia increases up to age of 6, as in non-squinters, the trend back toward emmetropization occurs approximately 4 years later than it does in non-squinters.

c. Scobee (1951) classified a number of esotropes as follows: purely accommodative in origin, 15%; partially accommodative in origin, 66%; non-accommodative in origin, 19%. He found the following mean spherical equivalents for the errors of refraction: non-accommodative, +1.18 D. hyperopia; partially accommodative, +3.30 D.; accommodative, + 4.01 D. He stated that by the age of 2½ years, the retinal development was sufficient to warrant a satisfactory reward for accommodative effort, and that the appearance of convergence strabismus at this age was frequent.

3. Over the years various investigators have placed the origin of strabimus as due to predominant elasticity of one group of muscles as compared to the antagonists (Graefe, 1898); to topographic or anatomic factors (Stilling, 1905; Landolt, 1886); and to interference of the higher centers controlling binocular vision or fusion (Parinaud, 1900; Worth, 1903).

4. *Chavasse* believed the causes due to deficient ontological development of the basic underlying reflexes. As summarized by Duke-Elder (1949), his premise is as follows:

a. Development dissociations of the binocular reflexes

(1) Failure in the development of the secondary fixation reflexes due to:

(a) Failure of the disjunctive fixation reflexes, evidenced in deficiency of convergence and periodic divergent squint.

(b) Failure of the corrective fusion reflexes, resulting in heterophorias.

(c) Failure of the conjugate fixation reflexes, resulting in conjugate deviations.

(2) Failure in the development of conjugate movements, resulting in congenital oculomotor palsy.

(3) Failure in the development of fixation, resulting in congenital nystagmus.

b. Acquired dissociations due to:

(1) Disruptions of the peripheral oculomotor mechanism, resulting in noncomitant strabismus.

(2) Disruptions of the central oculomotor mechanism, resulting in conjugate deviations.

(3) Disruptions of the postural or fixation mechanisms, resulting in acquired nystagmus.

c. Certain obstacles impaired or interfered with proper development of function:

(1) Optical – such as unequal ocular images, occlusion of one eye in infancy, opacities in the media, etc.

(2) Sensory – such as macular failure, lesions in the retino-cerebral pathway, etc.

(3) Motor – affecting the pathways and reflexes:

(a) static or anatomic – congenital orbital defects, tumors in orbit, muscle structural anomalies;

(b) kinetic – involvements of the accommodative-convergence relationship;

(c) neurogenic – lesions of nerves and centers;

(4) central or psychological – absence of fusion center, hyperexcitability, hysteria, psychopathic squints, etc.

5. *Skeffington* (1953) postulates an organismic theory of strabismus etiology.

a. Binocular vision, the preferred "gene matrixed performance" of the growing child, while possibly affected by anomalous biochemical pathological processes, is affected by "stresses of culture" so that "ineffective construction results," causing strabismus.

(1) The importance of ontological sequence and timing and that of performance at various stages of development is stressed. The latter is highly subject to environmental influence.

(2) Accommodation (organismically titled "identification") and convergence (identified as "centering") are developed and linked according to a gene matrix sequence. Active touch assists these ocular functions in fabricating the binocular space world, helping to form a "total action system."

(3) A deprivation in culture affecting the relation of the visual system input to that of the kinesthetic, haptic, and vestibular input of the total system, interrrupts the sequential process of "elaboration of the fusion of the retinal gradients" while "maturation progressions of other bodily operations continue."

(4) Such asynchrony, if too pronounced, makes "matching of gradient distribution impossible" and convergent squint supplies a simple solution for avoiding the problem.

b. Divergent strabismus, he postulates, occurs characteristically at school age due to influences of the "socially compulsive near-centered task." The stress causes the child to center (converge) nearer than identification (accommodation) resulting in esophoria.

(1) If this over-centering drive is not blocked, esotropia will result if binocular function is dissociated. This is atypical.

(2) The more common reaction is predicated as an attempt to block the centering innervation by negative relative convergence and that pattern is then transferred to the far-point.

(a) The resulting stress in attempting to match the differences in information provided by centering as compared to identification causes the abandonment of the matching of the two retinal gradients, improving "the processing of more complex data gathering demands" and through divergence, projecting "the demand for avoidance" to the far-point.

(b) At farpoint, a tendency to over-accommodate would result in myopia, while under-convergence would result in far exotropia. Thus both myopia and exotropia are two different reactions to the same fundamental problem, near esophoria.

[1] Thus, the rationale of treatment for both convergent and divergent strabismus calls for plus lenses at the near point.

c. *Restoration of binocular function*

(1) For both convergent and divergent strabismus, the following procedure is advised:

(a) The studied use of convex lenses for nearpoint.

(b) The development of "basic substrates of performance, i.e., adequate monocular centering and identification skills along with basic photostatic and photo-postural bilateral performance skills."

(c) Stimulation of the periphery and elaboration of binocular ground initially, followed by the use of emergent figure.

(d) Employing bilateral "active touch" in which limbs and eyes can participate.

(2) Once the organism is capable of utilizing and integrating these fundamental skills with visual performance, the more traditional building of fusion quality and amplitude, vergence breaks and recovery skills, and hand-eye coordination is undertaken.

6. *Scobee* (1952) considers the causation of strabismus from the following viewpoint:

a. Strabismus is caused by any of the following variables:

(1) *Innervational* – in which the convergence mechanism is either excessively or insufficiently activated and not properly controlled by the later developed fusional controls, due to interference with either the convergence center or higher centers.

(2) *Accommodative* – in which the accommodative center reflexly affects the convergence control.

(3) *Mechanical* – in which the relaxation of the antagonist is affected or interfered with by either muscular structural defects or obstacles.

(4) *Functional* – the innervational supply is altered due to psychogenic causes.

b. In addition, either sensory or motor obstacles may be involved:

(1) *Sensory* – the use of one eye, refractive errors, anisometropia, media opacities, lesions of the retina or pathways may interfere with proper development.

(2) *Motor* – anatomic factors, traumas to muscles, pathways or higher centers, etc.

c. The combination of the four factors and two obstacles provide six variables which may induce a strabismus. Most squints begin because of one of the factors and then involve some of the others.

7. *Bielschowsky* (1940) summarized the causes as follows:

a. *Mechanical causes*

(1) The physical relationship of the bulbi and their adnexa.

(2) The physical qualities, such as length, elasticity, insertion, volume of tissue of the adnexa.

(3) The size and form of the bulbi and orbits.

b. *Motor conditions* due to excessive or spastic innervation, such as Donders proposed, or due to irritation of the centers.

c. *A combination* of mechanical and motor factors.

d. So long as the fusion faculty is sufficiently strong to hold single vision, the above factors will not produce more than a latent squint or phoria. Bielchowsky also believed that a heriditary or congenital disposition was indicated. He notes that any disturbance of the fusion faculty, produced commonly by childhood diseases, may serve to disrupt it and to result in squint.

8. *Adler* (1953) briefly combines the various causes into two origins:

a. *Incomitant types* – due to disturbances of the nuclear and supranuclear pathways.

b. *Comitant types* – due to involvements of the supranuclear mechanisms controlling the vergences.

c. All true comitant squints are innervational in origin and due to a failure of either the convergence or divergence mechanisms.

9. It may be observed that the various conditions cited are all interferences in the objective of single and properly projected vision, and that the concept of uniocularity as a resort to avoid diplopia when fusion is impossible includes in principle all the particular causes noted, whether these be:

a. *Mechanical defects* of positioning which interfere with appropriate presentation of corresponding maculae.

b. *Innervational irregularities* which make the proper presentation difficult, fatiguing or erratic.

c. Disturbances of the *higher centers* which interfere with function.

d. *Sensory incongruities* such as differently focused images in the two eyes, size disparities, etc., which make fusion impossible or difficult.

(1) This premise holds that the deviation is a result of either a conscious turning of the eye to eliminate stimulation which elicits diplopia of a common object in the same spatial plane, or permits a latent imbalance such as a phoria to become manifest.

B. Development and Course of Strabismus

1. *Age of onset*

a. *Esotropia* is usually manifested in the early years of life, except in those forms exhibited as non-comitant types and due to pathological or traumatic sources. Scobee (1951) in a study of 558 cases reports the following distribution of age of origin:

(1) Table XXIX-2

Age	% cases incident	Age	% cases incident
birth	*27.6*	*6 years*	*2.1*
1 year	*20.6*	*7 years*	*1.1*
2 years	*16.6*	*8 years*	*.7*
3 years	*15.0*	*9 years*	*.4*
4 years	*8.7*	*10 years*	*.2*
5 years	*4.0*		

b. Keiner (1951) gives the following tabulation determined upon 656 patients:

(1) Table XXIX-3

Age	% cases incident	Age	% cases incident
under 6 months	*35*	*2-3 years*	*12*
6 mos.-1 year	*19*	*3-4 years*	*6*
1-2 years	*24*	*4-6 years*	*4*

c. Both tabulations indicate that the chief period of incidence is up to 2-3 years of age, and that hereditary factors may be considered significant. Keiner concludes that fully 50% of all cases are due to hereditary factors. Scobee places the percent of cases with familial significance as 41%. Scobee also noted that the highest incidence is at birth. He reported that whereas 3% of all infants are premature, 13.5% of the strabismus cases were premature. He also reported a correlation between the length of labor and the onset of strabismus, noting that the longer the labor, the earlier the age at which strabismus was manifest. Scobee intimated that injuries during the period of birth might be of prime importance in the etiology of strabismus. Schlossman and Priestley (1952) also investigated the hereditary aspect of strabismus, and report that 47.5% of all cases belonged to families in which two or more members also exhibited strabismus. Such familial strabismus exhibited no correlation with hyperopia alone, anisometropia, defective fusion faculties, or anatomic anomalies as potential causes.

d. The findings of Frandsen (1960) in an epidemiological study of strabismus in Denmark differ from those of Scobee and Keiner. She found only 15% of strabismus to be congenital and the age of six to seven to be the time when the sample showed the most strabismus, i.e.,

7%. Exotropia was revealed to usually exhibit a later onset than did esotropia, with the former exhibiting its greatest period of onset at the ages of five to eight, while the latter showed its greatest onset between the ages of two to five.

2. *Course of onset*

a. Chavasse (1939) described a model history of the onset:

(1) At birth neither accommodation nor visual acuity are developed so that an accommodative cause cannot be ascribed to a heterotropia present at birth.

(2) As accommodation and visual acuity develop, the mildly hyperopic child is enabled to compensate for the refractive discrepancy without affecting convergence markedly, while the extremely hyperopic child discerns no need for accommodation since good acuity has never been experienced. Both the moderate and moderately high hyperope may utilize the newly developed accommodation faculty, and since neither the fusional nor accommodative-convergence reflexes are as yet fully developed or controlled, an accommodative squint may appear.

(a) The hyperope with a small amount of error may nonetheless also develop a squint if the habit of holding objects exceedingly near is habitually employed, due to the not fully realized visual acuity, and if the habit of employing excessive accommodation becomes fixed.

(3) The remaining types of strabismus are due to emotional instability, a poorly developed fusional reflex, anatomic anomalies, and so forth.

(4) The marked myope, as the marked hyperope, is unlikely to develop strabismus.

(5), The moderate myope is unable to see clearly at distance, and may develop the habit of continuing his near-point convergence for all distances of fixation beyond his far-point, developing the so-called *esotropia of congenital myopia.*

(6) The myopia which is developed during growth induces a relaxation of convergence associated with the attempt to relax accommodation, and develops a habitual exophoria which may, because of other interferences, become the *exotropia of acquired myopia.*

b. Scobee (1951) notes that almost 66% of all esotropes exhibit some accommodative factor, although these are not all solely due to accommodative effort. He also notes that a vertical paretic involvement accompanied 43% of 456 esotropic patients, and that these were distributed as follows: the vertical involvements were found in 21% of purely accommodative esotropes; in 45% of partly accommodative esotropes; and in 49% of non-accommodative esotropes, an incidence of vertical components almost twice that present in purely accommodative cases. Other anomalies, such as thickened, fused, or misinserted check ligaments, thickened intramuscular membranes, abnormal muscular insertions and the like, were exhibited in 51.4% of all cases, but in almost 90% of the non-accommodative types, and 43.1% of the partially accommodative types.

c. Keiner (1951) concludes that all children are born without the later phylogenetic reflexes (see, however, Section II, 5 and 6 of this chapter), and that Hering's law of concomitant movements does not apply to the newly born. He presumes that hormonal influences retard the myelination and create disturbances of the optomotor reflexes.

3. *Progress*

a. Strabismus is usually latent in the early stages. As difficulty with fusion or innervational or other causes make the obtaining of single vision binocularly more difficult one eye may deviate under fatigue or stress. During this stage the squint is occasional. Frequent lapses of this order usually precede the onset of a constant deviation. The hyperope whose fusion faculty is deficient may exhibit excess convergence due to accommodation at far upon occasion, or the myope whose accommodative-convergence is not employed may exhibit divergent lapses at near when the fusional reserve is exhausted.

b. Sometimes physical or psychic debilitation may reduce the fusional compensation sufficiently to bring on a continuous manifestation of the latent squint. Sudden fright, diseases of childhood, particularly measles and whooping cough, and convulsions often precede the exhibition of continuous strabismus. These usually produce unilateral rather than alternating squints. Where such happenings do not precede the squint, discomfort occasioned by fusional effort may cause a relinquishment of the binocular pattern in favor of the monocular one.

c. As the squint persists, several secondary effects occur which alter the original appearance of the deviation.

(1) Increased angle of the strabismus

(a) This is partially due to relaxation over a period of time of the original fusional innervation, as is demonstrated by occlusion of one eye in heterophoria, and partially due to secondary changes of the structures of the orbit. As the squinting position is maintained, the relative position of the muscles and adnexa are stabilized under a new kinesthetic sense. In addition, the structures which are constricted tend to shrink while those expanded tend to assume a stretched or laxer tonic position. Wilkinson (1927) reports that actual shrinkages of the check ligaments occur, which sometimes maintain the angle of deviation even after the innervational disturbance has been remedied.

(2) Sensory changes such as suppression have already been noted.

(3) Purposive strabismus

(a) The squinting eye may be deviated in excess to move the confusing image even farther from the fovea and make suppression easier. In some cases the movement of the squinting eye follows the order of fusional movements except that the suppression area is presented to the target rather than a corresponding point. Charnwood (1948) reports three such cases in low amounts of squint and entitles the condition *Purposive Strabismus*.

[1] Another form of purposeful deviation is described by Swan (1948) as the *Blind-Spot Syndrome.* This is exhibited by accommodative estropes in which the refraction alleviates only part of the deviation, or by anomalous corresponders or suppressors under occlusion who have their habitual pattern of achieving single vision disrupted. The angle of squint usually falls between 12-18° of esotropia, so that the blind spot of the deviated eye is placed in correspondence with the fovea of the fixing eye. The condition is discernible by binocular field charts, or by viewing the deviated eye with an ophthalmoscope at a distance of 6 to 10 inches from the eye. It will be recalled that few cases of anomalous correspondence are found in squints of this degree, the blind-spot apparently sufficing instead.

C. Classification of Strabismus

1. *By the nature of the deviation*

   a. Concomitant, comitant, or functional – in which the versions of the two eyes are equal in all directions, indicating no interference with the yoked muscle action.

   b. Paralytic, paretic, nonconcomitant or spastic – in which both eyes do not exhibit equal binocular versional movements when moving together.

2. *By behavior*

   a. Fixed – in which the angle of deviation does not vary significantly in amount.

   b. Variable – in which the angle of deviation varies during the same examination.

3. *By appearance*

   a. Manifest

   b. Latent – heterophoria

   c. Apparent or pseudo – a false appearance of strabismus due to a large angle gamma or large epicanthal folds

   d. Spurious – the incoordinated dissociations of infancy before binocular vision is developed

4. *By time (frequency or periodicity)*

   a. Constant, continuous, permanent or absolute – present at all times

   b. Intermittent or occasional – manifested irregularly

   c. Relative or periodic – manifested only in specific relation to a given condition

      (1) Directly periodic – in which the deviation is greater at near than at far.

      (2) Inversely periodic – in which the deviation is greater at far than at near.

5. *By eye (variety of fixation)*

   a. Monocular or unilateral – the same eye is always deviated.

   b. Alternate or bilateral – either eye assumes the fixation while the other deviates.

6. *By direction*

   a. Esotropia, convergent, internal or medial – inward

   b. Exotropia, divergent, external or temporal – outward

   c. Hypertropia, sursumvergent, elevated – one eye up

   d. Hypotropia, deorsumvergent, depressed – one eye down

   e. Catatropic – both eyes down

f. Anatropic – both eyes up

g. Cyclotropic – vertical axis of eye rotated from vertical position

(1) Excyclo or positive - top of axis out

(2) Encylo or negative – top of axis in

h. Braids – both eyes turn up and in

D. Strabismus Related to the Total Action System

1. A number of observers have postulated concepts based upon their clinical experience with the interrelations of vision with the other sense modalities and motor responses. These are described by the stipulations contained in the following subsections.

2. *Vision and the other senses*

a. Not only is a relationship between vision and the other sensory and motor mechanisms stipulated, but the input data for vision and audition are conceived to achieve significance only after they are matched with other input data such as those derived from kinesthetic, proprioceptive, and postural sources (Woolf, 1965). These latter are presumed to develop earlier chronologically, but the question of which is the standard in maturity is not as essential as matching both input systems. Failure to do so may result in "distress in spatial orientation and higher perceptual abilities" (Arner, 1965).

3. *Vision and motor systems*

a. The establishment of an intimate relationship between the visual and motor system of the child during the course of their development was further postulated by Gesell, Ilg, and Bullis (1950) based upon their observations. Correlated refinement of the postural set of the organism, and current and antecedent motor factors were judged to play prominent roles in visual perception. The significance of these mechanisms in relation to visual perception and meaning has been restated by Montessori (1966), among others. Bartley (1962) notes that while this relationship has been long assumed, it has only been recently studied effectively. From his own investigations, Bartley finds that effective visual perception of space and accurate, visually-guided performance in space are not "entirely dependent on specific and rigid optical properties of the photic input."

(1) Held and Hein (1963) demonstrated that active movement of the subject proved useful and effective in perceptual adaptation to changed or distorted stimulus conditions. Held and Freedman (1963) qualifyingly state that "the maintenance and development of sensory-guided behavior depend in part upon bodily movement in the normal environment," and conclude that stable functioning of the plastic system of coordination is dependent upon ordered information in the motor-sensory feedback loop.

(2) Smith, Gould, and Wargo (1963), in a series of experiments relating movement, visual perception, and learning, conclude that all the major characteristics of vision are ascribed *not* to the receptor, the motor system, or to learning, but to the spatial or geometric properties of neural feedback control systems linking the sensory and motor systems. The "neurogeometric theory" which they derive from these findings holds that the visual perception of space, color, and motion are inseparable aspects of the same process, i.e., "the dynamic sensory-feedback neuro-motor mechanisms that relate the spatial congruence of the retinal and motor surfaces of the body."

4. *Relation to binocular problems and strabismus*

a. The general relationship between vision, the oculomotor system, postural and vestibular mechanisms, and movement, is extended to the development of strabismus.

(1) Gesell, Ilg, and Bullis (1950), note the varying and rhythmic shifts in growth and dominance of various muscle systems in the growing child, and the associated variations in general coordination which may result from them. They propose that such lapses in coordination of hand and eye, posture, or motor ability may be precursers of a manifest strabismus at a later date. Recognition of the potential squinter upon the basis of such developmental indications, and possible early treatment of the developmental defect is proposed as a means of preventing the emergence of the strabismus at a later time.

(2) Flax (1963) also strongly advocated and supported the association of strabismus to distortion in the early childhood developmental sequence. He commented on the frequency with which omission of crawling or of highly atypical crawling is reported among esotropic children (although no statistical significance has been given for the difference between such frequency in squinting and non-squinting children).

(3) Weinstein (1963) postulated a human ontogenetic developmental sequence and hierarchy involving the relationship of the motor activities and perception, in similarly supporting the concept stated by Gesell, et. al., and Flax.

(a) From this concept he considers that lags in development which may produce symptoms or visual problems may be revealed by applicable developmental tests but may remain undisclosed when classical visual test methods are used.

b. The utilization of these concepts broadens the base upon which treatment has been organized (Flax, 1963). Some precepts drawn from these premises are summarized as follows:

(1) Peripheral areas are more related to postural activities and using central stimulation alone will generally not achieve integration of visual cues with other spatial orientation cues.

(2) Instruments which confine or restrict the visual field to a central area will have limited success.

(3) Surgery which interrupts the habitual relationship of visual posture and space which has been developed in association with cues from other senses, may so disturb perceptual matching that binocular fixation remains absent and the eyes perform ordinarily as if still strabismic.

(4) Monocular procedures should precede binocular ones in training not only because they teach central fixation or hand and eye coordination, but because the matching of visuo-motor direction and spatial values with other sensory systems and bodily kinesthetics is easier for each eye treated individually. The association of each eye, individually, with such a factor tends to simplify the process of matching the functions of both eyes to each other.

REFERENCES

Adler, E. (1953): Pathologic Physiology of Strabismus. Arch. Oph., 50: 19.

Allen, M. (1966): The Bartley Phenomenon and Visual Rehabilitation – A Home Training Technique. Opt. Weekly, 57, (30): 21.

Alpern, M. Flitman, D. and Joseph, R. (1960): Centrally Fixed Flicker Thresholds in Amblyopia. A.J. Oph., 49: 1194.

Alpern, M.; Petrauskas, R.; Sandall, G. and Vorenkamp, R. (1967): Recent Experiments on the Physiology of Strabismus Amblyopia. Am. Orth. J. 17: 62.

Ammann, E. (1921): Einige Beobachtungen bei den Funktionsprufen in der Sprechstunde "Zentralen Sehen," Sehen der Amblyopen. Klin Monats fur Augenheilkunde, 66: 564.

Arner, R. (1965): A Rationale for Developmental Testing and Training. Section on Children's Visual Care and Guidance, Optometric Extension Program Duncan, Oklahoma.

Bangerter, A. (1955): Amblyopiebehandlung, Basel-New York, S. Karger, ed., 2.

Bartley, S.H. (1962): The Human Organism As A Person. Chilton, New York., p. 127.

Bielschowsky, A. (1935): Congenital and Acquired Deficiencies of Fusion. A.J. Oph., 18: 925.

Bielschowsky, A. (1940): Lectures on Motor Anomalies. Dartmouth College Publications. Hanover, N.H.

Boeder, P. (1964): Anomalous Correspondence Refuted. A.J. Oph., 58: 366.

Boeder, P. (1966): Single Binocular Vision in Strabismus. A.J. Oph., 61: 78.

Boucher, J. (1967): Common Visual Direction Horopters in Exotropes with Anomalous Correspondence. A.A.A.O., 44: 547.

Bower, T.G.R. (1965): Stimulus Variables Determining Space Perception in Infants. Science, 149: 88.

Bower, T.G.R. (1966): The Visual World of Infants. Reprint No. 502, Scientific American, No. 6., p. 80.

**Brock, F. (1939): Anomalous Projection in Squint. A.A.A.O., 16: 201.*

Brock, F. (1941): Conditioning the Squinter to Normal Visual Habits, Opt. Weekly, 32: 819.

Brock, F. (1952): Visual Training, concl. Opt. Weekly, 43: 1683.

Brock, F. (1955): Visual Training Part III. Opt. Weekly, 46: 391, 557, 763, 895, 1139, 1321, 1601, 1979.

Brown, E. (1950): Comparison of Refraction of Strabismic Eyes With That of Non-Strabismic Eyes From Birth to Twenty Fifth Year. Arch. Oph., 44: 357.

Burian, H. (1941): Fusional Movements in Permanent Strabismus. Arch. Oph., 26: 626.

Burian, H. (1947): Sensorial Retinal Relationship in Concomitant Strabismus. Arch. Oph. 37: 336, 504, 618.

Burian, H. (1966): Occlusion Amblyopia and the Development of Eccentric Fixation in Occluded Eyes. A.J. Oph., 62: 1161.

Caloroso, E. & Flom, M.C. (1969): Influence of Luminance On Visual Acuity in Amblyopia, A.A.A.O., 46: 189.

Charnwood, Lord (1948): Purposive Strabismus. A.A.A.O., 25: 117.

Chavasse, F. (1939): Worth's Squint. P. Blakiston, Phila.

Chodroff, M. (1947): Squint – The Psycho-Physiological Aspects Involved in its Treatment. A.A.A.O., 24: 433.

Cuppers, C. (1956): Moderne Schielbehandlung, Klin. Monatsbl. F. Augenh., 129: 579.

Dayton, G.O.; Jansen, G. & Jones, M. (1961): Abstract. Invest. Oph., 1 (3): 414.

Dayton, G.O.; Jones, M.H.; Aiu, P.; Rawson, R.A.; Steele, B. & Rose, M. (1964a): Developmental Study of Coordinated Eye Movements in the Human Infant, I. Arch. Oph., 71: 865.

Dayton, G.O., et al. (1964b): Developmental Study of Coordinate Eye Movements in the Human Infant, II. Arch. Oph., 71: 871.

Duke-Elder, W. (1949): Textbook of Ophthalmology. C.V. Mosby Co., St. Louis.

Dunnewold, C.J. (1967): "On the Campbell and Stiles-Crawford Effects and Their Clinical Importance. Thesis. Rijksuniversiteit Utrecht 1964 (cited by Alpern, et al. 1967).

Enoch, J. (1957): Amblyopia and the Stiles-Crawford Effect. A.A.A.O., 34: 298.

Enoch, J. (1959a): Further Studies on the Relationship Between Amblyopia and the Stiles-Crawford Effect. A.A.A.O., 36: 111.

Enoch, J. (1959b): Receptor Amblyopia, A.J. Oph., 481 (3, pt. 2): 262.

Enoch, J.M. (1965): An Approach Toward the Study of Retinal Receptor Optics. A.A.A.O., 42: 63.

Enos, M. (1950): Anomalous Correspondence. A.J. Oph., 33: 1907.

Fantz, R.L. (1961): Scientific American. Reprint No. 204, 5.

Fisher, H. and Ludlam, W. (1963): An Approach to Measuring Aniseikonia in Non-Fusion Strabismus – A Preliminary Report. A.A.A.O., 40: 653.

Flax, N. (1963): New Concepts of the Central or Binocular Deviations. J.A.O.A., 34: 451.

Flom, M.C. and Weymouth, F.W. (1961): Centricity of Maxwell's Spot in Strabismus and Amblyopia. Arch. Oph., 66: 260.

,Flom, M.; Weymouth, F. and Kahneman, D. (1963): Visual Resolution and Contour Interaction. J.O.S.A., 53: 1026.

Flom, M.C. and Neumaier, R.W. (1966): Prevalence of Amblyopia. Public Health Reports, 81: 4, April.

Flom, M. and Kerr, K. (1967): Determination of Retinal Correspondence-Multiple Testing Results and the Depth of Anomaly Concept, Arch. Oph., 77: 200.

Frandsen, A.D. (1960): Occurrence of Squint, Acta Ophthalmologica, (Kbh.) Supp., 62, 38: 158.

Gesell, A.; Ilg, F. and Bullis, G. (1950): Vision: Its Development in Infant and Child, 3rd printing, Paule Hoeber, New York.

**Getman, G. and Kane, E. (1964): The Psychology of Readiness. Programs to Accelerate School Success Pass, P.O. Box 1004, Minneapolis.*

Goldschmidt, M. (1950): A New Test for Function of the Macula Lutea. Arch. Oph., 44: 129.

Goldstein, J.; Clahane, A. and Sanfilippo, S. (1966): The Role of the Periphery in Binocular Vision. A.J. Oph., 62: 702.

Gording, E.J. (1951): A Report on Haidinger Brushes, A.A.A.O., 27: 604.

Graefe (1898): Cited by Bruce. Arch. Oph. 1935, 13: 639.

Grosvenor, T. (1957): The Effect of Duration and Background Luminance Upon the Brightness Discrimination of an Amblyope. A.A.A.O., 34: 639.

Hallett, J.W. (1951): Amblyopia Independent of Usual Associated Conditions. Arch. Oph., 45: 64.

**Harmon, D. (1958): Notes on a Dynamic Theory of Vision. Movement, Posture and Vision, 3rd revision, Published by author, Austin, Texas, 1.*

Haynes, H.; White, B. and Held, R. (1965): Visual Accommodation in Human Infants. Science, 148: 528.

Held, R. and Hein, A. (1963): A Movement Produced Stimulation in the Development of Visually Guided Behavior. Jour. Comp. and Physiological Psych., 56: 872.

**Held, R. and Freedman, S. (1963): Plasticity in Human Sensorimotor Control. Science, 142 (3591): 455.*

Jaffee, N. (1953): Anomalous Projection. A.J. Oph., 36: 829.

Jampolsky, A. (1958): Characteristics of Suppression in Strabismus, Arch. Oph., 54: 683.

Kaufman, L. (1963): On the Spread of Suppression and Binocular Rivalry. Vision Research, 3: 401.

Kavner, R. and Suchoff, I. (1966): Pleoptics Handbook. Optometric Center of New York, N.Y.

Kiff, R.D. and Lepard, C. (1966): Visual Response of Premature Infants. Arch. Oph., 75: 631.

Keiner, G. (1951): New Viewpoints on the Origin of Squint: A Clinical and Statistical Study of its Nature, Cause and Therapy. The Hague, Martinus Nijhoff.

Lawwill, T. (1966): The Fixation Pattern of the Light-Adapted and Dark-Adapted Amblyopic Eye. A.J. Oph., 61: 1416.

Lawwill, T. and Burian, H. (1966): Luminance, Contrast Function and Visual Acuity in Functional Amblyopia. A.J. Oph., 62: 511.

Lehmann, D. and Fender, D.H. (1968): Component Analysis of Human Averaged Evoked Potentials: Dichoptic Stimuli Using Different Target Structure. Electroenceph. Clin. Neurophysiol., Elsevier Pub. Co., Amsterdam.

Ling, B.C. (1942): A Genetic Study of Sustained Visual Fixation and Associated Behavior in the Human Infant from Birth to Six Months. J. Genet. Psych., Dec.

Lombroso, C.T.; Duffy, F.H. and Robb, R.M. (1969): Selective Suppression of Cerebral Evoked Potentials to Patterned Light in Amblyopia Exanopsia. Electroenceph. Clin. Neurophysiol., Elsevier Pub. Co., Amsterdam, 27.

Ludlam, W.M. and Pierce, J.: Clinical Techniques for Strabismus Training, The Professional Press, Chicago (in preparation).

Ludlam, W.M. and Wittenberg, S. (1966): The Effect of Measuring Corneal Toroidicity With Reference to the Line of Sight, Br. J. Physiol. Opt., 23: 178.

Ludvigh, E.; McKinnon, P. and Zaitzeff, L. (1965): Relative Effectivity of Foveal and Parafoveal Stimuli in Eliciting Fusion Movements. Arch. Oph. 73: 115.

Lyle, T. and Foley, J. (1955): Subnormal Binocular Vision With Special Reference to Peripheral Fusion. Br.J. Oph., 39: 474.

Marshall, R.L. and Flom, M.C. (1970): Amblyopia, Visual Acuity, and the Stiles-Crawford Effect. A.A.A.O., 42: 81.

Miller, E. (1954): The Nature and Cause of Impaired Vision in the Amblyopic Eye of a Squinter. A.A.A.O., 31: 615.

Montessori, M. (1966): A Montessori Handbook. Edited by R.C. Orem, Capricorn Books, N.Y., II, Movement in Education. p. 57.

Morgan, W. (1948): Methods Used in the Treatment of Squint. A.A.A.O., 25: 57.

Morgan, M. (1961): Anomalous Correspondence Interpreted as a Motor Phenomonon. A.A.A.O., 38: 131.

Murroughs, T. (1957): A Clinical Guide to Amblyopia Therapy. Committee on Visual Problems in Schools, A.O.A., St. Louis.

Parinaud, M. (1900): The Ocular Manifestations of Hysteria, in Morris, W.F. & Oliver, C.A.: System of Diseases of the Eye, Lippincott, Phila.

Pascal, J. (1953): Normal and Anomalous Correspondence-Need for Differentiation. O.J.R.O., 90 (8): 29.

Peckham, R.M. (1937): The Diagnostic Difference Between Correctible and Non-Correctible Amblyopia. Clinical Research Report No. 2, Optometric Research Institute, Detroit, Michigan.

Perry, N.W. and Childers, D.G. (1969): Cortical Potentials in Normal and Amblyopic Binocular Vision. In Advances in Electrophysiology and Pathology of the Visual System, 6th ISCERG Symposium (ed. by E. Schmoger), Thieme, Leipzig.

**Pugh, M. (1954): Foveal Vision in Amblyopia. Br.J. Oph., 38: 321.*

Rodger, F.C. (1952): Nutritional Amblyopia. Arch. Oph., 47: 5.

Schapero, M.; Cline, H. and Hofstetter, H.A. (1960): Dictionary of Visual Science, Chilton Book Co. Philadelphia.

Schapero, M. (1971): Amblyopia. Chilton Books Co., Philadelphia.

Schlossman and Priestly, B. (1952): Role of Heredity in Etiology and Treatment of Strabismus. Arch. Oph., 47: 1.

Scobee, R. (1951): Esotropia. A.J. Oph., 34: 817.

Scobee, R.G. (1952): The Oculorotary Muscles, 2nd ed., The C.V. Mosby Co., St. Louis.

Shipley, T. (1969): The Visually Evoked Occipitogram in Strabismic Amblyopia Under Direct-view Ophthalmoscopy. J. Ped. Oph., 6: 97.

**Skeffington, A. (1953): Squint: Practical Applied Optometry – Optometric Extension Program Papers. Duncan, Oklahoma, 25 (4): 31.*

Skeffington, A.: The Role of the Strabismic in the Lens Equation. Optometric Extension Program Papers, Duncan, Oklahoma, 35 (9): 61.

Smith, K.U.; Gould, J. and Wargo, L. (1963): Sensory Feedback Analysis of Visual Behavior: A New Theoretical-Experimental Foundation of Physiological Optics. A.A.A.O., 40: 365.

Smith, W. (1935): A Basic Technique in Orthoptics. A.A.A.O., 12: 224, 321, 394, 473.

Smith, W. (1947): Clinical Procedures in Orthoptics. O.J.R.O., 84 (1): 33 and cont. 24, issues.

Smith, W. (1961): The Use of Pleoptics in Orthoptics, A.A.A.O., 38: 28.

Spencer, J. (1967): An Investigation of Maxwells Spot. Br.J. Physiol. Opt., 24: 103.

Stuart, J. and Burian, H. (1962): A Study of Separation Difficulty. A.J. Oph., 53: 471.

Swan, K. (1948): The Blindspot Syndrome. Arch. Oph., 40: 371.

**Verhoeff, F. (1938): Anomalous Projection and Other Visual Phenomena Associated with Strabismus. Arch. Oph., 19: 663.*

Von Noorden, G. and Burian, H. (1958): An Electo-Ophthalmographic Study of the Behavior of the Fixation of Amblyopic Eyes in Light and Dark-Adapted State. A.J. Oph., 46: 68.

Von Noorden, G. and Burian, H. (1959): Visual Acuity in Normal and Amblyopic Patients Under Reduced Illumination, Part 1. Arch. Oph., 61: 58.

Von Noorden, G. and Leffler, M. (1966): Visual Acuity in Strabismic Amblyopia Under Monocular and Binocular Conditions. Arch. Oph., 76: 172.

**Von Noorden, G. and Mackensen, G. (1962a): Pursuit Movements of Normal and Amblyopic Eyes: 1. Physiology of Pursuit Movements. A.J. Oph., 53: 325.*

**Von Noorden, G. and Mackensen, G. (1962b): Pursuit Movements of Normal and Amblyopic Eyes: 2. Pursuit Movements in Amblyopic Patients. A.J. Oph., 53: 477.*

Von Noorden, G.E. & Mackensen, G. (1962c): Pursuit Movements of Normal and Amblyopic Eyes. 3. Phenomonology of Eccentric Fixation. A.J. Oph., 53: 642.

Von Noorden, G. (1967): Classification of Amblyopia. A.J. Oph., 63: 238.

Wald, G. and Burian, H. (1944): The Dissociation of Form and Light Perception in Strabismic Amblyopia. A.J. Oph., 27: 950.

Walls, G. (1951): The Problem of Visual Direction. A.A.A.O., 28: 55, 115, 173.

Weinstein, M. (1963): Perceptual Interferences in Normal Binocular Development. J.A.O.A., 34: 455.

Wertheimer, M. (1961): Psychomotor Coordination of Auditory and Visual Space at Birth. Science, 134 (3491): 1692.

Weymouth, F. (1963): Visual Acuity of Children. In Vision in Children, Chilton, Philadelphia. p. 138.

Wiesel, T. and Hubel, D. (1963): Single Cell Responses in Striate Cortex of Kittens Deprived of Vision in one Eye. Jour. Neurophys., 26: 1003.

Wilkinson, O. (1927): Strabismus. C.V. Mosby Co., St. Louis.

Woolf, D. (1965): Kinesiology Related to Vision. J.A.O.A., 36: 123.

Worth, C. (1903): Squint. P. Blakiston's Son Co.

Yasuna, E.R. (1951): Hysterical Amblyopia in Children and Young Adults. Arch. Oph., 45: 70.

Strabismus/Measurement and Diagnostic Testing 30

I. INTRODUCTION

A. The operation of the ocular neuromuscular control system is not completely understood at the present time.

1. Adler (1965) points out that nuclear or infranuclear lesions will produce incomitant strabismus, but that for concomitant strabismus, "Some pathologic process has disturbed the normal vergence mechanism which lies above the level of the nuclei of the oculomotor nerves. It is therefore a supranuclear lesion." The variety, extent and direction of the deviation exhibited would, following this premise, depend primarily upon the nature, location and level of the defect within the oculomotor apparatus.

a. The perceptual adaptations made by the strabismic individual in attempting to obtain valid visual information from his surround in the presence of his strabismic condition would be secondary to this basic cause.

2. While it is possible that the underlying primary etiology of a given concomitant strabismus may be due to neurological and innervational factors in the supranuclear oculomotor control system, it is also possible that *refractive anomalies, accommodative convergence problems, and aniseikonia* may have precluded an effective binocular relationship. The strabismus may serve only as a "defense mechanism" secondary to these primary problems. Thus, a strabismus may represent a symptom of a more basic problem as well as being a primary problem in itself.

a. Morgan (1963), for example, points out that:

(1) "One of the most common causes of binocular anomalies is an unfortunate and

apparently chance association of an abnormal accommodative convergence relationship with an intermediate degree of ametropia. This may be the basic cause or a contributing cause in as high as 60 percent of all convergent squinters" (Adler and Jackson, 1947).

(2) "Obviously, many concomitant motor anomalies cannot be due to this so-called accommodative factor. Practically every possible combination of etiological factors has been proposed to account for binocular anomalies. Unfortunately, in at least 50 percent of the cases the basic underlying cause cannot be identified."

B. The measurement and diagnostic testing of a strabismic individual serve a number of purposes:

1. To ascertain the presence of an anomaly.

2. To assess the abnormal strabismus adaptations of the patient and evaluate them towards the prognosis and recommendations deemed applicable.

3. To assess the interest and cooperation of the patient in testing-training procedures.

4. To locate the areas of normal or near-normal visual and oculomotor abilities from which one might begin a program of visual training.

II. TESTS MEASURING AND CLASSIFYING THE STRABISMUS

A. The Tests of the concomitant squinter can be divided into the following categories:

1. *Tests Measuring the Size of the Deviation*

a. Historically, the precise measurement of the size of the angle of the deviation in strabismus was important whether surgical or non-surgical methods of strabismus therapy were used. In surgery it was assumed that some relationship existed between the magnitude of the deviation angle and the amount of surgery to be performed.

(1) Scobee (1951) and others do not agree with this thesis and he states that:

(a) "A general conclusion is easily drawn. On the average, if two patients with esotropia, one having 15° and the other having 30° of deviation, are subjected to the same operation, the first will have about 15° of correction while the second will have about 30° of correction." And he concludes:

(b) "The amount of surgical correction obtained in a patient with esotropia is usually directly proportional to the deviation present before surgery and is not particularly related to the amount of surgery performed as measured in millimeters."

b. *Traditional orthoptic techniques* made use of instrumentation in which training was essentially performed at the objective angle of squint and, if fusion and stereopsis were obtained, ranges of motor fusion were extended until the strabismic could maintain alignment at the orthotropic position in the instrument. Transfer of this newly-learned neuromuscular skill was then attempted into everyday visual activities in "real" space with the support of prism worn in spectacles. The approach produced some good results but transfer of the neuromuscular skills learned in the instrument to space was slow and difficult. Therefore, the "objective angle" approach has less importance in non-surgical strabismus *therapy* than formerly. The measurement of this angle however has value in classification, prognosis and description of the status of a given strabismic.

(1) The measurement of the angle of deviation is an important aspect of the diagnosis and prognosis of the strabismus especially in its use in differentiating concomitant from non-comitant squint. Various methods for arriving at a precise measurement have been developed, the more common of which are considered below.

(a) The reader should be reminded at the outset that the primary angle deviation is defined as the angle by which the line of sight or other axis of reference of the deviating eye fails to intersect the object of *fixation.*

c. *Techniques of Measurement*

(1) Duane's Alternate Cover Test

(a) Duane's Cover Test can be used to measure a strabismus in the same manner as one customarily uses it to measure a phoria.

(b) The normally strabismic eye is occluded and the patient is requested to attend the fixation target.

(c) The occluder is then moved quickly from the strabismic to the normally fixating eye.

[1] The direction and magnitude of movement of the usually deviating eye are noted.

(d) Prism with the base corresponding to the direction of squint is placed before the strabismic eye, e.g., base out for esotropia, and the test repeated.

[1] The prism is increased in amount at each repetition of the test until no motion of the deviating eye is required to pick up fixation when the good eye is covered.

[2] Prism is increased beyond the point until a *reverse* in the direction of motion is observed.

[3] That amount of prism less 2^{∇} represents the amount of deviation.

(e) The test described measures the *primary* strabismic deviation. The *secondary* deviation may be measured by the same technique but using the strabismic eye as the original fixating one.

(f) The test is carried out both with and without the refractive correction before the eyes for both a distant and near fixation point. The efficacy of the lenses in changing the angle and an estimate of the ACA ratio may be obtained.

(g) As observed in previous chapters, Ludvigh (1949) reported that 2^{∇} was the limiting discernible discrepancy by this method. A ± estimate for accuracy may be attempted by noting the last amount of prism before neutralization of movement occurs and then the amount which first changes the direction of motion after the neutralization.

[1] White reported that the test was very delicate and quite tedious and useless unless patient cooperation was readily granted (Sloane, 1951).

(h) Scobee (1952) suggests that deviations as small as $\frac{1}{2}^{\nabla}$ can be discerned by using this method if the patient is requested to observe and report the "Phi phenomenon," in which the object of fixation appears to move when the eye is alternately covered and uncovered in rapid succession.

(i) It should be noted that continued alternate cover test movements, utilizing correcting prism to neutralize the movement, may produce a larger angle than that habitually exhibited by the strabismic, so that on cessation of the alternate cover movements the angle reduces to less than the value of the neutralizing prism in place.

[1] The subjective response by the patient of diplopia at the neutralization points may be erroneously interpreted as that of anomalous correspondence if this factor is not guarded against.

(j) The reader should be reminded that for a valid determination of the magnitude of the strabismus deviation using a cover test, the presence of *central fixation* in each eye must be established.

(2) Hirschberg's Approximate Method (Wilkinson, 1927)

(a) Hirschberg's method provides a quick but not too accurate means of estimating the amount of deviation with a minimum of equipment. As will be seen, the principle involved is used in other more precise methods. This approach finds its greatest utility in examining infants where a minimum of cooperation and no verbal reply can be expected.

(b) If a light source is held directly before the patient and the patient's good eye fixates the source, the examiner will notice a reflection of the source in both the fixing and deviated corneas. If no squint is apparent, the reflection of the source in each eye will occupy the same relative corneal position. With a squint, the reflection in the non-fixing eye will appear displaced from that position in accordance with the amount and direction of the squint.

[1] The radius of the cornea is approximately 7 millimeters. Each millimeter of displacement of the reflex from the center is equivalent to roughly 8°. A reflex seen at the margin of the pupil would equal a deviation of from 12-15° (20-27 ▿); one located between the pupil and the limbus, 25° (46▿); one at the limbus, 45° (100▿) (Morgan, 1948). A PD rule can be used with the test for greater accuracy of estimation, although a possible error of 7-8° exists at best (Scobee 1952).

[2] While this method is of some use in noting whether the strabismus is exceptionally large in extent, it is not sufficiently reliable to be of value for either diagnostic or prognostic purposes. It can be used to determine the existence of strabismus in doubtful instances.

(c) Krimsky (1943) utilized a modification of Hirschberg's method.

[1] He introduced prisms before the fixating eye until the corneal reflex of the deviating eye was properly aligned.

[2] The principal difficulty of this method, as well as of others using measuring prisms, as pointed out by Scobee (1952), is the discrepancy between the measuring prism power and the actual deviation. Also, as is obvious, the effective power of a prism varies with the fixation distance and the distance of the prism to the center of rotation of the eye.

[3] This approach finds its greatest utility in examining infants where a minimum of cooperation is expected. It is also important where fixation is unsteady or eccentric.

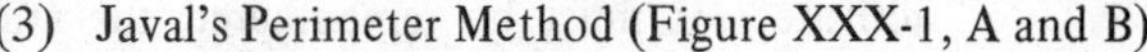

(3) Javal's Perimeter Method (Figure XXX-1, A and B)

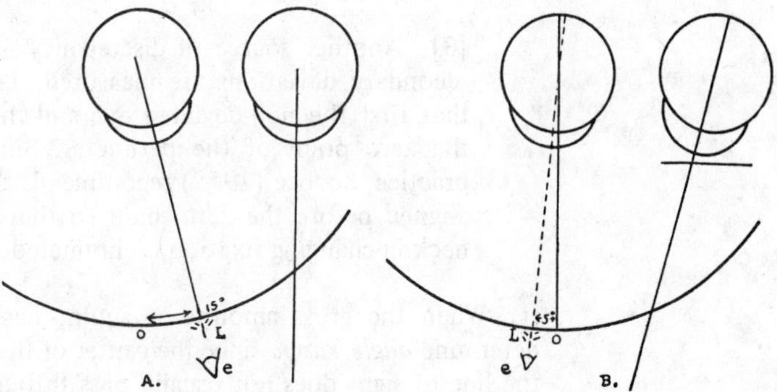

Figure XXX-1. Measurement of deviation by perimeter method. (A) and (B) Javal's method: (A) measuring gross angle of squint; (B) measuring angle kappa.

(a) An adaptation of the same principle upon a more reliable scale is made by Javal. This approach, as well as that previously suggested by Krimsky, can supply a better estimate of the squint angle measurement than a cover test when central fixation in one eye is lacking.

(b) The patient is seated in proper position before an arc perimeter without illumination arm or protractor, but with the head so elevated that the lines of sight, when directed towards the distance in the primary position, pass just above the upper rim of the arc. The deviating eye is before the fixation point of the perimeter.

(c) A target of fixation, which can be at any distance, is placed so that the line of sight of the deviating eye would pass directly above the fixation point or 0 mark of the perimeter if the eye were straight.

(d) The examiner holds a light source, such as the exposed bulb of an ophthalmoscope, against the back of the perimeter arc so that the light shines upon the cornea of the deviated eye. His own eye is placed along a line joining the cornea and the light source so that he is able to see the reflection of the source in the cornea by looking just above the source itself.

(e) With the patient maintaining fixation upon the original target with the good eye, the examiner moves both the light source and his eye along the arc until he finds the reflection of the light centered in the cornea of the deviating eye. The position of the source on the arc can be read in degrees and gives the *habitual deviation* of the eye.

[1] The technique may be used to measure the angle of deviation at any point by placing the fixation target at the distance desired. In convergent strabismus, however, there is a prospect that the examiner's head may pass before the line of sight of the good eye.

[2] Many modern perimeters are so constructed that it is difficult to align the patient's fixation above the arc of the perimeter without introducing a vertical component to the lines of sight. If the fixation point of the perimeter is used instead (1/3 meter), and accommodation is activated, it must be remembered that the angle of deviation will be altered by the ACA ratio, and will be approximately 12 Δ different (Morgan, 1948).

[3] Another source of discrepancy is introduced when the primary and secondary deviations are measured. The patient should be readjusted so that first the non-deviated eye and then the deviated eye is aligned with the zero point of the perimeter. Since this is seldom done, in actual practice, Scobee (1952) recommends that the sagittal plane of the head be aligned before the zero mark so that the effect of turning the head and neck in changing fixation is eliminated.

(f) When the gross amount of squint has been measured, it is necessary to determine *angle kappa* since the center of the cornea was used as a criterion, and the line of sight does not usually pass through the center of the cornea. This is done by occluding the good eye and having the patient fix with the squinting eye upon the 0 marker of the perimeter arc. If projection is normal, this will align the line of sight of that eye with the 0 point. The examiner then again aligns the light reflection, his eye, and the source so that the reflection appears in the center of the cornea. The position of the source on the arc when this is achieved measures angle kappa.

[1] *Angle Kappa* is defined as the angle between the pupillary axis (a line perpendicular to the cornea and passing through the center of the cornea) and the visual line (the line from the point of fixation, through the nodal points, to the fovea). This angle can actually be measured only at the anterior nodal point. What is measured clinically is an angle at the center of the entrance pupil between the pupillary and visual lines, which Fry has labeled *Angle Lambda.* It is this angle, which is erroneously called Angle Kappa, which is utilized in strabismometry; but fortunately, the difference in amount, for practical purposes, is relatively insignificant.

[2] If Angle Kappa is positive, meaning that the line of sight passes somewhat nasally to the center of the cornea, it is added to the gross amount in convergent strabismus and subtracted from the gross amount in divergent strabismus.

[3] If it is negative, it is added or subtracted in a reverse fashion from that described above.

(4) Charpentier's Method (Figure XXX-1, C and D)

(a) Because, in small angles of strabismus, the light source and examiner's head proved distracting or occluded the fixation target, Charpentier added a modification which is serviceable for smaller angles of deviation or for measuring angle kappa.

(b) Following the procedure of Javal, Charpentier digressed only in that he left the light source fixed at the 0 point of the perimeter and moved his head along the arc until he sighted the reflection in the center of the cornea. This position is obviously twice the actual angle of strabismus and not only eliminates the obstruction of the head by moving it twice as far along the perimeter but halves the possible error. Where the examiner stops is twice the deviation, and an error of a few degrees is reduced by half in computing the gross squint. In higher degrees of squint, however, the examiner is moved to so lateral a position that he finds it difficult to estimate the exact center of the cornea.

(c) Angle Kappa is measured by Charpentier in much the same manner as by Javal but with the light source fixed at the zero point while the examiner's eye follows the arc. Half the amount found represents the actual Angle Kappa.

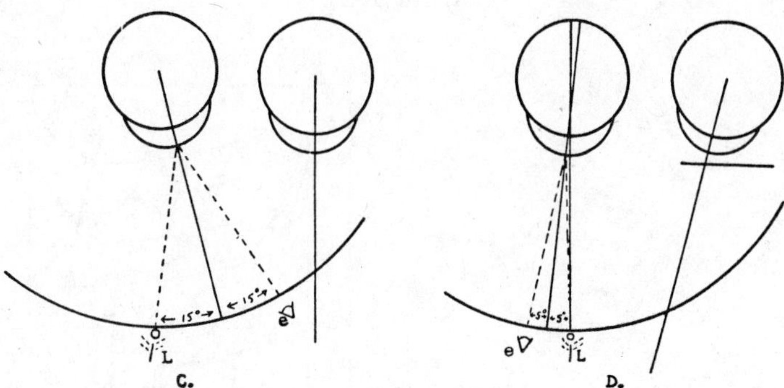

Figure XXX-1. (C) and (D) Charpentier's method: (C) gross angle of squint; (D) Angle Kappa. *L* light source of corneal reflection; *e* examiner's eye.

(5) Lancaster (1939)

(a) Lancaster employed a subjective means of measuring the deviation. In all cases, the test measures the subjective angle of the strabismus, but where normal correspondence exists, it becomes a bifoveal test. Both the foveas of the fixating and squinting eyes are then involved.

[1] In contrast to the usual crossed diplopia expected in strabismus, the position of the targets on the Lancaster screen agree with the direction of deviation, the images of the eyes appearing crossed in esotropia and uncrossed in exotropia when the retinal correspondence is normal.

(b) Lancaster used a white tangent screen at a 2 meter distance. The screen was graphed into boxes of 7 cm. size, approximating 2° or 4$^{\Delta}$ each, and extending to a total of 16° to each side of the median. If a larger deviation was involved the test could be made at a 1 meter distance, in which case the values doubled. While Lancaster recognized that the tangent involved should require extension of the size of the boxes as the chart extended peripherally, he maintained that the discrepancy was not important for practical and comparative purposes.

(c) The patient wore a pair of goggles consisting of one red and one green lens. The examiner held a light source which projected a green streak on the screen, while the patient held a light source which projected a red streak of equal dimension on the screen. The examiner projected the green streak to the various parts of the field and the patient attempted to cover the green streak with the red one. The actual discrepancy between the two on the screen indicated the extent of deviation.

(d) If a greater discrepancy was involved, or the limit of fixation was to be extended, the patient's head could be deviated. Also, the secondary deviations could be measured by exchanging the light sources with the patient. The linear target allowed the existence of torsion to be demonstrated.

(6) Hess Screen Test (1908)

(a) In still another variation, Hess employed a black tangent chart. The chart is divided by red lines into small sections of 10° separation. These are based upon true tangents, and the lines are curved and bow towards the center (see Figure XXX-2).

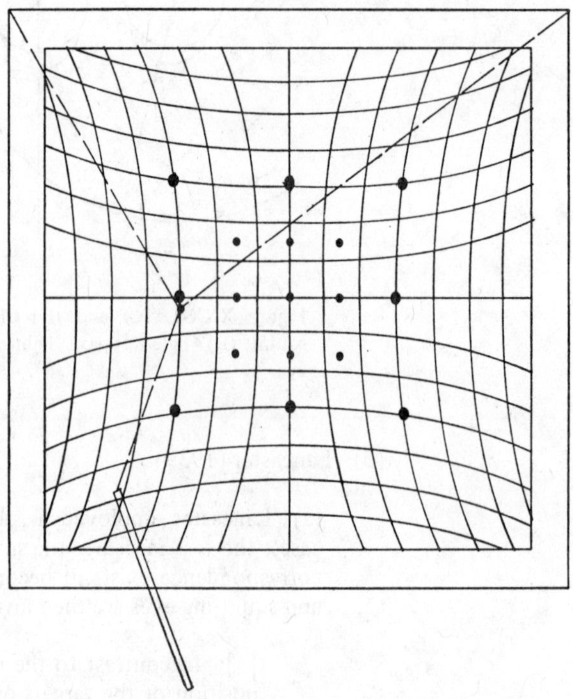

Figure XXX-2. Hess Screen. Solid lines indicate tangent markings in red. Dots are red, and indicate intersections of 15 and 30 degrees with vertical and horizontal markers. Dashes indicate green thread attached to wand.

[1] At the respective positions on the lines in the eight major meridians are small red dots indicating positions 15 and 30 degrees from the fixation point. Two small green threads extend from the upper corners and meet a third green thread which originates on the end of a pointer. The three threads form a figure similar to the letter, Y.

[2] By moving the pointer, the threads can be positioned so that any one of the red dots is enclosed in the crotch of the Y. The patient wears a pair of red-green goggles, so that one eye sees the red dots, and the other the green threads.

[3] The patient encloses each of the red dots in the Y, and the position of the Y is noted on a recording chart which is a copy of the screen. By reversing the goggles, the secondary deviation can be measured. Also by

tilting the head, the effective angle can be altered for extreme peripheral rotations of the eye.

[4] A comparison of the primary field and secondary field is immediately obvious upon completion of the test. (The fields are joined together like the limiting points of a visual field chart.)

(7) Anderson used a projected chart of similar design. Burian employed polaroid filters and projected a horizontal calibrated line to be seen by one eye and a vertical one to be seen by the other.

(8) Phorometer, Tropometer, Amblyoscope, etc.

(a) Any device which indicates an angle of deviation and which is usable for the measurement of a phoria, such as the Maddox rod tests on a phorometer, or the rotoscope or similar instrument, can be used to estimate the angle of deviation if suppression is not invoked. With the major amblyoscope, the corneas can be seen and the deviation measured objectively. Polaroid filters, colored lenses, and similar dissociating elements may be added to the devices to accomplish the dissociation and create diplopia.

(9) Other methods not presently in general use, but which have been of historical interest, are:

(a) Maddox's Tangent (Figure XXX-3)

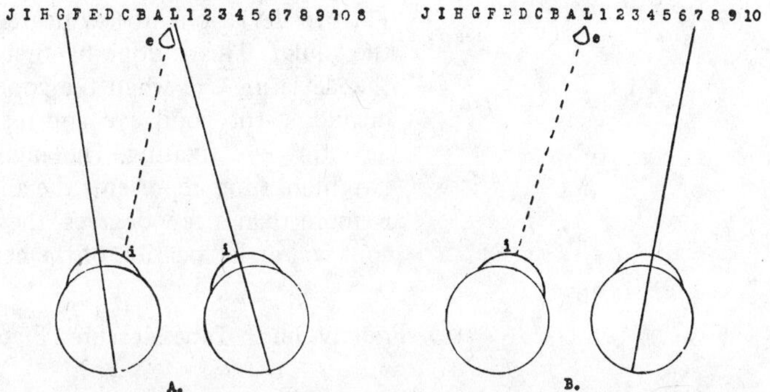

Figure XXX-3. Maddox tangent. (A) Shows images on both corneas when good eye fixates light at center of scale. (B) Shows image on cornea of deviating eye in same position as seen in (A) on good eye. Good eye fixates at 7, indicating amount of deviation. *L* light source; *e* examiner's eye; *i* image of *L* on cornea.

[1] Maddox used a tangent method of measuring the deviation. A scale is marked upon a wall or rod in either degrees or prism diopters and placed at a height just above the examiner's head. A small light source occupies the center of the scale.

[2] The examiner stands just beneath the scale and faces the patient, who in turn looks at the scale with his good eye. As he does so, the examiner observes the position of the reflection of the source in the cornea of the good eye when the patient is requested to observe the light.

[3] The patient is then directed to look at a figure to either side of the

scale and the examiner notes the reflection of the light in the cornea of the deviated eye. When the fixing eye observes a figure which corresponds to the amount of strabismus, the examiner will find the reflection of the light in the poor eye occupies the same relative corneal position as it did in the cornea of the good eye when that eye fixed the light.

[4] Maddox also used the tangent for a subjective evaluation of the deviation. The tangent contained a vertical scale as well as a horizontal one, forming a cross on the wall, with the small light occupying the center of the cross. The technique is almost identical with that popularized by Bielschowsky.

[a] The extent of deviation in the nine fields of fixation could be measured by having the patient tilt the head so that the eyes faced the cross in the desired fixation position.

[5] Sloane (1951) offered a portable version of the Maddox Tangent. The screen consisted of transparent plastic which could be held by a handle at a desired distance. A cross, calibrated in prism diopters, was in the center of the screen, at which a fixation light appeared. The observer stood behind the screen, which he held, and viewed the subject's eyes through it.

(b) Lloyd's Campimeter

[1] In deviations of low degree, the campimeter can be used to measure the squint. This is done by first charting the position of the blind spot of the deviating eye when the good eye fixates the fixation point, and then occluding the good eye and recharting the blind spot with the originally deviating eye fixating. The angular difference between the centers of the two blind spots represents the angle of deviation. However, if the deviation is more than a few degrees, the tangent projection of the displaced blind spot will make location of the center very difficult.

(c) Priestly-Smith Tape Measure (Figure XXX-4)

[1] Priestley-Smith used a set of tapes designed as follows: one tape contained a ring at one end which was placed against the cheek of the patient and encircled the deviating eye. The tape was held taut by the examiner, who stood directly before the patient, facing him. The other end of the tape contained a small ring through which a light, or instrument containing a light, was placed. Attached to this latter ring was a second tape calibrated in either degrees or prism diopters in accordance with the length of the first tape. (A one meter tape would represent one prism diopter per centimeter on the second or measuring tape.)

[2] With the first tape held taut, stabilizing the distance, the examiner observed the reflection of the source in the cornea of the fixing eye when that eye fixed the light. He then passed his hand along the second or measuring tape, extending it at right angles to the first tape. The patient was requested to follow the visible thumb as it moved along the second tape and the examiner meanwhile noted the reflection of the light source in the deviating cornea.

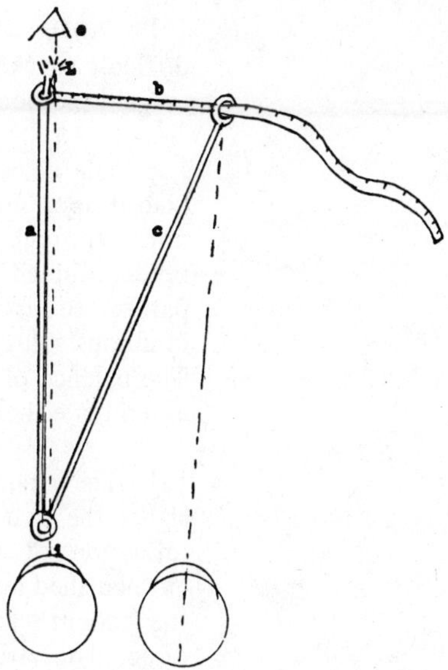

Figure XXX-4. Priestley-Smith tape measure. Examiner's eye, *e*, sights image, *i*, of light source. *L*, in center of deviating eye's cornea as good eye fixates upon ring moving along measuring tape. Tape *a* fixation distance tape; tape *b*, calibrated measuring tape, tape *c*, Holzer's tape modifying the original Priestley-Smith tape measure.

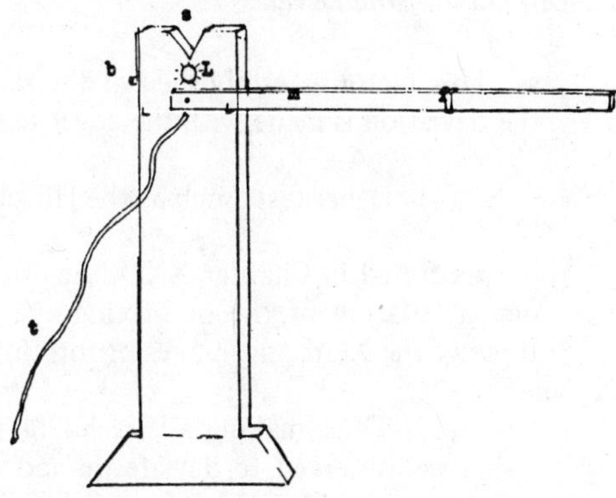

Figure XXX-5. Worth's Devionometer. The Worth portable version of the Maddox tangent. *s* sighting aperture for examiner's eye; *L* light source; *m* measuring tangent; *f* movable fixation target for good eye; *b* light control; *t* tape for stabilizing measuring distance.

[3] The position of the thumb along the measuring tape when the reflection approximated that first noted in the good eye indicated the extent of deviation. It will be observed that this method is a portable variation of the Maddox tangent.

(d) Worth's Devionometer (1903) (Figure XXX-5)

[1] Worth, who worked with many children, found the above methods difficult to execute and developed a portable device based on Maddox's tangent method which lent itself to more facile operation.

[2] The device consists of a vertical upright upon a base which can be placed upon an adjustable instrument table. At the top of the upright is a notch through which the examiner can sight the patient's eye. A cord of predetermined length is attached and is extended to the cheek of the patient to assure the testing distance. Imbedded in the upright is a luminous source which can be turned on and off when a button is pressed. The balance of the device consists of a lateral arm which can be rotated to extend in either lateral direction.

[3] The examiner takes a position behind the upright so that his eye sights the eye of the patient who faces him. After noting the corneal reflection of the source of light, just as Maddox did, the light is extinguished and a small metal clasp is moved along the lateral arm while the patient's good eye follows it. When the deviated eye appears to be directed towards the notch, the light is flashed on and the examiner notes the reflection in the cornea. The lateral arm is calibrated to indicate the angle of squint.

[4] The device has the advantage of removing the light which might distract children, and also of permitting a noise to be made by the clasp against the arm to attract a child's fixation. By alternating rattling the clasp and flashing the light, the squint can be measured with even a recalcitrant, confused or frightened child.

2. *Direction of the Deviation*

a. This factor is established at the same time that the determination of the magnitude of the deviation is made with the cover test.

(1) Other tests such as the Hirschberg test may also be used.

b. As stated in Chapter XXIX the direction of a strabismic deviation can be described as an ocular rotation of the non-fixing eye with respect to the fixing eye about one, two or all three of the X, Y, and Z axes of rotation.

(1) Thus, making a Hirschberg Test assessment of a condition in which the right eye was observed to deviate up and out (reflex down and in) relative to its fellow fixing eye would be said to be a right-hyper-exo deviation.

(a) The presence of even a large cyclotropia-component is impossible to detect using this method.

c. With the *Alternate Cover Test,* the direction of the imbalance is interpreted as being *opposite to the corrective fixation movement* observed when the eye is uncovered. A down movement would occur in the case of a hyper-deviation, a medial or inward movement is exhibited in exotropia and an inward wheel rotation can be observed in an excyclotropia.

(1) Thus, for example a left eye is observed by the examiner to move down, toward the midline and to spin in a clockwise direction as the cover is moved to the right eye.

(a) From such a move the condition would be interpreted as a left-hyper-exo-encyclo deviation.

(2) In all strabismus cases the entire movement sequence should be observed since an overcompensation usually is made followed by a corrective movement. This is particularly important in post-surgical cases.

d. A surgically aligned former esotrope, on alternate cover, may make an erroneous or paradoxical "out" movement of the size of the former deviation followed by a corrective "in" movement of the same size. This phenomenon generally decreases or disappears as the test is repeated.

e. Cover-Uncover Test

(1) This test is used to differentiate manifest strabismus from heterophoria.

(2) The test is performed in a manner similar to its performance when testing for phorias.

(a) Flom (1956) gives the following description of the analysis of the test: "If on covering each eye in turn, no movement of the fellow eye occurs, then a phoria is indicated provided that the Angles Kappa are equal and no eccentric fixation is present. If there is an eccentric fixation (e.g., Angles Kappa are unequal) and no movement of either eye is detected, then a strabismus with an angle of deviation equal to the degree of eccentric fixation is probably present. The fact that no movement for either eye with the unilateral cover test can still denote the presence of a strabismus emphasizes that Angle Kappa must be determined for each eye before the cover-uncover test can be interpreted correctly."

(3) In a condition of phoria, the occluded eye will assume the position of rest behind the occluder and resume the fixation position when the occluder is removed. In strabismus the deviating eye will make no motion if occluded, but will make a motion to fixate if the good or fixing eye is occluded. If the squint is alternating, the previously deviated eye will hold its fixation when occlusion is removed, but if it is uniocular, the fixing eye will resume its fixation upon removal of the occlusion and the deviating eye will concomitantly resume its angle of squint. Thus, two motions, one upon occlusion and one upon exposure, enable a differentiation to be made as follows:

(a) **Table XXX-1**

	Upon Occlusion		**Upon Exposure**		**Interpretation**
	occluded eye	**other eye**	**occluded eye**	**other eye**	
(a)	moves out	no motion	moves in	no motion	exophoria
(b)	moves in	no motion	moves out	no motion	esophoria
(c)	moves out	no motion	no motion	no motion	esotropia–occasional
(d)	moves in	no motion	no motion	no motion	esotropia–occasional
(e)	moves out	moves in	moves in	moves out	exotropia–continuous of unoccluded eye
(f)	moves in	moves out	moves out	moves in	esotropia–continuous of unoccluded eye
(g)	moves out	moves in	no motion	no motion	exotropia–alternating
(h)	moves in	moves out	no motion	no motion	esotropia–alternating
(i)	no motion	no motion	no motion	no motion	may have occluded the strabismic eye. If repetition upon other eye reveals same result, orthophoria

(4) As in the case of the alternating cover test previously mentioned, the patient is asked to report his subjective impression of the movement of the target after each cover-uncover.

3. *Time or Periodicity of the Strabismus*

a. *Frequency* relates to the amount of time which an eye is deviated. The category has been subdivided into:

(1) *Constant,* in which the strabismus is present at all times.

(2) *Intermittent or occasional* in which the strabismus is manifested, irregularly and unpredictably.

(a) Flom (1954) classifies the time of strabismus into constant and occasional, and classifies occasional, in turn, into periodic and intermittent.

(b) Clinical studies of large samples of strabismics have shown (Flom, 1954; Schlossman and Boruchoff, 1955; and Ludlam and Kleinman, 1965) that exotropes tend to be non-constant strabismics (80%) whereas esotropes tend to be constant (75%).

(3) The category into which an individual strabismic fits at any given period can be established by observation. This category may be changed from constant to intermittent by therapy (surgery, training or refractive correction) or may retrogress from intermittent to constant through neglect and the passage of time.

b. *Periodicity* refers to a strabismus which is manifested only in specific conditions, i.e., a fixation distance or field of gaze. With regard to distance the condition may be classified as either:

(1) *Directly periodic* in which the deviation is greater at near than at far. An example is an esotrope with a high ACA ratio or exotrope with a low ACA ratio.

(2) *Inversely periodic* in which the deviation is greater at far than at near. A well known example in this category is the divergence excess where the exotropia is manifested at distance fixation but not for near.

(3) The periodic strabismus can be clinically classified by performing a cover test for both distance and near fixation and by observation.

(4) The "A" and "V" syndromes are instances of relatively large changes in a horizontal deviation which occur with elevated or depressed gaze and are covered in detail under vertical incomitance in Chapter XXXI.

4. *Laterality*

a. The pattern of fixation may be characterized as:

(1) *Unilateral* – the same eye engages in fixation at all times and at all distances.

(2) *Alternating* – either eye may assume fixation while the other deviates. This pattern may take several forms:

(a) *Essential alternation* – the strabismic consciously chooses the eye with which he wishes to fixate.

(b) *Midline alternation* – the eyes alternate "automatically" when a pursuit movement or series of saccades, such as in reading a line of print, causes the then fixing eye to cross the midline.

(c) *Alternation with respect to distance* – in this category the typical pattern is to utilize one eye almost exclusively for distance fixation and to use the other for near point fixation. Usually, but not always, such a pattern is accompanied by anisometropia, and/or differences in accommodative facility between the two eyes.

(d) *Random or accidental alternation* – alternation occurs in no apparently systematic fashion related to field, fixation distance or volition.

(e) Clinical classification is carried out by observation, if the patient has a large angle, but for smaller angles, objective and subjective cover tests and subjective reports by the strabismic while wearing anaglyph glasses are more effective.

5. *Behavior of the Strabismus Angle*

a. The size of the deviation for a fixed distance of the object of regard may vary with time, illness, hunger, emotional state, fatigue, visual task, or viewing distance. This behavior classification is subdivided as follows:

(1) *Fixed* – in which the angle of deviation remains substantially unchanged under all conditions.

(2) *Variable* – in which the angle of deviation varies during the examination or is reported to vary because of one or more of the factors just enumerated.

(a) The presence of a variable angle, all other factors being equal, is generally held to be a favorable factor in the prognosis and treatment of a given strabismus.

III. MONOCULAR SENSORY AND MOTOR TESTING

A. Integrity of function of the pathways in the macular area

1. This function is generally tested in depth when the best corrected monocular acuities differ by more than one line. The poorer central acuity is usually, but not always, found in the deviating eye of a unilateral strabismus. The following tests are usually performed:

a. *Haidinger's Brush Test*

(1) Using any one of several available instruments, e.g., Koordinator and Macula Integrity Tester, the subject is asked to view, monocularly, the rotating polaroid with the eye exhibiting better acuity.

(2) Once the entoptic "rotating propeller" or Haidinger Brush has been observed, the suspect eye is exposed and the better one occluded. The patient is again asked to report the appearance and position of the propeller.

(3) If the cellophane filter supplied with the instrument is interposed before the eye, the observed direction of rotation should appear reversed.

(4) Although visible without an Rx (depending on acuity – see below), the effect may be enhanced by a strong plus lens which blurs the surround.

(5) Where the image is not seen initially, bringing the patient closer to the target may help by enlarging the image and either thereby improving the acuity, or in case of eccentric fixation, overlapping the foveal area.

(a) Sloan and Naquin (1955), as reported below, found that in amblyopia exanopsia, where the scotoma was small enough so that some portion of the brush could be recognized perimacularly, the patient was able to report the phenomenon accurately.

(6) Goldschmidt (1950) held that the inability to see the brushes in a condition of amblyopia ex anopsia offered a poor prognosis for improvement following occlusion of the other eye. Forster (1954) considered it chiefly useful for indicating the existence of pathology of the macular area in those cases in which the ophthalmoscope could not be used. He found it limited to better than 20/60 acuity.

(a) Sloan and Naquin (1955) made a study of the use of the technique in a variety of pathological and non-pathological cases. They concluded the test was only of limited diagnostic value.

[1] The technique appeared mainly useful for differentiating macular from optic nerve lesions where unsteady fixation prevents accurate central scotometry.

[a] In central lesions the spokes were absent if acuity was less than 20/100 whether the lesion was macular or in the pathways.

[2] The size of the central lesion was the important factor in whether the brushes were seen or not, rather than its density.

[3] In amblyopia ex anopsia, the central scotoma was generally smaller than in disease, and the brushes were seen partially (but identifiably so) or perimacularly.

[4] The subject must not wear contact lenses, plastic spectacle lenses, or safety glasses, which materials might be bi-refringent and alter the brush appearance or even eliminate its presence.

b. *Maxwell Spot*

(1) Like the Haidinger Brush test, the Maxwell spot test is another entoptic phenomenon which has been offered as a means of distinguishing between pathological and non-pathological affectations of the fovea, perifoveal regions and their pathways.

(2) The test is performed similarly to the Haidinger Brush test but a purple filter (wratten No. 2387) is used, and a red spot on a purple background should be observed. With any blue filter, a dark (shadow-like) spot on a blue background may be visible.

(3) Not every subject sees either of the entoptic phenomenon described but some may see one of them and not the other.

(4) Sloan and Naquin (1955) believe that the Maxwell Spot test and the Haidinger Brush test involve the same visual mechanism, one by means of unpolarized light and one by means of polarized light.

c. *Brock Posture Box* (Brock, 1962)

(1) This is an anaglyphic approach to testing macular integrity with the measured eye stabilized by means of contralateral fixation of the preferred eye.

(a) A red filter is placed before the eye to be tested and a green filter is placed in front of the fellow eye. A red grid, visible to the eye behind the green filter can be used to locate the approximate position of the visual axis of the deviating eye under test.

[1] This can be confirmed by the cover test, if desired.

(b) The red light, visible only to the eye under test is then slowly moved in visual space corresponding to the macular area of the eye under test, along horizontal, vertical, and oblique meridians.

(c) The patient is asked to report whether the circular red light disappears, dims, is deformed, or if parts or sectors are missing.

(2) Some reports indicate that such responses correlate with distortion or missing sectors reported during the Haidinger Brush or Maxwell Spot tests, and assume such reports to indicate a lack of neurological integrity of the retinal pathways. Training of amblyopia has resulted in a "cut-off" point (usually 20/50) at which improvement of acuity ceases.

(a) This conclusion is challenged by others who consider the indication essentially one of suppression, and do not agree that the Brock Test differentiates foveal suppression from foveal scotoma with any greater proficiency than does the Stereocampimeter, also often used to chart central scotomas, despite a professed greater contrast between target and ground in the Brock Test.

B. Centration and Steadiness of Fixation

1. As described in Chapter XXIX the presence of eccentric and unsteady fixation has been shown to be strongly related to the occurrence of functional amblyopia in strabismus.

2. *Steadiness of fixation* may be assessed externally with an ophthalmometer or slit lamp biomicroscope *while* the eye under observation is attempting to fixate. This quality of fixation may also be observed by utilizing a *measuring ophthalmoscope or Visuskop.*

a. The patient is asked to view with his non-preferred eye (the other eye being occluded) a small target (e.g., star or square) projected on the fundus. The examiner directly views the fundus and objectively estimates the steadiness of the fixation by fundus movements relative to the projected fixation target (or fundus vessel movements if these are easier to observe).

b. For comparison, the non-amblyopic or habitually fixating eye may be similarly observed for steadiness of fixation. It is not usual for the patient to be subjectively aware of the wavering fixation movements either through kinesthetic or visual sensations.

3. *Centration of fixation* may be gauged by both objective and subjective means.

a. The *objective techniques* are accomplished with a Visuskop as before, but the examiner observes instead the "average" fundus position of the fixated projected target, with relation to the foveal reflex.

(1) This can be determined by an experienced examiner on most amblyopes with a precision of 2^{Δ} to 3^{Δ}.

(2) Mydriasis is helpful in most cases but is usually not essential.

(3) It should be pointed out that although the test is called "objective" because of the examiner's part in observing the placement of the projected spot on the fundus, the results can be no better than the subject's cooperation in fixating or attempting to fixate the target.

b. There are several types of *"purely" subjective tests* for assessing centration of fixation:

(1) *Macula indicator or cue tests,* i.e., Maxwell Spot and Haidinger Brush

(a) A fixation target is viewed by the patient with each eye in turn and the spatial relationship of the projected entoptic phenomenon to the fixation target is reported. Thus, measurements can be made at various distances and compared for reliability.

(b) As mentioned in the previous chapter, Flom and Weymouth (1961) found a linear correlation of +0.94 between measured acuity and eccentric fixation as determined by the Maxwell spot displacement method.

(2) The *Brock after-image transfer test* can also be used to assess eccentricity of fixation. A vertical line after-image is impressed on the fovea of the habitually fixing eye and the "transferred" after-image is projected to a grid with a central dot. The displacement of the projected "transferred" after-image from the dot fixated by the amblyopic eye provides an estimate of the degree of eccentric fixation present.

(a) The results of this test may be influenced by the presence of anomalous retinal correspondence.

(3) *Maze Tracing*

(a) The patient is asked to trace a line maze with his amblyopic eye covered and then a different one with his amblyopic eye fixating, each time tracing with the same hand.

(b) An example of a typical performance is shown in Figure XXIX-6.

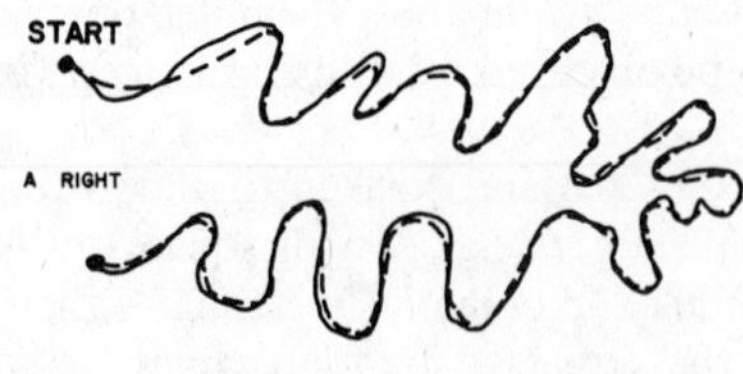

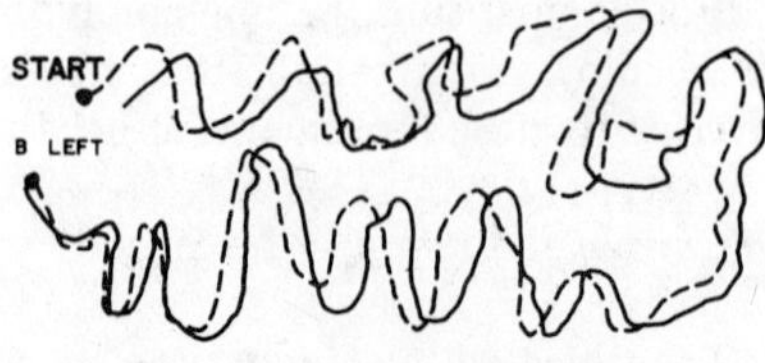

Figure XXX-6. Demonstration of Line Maze Tracing by patient using right hand. A centrally fixating right eye. B eccentrically fixating left eye.

(c) The amblyopic left eye exhibits a consistent bias to the right (historically known as "past pointing") which demonstrates a nasal eccentric fixation of this left eye.

(d) Similar demonstrations of this phenomenon by an amblyopic eccentric fixator can be exhibited in rolling a ball at an object, games of horseshoes or quoits, picking up eyeglass screws with tweezers, filling in hollow letters in the newspaper and "stick and soda straw" tests.

C. The presence of the "Fixation Reflex "

1. Central fixation is the ability to place and maintain the retinal image of an object on the fovea. The *"fixation reflex"* is the ability of an individual to act on the feedback information to recenter the image on the fovea whenever it departs. Testing this function for stationary targets has already been described under *Centration and Steadiness of Fixation.*

2. Three types of tests are generally conducted where motion is involved.

a. *Smooth pursuit movements*

(1) The subject holds his head steady and is directed to follow or 'track' a smoothly moving target, such as a penlight, first with one eye and then the other.

(2) The examiner notes the ability to stay on target and counts the number of overshoots and undershoots. He also notes the extent of head and torso movements used to carry out this "tracking" task.

b. *Discrete jumps or "saccadic" movements*

(1) In this test, the subject is directed to change fixation in vertical, horizontal and oblique meridians, first with one eye occluded and then the other.

(2) The ease and speed with which the patient gives up fixation of one object and the speed and smoothness with which he travels to and takes up fixation on the new target is observed.

(3) Head and torso movements which participate in and detract from the act are again noted. The performances of the two eyes are compared.

c. *The Prism Jump or Saccades*

(1) This is a test in which a loose prism of 25-30$^{\Delta}$ is abruptly introduced before each eye monocularly while a light is fixated, and the ease and speed with which fixation is re-established, as well as the ability of the patient to perceive the movement, are noted. This is a variation of the saccadic movement test because in the prism jump test the entire visual frame of reference (both target and background) is shifted. Generally, strabismics find it a more difficult test, particularly in the meridian of deviation. If the refixation is observed to be carried out smoothly and quickly, a prism of decreased power, e.g., 15$^{\Delta}$, is introduced, and the patient's eye movements again observed. The prism is reduced as long as correct refixation movements are made to a minimum power of 2$^{\Delta}$.

D. Monocular Field of Gaze

1. Testing of the monocular fields of gaze should be undertaken not only to identify complete limitations of movements, but to note also the quality of the movement, the tendency to use head

and body movements to compensate, subjective reports of pulling and even pain in some directions, and any differences in the performances of the two eyes.

a. In testing the habitually deviating eye of a unilateral strabismus, one generally finds a poorer quality of performance and sometimes even a limitation of gaze in the direction opposite the deviation.

(1) Thus for example, abduction and supra-abduction are usually the poorest fields of action in the squinting eye of concomitant unilateral esotropes.

E. Accommodative Rock or Facility

1. The monocular speeds and amplitudes of accommodative rock are compared. The test is performed at the subject's habitual reading distance of from 13 to 20 inches. A range of lenses from +1.50 D. to –2.00 D. should still permit clear vision.

a. Normal response time for adolescent and young adults to clear from one lens to the other, with ametropia corrected, should be less than 5 seconds. There should be less than ½ second differential between the two eyes.

b. In the case of marked amblyopia it has been assumed that there is usually little or no direct accommodative response to either plus or minus lenses.

c. In alternating strabismics who habitually fixate with one eye at a distance and the other at near, substantial difference in accommodative facility is also usually found.

IV. BINOCULAR SENSORY AND MOTOR TESTING

A. Once the integrity and centration of monocular fixation in each eye has been tested and found to be normal, a meaningful analysis of binocular function can be undertaken.

1. The presence of eccentric fixation must be considered in any investigation of a "correspondency system organized about the foveas" (Morgan, 1963), and subjective evaluation of such a system is subject to invalidity. However, the binocular Visuscope Test does enable an objective evaluation to be made.

a. Similarly, attempts to train binocularity have been viewed as potentially harmful to the achievement of binocular integration, fusion and stereopsis. Flom comments, however, that with normal retinal correspondence and eccentric fixation, binocularity may still be trained. This section includes the following classes of tests:

B. Binocular Color "Luster"

1. This is the most primordial and basic subjective binocular sensory test of strabismus where the input of each eye differs only with respect to wavelength or intensity, form differences being absent. The color differences can be presented:

a. *In space* at the centration point (point in visual space where the two visual axes cross) using colored anaglyph glasses. Care should be taken to use an evenly illuminated white surface free from shadows and borders in the binocular field.

(1) If the centration point is very close to the patient, or non-existent as in constant exotropia or hypertropia, prism should be used to establish one at a convenient distance.

(2) Any report of a true color mixture indicates at least primordial binocularity.

(3) The perceived color mixture may be named almost any color by the patient and all are acceptable if they meet three criteria:

(a) That the mixture not look the same as the color seen by either eye alone.

(b) That the two colors comprising the mixture appear to be in the same plane.

(c) That the mixed color be seen over the entire *binocular* field excepting the occurrence of normal binocular rivalry effects in which rhythmic changes in the balance of the color mixture occur in small areas. Such effects can be observed by any normal observer.

[1] One must guard against accepting a split-field response as luster.

[2] Here both colors are seen simultaneously but each in half of a divided field.

[3] This response is a classic manifestation of anomalous correspondence.

[4] If luster cannot be exhibited with the anaglyph glasses on one way, they should be reversed because the filter densities may not be well matched, and the trial repeated under this new condition.

(a) Rapidly blinking the eyes and slowly moving the head toward and away from the viewing surface also help to elicit the effect.

2. *In various instruments* such as stereoscopes, cheiroscopes and amblyoscopes, large, plain colored slides can be centered approximately along the visual axes (at the objective angle of squint) and the illumination level varied. Flashing, moving, oscillating and flickering may also be used to help elicit the luster response.

3. Any *true luster* response (i.e., which features a mixture of the two colors) indicates that the basic neurology necessary to enable at least some binocularity is present. Unless and until a luster response can be demonstrated, the breaking down of strabismic perceptual adaptations should be approached with caution.

C. Anomalous Correspondence (ARC)

1. Because of the importance of the prospect of anomalous correspondence, it is advisable to determine early whether correspondence exists. Over the years there has been considerable confusion in the differential diagnosis of eccentric fixation from anomalous correspondence. Since eccentric fixation is a monocular (usually unilateral) anomaly, its presence precludes a valid diagnosis of ARC. Thus, diagnosis of ARC, like the measurement of the size of the angle of deviation using the cover test, can only be validly made in the presence of central fixation in each eye. There are several widely used methods for testing this anomaly:

2. *After-Image Test*

a. The Hering or Bielschowsky (1937) after-image test is a simple and effective device for determining the retinal correspondence.

b. The device consists of a bright lumi-line filament with an opaque band covering its center, which serves as a fixation target.

c. Flom and Kerr (1967) describe the following effective technique:

(1) The subject fixates the center of a horizontal lumi-line filament with the preferred eye for 30 seconds from a distance of one meter.

(2) He then fixates the center of a vertical filament with the non-preferred eye for twenty seconds.

(3) He next views a silvered screen at one meter distance that is diffused and intermittently lighted to balance and stabilize the appearance of the after-images.

(a) In their study, Flom and Kerr rotated the position of the subject 180° in moving from the horizontal to the vertical filament and then another 90° to the screen. This was so that no suggestion that a cross was expected should be presented by the two after-images. Since few offices will employ such elaborate equipment, the lumi-line filament is usually designed so it can be rotated from a horizontal to a vertical presentation while the subject remains in a constant position.

(4) The preferred eye fixates a small spot on the screen, in the primary position.

(5) The *perceived position* of the vertical after-image is indicated by moving a fiducial mark so that it seems to coincide with the after-image, and the deviation of the projected image from the fixation spot is read directly in prism diopters from an inconspicuous scale on the screen.

d. The reading is a direct measure of the angle of anomaly.

(1) If the correspondence is normal, the two lines will form a perfect cross at the fixation point.

(2) If the correspondence is anomalous, the two lines will be separated.

(3) If eccentric fixation exists, a cross may still be seen if the area stimulated by the vertical filament was that peripheral area whose directionalization coincided with that of the fovea of the non-affected eye.

(a) The presence of eccentric fixation must have been noted previously for the test to be correctly interpreted.

(b) The method of questioning is important in this test, because if the patient is merely requested to report the appearance of a cross, it is possible for the patient to note a cross and still have anomalous correspondence. This condition is illustrated in Figure XXX-7.

3. *Variations of the After-Image Test*

a. The after-image can also be impressed by a stroboscopic flash apparatus. This has the advantage of impressing a sharp high intensity after-image which lasts for twenty minutes and more, thus allowing more time to test responses (Trotter and Stromberg, 1958).

(1) The flash technique has the disadvantage in that it is instantaneous. If the fixation of either eye wavers or is eccentric at the moment of flash, a diagnosis of ARC based upon a single report of the perceived relation of the horizontal and vertical after-images may be ambiguous or equivocal.

b. Parallel vertical after-image (Ronne and Rindziunski, 1953)

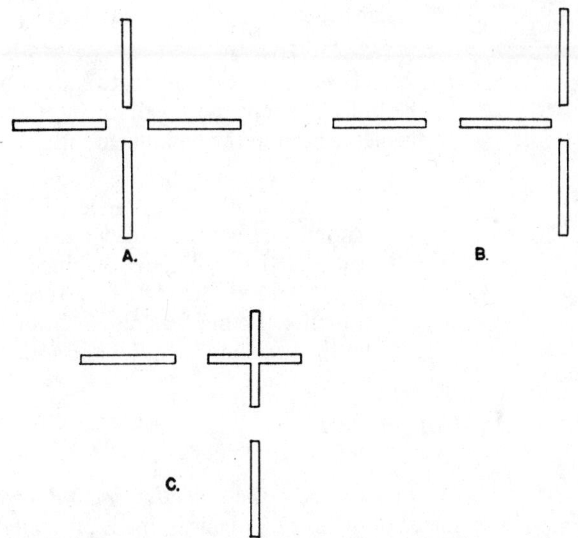

Figure XXX-7. After-Image Test. A. indicates projection of after-images where either normal correspondence or eccentric fixation exists. C. represents apparent cross when normal correspondence exists. B. represents anomalous correspondence, in a case of right constant exotropia, the vertical image being seen by the right eye, and the horizontal by the left eye; x measures the angle of anomaly. If x is greater than zero but less than the objective angle, the condition is unharmonious ARC; if it is equal to the objective angle, it is harmonious ARC.

(1) In this instance, instead of one horizontal and one vertical after-image, each eye has a vertical after-image impressed. It was found that many squinters who can perceive a perfect cross with horizontal-vertical after-images reported the two vertical lines separated by as much as 5 to 10 arc degrees.

(2) The authors suggest that this observation may have prognostic value in treating a given anomalous corresponder.

c. Prism-rack after-image test (Ronne and Rindziunski, 1953)

(1) After the two images are projected to the screen, a prism bar (prism rack) with horizontal prism is moved quickly to present increasing prismatic power before one of the patient's eyes. Some patients report a change in the separation of the projected after-images such that after-images originally separated (ARC) come partly or completely together during the movement of the prism bar.

(2) Since the "localization of the after-images on the retina is constant," these findings are explained on the basis of a "change in perception based on cortical process." The test is held to be especially valuable because "it can sometimes demonstrate that cases with which all other tests are obligatorily anomalous have some trace of normal correspondence."

d. It has been proposed by Ludlam (1967) that the after-image test be used to sample correspondence in the peripheral retina as well as at the macula as a prognostic aid in cases of ARC on the central after-image test.

(1) Additional fixation points at positions other than the center of the luminous bulb creating the after-image are provided.

(2) These are so located that fixation upon each of them in turn places the images of the bulb in a separate quadrant of the retina. It is important that they do not fall on the nerve head in the nasal quadrants.

(a) At an angular distance of 20° from the fovea, 10 of 24 esotropes exhibiting anomalous correspondence centrally on the after-image test reported a cross in each of the 4 oblique meridians measured (45°, 135°, 215°, and 315°), and in the 90° and the 270° meridians as well. A significantly higher incidence of functional cures was obtained for those patients not exhibiting an ARC response in the periphery than for those that did.

4. *Amblyoscope Test*

a. A comparison of the *objective and subjective angles* of deviation can be made by using a major amblyoscope. A vertical line is presented to one eye and a horizontal line to the other to attain an image similar to the after-image configurations. This is accomplished by neutralizing the movements made on alternate cover test. The *subjective angle* is determined by the position of the amblyoscope at which the cross is perceived.

(1) The subjective angle of directionalization, which this actually measures, is defined as the angular separation in subjective visual space between two diplopic images of a single object. The *angle of anomaly* is the difference between these two.

b. The advantage of this approach is its easy operation and the small amount of space taken up by the instrument.

c. Proximal convergence tends to reduce the values of exotropia measurements and increase the value of eso deviations over those measurements of the angle made in space.

(1) Since it affects both objective and subjective angles equally, however, the angle of anomaly is unaffected.

d. The position of a perceived cross (i.e., subjective angle) is not always found, since either suppression of one or the other eye may occur or a "jump" takes place at the cross-over point so that superimposition is not observed by the patient.

5. *Halldén's Test* (Halldén, 1952)

a. Halldén also used the after-image approach.

(1) A semi-circular annulus serves as a target for the after-image, while a spot or cross serves as the directly observed target.

b. Determination of the angle of anomaly (Figure XXX-8a).

(1) The target for the after-image is presented to the squinting eye.

(a) The after-image is projected to an aluminized screen at a known distance.

(2) By means of polarized filters, a spot of light (the measuring spot) is presented so that only the non-squinting eye perceives it.

(3) The patient is instructed to sight a fixation point on the screen, and to note when the measuring spot appears centered within the center of the after-image.

(4) The linear distance between the fixation point and the measuring spot on the screen (and the known distance of the screen from the eye) will denote the angle of anomaly.

(a) Usually a scale calculated for the test distance and denoting this angle is applied directly to the screen.

c. Determination of the Objective Angle (Figure XXX-8b).

(1) By rotating the polaroids, the measuring spot is now made visible only to the squinting eye.

(2) The test is repeated, and the distance between the fixation point and the measuring spot, again centered in the after-image, indicates the objective angle of squint.

d. Determination of the Subjective Angle (Figure XXX-8c).

(1) Instead of the previous fixation point, a projected cross, visible only to the non-squinting eye, is used for fixation. A projected spot, visible only to the squinting eye, is used as the measuring spot.

(2) The subject moves the measuring spot until it is centered directly in the cross.

(3) The distance between the measuring spot and the cross, on the screen, indicates the subjective angle of squint.

e. The Halldén Test provides a good laboratory method for determining the presence of ARC and the size of the objective and subjective angles and the angle of anomaly, but requires too much room for general clinical and office utilization.

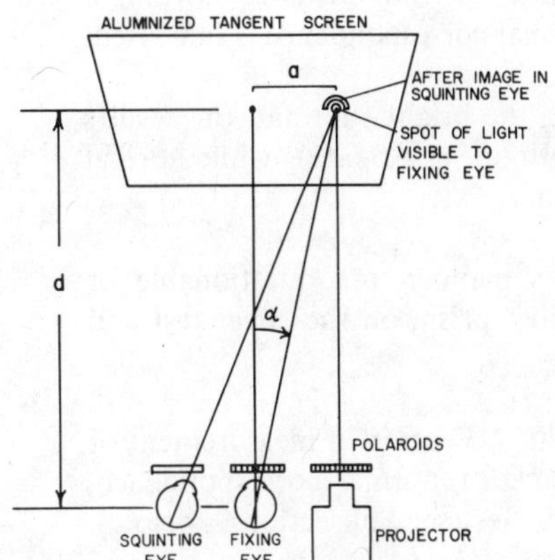

Figure XXX-8a. The projected spot of light is moved until the subject sees it in the center of the after-image; the distance *a* is a measure of the angle of anomaly *d* is the distance from the center of rotation of the two eyes, *L* is the angle of anomaly.

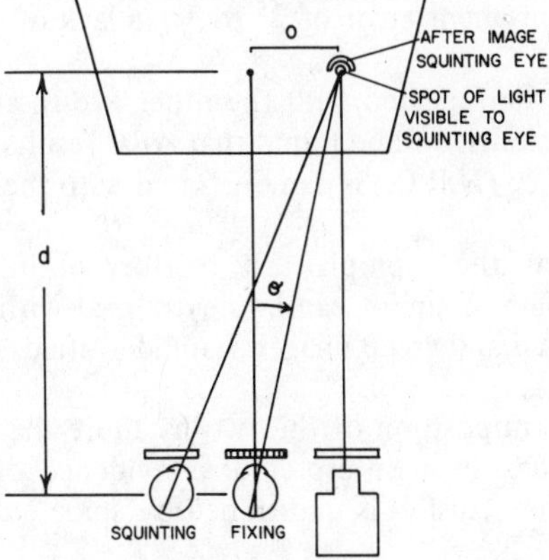

Figure XXX-8b. The projected spot of light is moved until the subject sees it in the center of the after-image; the distance *o* is a measure of the objective angle; σ is the objective angle; *d* is the distance from center of rotation of the eyes to the screen.

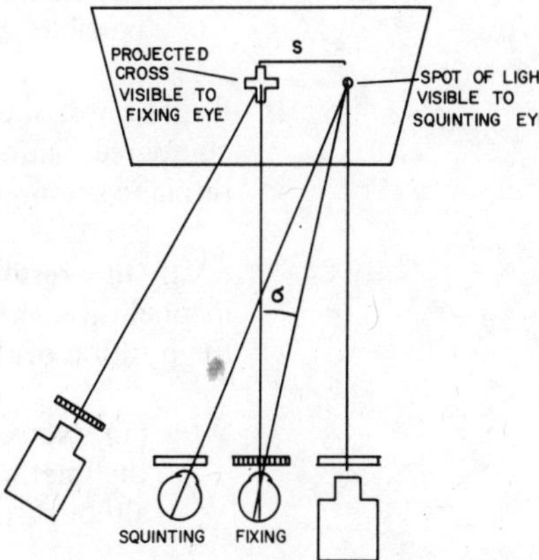

Figure XXX-8c. The projected spot of light is moved until the subject sees it in the center of the fixation-cross; the distance *s* is a measure of the subjective angle; σ is the subjective angle.

6. *Subjective Cover Test*

a. In the alternate cover test the subject with normal correspondence notices a movement of the fixated target as the uncovered deviating eye is exposed to the object of regard (the so-called Phi phenomenon). The direction of this movement should correspond to the direction and extent of the deviation, since the apparent movement results from stimulation of a series of retinal points while the eye moves to take up foveal fixation.

b. In anomalous correspondence this perceived movement either may not occur at all or is paradoxical, i.e., opposite to the expected direction.

(1) On some occasions, where constant unilateral strabismus exists, the Phi movement may be exhibited normally by the non-squinting eye upon re-fixation, and either be absent or paradoxical in nature when the squinting eye refixates.

(a) For young patients, this test is very difficult to interpret, and its use is therefore not ordinarily recommended for the preschool squinter.

7. *Diplopia Test*

a. The strabismic patient is required to view a single projected small bright spot in a dark room. A Worth 4 dot test target can also be used for fixation. If ARC is present or NRC with suppression, no diplopia is usually experienced.

b. Red-green anaglyph glasses are then worn by the patient and the patient again queried concerning diplopia. If none is present, loose prism is introduced base-down or base-up in amounts beginning at 10^{Δ} and increasing to 40^{Δ} if necessary.

c. Once the patient experiences diplopia, the direction and extent of diplopia separation are evaluated and compared with the size and direction of the angle measured on the cover test for the same distance.

(1) If the direction and amount of the diplopia does not agree with the angle as determined objectively by the cover test at the same fixation distance (within a possible measurement error of 2^{Δ} to 3^{Δ}), a lack of normal correspondence is indicated.

d. The test should be repeated with the other eye fixating the bright spot and the results compared. On occasion it will be found that ARC results with one eye fixating while normal retinal correspondence (N.R.C.) is demonstrated with the other.

e. If the results of the diplopia test, performed in this manner, are questionable or inconclusive, the angle of squint can be neutralized with loose prism on the cover test and the position of the red and green images again identified.

(1) Non-superimposition of the two by more than the 2-3^{Δ} error of measurement of the method has been interpreted as evidence of lack of normal correspondence, although this conclusion is questioned by some authorities (see Subsection 9, below).

8. *The Brock String Test*

a. This test is used to evaluate binocular correspondence at the near point. A string four feet long is fastened at one end, and is held along the midline firmly at the bridge of the nose. A fixation light is held at or within the centration point. The test is performed without red-green glasses unless deep suppression is evidenced at the near point. Answers indicating anomalous correspondence are:

(1) A single string down the midline, appearing as a mixture of red and green, with the fixation light split into red and green halves; or,

(2) The "inverted Y" where the string between the nose and the fixation light is seen split (NRC) but is perceived as single beyond the fixation light (ARC), thus forming the "Y."

9. *Bagolini-Čampobianco Striated Glass Test (Bagolini-Campobianco, 1965)*

a. This test makes use of plano lenses upon which tiny striations (.005 mm. in width) have been inscribed. These "leave the transparency of the glass and the visual acuity practically unaltered." A small fixation light viewed through these lenses "appears to be crossed by a weak luminous ray oriented perpendicularly to the striations on the glass," an effect quite similar to that produced by the well known Maddox groove. The lenses are oriented before each eye of the patient so that the axes of striations are: O.D., 45°; and O.S., 135°. The test is performed both at distance (20 feet) and at near (13 inches).

(1) The patient may experience suppression of one eye or the other, in which case only one oblique line corresponding to that seen by the non-suppressing eye is visualized.

(2) If the patient perceives the two oblique lines crossing at the fixated light, he has either harmonious ARC or NRC depending on whether a cover test shows him to be at that moment strabismic.

(3) The test, by avoiding dissociation, permits an investigation of correspondence under relatively normal visual conditions.

b. Its chief disadvantage according to Von Noorden and Maumenee (1967) is that it cannot be used to make a diagnosis of unharmonious anomalous retinal correspondence, and the quantitative determination with it of the angle of anomaly is difficult.

(1) Flom considers this an unwarranted criticism and points out that the test actually measures the subjective angle. By comparing this subjective angle with the angle of deviation, the angle of anomaly is determined, just as with the amblyoscope.

10. Opinion has been expressed that the employment of different tests, and the extent of agreement among them might indicate the "depth" of the anomaly (Burian, 1947), or some variant be disclosed in the condition which would provide a treatment opportunity by some special test or treatment approach. Flom and Kerr (1967) evaluated this concept by utilizing five different test approaches upon a number of subjects. They concluded:

a. Measurement errors and unsteady eccentric fixation account for a large proportion of diagnostic disagreement of the five different tests for retinal correspondence used.

(1) The measurement of the angle of anomaly includes random error which is a function of the particular test and reflects the naivete or sophistication of the patient.

(2) Unsteady fixation is a common and added source of error.

b. The regular range of measurement error is on the order of $\pm 3^{\nabla}$.

(1) A larger than average measurement error may appear to indicate anomalous correspondence even when normal correspondence exists.

(2) If the true angle of anomaly is small or zero, the combination of errors may lead to a misdiagnosis.

c. A change in the relative position of the two eyes also introduces disagreement for different tests.

(1) If the eyes change from a squint in one test to binocular fixation in another, a judgment of anomalous correspondence in the first and normal correspondence in the second may be made.

(a) ARC may be latent in periodic squints when binocular fixation occurs.

(2) Changes in the angle of squint between two measurements may lead to a conclusion of ARC.

d. Of a total sample of 93 subjects, only 17 showed ARC on all tests and 16 showed NRC on all tests. Thus, 60 subjects showed diagnostic disagreement among the the battery of five tests administered. From this it can be inferred that the diagnosis of ARC in a given strabismus patient is most difficult. Flom and Kerr have detailed many of the reasons why this is so.

e. Since the final results of treating the 93 patients were not reported nor related to the number of tests in which ARC was found, no conclusion can be drawn as to the relative difficulty of treating the patient with the largest number of tests indicating ARC or those showing wide diagnostic disagreement. Thus, the "depth of anomaly" principle which relates the number of tests which show ARC responses to the difficulty in treatment, while brought under serious question, has not yet been disproved.

D. Binocularity at the Centration Point

1. This test is necessary only for constant esotropes since hypertropes and constant exotropes have no centration point and intermittent esotropes and exotropes have at least occasional fusion.

2. The centration point has been defined earlier as the physical point in space at which the visual axes cross. A penlight may be held at this point, and bi-fixation behavior of the two foveas may be tested in space, and the presence of diplopia investigated.

a. If none is reported, the light is moved in and out along the patient's midline while the clinician searches for any fixation or binocular tracking behavior on the part of the patient.

3. If suppression of one eye is demonstrated, the red green glasses test for "luster" should be attempted. A very unusual response is an "avoidance" reaction where the eyes actively avoid bifixation, usually by turning farther inwards.

4. If no tracking response can be demonstrated, a 5^{Δ} loose prism, base-out, is introduced before either eye and a diplopia and fusion recovery response is solicited.

a. A demonstration of a positive movement to attain fusion is a good prognostic sign.

E. Physiological Diplopia (Simultaneous Perception Without Superimposition)

1. A second (extra-horopteral) light at some greater distance (3-4 feet) than the light at the centration point is added to the test situation. While the strabismic continues to observe the light at the centration point, he is queried as to the presence of a double light (homonymous or uncrossed diplopia) at the further distance.

a. If no response is obtained, red-green glasses, and then if necessary, prism, can be used to bring about the physiological diplopia response at both distance and near.

b. Hopefully, single fused imagery of the fixation light with a double percept of the distant non-fixated light, may finally be attained, and even fusion of the distant light attempted.

F. Range and Quality of Fusion

1. Worth (Chavasse, 1939) proposed what he felt were the three graded or ordered states of the development of binocular vision as:

a. *First degree* or simultaneous binocular perception
b. *Second degree* or flat fusion with range
c. *Third degree* or stereopsis

2. The order as presented by Worth is not necessarily the hierarchical steps of natural development in normal individuals and is definitely not the order in which strabismics undergoing training acquire binocular skills most easily.

3. In part D of this section, testing of binocularity at the centration point, the evaluation was made of simultaneous binocular perception at a very special point in space. This function, as well as the two "higher" levels can also be measured in various instruments such as the stereoscope, amblyoscope and cheiroscope. All of these instruments have in common the separation of the two visual fields by a septum or tubes so that the targets presented before each eye may be manipulated independently.

a. To *evaluate first degree fusion* or *simultaneous macular perception* with an instrument, two dissimilar targets are placed in the instrument set at the objective angle of squint. The strabismic is asked to attempt to perceive both superimposed, i.e., to perceive the two targets in a single egocentric direction. Many stereoscope targets such as the ball and hoop, cat and fence, etc., are designed to both ascertain and develop this faculty. Flashing, blinking, oscillating the target and changing the relative levels of illumination before the two eyes is often helpful in bringing about this result.

b. Simultaneous perception targets which, when superimposed, have no crossing borders, such as a small square within a circle, or the hands superimposed on a clock face, are much more amenable to being perceived simultaneously by a suppressing strabismic than targets with overlapping lines or crossing contours, such as a lion in a cage or a baby in a crib with bars.

c. The anomalous projector or the sufferer from horror fusionis will reject or fail to demonstrate even this faculty. In severe cases of suppression, the presence of two macular targets will also induce suppression. Even simpler targets designed to merely elicit simultaneous macular perception are sometimes necessary, such as two differently colored circles or squares presenting colored backgrounds without perceptual details.

4. *Second Degree or Flat fusion* is the ability to fuse identical targets presented to each eye, (a condition normally encountered at very large viewing distances compared to the interpupillary distance). The targets are identical except for non-fusible areas called controls which are used to differentiate fusion from suppression. In targets of better design there are several sets of controls; larger and smaller, nearer and further from the fusible targets and situated in different meridians.

a. *Initial fusion* responses by a strabismic at the objective angle in an instrument often will be accompanied by suppression of some but not all of the controls.

b. *Fusion range* or amplitude of motor fusion is the extent of convergence or divergence which the patient can or will exert in order to maintain fusion. This measurement has traditionally been made in instruments such as an amblyoscope or stereoscope.

c. In testing for the extent of suppression, the actual size and extent of the suppression area can be charted by a binocular field testing device similar to the technique used to graph a central pathological scotoma. The severity of the suppression may not, however, be reflected in the physical dimensions. Testing may be performed in a stereoscope by the presentation of targets passing gradually through the various degrees of fusion from stereopsis down. Most squinters will reveal some element of first degree fusion, dependent upon how different the targets are. An important objective is to determine some stage at which simultaneous perception can be elicited from both maculae. Variations in color, intensity of illumination, and even some displacement of the target in the suppression area may be required to elicit any response, as may intermittent or so-called flash presentation of the targets. Motion of the targets is also frequently used. The farther from the normal presentation of identical targets exposed under identical conditions the examiner must proceed to elicit simultaneous vision, the more absolute is the suppression.

d. *The Javal grid* is a useful device for demonstrating the existence of suppression at near point. It consists of several vertical bars placed so that portions of a printed page are exclusively obstructed for each eye. As the patient is requested to read the page, certain portions will be occluded from the habitually fixing eye. If the patient can read across the page, without moving his head, the other eye must have been used. Javal also found this device useful in breaking up suppressions during training.

5. *Third Degree Fusion or Stereopsis*

a. Since the two eyes do not view objects from the same viewing point, the retinal images differ slightly and these discrepancies serve as binocular cues to that perception of depth known as stereopsis.

b. This appreciation of stereoparallax is only one of the many cues to depth perception and in general one of the less important (especially at distances beyond arms length). However, stereoparallax can be introduced in drawings or photographs, and if its magnitude does not exceed the limits of fusion dictated by Panum's areas, the single percept obtained by the normal binocular observer will be perceived as tri-dimensional and appear to have depth or solidity. Because stereopsis can only be achieved in binocular vision and can be readily isolated from all the other monocular and binocular cues to depth, it is useful in training.

c. The targets traditionally employed in testing stereopsis have been divided into three classes relating to the size of the retinal area on which they are imaged:

(1) Macular
(2) Peri-macular
(3) Peripheral

d. *Testing of stereopsis* can be conducted both by using instruments such as the stereoscope or its derivations, and also in space using the dissociation provided by anaglyphic (such as polaroid) glasses. Evaluation of macular and perimacular stereopsis is usually performed at high levels of illumination in instruments, while the peripheral response, prevented by the small field of view allowed by most instrumentation, is tested in space. By moving the targets or parts of the targets in such manner as to increase the horizontal retinal image disparity angle, the apparent depth or relief is increased. This is most easily accomplished with polaroid or other anaglyphic techniques. In addition to perceived change in stereopsis, two other effects are found to be concomitant. These are:

(1) *Apparent size changes,* the so-called SILO (small in – large out) effect.

(a) The part of the stereo figure which appears to move closer appears to become smaller and that which recedes becomes larger.

(b) Wheatstone first described the SILO effect in 1852. In effect, it is similar to the changes in the projected after-image as the surface to which the image is projected is brought closer to the eye.

(c) Alpern (1962) offers an explanation of the effect which is summarized below:

[1] A change in the perceived size of objects relative to the retinal image size appears to produce a change in the stimulus for proximal convergence.

[a] "Proximal effects are a manifestation of a facilitation of fusional convergence induced by an awareness of nearness."

[b] "Proximal convergence is larger when the limit of positive fusional convergence is used as a criterion than when the limit of negative fusional convergence is used."

[2] Since changes in vergence are produced by size changes, an increase in convergence is continuously associated with a reduction of perceived image-size in the operation of size-constancy. By the constant association, the size constancy changes are firmly established (Liebowitz and Hartman, 1959), so that the presence of either process by itself serves as a stimulus for the elicitation of the other.

[3] Thus, "size changes induce vergence movements, and vergence movements are effective stimuli to induce size changes."

(2) *Paradoxical Parallax*

(a) Ordinarily, when an observer's head is shifted laterally, objects closer to him appear to move opposite (an "against" movement) to the direction of more distant objects.

[1] In the case of the variable stereo targets presented by anaglyphic methods the parallax effect observed is opposite to that just described. The nearer target is perceived by the subject to move "with" his lateral head movement while the more distant parts move "against" it.

[2] These additional phenomena may be used to help ensure the validity of the patient's stereo responses.

(b) Whether the measurements are performed in space or in instruments, control marks are usually employed to differentiate the trouble frequently encountered by the patient in manifesting stereoscopic awareness from that dictated by the presence of suppression. (See Figure XXX-9.)

[1] If the two figures are viewed either in a stereoscope or with convergence relaxed, and fusion occurs with a binocular observer, the circle is seen to "float" out in space at a perceived distance closer to the observer than the square. Even though each of the individual targets has the circle displaced nasally with respect to the center of the square, in the fused percept the floating circle is seen "centered" in the square background.

[2] It is important to confirm that this occurs while testing the strabismic patient's stereo response.

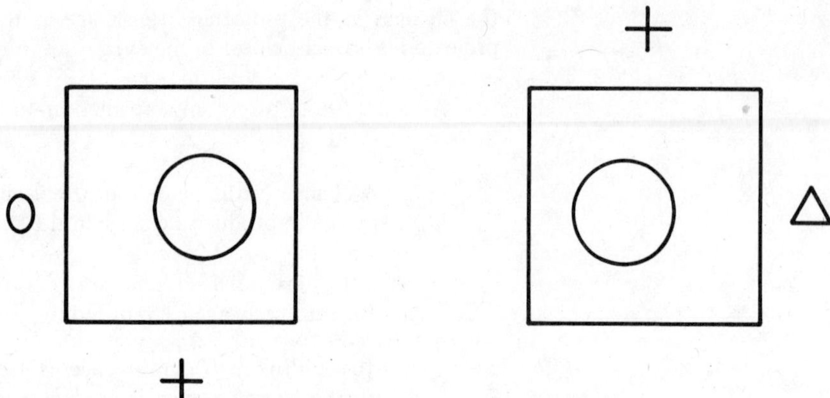

Figure XXX-9. A stereoscopic target with controls in both horizontal and vertical meridians.

(c) The means of testing for suppression or the state of fusion are also the means for improving and training quality of fusion. While the test procedure commonly begins at stereopsis and descends to the level manifested, the training procedure moves in a reverse direction with a target demanding constantly higher ability, as each successive one is mastered.

e. Julesz (1964 and 1968) utilized computer designed "random dot stereo-graphs" in which all the apparent monocular cues to depth had been eliminated, and which exhibited no shapes or contours when viewed with one eye but yielded predetermined shapes when seen with both eyes. These have been found to be useful in testing and training the faulty binocular apparatus in strabismus.

G. Binocular Field of Gaze (Comitancy of Deviation)

1. Once binocular function at a centration point (with the help of plus lenses or prism if need be) has been established along the midline, the lateral and vertical ranges of binocularity are tested.

a. The examiner's light is moved slowly from side to side, obliquely and then vertically to the six cardinal positions of gaze. Any departure of the centered corneal reflexes observed by the examiner or report of diplopia by the patient is recorded.

2. Limitations of gaze found in this testing procedure may not necessarily be due to innervational deficiencies. Other causes, such as fibrosis, orbital tumors, gaze palsies, and muscle malinsertion, as well as cheek ligament changes secondary to a long standing strabismus may also limit them. As will be discussed in the next chapter, ocular calisthenic exercises are frequently of help in reducing such limitations or incomitancies as may be due to the latter.

H. Binocular Accommodative Rock

1. The speed, amplitude and quality of the binocular accommodative facility may be evaluated by this procedure. Before employing this binocular test it is expected that speed, amplitude and quality of the monocular accommodative rock in each eye will have been found to be normal or trained to be so, and that the performance for each eye will be about equal. In order to have a truly valid evaluation of binocular accommodative rock (such as also holds in testing for NRA and PRA), the subject must have functional binocularity at the centration point or range and the test must be conducted at this point or range.

2. Using the same procedure as described for monocular rock testing, the patient is asked to clear the blurred targets as rapidly as he is able and in addition to report any diplopia. The examiner watches the patient's eyes to ascertain the continuation of bi-fixation throughout the test sequence. If the lenses through which clear vision was attained during monocular testing cannot be cleared during the binocular tests, the power is reduced until clear vision can be secured binocularly.

I. The AC/A Ratio in Strabismus

1. As mentioned earlier in this chapter, an abnormal relationship between accommodation and convergence is held to be a major cause of concomitant strabismus. Proper handling of the interaction of convergence and accommodation can constitute one of the major aids in achieving alignment of the visual axes and functional binocularity in concomitant strabismus. Thus, it is important that we be able to evaluate the status of the vergence-accommodation synkinesis, the so-called AC/A ratio. The ratio is the amount of change in vergence per unit change in accommodation and can usually be determined in one of two ways:

2. *Gradient*

a. *In space*

(1) The strabismic, with the ametropia corrected, is directed to fixate a target at, e.g., ½ meter. The target should have sufficient detail to serve as an effective accommodative stimulus (20/25 letter).

(2) A prism which neutralizes the patient's squint is applied during the alternate cover test.

(3) The power of the lens used to determine the gradient should be large enough to minimize the effect of measurement error on the determined ratio, and yet should fall within the habitual accommodative range.

(4) The cover test is then repeated after each change of the stimulus to accommodation.

(a) If the detail of the target is blurred, the range of accommodative response has been exceeded and lesser power is required for the test.

(5) The prism diopter difference between the cover test measurements is then divided by the dioptric value of the range of accommodative stimuli to yield the AC/A ratio.

(6) This approach has the advantage of minimum calculation with no necessity of inclusion of interpupillary distance measurements. It also provides a check on linearity of the accommodative response for both stimulation and relaxation of accommodation.

(7) The disadvantages are that the cover test neutralization point must usually be made through two pairs of glasses, i.e., the patient's own and the test lenses, and that it requires the performance and recording of the results of cover tests at 3 different distances.

b. *In instruments*

(1) The same test can be performed admirably in a major amblyoscope.

(2) The initial test is performed with the patient viewing slides containing

accommodative targets and –2.00 D. spheres in the amblyoscope's lens cells. Again the patient is urged to clear the detail for each set of lenses introduced.

(3) A "cover" test is performed by alternately blanking the illumination and changing the angle between the tubes until no motion occurs at the alternate blanking.

(a) Stimulus lens pairs of –0.50 D. and –3.50 D. power are then successively placed in the lens cells and the objective angle established for each.

(b) The difference in angles measured is again divided by 3.00 D. to give the AC/A ratio.

(c) An illustrative example would be:

[1] **Table XXX-2**

Added Lens Power	Angle of Deviation
–2.00 D.	32^{Δ} Base out
–0.50 D.	25^{Δ} Base out
–3.50 D.	43^{Δ} Base out

[2] The difference for the extreme ends of the range is $43^{\Delta} - 25^{\Delta} = 18^{\Delta}$ which divided by the accommodative stimulus range of 3D yields an AC/A ratio of 6/1.

[3] It should be noted, as is frequently the case, that the measured angle of deviation changes less for the relaxed accommodation (7^{Δ}) than for the stimulated condition (11^{Δ}).

3. *Change in Strabismus Angle – Different Distances*

a. In this method, the AC/A ratio in strabismus (or the heterophoria) is determined by measuring the change in the angle of deviation occurring between distance and near fixation. Again central fixation is prerequisite to the test's validity and the patient should be encouraged to respond to the changed stimulus condition by clearing the target detail. Cover Test measurement is made and recorded for fixation at 6 M and 1/3 M. The use of these distances also provides a 3.00 D. stimulus to accommodation. Since different test distances have been employed, the patient's P.D. now becomes a factor and must be considered.

b. Flom (1963) has presented a calculation which can be performed mentally during clinical procedure. His method is as follows:

(1) $PD + w\,(tn - tf) = ACA$.

(a) P.D. = patient's interpupillary distance in centimeters; w = near working distance in meters; tf = far cover test angle in $^{\Delta}$; tn = near cover test angle in $^{\Delta}$.

(2) Thus, an esotrope with P.D. of 65 mm., a 30^{∇} tropia at 6 meters, and a 45^{∇} tropia at 33 cms., will have the following ACA ratio:

(a) $6.5 + .33\,(45 - 30) = 11.5$.

4. On occasion, for either method, an obvious difference in angle will result depending upon which eye is fixating at a given moment. Such a difference could result from an inequality of accommodative response in the two eyes and can be evaluated by using the cover-uncover test successively on each eye. The unequal accommodative response could result from an unequal or

incomplete correction of the refractive error, which should be rechecked, or a true difference in accommodative response such as occurs in amblyopia cases, or merely be an indication of the existence of non-comitant strabismus.

V. PERCEPTUAL MOTOR AND INTERSENSORY TESTING IN STRABISMUS

A. As noted in the concluding section of the previous chapter, concepts have been offered relating the role played by vision as a primary source of sensory information and the motor and perceptual development of the individual. These not only relate faulty development of the latter with possible causation of the ocular anomaly, but also postulate that the interference with the normal bi-lateral visual input caused by strabismus and the attempts of the strabismic to produce harmony and unity in the visual percept of his surround should influence the motor and perceptual development of a child afflicted with strabismus. Such interference should be demonstrable and subject to attempts at evaluation.

B. One such assay consists of requiring the subject to perform an unstructured task involving bi-manual and bi-visual operation, and noting the general facility or quality of performance demonstrated, the type of visual monitoring used during the performance, and the nature of any postural shifts of the body made in carrying out the task.

1. One corollary assumption is that the better the quality of performance with the eye in the strabismic position, the poorer the prognosis, assuming that the better the task is performed, the more apparent harmony of perceptual approach the subject has achieved and the less the requirement for alteration in the existing established environmental adaptation. That this is necessarily so – i.e., that the prognosis is poorer where greater facility is exhibited by a strabismic – has not been accepted by all authorities, and publication of explicit evidence demonstrating the premise is yet awaited.

C. Perceptual Motor Testing In Strabismus

1. *Laterality and Directionality*

a. Problems in the awareness of right and left and in the development of a right-left gradient by which "concepts of the coordinates of space" are developed may be revealed by a series of tests.

b. The ability to "cross the midline" has been assumed (Kephart, 1958) to be related to the development of bilaterality (the awareness, use, and integration of both sides of the body). Opinion has been expressed that the development of binocularity is dependent upon, and should be preceded by, adequate development of bilaterality, and, that strabismus could be presumed to be among the results of mal-development or inadequate consummation of bilaterality.

c. In testing children with learning problems, a battery of tests are used to evaluate these above concepts, but for strabismus, two may suffice.

(1) *Drawing a circle with one hand*

(a) The patient is requested to draw a circle on the chalkboard.

(b) Factors noted are:

[1] The hand used; the size of the circle; and the likeness to a circle.

[2] The placement of the circle in respect to the patient's midline; and the tendency, if present, to move the body back and forth to avoid crossing the midline.

[3] Steadiness of motor control; and the use of vision to control the act.

(c) Roach and Kephart(1966) have rated the performance of this test in four categories, from best to worst, as follows:

[1] The circle is drawn in proper size, direction, position and shape.

[a] One added instruction to achieve size and position is permitted.

[2] A circle nearly correct in size, position and shape is achieved after two or three tries.

[a] The drawing must have crossed the midline, must attain the proper size, and must exhibit only minor errors in shape.

[3] An acceptable drawing is exhibited, but only with effort and marked difficulty. Also, the direction of drawing, if otherwise readily accomplished, is wrong for the subject's preferred hand.

[4] A circle of proper size, shape, and location cannot be produced; or, the midline cannot be crossed during drawing, and is avoided; or, confusion is displayed as to proper direction; or, the drawing exhibits distortion, especially a flat side to either side or the bottom.

(d) Where strabismus is present, the performance is frequently characterized by a circle drawn to one side of the midline, by head turning, and by "walking" with the circle.

[1] Upon completion of the task in this unstructured manner, the drawing is repeated around a dot placed on the board by the examiner at the subject's midline. The subject uses the other hand this time and keeps the feet still.

[2] The performances are compared, and a shift to bring the fixating eye in line with the midline is noted.

(2) *Drawing two circles simultaneously with both hands*

(a) The subject is required to take chalk in each hand and draw two circles at the same time.

(b) Factors noted include:

[1] Position of the drawings relative to each other and the subject; the relative sizes, and the degree to which each is circular.

[2] Direction of movement of the two hands, and the ability of moving both together at the same rate (synchrony, and steadiness of motor control).

[3] The use of vision to guide the hands.

(c) The performances of this task have likewise been rated from best to worst by Roach and Kephart (1966):

[1] Performance is smooth and certain.

[a] One additional directive is permitted to achieve size and position.

[2] Two or three trials are required to achieve the necessary production; or, the performance is halting or stiff.

[3] Extreme difficulty is exhibited at any part of the performance; or, the direction of the drawing is incorrect; or, the performance is not acceptable despite two or three trials.

[4] The task cannot be performed; or, drawings of acceptable size, shape and position are not attained; or, one hand only is attended to; or, the circles are distorted (flat) towards the center.

(3) The Roach-Kephart rating scale was established to grade subjects for performance in terms of school learning disability. In strabismus testing, some clinicians have noted that the better the performance with the eye in the strabismic position, the poorer the outlook for recovery of functional binocularity according to premises stated earlier; the reader is again cautioned that authorities are in disagreement with such hypotheses, and verification and evidence are still awaited.

(a) Strabismic patients often find it difficult to monitor two simultaneous motor tasks visually. The unilateral fixator will usually center attention upon the hand homolateral to the fixing eye, withdrawing visual attention from the other, and the circles drawn will often reflect this in size and shape difference.

[1] It should be pointed out that difficulty in monitoring two simultaneous motor tasks visually is not necessarily confined to strabismics, since many non-squinters also exhibit such difficulty. Whether this bears a relation in these cases to efficiency of binocular performance and coordination is not established.

[2] Similarly, all authorities are not in agreement that the difference in size and shape of the two circles need reflect only a visual preference. It is conjectured that the squinter (and non-squinter having trouble with dual monitoring) may essentially demonstrate a better drawing when performed by his "dominant" hand, and that this, most likely his writing hand, would perform more skillfully than the other in any case, even if both eyes were shut, or if each circle were drawn separately with full visual attention upon each.

(b) Alternators tend to shift attention from one hand to the other, losing synchrony.

[1] Tell-tale head movements and completion of one circle before the other are exhibited.

(c) Total avoidance of visual control, such as gazing away entirely or at a neutral point, is a more rarely exhibited response.

2. *Balance*

a. It is assumed that the demonstration of relative skill of balance indicates the extent of integration of the total body parts, and the association of the accustomed visual pattern, constituting one of the essentials of integration, would thereby be influential in the acquisition and development of balance. Some inkling of the strabismic integration might be revealed, therefore, by tests of balance.

(1) A 2″ x 4″ beam, twelve feet long is supported 4″ above the floor.

(2) The subject is required to walk forward and backward on the beam.

(a) The test is repeated with:

[1] The deviating eye closed

[2] Both eyes closed

[3] A prism before the deviating eye of the amount which neutralized the "flick" during the cover test

[4] Red-green glasses before the eyes

(b) The degree of visual component employed is judged by comparing these, and by noting how much anticipatory toe-exploration is performed before each step.

[1] The prognosis is assumed to be better (for reasons previously conjectured in other tests):

[a] The less vision employed for performance

[b] The more the perturbing factors (prism, occlusion, etc.) demean the performance

[c] The poorer the unhampered performance as revealed by balance, pauses, stepping off, unsteadiness, maintaining a dynamic body skew, head turn, etc.

D. Perturbation of the Strabismic Perceptual Adaptation

1. Although the state of testing gross motor and perceptual motor relationships in strabismus is not formalized and advanced, the following constitute some clinically derived rules of thumb and suggested techniques:

a. An essential proposition is "The better the patient performs with both eyes open in the strabismic posture, the more difficult it usually is to treat and 'cure' the condition."

(1) As noted earlier, this proposition is not accepted by all in the field of strabismus, and Flom, for one (personal communication, 1969), challenges it until evidence substantiating it is available.

2. Among the examples which explore the relationship are the following:

a. The patient is requested to stand on one leg and lean sideways while binocularity is evaluated.

(1) The patient is sometimes found to exhibit diplopia, luster, or even fusion in this position as compared to the alternation or suppression revealed when ordinarily standing or sitting; this is based upon the following postulates:

(a) It is assumed that some disorientation is created by the unsteadiness, and this may require increased attention to balancing and postural reflexes, which cannot be handled effectively at the sub-cortical level under the changed conditions.

(b) The changed stimulus to the vestibular mechanisms may also cause a counter-rolling reflex and thus possibly reduce the existing oculo-motor feedback supporting the anomalous strabismus adaptation.

(c) The fear of falling might bring about a change in the habitual angle of deviation, thereby altering the conditions under which the suppression was learned.

(d) In accordance with the first proposition, the more rapid and complete the breakdown of the strabismus perceptual adaptations, the better the prognosis.

(2) The patient is seated upon a swivel stool which is rotated rapidly several times until the patient is slightly dizzy.

(a) Frequently, a spontaneous breakdown of alternating or uniocular suppression takes place. Diplopia, which disappears as the dizziness does, may be reported.

(b) The rationale is similar to that offered for leaning plus the added influence of acceleration nystagmus.

(3) A child patient may be required to peer between his legs at a target.

(a) The inverted position may result in the disappearance of suppression, and is particularly likely if prism or red-green lenses are placed before the eyes during the test. (The introduction of the same devices while the subject is upright does not produce the same breakdown of strabismic perception.)

(b) While the same vestibular influences affecting the other tests apply here, Flom (personal communication, 1969) suggests that in some instances the result might be evidence of non-comitancy and the influence of a greater angle of deviation exhibited when the gaze is directed "up" between the legs.

E. Tests Applying to Paralytic Strabismus

1. Other tests, such as those measuring the deviation in different fields of view, the primary and secondary deviations, localization tests, and others of similar portent, intimately concerned with the differentiation of paralytic from concomitant strabismus, are discussed in the next chapter, XXXI, Paralytic Strabismus.

REFERENCES
Adler, F. (1945): Pathologic Physiology of Convergent Strabismus. Arch. Oph., 33
Adler, F. (1953): Pathologic Physiology of Strabismus, Arch. Oph., 50: 1.
Adler, F. (1965): Physiology Of The Eye With Clinical Applications, Mosby & Sons, St. Louis.
Alpern, M. (1962): Movement Of The Eye; in Davson: The Eye, vol. 3; Academic Press, N.Y., 3.
Bagolini, B. and Capobianco, N. (1965): Subjective Space in Comitant Squint. A. J. Oph., 59
Bielschowsky, A. (1937): Application of the After-Image Test in the Investigation of Squint. Arch. Oph., 17: 3
Bielschowsky, A. (1949): Lectures on Motor Anomalies, Dartmouth College, Hanover.
Brock, F. and Givner, I. (1952): Fixation Anomalies in Amblyopia. Arch. Oph., 47
Brock, F. (1953): Visual Training Part II. Opt. Weekly.
Brock, F. (1958): Visual Training, XXX, Part III, The Problems Pertaining to the Loss of Binocular Vision. Opt. Weekly, 47.

REFERENCES

*Adler, F. (1945): Pathologic Physiology of Convergent Strabismus. Arch. Oph., 33: 362.

*Adler, F. (1953): Pathology of Strabismus, Arch. Oph., 50: 19.

Adler, F. (1965): Physiology Of The Eye With Clinical Applications, Mosby & Sons, St. Louis.

Adler, F.H. & Jackson, F.E. (1947): Correlation Between Sensory and Motor Disturbance in Convergent Squint. Arch. Oph., 38: 289.

Alpern, M. (1962): Movement Of The Eye; in Davson: The Eye, Vol. 3; Academic Press, N.Y., 3.

Bagolini, B. and Capobianco, N. (1965): Subjective Space in Comitant Squint. A.J. Oph., 59: 430.

Bielschowsky, A. (1937): Application of the After-Image Test in the Investigation of Squint. Arch. Oph., 17: 408.

*Bielschowsky, A. (1949): Lectures on Motor Anomalies, Dartmouth College, Hanover.

*Brock, F. and Givner, I. (1952): Fixation Anomalies in Amblyopia. Arch. Oph., 47: 775.

Brock, F. (1952): Visual Training Part II. Opt. Weekly. 43: 191, 237, 1641, 1683.

*Brock, F. (1955): Visual Training, Part III, The Problems Pertaining to the Loss of Binocular Vision. Opt. Weekly. 46: 557, 763, 895, 1139, 1321, 1601, 1979.

Brock, F. (1962): A Clinical Measure of Fixation Disparities. J.A.O.A., 33: 497.

*Duane, A. (1919): The Basic Principles of Diagnosis in Motor Anomalies of the Eye. Arch. Oph., 48: 1.

*Duke-Elder, W. (1949): Text Book of Ophthalmology. Vol. IV. C.V. Mosby, St. Louis.

*Emsley, H. (1948): Visual Optics. Hatton Press, London.

*Flax, N. (1963): Prism Saccadic Training. Optical Journal and Review of Optometry, Vol. 100; (9): 31.

Flom, M. (1954): Strabismus and Orthoptics Study, a preliminary report (unpublished, prepared for the Research Projects Committee of the American Academy of Optometry.

Flom, M.C. (1956): A Minimum Strabismus Examination. J.A.O.A., 27: 11.

Flom, M.C. (1958): The Prognosis in Strabismus, A.A.A.O., 36: 509.

Flom, M.C. (1963): Treatment of Binocular Anomalies of Children, Vision of Children, ed. by M. Hirsch and R. Wick, Chilton Books, Phila.

Flom, M.C. and Kerr, K.E. (1967): Determination of Retinal Correspondence. Arch. Oph., 77: 200.

Flom, M. and Weymouth, F. (1961): Centricity of Maxwell's Spot in Strabismus and Amblyopia. Arch. Oph., 66: 260.

Forster, H.W., Jr. (1954): The Clinical Use of the Haidinger's Brushes Phenomena. A.J. Oph., 38: 161.

Goldschmidt, M. (1950): A New Test for the Function of the Macula. Lut., Arch. Oph., 44: 129.

Hallden, U. (1952): Fusional Phenomena in Anomalous Correspondence. Copenhagen Acta Ophthalmologica, Supp. 37.

Hess, W. (1908): Ein neue Untersuchungs methode bei Doppelbidern. Arch. Augenheilk, 62: 233.

*Hirschberg, J. (1881): On the Quantitative Analysis of Diplopic Strabismus. Med. J., 1: 5.

*Javal, E. (1896): Manuel Theorique et Proctique de Strabisme. Paris, Masson & Co.

Julesz, B. (1964): Binocular Depth Perception Without Familiarity Cues. Science, 145: (3630) 356.

Julesz, B. (1968): Experiment in Perception. Psychology Today, 2: 16.

Kephart, N.C. (1958): Visual Behavior of the Retarded Child, A.A.A.O., 35: 125.

Krimsky, E. (1943): The Fixational Corneal Light Reflexes as an Aid in Binocular Investigation. Trans. Amer. Acad. Oph., 47: 269.

Lancaster, W. (1939): Detecting, Measuring, Plotting and Interpreting Ocular Deviations. Trans. Sect. Oph., A.M.A. 22: 867.

Liebowitz, H. and Hartman, T. (1959): Magnitude of the Moon Illusion as a Function of the Eye of the Observer. Science, 130: 569.

Ludlam, W. (1967): A New Clinical Approach to Anomalous Correspondence. Paper read before the Section on Binocular Vision and Perception (Dec. 12, 1967), American Academy of Optometry Meeting, Chicago, Ill.

Ludlam, W. (in preparation): Clinical Techniques for Strabismus Training. Professional Press, Chicago.

Ludlam, W. and Kleinman, B. (1965): Long Range Results of Orthoptic Treatment of Strabismus. A.A.A.O., 42: 647.

Ludvigh, E. (1949): Amount of Eye Movement Objectively Perceptible to the Unaided Eye. A.J. Oph., 32: 659.

*Maddox, E. (1907): Tests and Studies of the Ocular Muscles. Keystone Pub. Co., Philadelphia.

Morgan, M. (1948): Methods Used in the Treatment of Squint. A.A.A.O., 25: 57.

Morgan, M. (1963): Anomalies of Binocular Vision, in Vision of Children, edited by Monroe Hirsch & Ralph Wick, Philadelphia, Chilton Books.

*Roach, E. and Kephart, N. (1966): The Purdue Perceptual – Motor Survey. Charles Merrill, Columbus, Ohio.

Ronne, G. and Rindziunski, E. (1953): The Diagnosis and Clinical Classification of Anomalous Correspondence. Acta Ophthalmologica, 31: 321.

Schlossman, A. and Boruchoff, S. (1955): Correction Between Physiologic and Clinical Aspects of Exotropia. A.J. Oph., 40: 53.

Scobee, R. (1951): Esotropia. A.J. Oph., 34: 817.

Scobee, R. (1952): The Oculatory Muscles. 2nd ed., C.V. Mosby, St. Louis.

Sloan, L.L. & Naquin, H.A. (1955): A Quantitative Test for Determining the Visibility of the Haidinger Brush: Clinical Application. A.J. Oph., 40: 393.

Sloane, A. (1951): Analysis of Methods for Measuring Diplopia Fields, Arch. Oph., 46: 277.

Trotter, R. and Stromberg, A. (1958): An Improvement on the After-Image Test. A.J. Oph., 46: 71.

Von Noorden, G. and Maumenee, A. (1967): Atlas of Strabismus, C.V. Mosby Co., St. Louis.

Wilkinson, O. (1927): Strabismus. C.V. Mosby Co., St. Louis.

*Worth, C. (1903): Squint, P. Blakiston Sons, London.

31 Paralytic Strabismus

I. INDICATIONS

A. A major objective in the analysis of strabismus is to differentiate the concomitant form from the non-comitant type. This differential diagnosis was reported to have been first introduced by Hippocrates (Wheeler, 1942). Concomitant strabismus may be corrected by refractive correction, orthoptics, surgery, or all of these, while the latter may require systemic and neurological treatment as well. Also, the causes of paralytic strabismus may be such that more than merely the ocular performance is involved or threatened. Many special tests and diagnostic techniques are designed to assist in the detection and treatment of this pathological form of strabismus.

B. Non-comitant strabismus is distinguished from the concomitant forms by characteristic indications involving the mode and appearance of the strabismus and the performance of the eyes. These indications are as follows:

1. Age and manner of onset
2. Diplopia
3. Vertigo
4. Head turn and tilt (torticollis)
5. False orientation
6. Limitation of the excursions
7. Comparison of the primary and secondary deviations

C. Most of the symptoms are associated with the limitation of movement of the eye and with the action and innervation of the muscles as a group. Before considering the symptoms in detail, it is essential that the laws of ocular motility which pertain to non-comitant strabismus be reviewed.

II. OCULAR MOTILITY

A. The Action of the Muscles (Figure XXXI-1)

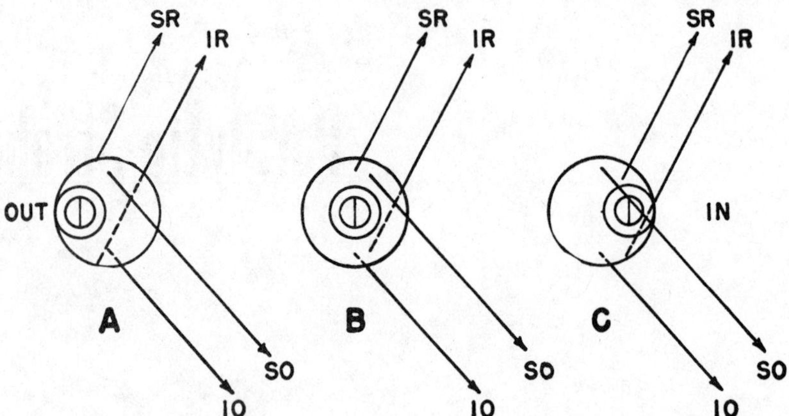

Figure XXXI-1 – Right eye as seen from above and in front, indicating lines of force of vertical ocular muscles. (A) When eye is turned outwards, showing increased potential vertical action of recti and torsional effect of the obliques. (B) When eye is straight ahead. (C) When eye is turned inwards, showing increased potential vertical action of obliques and torsional effect of the recti. *SR* superior rectus; *IR* inferior rectus; *SO* superior oblique; *IO* inferior oblique. Recti inserted at 27° and obliques at 51° to anterior-posterior axes.

1. The angles of the orbit and the angles traversed by the long axis of the various muscles in traveling from their origins to their insertions affect the action of each muscle in respect to the position of the eye when the eye is in the primary position and when it is turned in any secondary position. The rules governing the action of a muscle when the eye is in the primary position do not necessarily explain its action when the eye is rotated either laterally or vertically.

a. In the primary position, the *external and internal rectus,* assuming that the insertion of each is symmetrical to the horizontal plane of the eye, affect only simple lateral versions of the eye. If the eye is turned to the left or right, these muscles still affect only the lateral movements, but if the eye is elevated or depressed, they provide vertical and torsional effects that are in accordance with the direction in which the eye is turned.

(1) If the eye is elevated, the following occurs:

(a) The external rectus muscle will provide a supraduction action, and will add to the intorsion.

(b) The internal rectus will provide supraduction but add to the extorsion.

(2) If the eye is depressed, the following happens:

(a) The external rectus will provide infraduction but will add to the extorsion.

(b) The internal rectus will provide infraduction but will add to the intorsion.

b. The superior and inferior recti form an angle of about 27° with the visual line in the primary plane and travel from the nasal posterior part of the orbit forward and temporalwards.

(1) The contraction of the superior rectus will therefore result in three actions: primarily, that of elevation; secondarily, that of an inward pull; and thirdly, a torsional effect inclining the vertical axis with the top inwards. The inferior rectus will exert the same effect in its respective manner.

(2) If the eye is abducted sufficiently, the visual line will approach the plane of the muscles. Contraction of these muscles will now produce merely elevation or depression with the secondary and tertiary actions either reduced or eliminated.

(3) If the eye is adducted sufficiently, the line of sight may almost approach a position at right angles to the muscle plane. Contraction of these muscles will produce a very much reduced vertical or lateral action concurrent with a markedly increased torsional effect.

c. The *obliques* have their functional origins in the anterior and nasal portions of the orbit and follow a plane which extends posteriorly and temporalwards. The angle of their plane and the primary visual line is 50°.

(1) Contraction of the obliques with the eye in the primary position will also produce three movements: mainly torsion, to an extent greater than that produced by the recti; secondarily, vertical motion but less than that produced by the vertical recti; and third little or no lateral motion (abduction).

(2) If the eye is abducted, the torsional effect will be markedly increased, while the vertical and lateral effects will be diminished.

(3) If the eye is adducted, the vertical effect of the obliques will be increased, while the torsional and lateral effects will be diminished.

d. The cooperation of the recti and obliques permits elevation or depression or lateral movements with the eyes in either the primary or secondary position because as one set has its vertical effect reduced, the other has it increased, and the two sets balance the torsional effects in movements from the primary position. While it is common practice to speak of a single muscle turning the eye in a given direction or directions, in actual practice all muscles participate, some acting as agonists and some as antagonists.

(1) The variations in the effects of the different muscles in the group action produce the variations of the position of the eye in different quadrants of the field. To turn the eye down and out requires action of the inferior rectus, external rectus and superior oblique, with the major vertical action falling to the inferior rectus as the eye turns out. In turning inwards, the major vertical action falls to the superior oblique. Thus a paralysis of the superior oblique will not impede the depression of the eye in the lower temporal quadrant but will impede it in the lower nasal quadrant.

2. The action of the muscles can be summarized as in Table XXXI-1.

a. It will be noted that the torsional and other effects are balanced by agonistic and antagonist groups in each position. If any one muscle is cancelled out, the resultant dominant action which determines the position of the eye can be readily ascertained by noting in which column the effects no longer balance. Thus paralysis of the inferior oblique would ordinarily leave the eye turned in, down, and exhibiting minus torsion with the other eye in the primary position. The extremes would be the positions of the eye at which the visual line would be either parallel to or at right angles to the muscle planes. Since these positions would not be identical for both the recti and obliques, the effects indicated would not apply to both sets at the same time in equal amounts. At the extremes for the recti some of the other actions of the obliques would still be evident and vice versa. The "less" may be assumed to indicate merely reduced effect as compared to the effect in the primary position, just as the notation "more" is to be interpreted to indicate increased effect when compared to the effect in the primary position. The nature of the action is the same as that indicated in the primary position.

3. Pascal (1952) developed the so-called *"Benzene Ring"* schematic illustration of muscular activity (Figure XXXI-2).

Table XXXI-1

	In primary position			Adducted			Abducted		
Muscle	**Lat.**	**Vert.**	**Tors.**	**Lat.**	**Vert.**	**Tors.**	**Lat.**	**Vert.**	**Tors.**
Int. Rectus	*in*	*0*	*0*	*in*	*0*	*0*	*in*	*0*	*0*
Ext. Rectus	*out*	*0*	*0*	*out*	*0*	*0*	*out*	*0*	*0*
Sup. Rectus	*in*	*up*	*extort*	*less*	*less*	*more*	*less*	*more*	*less*
Inf. Rectus	*in*	*down*	*intort*	*less*	*less*	*more*	*less*	*more*	*less*
Sup. Oblique	*out*	*down*	*extort*	*less*	*more*	*less*	*less*	*less*	*more*
Inf. Oblique	*out*	*up*	*intort*	*less*	*more*	*less*	*less*	*less*	*more*

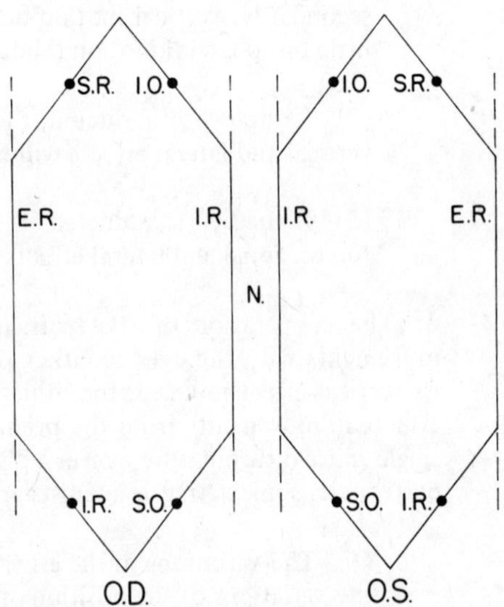

Figure XXXI-2 – Pascal's Benzene Rings. *O.D.* right eye of patient; *O.S.* left eye of patient; *N,* nose–viewed from in front. *S.R.*–superior rectus; *S.O.*–superior oblique; *E.R.*–external rectus; *I.R.*–internal rectus; *IfR.*–inferior rectus; *I.O.*–inferior oblique.

a. If the ring is considered as the action of the eye as seen from in front of the patient, so that the patient's right is the examiner's left, it will be noted that the following actions are readily determinable:

(1) *Primary action* is shown simply by the position of the correspondingly entitled limb of the ring. Thus, the primary action of the External Rectus is obviously temporalward while that of the Superior Rectus and Inferior Oblique can be seen to be elevated.

(2) *Secondary action* is indicated by the position of the dot on the limb in relation to the dotted extensions of the ring, and the slant of the limb itself.

(a) The *directional* secondary action of the Superior Rectus, for example, shows the dot on the limb, so entitled, to be nasalward of the dotted extension which forks away from its base. Thus, the secondary action of the Superior Rectus is to move the eye nasalward. The dot on the limb designated as the Superior Oblique is temporalward of the dotted line branching from its base so that the secondary action of that muscle is to move the eye temporalward.

(b) The *torsional* secondary action of the Superior Rectus is to slant the vertical meridan of the cornea identical with the slant of the limb on the Benzene Ring, or extorsion; while the slant of the Superior Oblique is likewise shown to be that of extorsion.

b. In addition, the Ring indicates the field of fixation in which the particular muscle exerts its greatest vertical action, so that the Inferior Rectus shows its most marked depressive effect when the eye is turned out, while the Superior Oblique shows the most marked vertical effect when the eye is turned in.

c. Finally, it must be remembered that the primary actions are most marked when the secondary ones are least effective, and the secondary ones most marked when the primary ones are least effective. The Inferior Rectus exerts the least vertical effect when the eye is already turned in, but exerts its greatest lateral and torsional effect in that position.

B. Innervation and Contraction

1. The fundamental law of ocular movements, *Hering's law*, states that both eyes are equally innervated during ocular movements and that two yoked muscles of the two eyes, when performing a conjunctive or disjunctive movement, receive equal innervation. This law is of specific pertinence when the paresis or palsy of an individual muscle is considered. If the maximum innervation were required to enable the eyes to reach the limits of the field of fixation, the fact that an eye accomplished this feat would be proof of the unimpaired motility of the eye. However, as Bielschowsky (1940) pointed out, only a contraction of a fourth of the length of the muscle was required to achieve the limit of the field (as compared to a reduction to half their length of the other muscles of the body by maximal innervation), so that only a moderate innervation was required to enable an unimpaired muscle to move the eye to the limits of the field. An impaired muscle could, thereby, still achieve the full rotation of the eye in response to an increased innervation.

a. An unusual aspect of the extraocular muscles is the fact that the movement of the eye is limited not by the total contractibility of the muscles but by the check ligaments.

2. The disclosure of impairment of a muscle of one eye only cannot be readily determined, except in cases of total paralysis, by a monocular test of the field of rotation. If the limits are tested binocularly, however, the moderate innervation which enables the unimpaired eye to reach the limits may be insufficient to permit the disabled eye to do so and the paretic eye will lag behind.

3. The muscles of each eye receive equal innervations whether these are voluntary, fusional, or vestibular. The voluntary command innervations arise from centers in the frontal lobe, while the centers in the occipital lobe probably are responsive to the fusional and other sensorial stimuli.

4. The organization of associated and antagonistic innervations can be readily determined by again referring to Pascal's Benzene Ring.

a. *Synergists* for a given movement in the same eye occupy the same relative positions on the ring, as the S.R. and I.O. for elevation, and the I.R. and S.O. for depression.

b. *Antagonists* in the same eye are shown by their relative positions, as the S.R. and I.R. for vertical movements, S.R. and S.O. for lateral, or S.R. and I.O. for torsional.

c. *Yoked* muscles of the two eyes occupy identical limbs on the rings for both eyes, as the S.R. of the right eye ring and the I.O. of the left eye ring.

d. *Crossed antagonists* comprise the antagonists of the yoked muscles, as the S.R. of the right eye and the S.O. of the left eye.

III. DEVIATION

A. If a muscle is paralyzed, the eye would be expected to turn in accordance with the resultant effectivities of the remaining muscles. However, the actual extent of the deviations may not be indicative of the extent of the paralysis. The original tonus of the muscles and the original position of rest of the eyes prior to the paralysis may influence the ultimate position. If a patient had been highly exophoric and suffered paresis of the external rectus, the eye might be almost straight or only slightly converged. Also, Bielschowsky believed that the location of the lesion producing the paralysis had some association with the extent of the deviation produced.

1. It should be emphasized that there may be present a limitation of gaze because of anatomic conditions in the orbit rather than for neurological or innervational reasons. Mark (1960) pointed out that faulty insertions or origins of the muscles, adhesions of Tenon's capsule and the surrounding fascia to the muscle sheath, and check ligament abnormalities all produced motility anomalies which he grouped under the label *"mechanical-anatomic factor."* These may be most difficult to differentiate from spasticity, paresis or paralysis of one or more of the extraocular muscles. These conditions are especially noticed in post-surgical strabismus cases where adhesions have formed at the site of the incision.

B. Secondary Contracture

1. Another effect which influences the extent of deviation is the action of the antagonist to the paralyzed muscle. As this muscle is relatively contracted due to the flaccidity of the paralyzed muscle, anatomical changes frequently take place which include shrinkage of the fascia and adnexa. Physiological changes in the tonus also occur. The additional tonus tends to increase the angle of deviation. Furthermore, the paresis may be cured or corrected, but the deviation often remains non-concomitant due to the secondary contracture.

a. The spasticity may be due to over-innervation of a muscle, creating a hyperirritability which results in an overaction to a normal amount of stimulation. Or the spasticity may be due to paralysis of the antagonistic muscle so that the spastic muscle acts constantly without the normal opposition. The former usually affects the yoke muscle in the other eye, since the paralyzed muscle may be receiving excessive innervation in an attempt to activate it. The latter usually occurs in the antagonist of the paretic muscle in the same eye. Thus, in many cases the effect of a paralysis of a given muscle in one eye is almost the same as a spasm of the yoke muscle in the other eye.

(1) The choice depends to some extent upon which eye the patient uses to fixate. If the eye with the paretic muscle is the fixing eye, the yoke muscle becomes spastic, but if the eye with the paretic muscle is the non-fixing eye, the direct antagonist usually becomes spastic.

(a) If the spasticity is due to yoking action, the deviation will disappear with cure of the paralysis but if it occurs in the antagonists, and this is maintained in a constant state of contracture, fibrosis of the tissues may occur, and the deviation will exist even after cure of the paralysis. Consequently, Scobee (1952) recommended that a prism over the fixing eye to prevent contracture of the affected eye's muscles by extending the ones tending to be spastic, may be useful in such cases. If the L.R. of the right eye were paralyzed, and a prism base out were placed before the left eye, the yoked stimulations would tend to be to the internal rectus of the left eye and external one of the right eye. The internal rectus of the right eye, which is ordinarily in danger of becoming spastic in such circumstances, would be inhibited.

C. As noted, the angle of strabismus may be influenced by the fact that the patient may frequently select the paretic eye for fixation and deviate the non-affected eye. As will be seen in discussing primary and secondary deviations, this exhibits an increased angle of deviation. This may be done because the patient has always used the affected eye as his dominant one, the vision of the paretic eye is better, or the increased separation of the diplopic images renders the diplopia less disturbing.

D. Mildly paretic conditions of the internal rectus may not result in a manifest strabismus because only a slight convergence effort may be needed to overcome the divergency. Slight paresis of the vertical muscles will, however, always be exhibited as a manifest deviation because the range of vertical fusional effort is very small.

IV. DIFFERENTIATING SYMPTOMS

A. Age of Onset

1. As previously considered, the concomitant strabismus usually develops because of structural or innervational or sensory interferences with the development of fusion. Since fusion is developed during the first years of life, strabismus due to such interference manifests itself early and the child learns to suppress or otherwise secure the single vision required.

a. In Chapter XXIX, the various age levels of the onset of strabismus were considered. It may be repeated that typical accommodative esotropia generally becomes manifest at the age of 2 to 4 years, while accommodative exotropia is revealed at the age of 5 to 7 years. The distribution of cases as totally accommodative, partially accommodative, and non-accommodative may also be recalled.

2. If some systemic disorder, cranial disturbance or traumatic involvement should impede the innervational pathways or affect the centers, and a paresis or paralysis of an ocular muscle occurs, a previously formed habit of seeing with both eyes may be interrupted because of the mechanical impediments suddenly introduced. Instead of the development of the squint from a latent through an intermittent to the constant phase such as is common to the concomitant esotrope, a sudden manifestation of strabismus will appear. As this is due to conditions which may affect the patient at any age of his life, the age and nature of the onset is usually directly indicative of the paralytic or non-paralytic nature of the strabismus.

a. The onset of strabismus at a relatively *mature age* and in a *sudden manifestation* is generally characteristic of the paralytic form.

b. In considering the chances for functional correction, the age of onset of a squint of a comitant form is usually related in that the later the onset, the better the chances. Flom (1963) reported the results of three investigators which bore this concept out, indicating "an increasing percentage of fusional correction with later age of onset, at least up to the age of 5 or 6 years." A similar association is held by many between the duration of the squint (from age of onset to age of treatment) and the prospects of correction. Flom noted that the complication of the problem by associated unfavorable conditions was held to be more likely the longer the duration of the condition, and that these were the factors which were considered to increase the unfavorable aspects.

(1) However, since the judgment of the onset of the strabismus often depends upon the parents, where children are concerned, and since these may misinterpret early

random vergence movements of the child's eyes as squint, unequal orbital formation or epicanthus, or on the other hand will totally ignore a concomitant squint in the early years because they never noticed the periodic stage, the sole reliance upon age of onset to distinguish the concomitant from the non-concomitant strabismus is fraught with error.

(2) In further contradiction is the condition of *congenital strabismus*, which may have been present from birth. If the deviation is of slight amount, it may not have been noticed by the parents until the child is of an age which would confuse its recorded onset with that of comitant strabismus.

(a) Scobee (1951) did assign some importance to a history of difficult delivery, particularly where instruments were used or deformation of the child's head occurred. This implied that a high association of trauma was incurred at that time with noncomitant strabismus.

3. Duke-Elder (1938) listed the following characteristics of congenital squints:

a. The squints are frequently alternating, with good visual acuity in both eyes, and an absence of a significant refractive anomoly.

b. Disturbing diplopia is frequently absent, and abnormal correspondence is often evident.

c. The deviation is of a stationary character, with an absence of secondary contracture.

d. Compensatory postural attitudes are adopted, and torticollis is evident if the cyclovertical function is affected.

e. Retraction is often evident.

B. Family History

1. The relation of origin to familial and hereditary influences has been noted in Chapter XXIX.

C. Diplopia

1. The concomitant strabismic usually develops the habit of suppression and amblyopia at the same early age at which the squint becomes manifested and during the period when the battle to secure single vision is under way. Such patients are either too young to report the state of vision accurately, or if older, have learned to suppress far enough back in their histories to have forgotten that diplopia existed.

2. The sufferer from a sudden paresis has, on the other hand, usually enjoyed single binocular vision and formed the normal habit of avoiding diplopia. The sudden deviation results in an immediate noticeable, annoying diplopia. The patient is usually old enough to be distinctly aware of it, and the happenstance is usually recent enough so that he can be fairly accurate in denying any previous intermittent diplopia. The persistence of the diplopia is sufficient to create great discomfort and may require temporary occlusion. If the paresis disappears and the normal binocular balance returns, the fusion generally automatically returns, but if secondary contracture develops and the deviation persists, the patient may either volitionally learn to increase the deviation to move the peripheral image farther from the fovea or may ultimately learn to suppress.

D. Vertigo

1. The patient who is a recent sufferer from palsy may suffer from vertigo due to two factors introduced by the new condition.

a. As an object traverses the motor field of vision, the double images will now separate or come together according to whether the object is in the field of action of the muscle or in the field of action of its unaffected antagonist. The patient seems to see an apparent movement of the secondary image as its distance from the primary image is greater or lesser.

b. The disturbance of the egocentric localization (absolute localization) of objects also produces vertigo. The nature of this disturbance is exhibited by false orientation.

E. False Orientation

1. If a patient suffering from paralysis of an ocular muscle is asked to point to an object which he fixates with his deviating eye while the good eye is occluded, he will, if a recent victim, usually point beyond the object towards the field of action of the paralyzed muscle. That is, if a patient suffering paralysis of the external rectus of the right eye is asked to point to an object to the right while using only the right eye, he will point to the right of the actual object, or towards the field of action of the paralyzed external rectus. This phenomenon has been traditionally and historically noted as *past pointing.*

a. The error in projection is due to the fact that the habitual egocentric localization of objects in space is dependent in part, upon the correlation of the innervation of the ocular muscles and their effects or, the comparison of the parametric feedback (proprioceptive impressions) from the unaffected eye which is habitually used to govern the location of objects (Ludvigh, 1952). As had been previously noted, if the unsound eye is required to fixate, an excess beyond the customary innervation will be required to straighten that eye. The yoked muscle or internal rectus of the sound eye will also equally receive this excess innervation and will actually be turned toward the right. The patient accustomed to judging by the position of the sound eye will, even though that eye is occluded, locate the object in line with the new position of the sound eye (Figure XXXI-3). This condition is usually manifested only in the early stages of the paretic condition.

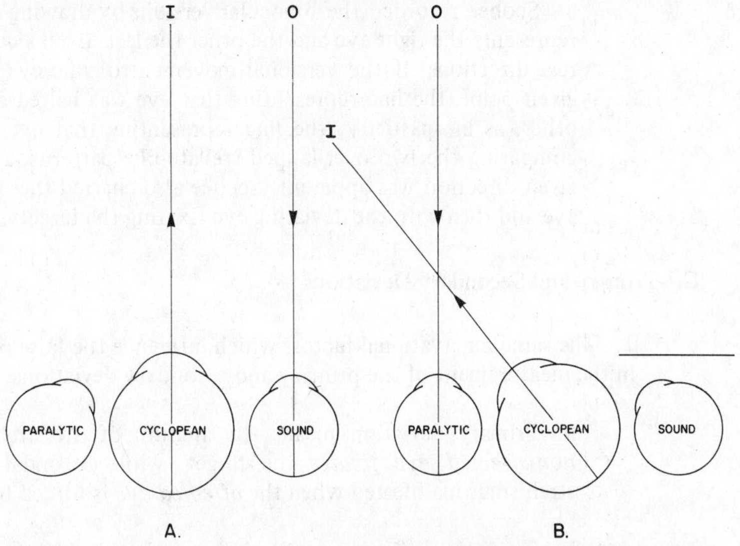

Figure XXXI-3 – (A) Fixation with sound eye. (B) Projection of paralytic eye when sound eye is occluded, demonstrating kinesthetic association with sound eye. *O* object; *I* image localization.

b. In a similar manner, if the patient habitually has used the paretic eye for fixation, a spastic form of projection is manifested. In this case, the patient has learned to associate the excess innervation of the affected eye with proper localization. If the same patient is now asked to point to the target while the normal eye, which was not habitually used, is exposed, less innervation will be required than was habitually needed for the affected eye; the occluded affected eye will not be fully turned towards the target by that innervation, and the patient will point short of the position of the object or to the left.

F. Limitations of the Excursion

1. As has been noted, monocular *ductions* of the eyes may reach to the normal limits of the field even in an affected eye, and therefore, cannot be solely relied upon as an indication of paralysis or noncomitance. However, Scobee measured the extent of duction in eight directions on the perimeter for each eye separately, recording both fields upon the same chart for an obvious indication of an actual limiting paralysis. Some allowances must be made for obstructions of the field by facial and orbital structures. The test was more precisely made by objectively centering the fixation light upon the corneas, than by relying upon subjective answers of the patient.

a. A lag of duction of one eye which is purely functional will usually disappear after 24-48 hours of occlusion but will persist if paralytic in origin.

2. In binocular rotations, since both eyes receive equal innervation, the sound eye will reach the limits of the field, while the affected eye lags behind, in the direction of action of the affected muscle which would require more innervation to attain the same point.

3. Similarly, if the condition is spastic, the affected eye will precede the sound one.

4. Whereas, in concomitant strabismus the innervation is equally distributed to both eyes and produces equal rotations of the two eyes, maintaining a consistent angle of strabismus in most parts of the field. In any non-comitant strabismus the angle of deviation varies in different parts of the field, increasing in amount as the field of action of the paralyzed muscle is entered and decreasing in amount as the field of action of the unimpaired antagonist is entered.

a. Scobee recorded the binocular versions by drawing a series of parallel lines, one of which represents the right eye and the other the left, from a central point towards each of the eight test directions. If the versional movement of one eye lagged behind that of the other at a given point, the line representing that eye was halted at that point. If one eye exceeded the other, as in spasticity, the line representing that eye extended farther than the other. By comparing the two over-lapped stellate-like patterns, a ready evidence of deficiency in any given direction was apparent. Scobee also charted these fields with first the habitually fixing eye and then with the deviating eye fixating the targets, and compared the two charts.

G. Primary and Secondary Deviations

1. The same innervational factors which influence the false orientation of objects are also revealed in the measurement of the primary and secondary deviations.

a. Primary deviation means the amount of the strabismus which is measured when the *non-affected eye fixates* the target, while secondary deviation means the amount of strabismus mainfested when the *affected eye* is forced to fixate the target.

b. To avoid difficulty, a red glass or other device of similar distinguishment is used before the fixing eye, so that the patient can be directed to fix the red light, for example. In Bielschowsky's technique this merely requires transference of the red glass from one eye to the other.

2. With the good eye fixing, the deviation of the affected eye is measured for the primary deviation.

3. When the affected eye is required to fixate, more innervation is needed to rotate the eye towards the target than was needed for the sound eye. Since both eyes receive equal innervation, the good eye is rotated even farther than the original angle of squint. The secondary deviation, therefore, exceeds the primary in paralytic strabismus (Figure XXXI-4). This manifestation is of itself a substantiation of Hering's law of equal ocular innervation.

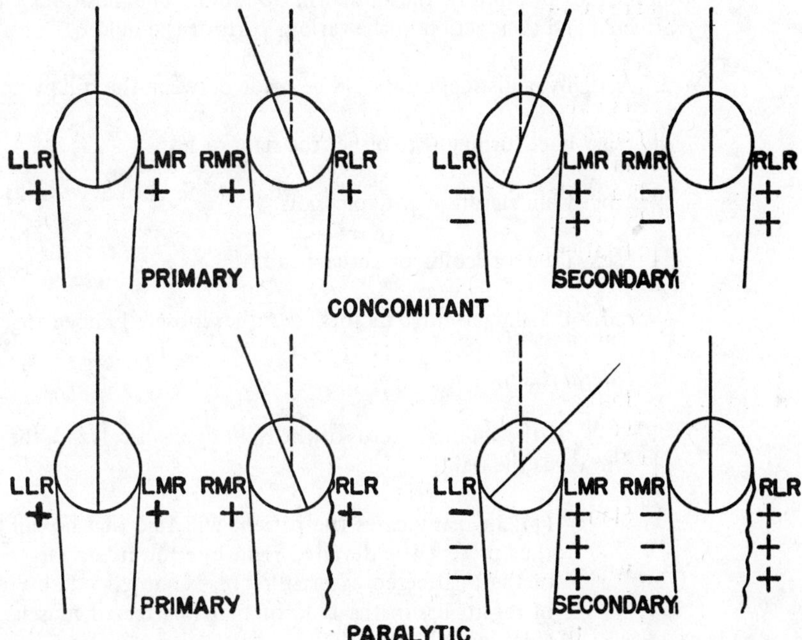

Figure XXXI-4 – Comparison of primary and secondary deviations of concomitant and paralytic squint. Right lateral rectus of right eye paretic. Excessive dextroversion innervation required to bring right eye straight due to paretic *RLR*, produces excessive dextroversion of the left eye.

4. In contrast, since the action of the respective muscles of the concomitant squint are equal for both the sound and deviated eye, the primary and secondary deviations will be equal.

a. It should be pointed out that in the case of anisometropic hyperopes these tests should be performed with refractive correction in place. The unequal accommodative effort to clear the target for first one eye and then the other, especially if the ACA ratio is high, will produce an apparent but erroneous diagnosis of incomitancy and a large difference in the primary and secondary deviation measurements. If a gross accommodative stimulus is used with an uncorrected isometropic high hyperope, who attempts accommodation with one eye and relaxes with the other, a similarly erroneous diagnosis can be unwittingly made.

(1) A potential error also exists in the corrected anisometrope, if the degree of anisometropia is of a marked amount. If one eye is directed to fixate in an extreme direction of gaze and then the other is likewise required to do so, each of the correcting lenses will induce prismatic effect in accord with its power in the meridian involved. Thus, each eye might be required to perform a different angle of rotation not in response to non-comitancy but to the difference in line of fixation produced by the prismatic effect of the respective lenses.

5. In spastic paralysis, in which the yoked muscle has become spastic or hyperirritable, and

responds more highly to normal innervation, or in which the antagonist has become spastic, the primary deviation may exceed the secondary, since less innervation may be required for ordinary primary fixation by the yoked muscle while the antagonist responds to a greater extent than the paralysis warrants.

H. Head and Face Turning, Tilting, and Torticollis

1. In almost all cases in which binocular vision has been retained in a certain part of the field, an anomalous position of the head will be found. This position will vary with the particular muscles affected and their action in the various parts of the field.

2. Actually, a distinction should be made between the following factors:

   a. Face turning – to either the right or left

   b. Chin elevation or depression

   c. True torticollis, or actual head tilt

   d. Usually, all three factors are rather loosely lumped together under the title of torticollis.

3. *Lateral Recti*

   a. If the internal rectus of the right eye is paralyzed, the right eye will deviate outwards or towards the right.

      (1) In many cases the patient will find that he can turn his head towards the left and thus present the deviated right eye towards a target lying in front of him. The action of the unaffected external rectus is normal, and by rotating his head so that the object of regard lies in the field of that unaffected muscle, he may be able to secure fusion (Figure XXXI-5).

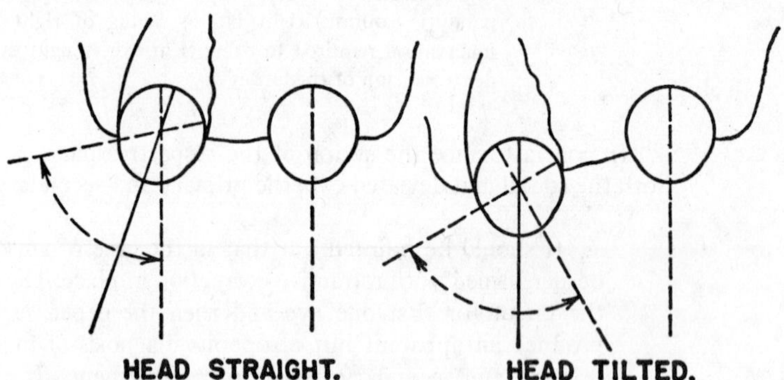

Figure XXXI-5 – Tilting of the head in paralysis of the right medial rectus. Head tilted to the left, in the direction of the affected muscle, to bring the useful field of action of the unaffected right lateral rectus in front of the patient. Dotted line arcs connecting arrow heads indicate field of action of right lateral rectus.

      (2) Should secondary contracture of the external rectus have taken place, however, the turning of the head towards the left may not reduce the deviation. In such cases, if the deviation is not too great, the patient may prefer to tilt his head back, forcing a depression of the eyes. This depression is associated with convergence just as an elevation is associated with divergence. The action of the vertical muscles is thus utilized to assist the deficient lateral muscles.

4. *Vertical Muscles*

a. If the vertical or oblique muscles are involved, the tilting of the head is much more complex.

b. If both elevators or both depressors of an eye are involved, the horizontal and torsional effects are neutralized and the position of the head may be a simple tilting backwards or forwards.

c. If an individual vertical muscle is involved, however, the position of the head is seldom in accordance with the above.

(1) If a single vertical rectus muscle is involved, such as the superior rectus or the inferior rectus, the head may be simply turned so that the affected eye is turned in. This may seem unusual for vertical deficiency, but if secondary action of the vertical muscles is recalled, it will be remembered that the vertical action of superior and inferior recti is increased as the eye is abducted, and decreased as it is adducted. By turning the head so that the affected eye is turned inwards, the vertical action is reduced to a minimum, and the eyes can be held upon equal planes by the increased vertical action of the unaffected obliques.

(2) If a single oblique muscle is affected, the head will be tilted to minimize the cyclo-torsional effect of the oblique muscle. The turn may also place the eye in a relatively outward or abducted position, reducing the vertical effect of the oblique.

d. The dominant influence in the tilting of the head is the matter of maintaining parallelism of the vertical axes of the cornea, and avoiding the effects of cyclotorsion. Where fusion is still possible by turning the head so that the eyes are directed towards fields of action of the nonparalytic muscles, the tilt will be of such an order as to align the corneal meridians.

(1) Head tilt is most commonly found when the superior or inferior oblique is involved, and in such cases is usually towards the shoulder of the same side as the affected muscle; it is also found, much more rarely, when the superior or inferior rectus is involved, and in such cases the tilt is toward the shoulder of the side opposite to the affected muscle.

(2) The face is always turned in the direction of action of the affected muscle.

(3) The tilt is always greater in an involvement of the obliques than of the recti.

(4) The Pascal Benzene Ring can be used to indicate the head tilt by considering the vertical axis of the face plane as a line corresponding to the limb of the affected muscle. It will be noted that the limb representing the S.R. of one eye tilts so that its top is toward the opposite side of the unaffected eye. For the face turn, the face is turned in the direction of the limb representing the affected muscle in the Ring, as up and to the right for S.R. paralysis, or down and to the left for S.O. paralysis.

5. The various head tilting positions will be altered in accordance with the degree of the deviation and the onset of secondary contracture.

V. DIFFERENTIATION OF THE AFFECTED MUSCLE

A. The recognition of the eye and muscle involved is usually determined upon the basis of tests. Since the affected muscle will lag behind its unaffected functional counterpart in the customary versional movements, an image of an object being viewed will appear farther away from the image of the same object as seen by the intact eye when the target is moved into the field of action of the paralyzed muscle.

1. If doubt exists as to the eye affected, it will be noted that the separation of the diplopia images increases as the target is moved in the direction occupied by the image of the affected eye. For example, a target presented to a divergent paralytic strabismus of the right eye will be seen as two targets, the image seen by the divergent right eye falling to the left of the image seen by the unaffected left eye. If the target is moved towards the right, the two images will appear closer together as the target enters the field of the uninvolved lateral rectus of the right eye. But if the target is moved towards the left or into the field of action of the affected medial rectus of the right eye, the diplopic separation will increase. Thus, if a red glass is placed before one eye and the patient is asked to report which of the targets, the red or the white, appears to the left, and *movement of the target in the direction of one of them increases the distance between them, the eye seeing that target is the affected eye* (Figure XXXI-6).

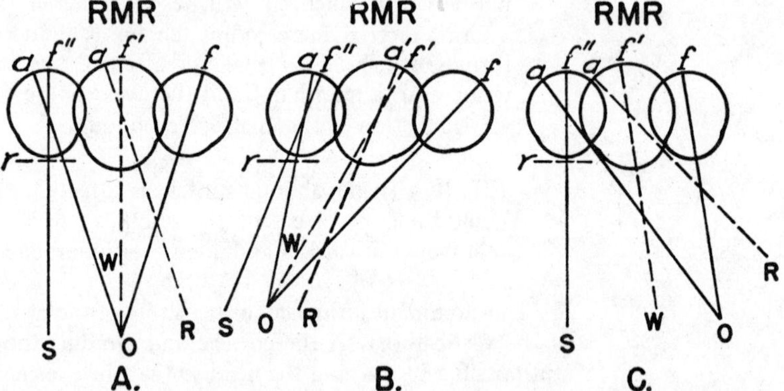

Figure XXXI-6 – Increase in diplopia separation as object is moved towards image of affected eye and into field of action of affected muscle. (A) Paralysis of the medial rectus of the right eye produces crossed diplopia, as shown by cyclopean eye. Red glass in front of right eye produces red image, *R*, seen by patient to his left. (B) As object, *O*, is moved in the direction of the image of the left eye, *W*, the diplopia decreases, as the field of action of the unaffected lateral rectus is entered. (C) If the object, *O*, is moved towards the left, or in the direction of the image of the right eye, *R*, the right eye lags farther and farther behind as the field of action of the paralyzed medial rectus is entered, and the extent of diplopia increases. *f* fovea of unaffected eye; *f'* fovea of cyclopean eye; *f''* fovea of affected eye; *O* object; *R* red image seen by right eye; *W* white image seen by left eye; *f''S* line of sight of paralyzed eye; *a* area stimulated by *O* in paralytic eye.

a. In all diplopia tests it must be remembered that the more peripheral image always belongs to the affected eye.

b. If secondary contracture has taken place, particularly in vertical deviations, the image separation may be constant throughout the field and more detailed investigation will be required.

2. Once the eye has been determined, the identification of the muscle involved is similarly dependent upon the elements of projection. *The muscle affected is that in whose field of action movement of the target produces an increase in diplopia.* If the right eye has a paralyzed muscle and a red glass is placed before it, the patient will report both a white and red image. If diplopia increases when the target is moved nasalward and decreases when it is moved temporalwards, the images move apart when the field of action of the internal rectus was entered, indicating that the muscle is involved. If the same test is made for a concomitant strabismus, the extent of diplopia will remain essentially constant in either direction.

B. The principles of projection and muscle action employed in distinguishing the specific muscles involved are based upon fundamentals similar to those applied to the simple lateral motions in the primary and horizontal planes. Since the vertical muscles comprise several effects, the projection test cannot be made as simply as has been described. In order to indicate both the lateral, vertical, and torsional effects, it is necessary to use a target which will exhibit inclination. The target generally consists of a line, placed either vertically, as is commonly done in this county, or horizontally, as is commonly done in Europe. Bielschowsky preferred the horizontal line because the position of the vertical line's inclination apparently varied with differing muscles according to whether crossed or uncrossed diplopia was manifested. Figure XXXI-7 demonstrates the diplopia field when a horizonatal line is used. The figure, as do most such charts, refers to the unifoveal-extrafoveal projection methods, and does not represent the appearance of the targets when tested by Lancaster's bifoveal method which tests projection rather than diplopia.

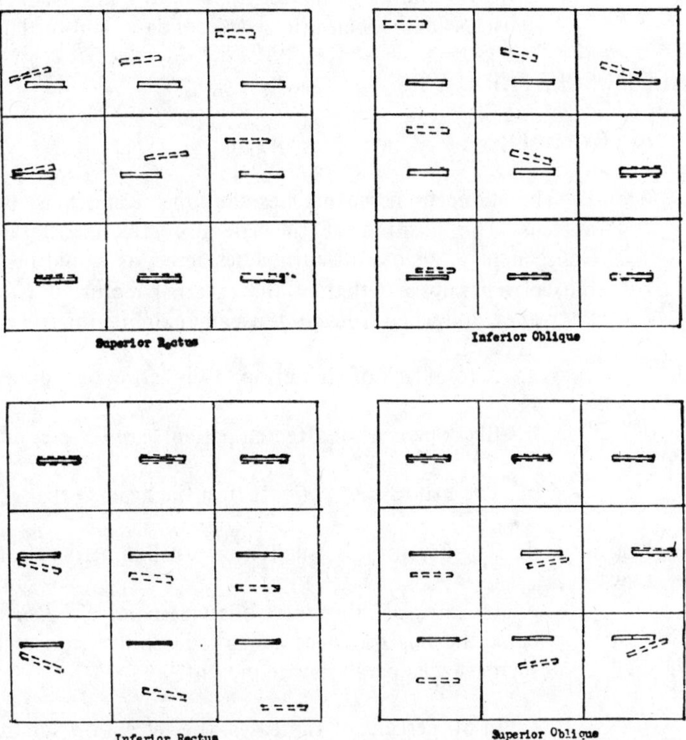

Figure XXXI-7 – Mnemonics of paralytic strabismus by Franceschetti's horizontal line technique (after Bielschowsky). Dotted image represents image of paralyzed right eye for each vertical muscle. Note the vertical discrepancy decreases for the recti as eye is adverted, and for the obliques as eye is abverted while torsional effects increase in reverse.

1. The examination is conducted by presentation of the target in nine different aspects of the field, three while the eyes are elevated, three while the eyes are level, and three while the eyes are depressed. In each position the eyes are turned to the right, straight ahead and to the left. A red glass may be used over one eye to differentiate the two targets. The patient is asked to draw the position of the two images or otherwise describe them. The examination may also be performed by having the target fixed directly before the patient and by moving the patient's head so that the eyes are turned toward the various portions of the field. Torticollis and other anomalous head positions must be avoided except as the position of the targets require.

2. Since the action of the vertical muscles varies as the eyes are abverted or adverted, the vertical

discrepancy between the targets will vary, as will the lateral and torsional effects. Likewise, the variations will increase or decrease as the eyes are elevated or depressed according to the primary action of the affected muscle. Figure XXXI–7 shows the typical relative positions of the horizontal lines for paralysis of each of the four elevators and depressors.

a. The position of the false image will be indicated on the Benzene Ring by noting that the slope of the limb of the muscle affected corresponds to the slant of the false image of the horizontal line as shown in Figure XXXI-7. If the Benzene Ring is drawn so that the right and left are reversed and represented as if seen from behind the patient, the new positions of the corresponding limbs will represent the slant of the false image and its position when a vertical line target is used.

b. It should be pointed out that the Benzene Ring is merely an additional mnemonic, and gives no more information than does a knowledge of the angles of insertion of the various muscles and of their primary, secondary, and tertiary actions.

VI. SINGLE MUSCLE PARALYSIS

A. External Rectus

1. The abducens nerve pursues the longest and most isolated course and has its own individual nucleus. The position of the lateral rectus muscle is also the most exposed in the orbit. Consequently, almost all authorities agree, as would be indicated, that the *most prevalent single* muscular paralysis is that of the external rectus. It is also among the most frequent congenital anomalies, and when *congenital* usually exhibits the following characteristics:

a. A total lack of abduction of the left eye is found in over 60% of the cases.

b. Sixty percent of affected patients are female.

c. The majority of patients turn the head so that single binocular vision is maintained.

d. The deviation is usually very small in marked contrast to the total paralysis.

e. In cases of congenital bilateral paralysis, *Bell's phenomenon,* in which an attempt to close the lids produces a marked supraversion of both eyes, and other congenital defects, such as facial paralysis, are present.

f. In 50 percent of the cases, the retraction syndrome is also present as an accompaniment of a deficiency of abduction.

(1) The *Duane Retraction Syndrome* consists of the following signs:

(a) An eso-deviation in the primary position.

(b) Restriction abolition of abduction of one, but rarely both, eyes.

(c) Slight restriction of the adduction of the affected eye.

(d) Attempted adduction results in retraction of the eye into the orbit.

(e) A pseudo-ptosis results from retraction of the globe upon attempted adduction.

(f) In marked cases, the ability of the affected eye to respond to convergence is affected.

B. Superior Oblique

1. While many authorities maintain that the superior oblique is not as commonly affected as other muscles, Bielschowsky believed that its occurrence was half that of paralysis of the external rectus, but that its manifestation was often confused with superior rectus paralysis of the other eye. Like the abducens, the trochlearis pursues an isolated course and has an individual nucleus. The most striking indication of superior (or inferior) oblique paralysis is *torticollis,* in which the head is tilted towards one shoulder.

a. It had been supposed that this was done to eliminate the vertical discrepancy of the two eyes by bringing them to the same level by tilt of the head. However, a convergent movement would still be required to equalize the horizontal discrepancy and it can be seen that action of the lateral muscles would not move the eyes on a horizontal plane with the head tilted.

b. If the head is tilted, vestibular reflex innervation produces a parallel rotation of the eyes. Such a movement could only be performed by a combined action of the inferior rectus and inferior oblique of one eye and the superior rectus and the superior oblique of the other. If the head is tilted towards the sound side, a paralyzed superior oblique will not be required to perform parallel rotations, and the eyes will not deviate.

(1) For example, let it be assumed that a condition of paralysis of the right trochlear nerve existed (Bielschowsky, 1940).

(a) If the head is tilted towards the right shoulder vestibular excitation is involved, provided those muscles that turn the eyes in, do so in a parallel rotary motion to the left.

[1] This motion is produced in the left eye by the two inferior muscles, and in the right eye by the two superior muscles.

[2] The paralyzed right superior oblique muscle cannot compensate for the elevating and adducting component of the right superior rectus, and a vertical and lateral deviation results.

(b) If the head is tilted towards the left shoulder, vestibular excitation involves the muscles which turn the eyes in a parallel rotary motion to the right.

[1] Since the inferior muscles of the right eye and superior ones of the left are involved, and the paralyzed muscle is not concerned, no deviation occurs.

(c) This principle is the basis of Bielschowsky's Head Tilt Test, described below.

c. This tilting is apparently confined only to paralysis of the oblique, although the action of the vertical recti would also imply that tilting is necessary if one of them is paralyzed.

2. Where secondary contraction of the inferior oblique has replaced the inital superior oblique paralysis, the patient may not exhibit a typical variation in vertical discrepancy if the eye is adducted into the main field of vertical action of the superior oblique.

a. In such cases, the discrepancy will increase as if the superior rectus of the other eye were involved, and thus make a more difficult decision as to which eye and which muscle is involved.

3. It has also been postulated that the tilt could be caused by spastic over-action of the superior oblique in conjunction with a paralyzed superior rectus muscle. However, Giotta (1950) in a study of such conditions, maintains that the tilt is never associated with anything but a weakened superior oblique muscle.

4. Bielschowsky spent much effort devising means of differentiating the muscle involved. Two methods bearing his name are as follows:

a. *Bielschowsky's Sign*

(1) As explained, if the superior oblique is the paralyzed muscle, the head will be tilted towards the opposite side so that the torsional ability of the affected superior oblique is not required to maintain verticality of the retinal meridian.

(a) If the head is held in the primary position, or is forcibly tilted in the direction of the affected muscle (towards the left if left superior obliqe is the affected muscle, for example), the involved muscle is now required to help maintain verticality.

(b) Since it is deficient in this action, the superior rectus of that eye is employed to attain the needed intorsion, but this muscle also elevates the eye.

(c) Thus, an increased hyperdeviation is noted when the head is tilted in the direction of the affected superior oblique.

[1] In paralysis of left superior oblique, with head tilted to left, the left eye deviates upward to an increased extent.

[2] In paralysis of right superior oblique, the right eye deviates upward to an increased extent if the head is forcibly tilted to the right.

(d) Since such compensatory actions are not required when the head is tilted opposite, less or no such deviation is noted.

b. *Bielschowsky Subjective Head Tilt Test*

(1) The apparatus consists of a piece of white cardboard upon which appears a horizontal black stripe. This card is attached to a rod, which is 75 cm. long, in such a way that the stripe is viewed by the eyes when the other end of the rod is held by a bite plate between the patient's teeth. The rod passes through a tubular holder which the patient holds in his hand, and the card, rod and bite plate will all rotate together through the same axis and angle as the patient's head tilts.

(2) A patient with a trochlear palsy will see, while his head is erect, two images of the black stripe, the image of the affected eye being below that seen by the unaffected eye, and tilted so that the left ends converge if left troclear nerve palsy exists, or converging at the right end, if right trochlear nerve palsy exists.

(3) If the head is tilted in the same direction as the palsied nerve, both the vertical separation and tilt of the two lines increases.

(4) If the head is tilted opposite to the direction of the palsied nerve, the two images may fuse or become more nearly parallel and closer together vertically.

c. Since the major association of head tilt is with paresis of the superior oblique, both forms of the test tend to indicate which eye's muscle is involved. However, it should be remembered that similar reactions may be obtained with overaction contractures of the oblique muscles, and even occasionally with vertical rectus muscle anomalies (Jampolsky, 1964).

C. Oculo-motor Paralysis

1. *Paralysis of the individual muscles* innervated by the third nerve is relatively rare.

a. The most *frequent condition* is that of *superior rectus* paralysis which is most often congenital in origin and combined with paralysis of the levator palpebrarum.

b. That of the inferior oblique is extremely rare, as is that of the inferior rectus.

c. The internal rectus is involved in the function of convergence as well as in adversion. Paralysis may occur in either function, although paralysis of both without involvement of the other third nerve muscles is rare. The eye may be directed to the primary position by a convergence effort which, while not activating the internal rectus, will inhibit the tonus of the external rectus sufficiently to allow the eye to assume the primary position.

d. The most frequently isolated paralytic condition of the third nerve is that of the levator, producing ptosis. This can be differentiated from spastic ptosis due to contraction of the orbicularis, by the flaccidity of the lid and its non-resistance to elevation mechanically. The latter also exhibits a raised condition of the lower lid and a wrinkling of the brow.

2. *Total oculo-motor paralysis* exhibits a characteristic appearance.

a. The pupil is dilated and accommodation is paralyzed.
b. The eye is usually turned down and out.
c. The loss of the retracting component of most of the muscles results in a marked exophthalmos.

3. *Strabismus Fixus*

a. A congenital condition in which both eyes are turned in, and the head must be turned to fixate, is known as Strabismus Fixus. The external recti are unable to abduct either eye, while the eye as a whole is retracted into the orbit. Vision is usually equal in both eyes. The internal recti and the check ligaments may be fibrous or elastic, in which latter case, surgical intervention may be helpful.

D. Combined Paralysis

1. Some investigators have reported a high incidence of vertical deviation in association with lateral squints. Scobee (1951) found 296 of 698 cases, or 42.4%, which had one or more vertical muscles involved along with a lateral strabismus. These grouped as follows:

a. *Unilateral*

(1) Superior Rectus	81
(2) Inferior Rectus	43
(3) Superior Oblique	32
(4) Inferior Oblique	4

b. *Bilateral*

(1) Both Superior Obliques	18
(2) Both Inferior Recti	16

(3) Both Superior Recti 10
(4) Both Inferior Obliques 1

c. *Compound*

(1) Both depressors (S.O. and I.R.) same eye 45
(2) Both elevators (S.R. and I.Q.) same eye 18
(3) S.R. one eye, I.R. other eye 15
(4) S.O. and S.R. same eye 5
(5) S.O. and I.R. same eye 4
(6) Miscellaneous 4

2. Scobee further stated that he did not believe that vertical or torsional tropias could be truly comitant.

3. In a study of esotropia, Scobee (1951) found 43% of 457 patients with a vertical or paretic component. By surgical means alone he was able to restore fusion to 46.5% of the cases without the vertical component, but to only 23.6% of those with the vertical component.

4. Urist (1951) cited the following findings for the extent of vertical association with lateral squints: Bielschowsky – 45%; Pugh – 42%; Dunnington and Regan – 50%; Enos – 60%. Urist found a vertical component in 79% of 615 cases, but differed in considering some 50% to fall into several categories in which the vertical element was secondary to the lateral one, rather than the basic cause of the lateral one. These categories are as follows:

a. *Group 1*

(1) Esotropia with bilateral elevation in adduction
(2) Esotropia greater at near and down
(3) Right hypertropia when deviated to the left, left hypertropia when deviated to the right
(4) Convergence good

b. *Group 2*

(1) Esotropia with bilateral depression in adduction
(2) Esotropia greater at far and up
(3) Right hypertropia to the right, and left hypertropia to the left
(4) Convergence good to fair

c. *Group 3*

(1) Esotropia with bilateral elevation in adduction
(2) Exotropia greater at far and up
(3) Right hypertropia to left, left hypertropia to right
(4) Convergence good

d. *Group 4*

(1) Exotropia with bilateral elevation in adduction
(2) Exotropia greater at near and down
(3) Right hypertropia to right, left hypertropia to left
(4) Convergence poor

5. Two of three recent strabismus samples show distinctly smaller numbers of significant vertical deviations than those quoted by Urist.

a. Flom (1954) found 20% of his sample of 68 exotropes to have a hyper component of 3Δ or more of vertical deviation. Ludlam (1961), of a total sample of 284 strabismics, found a vertical component of 2Δ or more in 28% of his 172 esotropes and in 32% of his 112 exotropes. Fletcher and Silverman (1966) found that 46% of 748 esodeviations had associated vertical anomalies while 40% of 326 exodeviations had vertical components.

b. Fletcher, et al. (1965), in an earlier study in which the reliability of recorded data in clinical strabismus research on patients 5 years to 21 years of age was investigated, explained some of the variability when she noted that agreement between two experienced examiners occurred on independent measurements of vertical deviation in only 68% of 107 patients. Poor attention span, lack of fixation, the presence of eccentric fixation, the frequency of occurrence of post-operative vertical componentss, improper adjustment of eye glasses, the difficulty in spotting small vertical movements by the examiner on the cover test, and the use of differing criteria (note 2Δ by Ludlam, 3Δ by Flom and unstated by the others) all went to make the data presented inconclusive as to the actual number of significant vertical components actually present in the strabismus population before treatment.

E. The A and V Pattern

1. Although Duane had noted differences in the horizontal angle of strabismus in upward and downward gaze, it was half a century later that Urrets-Zabalia (1948) and Urist (1951) discussed the condition which became known as the A-V syndrome. Since "syndrome" was not actually fulfilled, Costenbader (1964) suggested that A-V "Pattern" be used.

a. "When there is a more divergent position in elevation than in depression, or more convergence in depression than in elevation, the configuration resembles the letter V" (Albert, 1966). The reverse conditions simulated the letter A. If the divergence was greater in both the elevated and depressed positions than in the primary position, the letter X denoted the pattern.

(1) The condition may be present in either form for either esotropia or exotropia.

b. Costenbader (1958) used the term "vertical incomitance" in discussing these conditions, but as was apparent, it was the horizontal deviation which varied at different vertical levels.

c. Stanworth (1968) reported that various estimates of occurrence range from 12 to 40% of all strabismus.

2. The question of the primary cause has not been ascertained satisfactorily. Several different concepts of the etiology have been presented.

a. Overaction or underaction of the vertical muscles are assumed responsible by one school of thought.

(1) The A pattern is associated with overaction of the superior obliques, underaction of the inferior obliques, or both.

(a) The converse may also be seen, exhibiting A patterns with underaction of the superior obliques.

(2) The V pattern is associated with the opposite, i.e., underaction of the superior obliques, overaction of the inferior obliques, or both.

(a) The converse is sometimes found in this instance, also.

(3) Similarly, the vertical recti are assigned the cause, the superior recti being responsible for anomalies in the superior field, and the inferior recti those in the depressed field.

(4) A combination of recti and oblique malfunction might also be responsible.

(5) Gobin (1964) offered the concept that the phenomena were secondary torsional effects resulting from compensatory actions of the obliques in their efforts to correct or eliminate cyclo-rotary activity.

b. Urist (1951) held that the horizontal recti were responsible. The incomitance was based on imbalance of the horizontal recti which exaggerated the normal tendencies toward increased exodeviation upon elevation of the gaze and towards increased esodeviation upon depression.

(1) Stanworth (1968) pointed out the frequent occurrence of compensatory chin elevation in A esophoria and V exophoria, and chin depression in V esophoria and A exophoria.

c. The condition may be due to a combination of both vertical and horizontal recti malfunction. Breinin (1961) reported that electromyographic findings showed altered firing of both the horizontal and vertical recti, as the deviating eye moved into an oblique position.

d. Hoyt and Nachtigaller (1965) presented evidence to support the concept that anomalies of distribution of branches of the motor nerves may have been a factor in the genesis of A-V patterns.

3. *Treatment*

a. Since A and V effects are reported to occur so frequently and can have such an important bearing on the results of therapy in strabismus, it is important that measurements of the angle of deviation in the straight ahead, upward, and downward positions of gaze, be made a routine part of the strabismus examination. Dunlap (1961) suggested that the fixation target utilized should be "an accommodation symbol of appropriate size rather than the usual fixation light," both to standardize measurements, and to eliminate accommodative variation which might, for example, "produce a false V esotropia."

b. Reports of various attempts at surgical correction by Von Noorden and Olsen (1965), McNeer and Jampolsky (1965) and Urist (1968) have produced indifferent results since different criteria have been employed to judge the outcomes.

c. Ludlam claimed that when the A and V phenomena have total action of less than 15_{Δ}, from the primary position, building cover-uncover-recovery ranges into the affected area, developing accommodative facility while viewing in this area of gaze, and developing jump duction amplitudes have met with moderate success in allowing the patient to control the deviation and retain single binocular vision in all fields of gaze.

VII. CAUSES OF PARALYSIS

A. The specific organic causes of a paralytic condition involve diagnostic procedures beyond the scope of this text. However, the general causes of paralysis can be briefly summarized in a causal relationship to the types of paralyses involved.

1. The causes of paralysis are usually either congenital, in which case a deformation of the nerve

pathways, or abnormal development of the muscular tissue, or one of the adnexa are primarily at fault, or they may be due to the action of systemic pathology inducing lesions in the neurologic processes, tumors, hemorrhages, and traumatic interferences with either the muscles, or the neural paths or the centers.

2. The *most frequent causes* are generally given as follows:

   a. Syphilis and tabes, sclerosis, trauma, vascular disorders and meningitis

3. Hemorrhages, embolism, diphtheria, and trauma are usually *suddenly developing causes.*

B. The location of the lesion or tumor is of significance in the order of the paralysis. Lesions may be located along any part of the neural pathway, along connecting fibers between centers, and in the orbit. They are ordinarily grossly classified as follows:

1. *Orbital or Peripheral*

   a. Such involvements are usually either congenital, such as absence of elastic muscle tissue, or traumatic in origin. Usually the effect is unilateral and often only one muscle is involved. Usually the iris and ciliary are not involved unless a severe trauma is the cause.

2. *Central Lesions may be:*

   a. *Basal,* involving the course of the nerve trunk. If the third nerve is involved, usually more than one muscle is affected. The condition is unilateral. Other nerves may become involved.

   b. *Nuclear,* meaning that both eyes may be involved as well as other than ocular muscles. Usually vestibular and convergence reflexes are also affected.

   c. *Supranuclear,* meaning that the pathways connecting the centers of ocular movement are concerned. Such conditions are almost always bilateral and may involve the vestibular, cortical or sub-cortical pathways.

   d. *Cortical* meaning that the centers of volitional movement are involved, producing a bilateral deviation which does not affect the reflexes of the lower centers.

C. The paralysis may disappear of its own volition, may be permanent or may be replaced by *spastic action* of the antagonist. The spastic condition resembles the paralytic one except that the condition is usually temporary unless secondary contracture takes place, and the deviation is not consistent. Spastic paralysis may be differentiated from actual paresis by the fact that the tests indicating paralysis are reversed; that is, the projection undershoots the mark, the primary deviation exceeds the secondary, and the affected eye reaches the limits of the field first. The most characteristic symptom of spastic deviation is that the extent of deviation fluctuates from one time to the next.

D. *Congenital paralysis* may likewise be differentiated from acquired paralysis by indications which are obviously associated with the nature of the onset. The congenital case does not exhibit the variations in orientation, the difference in secondary and primary deviations and the secondary contracture as consistently as does the acquired type. Also, there is no history of spontaneous diplopia. The two eyes may move erratically in relation to each other, spasms of the paralyzed muscles may occur, and ptosis or nystagmus may be found.

VIII. SUPRANUCLEAR AND CORTICAL LESIONS (CONJUGATE DEVIATIONS) (Figure XXXI-8)

A. Supranuclear lesions can produce two kinds of oculomotor disorder:

1. *Concomitant strabismus* results if the lesion is in the supranuclear mechanism controlling *vergences* (Adler, 1953). Diplopia is usually experienced in this case.

2. *Paralysis* of associated muscles results in both eyes if the damage is in the area of the supranuclear mechanism having to do with *versions.* Diplopia is usually not experienced. The most common form of lateral deviation has been found to be due to lesions situated near the pons and the region of the fourth ventricle.

a. The eyes are deviated slightly towards one side and the head is turned to bring the object of regard into a position of view. Neither eye may be able to move beyond the midline or they may be equally limited if able to do so. The convergence is intact, indicating that the convergence center, the nucleus of the nerves, and the pathways are unaffected. The vestibular reflexes are also frequently found to be unaffected.

b. The vertical deviations are usually due to paralysis of elevation, next commonly both elevation and depression are paralyzed, and least commonly, depression alone. As in the lateral deviations, the patient can be forced to slowly follow a target into the paralyzed field or to respond to quick jerks of the head by means of a vestibular reflex.

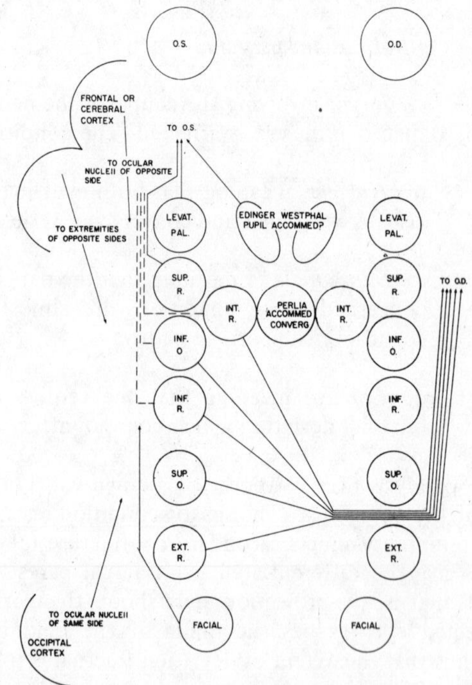

Figure XXXI-8 – Diagrammatic representation of nuclei and cortical centers in relation to conjugate deviations. Connections shown for left side only.

B. The tests for the vestibular and following reflexes, and for convergence are valuable in assisting in the location of the lesion. As long as the muscles respond to vestibular stimulation, the nerves, nuclei and pathways connecting them with the vestibular centers cannot be involved. The relation of the lesions to the nature of available eye movements can be summarized as follows:

1. Volitional movement is impossible, but there is following movement when attention is maintained and the vestibular reflexes are all undisturbed. The lesion is assumed to lie in the transcortical fibers connecting the frontal oculomotor centers and other parts of the cortex.

2. The volitional movements and the recovery or fixing movements are lost, but the following and vestibular movements are intact. The lesion is probably below the cortex in fibers to the nuclei.

3. The volitional fixing and following movements cannot be produced; only the vestibular remain intact. In lateral paralysis, convergence is still possible, while in vertical movements, Bell's phenomenon is possible. The lesion lies close above the nucleus but does not affect the posterior longitudinal balance.

4. None of the movements are possible, including convergence in lateral deviations or the Bell phenomenon in vertical ones. The longitudinal bundle or the nuclei themselves are involved.

5. None of the movements are possible and in addition a paralytic squint, diplopia, and other variations exist. An injury to the nucleus as well as a supra-nuclear involvement may exist.

C. Conjugate deviations, due to lesions in the cerebrum, usually manifest simultaneous deviation of both eyes. This is because the center stimulating voluntary muscular movements also inhibits the antagonistic muscles at the same time and by the same pathways and if the one set is paralyzed the other remains uninhibited. The differences between the cerebral lesions and pontine lesions of supranuclear type are summarized as follows:

Table XXXI-2

	Hemisphere	**Pontine**
Deviation	*Immediate, large, regular* *Duration short* *Toward side of lesion* *Usually due to stimulation*	*Rare and small* *Permanent* *Toward opposite side* *Usually due to paralysis*
Head turned	*In same direction as eyes*	*Opposite to eyes, usually not turned*
Associated paralysis	*Contralateral muscles* *Slight and transient*	*In direction of lesion* *Severe and permanent*
Associated muscles	*Symmetrical disturbance*	*Asymmetrical*
Facial nerve paralysis	*Collateral with eye muscles*	*If present, collateral*
Extremities paralyzed	*Collateral*	*If present, opposite*
Both hemispheres or side affected	*All movement restricted*	*Vertical movements unaffected*

IX. CONVERGENCE AND DIVERGENCE PARALYSIS

A. **Convergence paralysis** in which the eyes can perform the versional movements fully but convergence is absent would be due to a localized lesion of the convergence center in the region of the corpora quadrigemina.

1. Although a median center for convergence located in the Central Nucleus of Perlia has been postulated, Warwick's (1955) typographical study of the brains of 95 monkeys appeared to oppose this. In only a few monkeys was a recognizable nucleus found, and even in those, the nuclei contained "were not internuncial, and so could not constitute an integrative center." Since convergence involved a finely graded action between more than just the recti muscles, Warwick concludes that the Central Nucleus of Perlia could not serve as the center of convergence.

2. Bielschowsky believed that many cases of convergence paralysis were actually only cases of functional weakness of convergence. To be certain of actual convergence paralysis, he specified the following:

a. There must be symptoms of intracranial disease.

b. The paralysis must have occurred rather suddenly.

c. The signs and symptoms must be reasonably constant at different times.

d. The accommodation and pupillary responses should be producible without the corresponding convergence.

B. Much speculation has existed as to whether a true *divergence center* exists and whether divergence paralysis as such is possible.

1. Adler (1953) described electromyographic experiments on the lateral rectus muscle in which he and his associates, "recorded the changes in electrical potential and number of impulses discharged per second in this muscle in varying positions of gaze." On divergence following convergence, there was a "burst of impulses which precedes the actual movement of the eye by some milliseconds." Adler interpreted this finding as showing that the innervational activity produced, rather than was caused by, the eye movement. He felt he has proved that "during divergence from the convergent position the lateral rectus muscles are actively innervated. Divergence is due therefore to cocontraction of the lateral rectus muscles, with simultaneous inhibition of the medial rectus muscles." Although still not having demonstrated the existence of a divergence center, Adler concluded that a divergence *mechanism* existed.

2. Breinin and Moldaver (1955) also made use of electromyographic evidence in a patient with intermittent exotropia. They claimed that the result with this case "conclusively demonstrates that divergence is definitely associated with active innervation of the lateral recti." They further conclude, "The concept of divergence based solely on the inhibition of convergence and elasticity of the orbital tissues, fascia and muscles cannot be contenanced any longer."

3. Before any such complete generalization can be validly made, it would seem necessary to demonstrate the same kind of overt electrical activity during an active attempt at divergence, such as during abduction while attempting to fuse through a base-in prism.

4. It has been suggested that several different kinds of conditions may be interpreted as divergence paralysis. One is the case of abducens paralysis which vanishes and leaves a convergent strabismus due to secondary contracture. Another is spastic convergence action due to irritation of the convergence center. The third is the latent esophoria which becomes manifested as a convergent squint due to shock or illness. True divergent paralysis would present a condition similar to convergence paralysis in that the range of convergence would be limited in divergence paralysis outwards from the crossed position of the eyes rather than inward as in the other; and the field of fixation within the limits of the rotations be normal. As in convergence paralysis, it is essential that the angle of deviation be consistent.

X TREATMENT

A. Newly Acquired Incomitant Strabismus

1. Of all the patients seen those with newly acquired diplopia are in the most acute state of discomfort and anxiety. Having had the advantages of single binocular vision for many years, the disorientation, headache and vertigo associated with diplopia is naturally very alarming. Diplopia of sudden onset may be the result of an incomitant strabismus or can be caused by many other factors. Examples of such other factors have in the experience of the author been the following:

a. A side effect from a systemic medication.

b. Glasses tilted and in need of adjustment.

c. Recent change of spectacles which have omitted previously worn prism or the inadvertent inclusion of unwanted prism in a new pair of spectacles or recent replacement of a broken spectacle lens including unwanted prism.

d. Nose drops which affect accommodative innervation and reflexly change a previously high phoric condition into a manifest strabismus.

e. The after-effect of too much alcoholic intake.

f. Effect of chronic overwork or fatigue.

g. A result of 'whiplash' injuries from automobile accidents.

2. The patient is queried as to the orientation of the diplopic images and whether any head or body position seems to accentuate their occurrence or change their separation. A careful version test is performed with a light, the examiner watching the corneal reflexes, as well as listening to the subject's description of any changes in separation or relative position of the diplopic images.

a. If any incomitancy of apparently recent onset is evidenced, this sign is not to be taken lightly, and should be referred to a neurologist or neuro-ophthalmologist as the case warrants.

B. Incomitancy of Long Duration

1. Once the immediate threat of progressive, serious neurological pathology has been ruled out and the incomitancy has become 'stable' and chronic, the patient needs relief from the discomfort and a return of single binocular function as quickly as possible. The courses of treatment available are as follows:

a. Lenses
b. Prisms
c. Oculomotor calisthenics
d. Fusion training
e. Occlusion
f. Referral for surgery

2. *The use of lenses* should be aimed at the reflex manipulation of vergence, in horizontally acting paresis, to enlarge the useful zone of single binocular vision, which will reduce the extent of and the recourse of the patient to head turn or tilt, and to suppression to accomplish this. Thus, for example, if a paresis of a lateral rectus muscle is diagnosed, the use of maximum acceptable plus to inhibit convergence is needed, and for a medical rectus involvement, maximum minus to maximize convergence effects is necessary.

3. *Prisms* can be worn in spectacle corrections, used as fitovers and employed as aids in training versions and vergences. The fields of gaze most useful to the patient are the straight ahead field and that along the midline, especially below eye level.

a. The prescription of prisms is thus aimed at securing a maximum area of binocular single vision in these two fields with minimum head turn or tilt. If training is going on simultaneously, the prism may be prescribed in clip-on form with the idea of making changes in power, base-apex orientation, and/or distribution of prism between the two eyes.

b. When a supranuclear lesion affects conjugate gaze movements, the prism base is usually prescribed in the same direction in both eyes in order to extend a limited field of gaze. For example, base left O.U., in order to extend the left field of gaze for a given position of eyes and head.

(1) Diamond (1964) presented four case histories of incomitant ocular deviations which were corrected through the use of conjugate and oblique prism combinations. The aides resulted in relief of symptoms and sensorial reorientation of the frontal binocular field without anomalous head posture. His objective in using prism was to shift the entire binocular visual field "into an area of useful binocular fusion range" which will allow "a more comfortable ocular posture." Diamond listed four primary requisites for success of his method as follows:

(a) The presence of fairly stable and compulsive fusion.

(b) An intact binocular fusion field.

(c) The ability to overcome the deviation to some extent by anomalous head position.

(d) Satisfactory motivation and adaptability.

4. *Oculomotor calisthenics* have been recognized for some time as beneficial in cases of paretic oculomotor involvements (Smith, 1954). That the stimulation and use of muscles can restore at least some control of muscles to the cerebral centers is not a new idea to physiotherapy and has met with limited success in many and complete success in a few patients with oculomotor palsies. Since, as mentioned earlier, it is not always possible to make a definitive differential diagnosis between neurological disorders of the ocular muscles and mechanical-anatomical factors in the orbit, several weeks of ocular calisthenics may help in the diagnosis-prognosis of the condition. The following several types of calisthenics are generally utilized:

a. Monocular pursuit and saccadic movements into the field of the affected muscle with the head held still.

b. Binocular pursuit and saccadic movements into the affected field of gaze with the head held still.

c. Head swings, nods and rotations with eyes fixating a given object. The amplitude of the movements dependent on the ability of patient to maintain bifixation.

5. *Fusion training* also is found to be useful in enlarging the zone of binocular vision and should be employed in conjunction with the previously mentioned therapeutic approaches both with and without instruments and with and without moving targets. Small improvements over a longer time interval than that expected in orthoptic results with concomitant squint is the rule, but e.g., a 20° increase in the extent of binocular gaze in a given field with an accompanying decrease in head turn and body torque achieved in six months, may be an extremely important accomplishment for the happiness and well-being of the patient.

a. Guibor (1959) in his estimate of the efficacy of non-surgical treatment stated: "Non-surgical treatment of recent paralytic deviations in children is rarely discussed. Yet, such treatment achieves a satisfactory decrease in the deviation and an increase in the motor ability of the paretic eye."

6. *Occlusion* of one eye or one field has the most direct and immediate effect on diplopia. However, as Guibor (1959) warned: "Occlusion of the paralytic eye *always* makes the deviation resulting from the paresis worse, and permits a contracture of the antagonist of the paretic muscle

and an elongation of the paretic muscle itself. Occlusion of the paretic eye *always* increases problems encountered in treating paralyses." It can thus be seen that in prescribing occlusion, short term relief must be weighed against the long term disadvantages usually inherent in the procedure.

a. Occlusion of a portion of the field such as, the left temporal field, in a left lateral rectus palsy, often achieves an optimum functional result where symptoms, diplopia and head tilt are minimized. This can easily be accomplished by affixing adhesive tape to the rear side of the spectacle lens in the desired amount and position. The slight cosmetic stigma resulting from the appearance of the tape on the glasses and the additional head movement often required to scan a full field is only a relatively small price for the patient to pay for the comfort usually obtained with monocular partial field occlusion.

7. *Surgical results* depend on the nature of the cause of the incomitancy.

a. If the incomitant strabismus stems from an anatomical problem in the orbit such as faulty insertion of one or more of the extraocular muscles, incorrect check ligament attachment, or adhesion of a muscle to its sheath, to Tenon's capsule, or surrounding fascia, then surgical intervention can often restore comitancy.

(1) However, even in the case of the "sheath syndrome," Dunlap (1966) warns that, "Surgery in this condition is usually contraindicated if there is fusion in the forward and lower gazes without disfiguring head tilt. Even with surgery, prognosis should be very guarded. Our own overall results have been poor. Early surgical intervention (before age 10-12) is undesirable in most instances, as time alone may alter the defect."

b. If an "A" or "V" syndrome is present, which really presents a specious "vertical incomitancy," surgery for correction, at present, is still in the experimental stage. Studies of the results produced by the various types of surgical procedures advocated are just beginning to be reported (McNeer and Jampolsky, 1965; Von Noorden and Olson, 1965).

(1) Costenbader and Albert (1962) summarized their mixed results utilizing the various proposed surgical procedures as follows:

(a) "We have utilized the principles presented by Knapp (1959) for supra and infra placements of the horizontal rectus muscles for several years with minimal results. Somewhat better results have been obtained by the nasal or temporal placement of the vertical rectus muscle insertions as suggested by Miller (1960). Utilizing the suggestion of Urist (1951) for correction of the A-V syndromes has been variably effective in our hands and often is contraindicated in the consideration of other factors."

c. In congenital incomitancies, Dunlap (1966) warned against the uncertainties and dangers of early surgery for a wide variety of anatomical and neurological and etiological conditions. Costenbader and Albert (1962) stated that the horizontal incomitancies, "When there is a relatively small difference in the angle of squint between right and left gaze, good results are often obtained by the usual procedures for comitant strabismus. Surgery for profound paralysis of a horizontally acting muscle leaves much to be desired."

(1) They further state, "When a significant field of binocular single vision exists in the presence of a gross incomitancy, such as Duane's retraction syndrome or Brown's superior oblique sheath syndrome, no surgery should be performed unless an awkward head position is present."

(2) It should be noted that the very factors listed in this caveat against surgery are the

ones which Diamond (1964) found most important in securing a good result by the prescription of conjugate and oblique prisms.

d. In the surgical treatment for acquired incomitant imbalances, Dunlap (1966) cautioned "It is usually considered mandatory to wait at least six months in most patients with acquired imbalances if the cause cannot be found and the condition is not spontaneously improving. But in the few instances where the paralysis is known to be permanent and complete, early surgery is preferable so as to circumvent the development of secondary contracture."

e. Thus, in summary an incomitant squint of long standing should be referred for surgical interference only for reasons of extreme cosmetic disfigurement, that is, from the strabismus itself, the head position, or for bothersome diplopia and other symptomatology related to the non-comitant oculomotor condition. The more conservative approaches previously listed should be exhausted before surgery is entertained.

XI. CONCLUSION

A. The understanding of the symptoms and indications, and of the tests for recognizing the existence of paralytic strabismus fulfills only part of the responsibilities incurred in handling patients with incomitant strabismus. If, after careful testing and complete case history, an incomitant squint of recent onset can be identified, the patient should be referred to the neurologist or neuro-ophthalmologist where the actual diagnosis of the specific location of the lesion and the treatment to arrest or cure the condition can be undertaken. The value in discovering the paralytic origin of a strabismus of recent onset is that of early recognition of a central nervous system disorder which may endanger or involve more than merely the oculomotor system.

B. If, on the other hand, long standing incomitant strabismus is disclosed, and the patient is suffering from diplopia and/or limitation of field or gaze, a carefully planned and cautiously executed program of prescription of prism, full or partial occlusion and/or training may be undertaken. A patient well adapted to a long standing incomitant squint without symptoms should not be interfered with merely or solely because he has an identifiable condition.

C. Procedures for the determining of the existence of a paralysis should be performed as a regular routine in all cases of strabismus in order to avoid hasty and ill conceived attempts at therapy (both surgical and orthoptic) based on the false supposition of a *concomitant* ocular deviation. The presence of a paresis or paralysis greatly complicates the therapy and a complete cure is not usually to be expected no matter what treatment is undertaken, passive or active, conservative or radical. The best that can usually be achieved is a useful range of single binocular vision accompanied by a head turn or tilt, as well as compensating head movements when an object of interest cannot be tracked visually into the affected field.

REFERENCES

Adler, F. (1953): Pathologic Physiology of Strabismus, Arch. Oph., 50: 19.

Albert, D.G. (1966): Vertically Incomitant Horizontal Strabismus, I.O.C., Little, Brown, Co. Boston, 6: 3.

Barany, R. (1906): Untersuchungen Uber den vom Vestibularapparat des Ohres refeflektorisch ausgeloesten Rythmischn Nystagmus und seine Begleitererscheinungen. Monatschr. f. Ohren 40: 191.

Bielschowsky, A. (1940): Lectures on Motor Anomalies, Dartmouth College.

Breinen, G.M. (1961): Spectrum Analysis ·of the Extra Ocular Muscle Electromyograph. Arch. Oph. 16: 433.

Breinin, G. and Moldaver, J. (1955): Electromyography of the Human Extra-ocular Muscles I. Normal Kinesiology; Divergence Mechanism, Arch. Oph. 54: 200.

Costenbader, F. (1958): Clinical Course and Management of Esotropia. In Strabismus Ophthalmic Symposium II, James H. Allen, ed., C.V. Mosby, St. Louis.

Costenbader, F.D. (1964): Symposium: The "A" and "V" Patterns In Strabismus, Trans. Am Acad. Oph., 68: 354.

Costenbader, F. and Albert, D. (1962): Surgery of Strabismus, I.O.C., 2: 4, Dec.

Diamond, S. (1964): Conjugate and Oblique Prism Correction. A.J. Oph., 58: 89.

Duke-Elder, W. (1938): Textbook of Ophthalmology, C.V. Mosby Co., 1.

Dunlap, E. (1961): Present Status of the A and V Syndromes, A.J. Oph., 52: 396.

Dunlap, E. (1966): Complications in Strabismus Surgery, in Strabismus, I.O.C., 6: 3, Fall.

Fletcher, M. and Silverman, S. (1966): Strabismus. A. Summary of 1,110 Consecutive Cases. A.J. Oph., 61: 93.

Fletcher, M.; Silverman, S. and Abbott, W. (1965): Strabismus – Reliability of Recorded Data As Used in Clinical Research. A.J. Oph., 60: 1047.

Flom, M. (1954): The University of California Strabismus and Orthoptics Study Preliminary Report (Unpublished Paper presented before the A.A.A.O.

Flom, M.C. (1963): Treatment of Binocular Anomalies of Children, in Vision of Children (Hirsch & Wick); Chilton Books, Phila.

**Giotta, A.J. (1950): Differential Diagnosis of Paresis of the Superior Oblique and Superior Rectus Muscles. Observations in 6 Cases with Discussion of their Significance. Arch. Oph. 43: 1.*

Gobin, M. (1964): Anteroposition of the Inferior Oblique Muscle in Esotropia. Ophthalmologica, 148: 325.

Guibor, G. (1959): Squint and Allied Conditions, Grune and Stratton, New York.

Hoyt, W.F. & Nachtigaller, H. (1965): Anomalies of Oculomotor Nerves; Neuro-Anatomic Correlates of Paradoxical Innervation in Duane's Syndrome and Related Congenital Ocular Motor Disorders. A.J. Oph. 60: 443.

Jampolsky, A. (1964): Ocular Deviations, I.O.C., Little, Brown & Co., Boston, 4: 3.

Knapp, P. (1959): Vertically Incomitant Horizontal Strabismus; The So-Called (A) and (V) Syndromes; Trans. Am. Oph. Soc., 57: 666.

**Lancaster, W.B. (1941): Fifty Years Experience in Ocular Motility. A.J. Oph., 24: 488, 619, 741.*

Ludlam, W. (1961): Orthoptic Treatment of Strabismus, A.A.A.O., 38: 369.

Ludvigh, E. (1952): Control of Ocular Movements and Visual Interpretation of Environment, Arch. Oph., 48: 442.

**MacLean, A. (1963): The "A" and "V" Syndrone, Amer. Orth. J., 13: 122.*

Mark, M. (1960): The Mechanical-Anatomic Factor in Ocular Motor Affects. O.J.R.O., 97 (17): 35.

McNeer, K. and Jampolsky, A. (1965): An Evaluation of Underactive Inferior Oblique Muscles. A.J. Oph., 60: 114.

Miller, J. (1960): Vertical Recti Transplantation in the A and V Syndromes. Arch. Oph., 64: 175.

Pascal, J. (1952): Selected Studies in Visual Optics, The C.V. Mosby Co., St. Louis.

Scobee, R. (1951): Esotropia, Incidence, Etiology and Results of Therapy. A.J. Oph., 34: 817.

Scobee, R. (1952): The Oculorotary Muscles, C.V. Mosby Co., 1948; ibid, 2nd ed.

Smith, W. (1954): Clinical Orthoptic Procedure, 2nd ed., C.V. Mosby, St. Louis.

Stanworth, A. (1968): The A and V Phenomena. Brit. Orth. J., 25: 12.

Urist, M. (1951): Horizontal Squint With Secondary Vertical Deviations, Arch. Oph., 46: 245.

Urist, M. (1968): Recession and Upward Displacement of the Medical Rectus Muscles in A-Pattern Esotropia. A.J. Oph., 65: 769.

Urrets-Zavalia, A., Jr., (1948): cited in Albert, D.G., (1966).

Von Noorden, G. and Olson, C. (1965): Diagnosis and Surgical Management of Vertically Incomitant Horizontal Strabismus. A.J. Oph., 60: 434.

Warwick, R. (1955): The So Called Nucleus of Convergence. Brain, 78, Part I, 92.

Wheeler, M. (1942): The History of Orphthoptics. A.J. Oph., 25: 569.

Strabismus/Prognosis and Treatment and Results 32

I. TREATMENT

A. With the diagnostic testing completed and the relevant data gathered, a decision as to the form of treatment to be undertaken must be considered. At the present time there are four modes of attack which may be used separately or in combination in strabismus therapy. The squint condition may also be left alone so that a fifth choice, an option for no treatment, is available as well. These choices are:

1. Refractive
2. Pharmacological
3. Training
4. Surgical
5. Leave untreated

II. REFRACTIVE TREATMENT

A. Refractive Correction.

1. This method has been used with at least some success since 1801 when Erasmus Darwin recommended spectacles to correct "the inequality of force of the two eyes" in strabismus. The elucidation of the relationship between accommodation and convergence by Donders (1864) provided a rationale for the systematic application of lens therapy for both convergent and divergent strabismus.

a. Since that time, in addition to making use of accommodative-vergence to achieve alignment of the visual axes by adding plus lens power for esotropia and minus lens power for exotropia over the manifest correction lens, spectacle corrections have been employed to:

(1) *Equalize the ocular image differences* present in aniseikonia thus enabling fusion to come about.

(2) *Supply prismatic aid* in overcoming vertical deviations and small amounts of residual lateral imbalance not correctible by manipulation of the accommodative-convergence relationship. The practical limit is usually 12^{Δ} in each eye for reasons of weight, appearance and induced prism distortion.

(3) *Correct anisometropic* refractive errors.

(4) *Change the angle of deviation* in constant esotropes to attempt to interfere with the feedback reinforcement relationships of the extra ocular muscles in anomalous correspondence (Morgan, 1961). In addition, Rubin (1966) uses small prism "in reverse" in combination with graded occlusion for eccentric fixation cases to change the sensorimotor relationship and thus help to produce central fixation.

(5) The use of spherical and cylindrical spectacle lenses to change perceived and subjective space (Apell and Lowry, 1959) as, e.g., in changing a near working distance by the application of additional convex sphere.

(6) The use of bifocals in cases of divergence excess intermittent exotropia.

b. *Contact lenses* have been increasingly employed in refractive correction of strabismus because of: the cosmetic improvement they afford over the heavy spectacle lenses frequently needed, the better equalization of ocular image size they bring about in refractive anisometropia, and the reduction in unwanted prismatic effect frequently provided in spectacle corrections. Hermann (1966) points out, furthermore, that the use of contact lenses increases the potentially usable peripheral field thus providing additional opportunity for the development of peripheral fusion. Contact lenses do have a notable limitation, however, in that even small horizontal prism corrections are most difficult to fit and keep oriented satisfactorily except by the use of scleral lenses.

c. The rationale of refractive correction in strabismus differs from that traditionally employed for ametropia where the major objectives are generally the reduction of asthenopia and other symptoms, the improvement of acuity and enhancement of visual performance generally. In lens therapy for strabismus initial subjective acceptance is not the primary aim. If immediate followup training is not contemplated to attempt to bring about functional binocularity, the complete correction of a hyperopic refractive error which does not completely align the eyes may produce an invariant, although smaller, squint angle which enables the strabismic to more easily develop stronger perceptual adaptations such as anomalous correspondence. Thus, early complete correction of a hyperopic error which does not fully correct a convergent deviation and where immediate followup is not undertaken need not serve well towards the attainment of functional binocularity. In a second example, full correction of the anisometropia commonly found in cases of amblyopia may also not be in the interest of full recovery of central fixation and accommodation in functional amblyopia. The direct accommodative reflex is often absent or markedly deficient in an amblyopic eye and in the author's experience, constant wear of a full plus prescription tends to inhibit the eventual normalization of the direct accommodative response in that eye. In addition the full prescription of an anisometropic difference often raises potential obstacles to fusion both in the form of unwanted prism which varies with the position of gaze and spectacle magnification which induces aniseikonia.

d. Refractive corrections exhibit several other benefits in the treatment of squint.

(1) They may help to provide, in addition to clear and equal images in the two eyes, the advantage of equal image *quality*. Thus, "similarity of sharpness of the retinal images" obtained by prescription of even small optical corrections may assist in preventing suppression of one ocular image, thus improving the quality of sensory fusion and providing a "stronger stimulus to reflex vergence" (Flom, 1963).

(2) Spectacles or contact lenses worn full time also contribute a continuous influence on the strabismus deviation through accommodative vergence while other forms of therapy, such as training, pharmacology, and surgery, vary in effectiveness from the time of their application.

2. *Side Effects and Complications*

a. Although refractive correction is used regularly and successfully in concert with the other types of therapy to be described it is only occasionally employed as a sole therapeutic measure in strabismus. Spectacle correction in strabismus has been known on occasion to produce temporary annoyances such as:

(1) asthenopia and dizziness
(2) spatial distortions
(3) diplopia
(4) nausea
(5) blurred vision

III. PHARMACOLOGICAL METHODS

A. Cycloplegics

1. *Homatropine,* and *atropine* and its derivatives have been in use for some time to measure what is alluded to as the "full" hyperopic error, or the refractive component in accommodative esotropia, and used in the non-amblyopic eye for periods of several months in the treatment of amblyopia. The prolonged use of such drugs to maintain alignment while occasionally advocated has been only seldom employed (Guibor, 1959), because of the loss of the accommodative function, the widely dilated pupils and the possibility of systemic and ocular side effects on intraocular pressure, digestion and circulation.

B. Miotics

1. *Pilocarpine,* a miotic whose action is directly on the motor end plates of both the iris and ciliary muscle, has been occasionally used since first reported by Javal (1896) as a temporary measure to allow accommodative esotropes to remove their glasses without squinting.

a. Edwards (1958) reports that of a sample of 30 strabismic patients, who had been given pilocarpine treatment a sufficient length of time to enable a conclusion to be drawn, nine showed some improvement. Of those not improving, five stopped the drops because of "headaches, hives or parental indifference." The specifics of the improvement were not described.

b. Breinin, Chin and Ripps (1966) after observing that pilocarpine and eserine act directly on the ciliary muscle to produce an accommodative spasm, state:

(1) "Except for correcting a hyperopic error or making the patient somewhat myopic for distance and thereby reducing the accommodative requirement at near, these drugs are relatively inefficient as therapeutic agents."

2. Recently, topically applied, long-acting cholinesterase inhibitors such as diisopropyl fluorophosphate (DFP) and echothiophate iodide (Phospholine Iodide) have been employed increasingly in the treatment of young accommodative esotropes. Since one of the actions exerted by these drugs is a parasympathomimetic type of effect on the pupil they have been termed miotics.

a. Although the precise action of these drugs is not known completely, they are known to form an irreversible reaction with cholinesterase which results in its deactivation and hence causes a locally unopposed contraction of the iris and ciliary sphincters. The results of experimental work on the cat by Ripps, Breinin and Baum (1961) indicate that these drugs facilitate neuro-muscular transmission so that a lower level of innervation is necessary to attain a given amount of accommodation. This then is thought to activate less reflex convergence and so a lower AC/A ratio is obtained.

(1) Breinin, Chin and Ripps (1966) for example, report one case in which a 13/1 AC/A ratio was reduced to 3/1 in 5 weeks with treatment by 0.12% Phospholine Iodide combined with phenyepherine. Breinin, Chin and Ripps (1966) point out the difference between the action of convex lenses and miotics as follows:

(a) "It should be noted that whereas lenses cause the patient to use less accommodation, the normal dioptric amount of accommodation is required of patients on anticholinisterases; only the innervational requirement to achieve this degree of accommodation has been reduced."

b. Since D.F.P. and phospholine iodide permanently deactivate cholinesterase, it takes some time before sufficient cholinesterase can be drawn from other parts of the body or regenerated at its site of action in the ciliary muscle so that the effect on accommodation may last anywhere from 12 hours to one week.

c. Abraham (1949) was the first to report on the use of cholinesterase inhibitor miotics in strabismus and detailed his results of a sample of 46 esotropes. Since that time a number of other investigators have reported results which will be covered under the section "Results of Treatment."

d. Although it is generally agreed that the various miotic drugs previously described are especially useful in diagnostic testing in all accommodative esotropias and for the specific treatment of "convergence excess" types of high ACA ratio esotropes, various other uses have been suggested:

(1) *Functional amblyopia*

(a) Abraham (1949) and (1961) and Johnson and Antuna (1965) have made use of miotics in treating amblyopic eyes. Abraham uses "time honored and effective means of successfully treating amblyopia" in conjunction with a miotic instilled only in the amblyopic eye: and reports increased facility of accommodation in the amblyopic eyes. He believes the miotic is acting to "equalize the tone of the ciliary muscles" of each eye and thus will result in improved acuity.

(b) Johnson and Antuna, on the other hand, use atropine in the non-amblyopic eye and a miotic in the amblyopic eye. They advise daily instillations of each medication and forbid use of glasses during the treatment. The authors report their highest rate of success in patients with anisometropic hyperopia of four to six diopters. They feel that the major factor in achieving improvement in acuity, especially in anisometropia, is that the "ciliary muscle spasm induces myopia," where patients "exhibited a prolonged decrease in hyperopia which greatly facilitated image size equalization and decreased aniseikonia."

[1] Large improvements in vision are reported as being often obtained in one or two months by this method.

(2) *Convergent strabismus of early onset*

(a) Birnbaum (1963) in an article reviewing the field to that date states:

[1] "It seems to me that while miotics may be useful in conjunction with other forms of therapy in strabismus, their prime use and greatest benefit lies in the treatment of esotropia in children too young to undergo orthoptic treatment, in order to prevent amblyopia and anomalous retinal correspondence. If not completely successful in these cases, miotics might at least prevent further deterioration until orthoptic training could be instituted."

(b) Abraham (1961) agrees stating:

[1] "Miotics may be used in younger patients when the use of glasses is not desired by the parents or patient, or where prescribing of glasses would be dangerous, if not impractical. The use of miotics in such cases can help long before the abnormal pattern has become entrenched."

(3) *To overcome residual deviations after surgery*

(a) This use is very popular but is generally only effective where moderate hyperopia or hyperopic anisometropia is present.

(b) Wheeler and Moore (1964) however, report that in 4 of 12 patients in their "non-accommodative group" of post-surgical esotropes, the decrease in residual deviation with a combination of D.F.P. and glasses or D.F.P. alone "was significant enough to warrant continuation of D.F.P. for treatment."

(c) Chamberlain and Caldwell (1965) also report the successful use of miotics with surgically overcorrected exotropes.

[1] A trial use of several weeks is generally indicated.

(4) *The combined use of miotics with glasses*

(a) Most authors have reported their measurement of the acuity and the deviation with glasses alone, with a miotic alone, and with a combination of the two. The expected contribution of the miotic is usually greatest at nearpoint.

[1] Breinin, Chin and Ripps (1966) observe that, ". . . one often finds that the combination of miotics and plus lenses works better than either method alone."

[2] Chamberlain and Caldwell on the basis of experience with 36 esotropes over three years state, "It is our impression that a number of patients show a more satisfactory response with both lenses and miotics than when using glasses alone or only the medication."

[a] They emphasize the importance of using specific criteria for prolonged treatment and suggest that the patient should demonstrate "at least gross fusion while using the drug." In addition they emphasize close supervision at regular intervals to detect signs of side effects.

(5) *Substitution for glasses*

(a) Several writers have recommended that especially in low degrees of hypermetropia drops may be used instead of glasses, usually on a short term basis, as for example, "to maintain alignment while swimming during the summer" (Chamberlain and Caldwell, 1965), and for various social occasions.

(b) Miotics have also been recommended as a substitute for bifocals in cases of esotropia with a high AC/A ratio.

[1] Cooper (1963) observes that although miotics have been "recommended as a substitute for glasses and particularly as a substitute for bifocals, they do not always work." He suggests that the results are more satisfactory when the miotic acts as "an adjunct to, rather than a substitute for glasses." He points out that patients on Floropryl must be checked much more frequently than those wearing glasses or bifocals.

(c) Koskinen (1957) concludes that, "treatment with miotics is a welcome addition to the treatments of periodic, convergent strabismus of small children when it is not desirable to give glasses."

(6) *Pharmacological training*

(a) Abraham (1961) Parks (1958) Hill and Stromberg (1962) and Breinin, Chin and Ripps (1966) have stressed the importance of the gradual withdrawal of the miotic once fusion has been achieved so that the fusional divergence amplitude is slowly increased.

[1] Parks (1958) notes: "As the isoflurophate effect wears off an increasing amount of accommodation innervation is necessary to assure a sharp image, which is associated with a like increase in the accommodative convergence innervation. The alert child, with good binocular visual ability, will subconsciously apply progressively more fusional divergence to counter the increasing 'eso' in an attempt to maintain fusion."

[a] "This cycle, repeated day after day insidiously increases the fusional divergence amplitude."

[2] Sloan, Sears and Jablonski (1960) utilizing *subjective* phoria measurements on 15 patients found that during the course of regular instillation of the miotic a significant number demonstrated decrease in the AC/A ratio. After cessation of the use of the drug: "There was gradual return to the previous level."

[a] "Although the decrease in AC/A ratio was in some instances maintained for several weeks after cessation of therapy, in every case it rose eventually to a value as high or almost as high as that observed prior to therapy."

[b] These findings thus, differ from those previously stated by Park.

[3] Birnbaum (1963) after reviewing the conflicting results noted above, concludes, "There are considerable differences of opinion and conflicting reports relating to the extent of lasting change in the accommodative-convergence relationship."

[a] "It appears likely that any permanent change in the accom-

modation-convergence relationship, in the fusional divergence, or in the esotropia, occurs as a result of a sort of training procedure: that is, as the miotics are gradually withdrawn or their effects gradually wear off, the patient is faced with a constantly increasing need to decrease convergence in order to maintain single binocular vision."

[b] He continues: "This is very similar in many ways to the situation set up in the orthoptic treatment of strabismus."

C. Side Effects

1. The use of these drugs has been accompanied by a number of reported undesirable ocular and systemic side effects.

a. *Ocular side effects*

(1) The most widespread of these effects are the so-called *iris nodules or iris cysts.*

(a) The earlier investigators found them to occur after one to forty weeks of treatment, (Abraham, 1954), in 50% or more of the cases in which miotic drops were instilled daily for periods of a month or longer (Miller, 1960), (Chin et al. 1964). They usually shrivel up within 2 to 42 weeks after discontinuance of the drug (Knapp and Campobianco, 1956), although Abraham (1961) reports that the residual "tags" have been observed seven and eight years after the onset of the original iris nodules.

(b) They have been dismissed by some as "harmless" although little is known of their etiology or nature.

[1] In one case, an eye being treated for congenital glaucoma with miotics was enucleated after the appearance of these cysts because of suspected "malignant melanoma" (Christensen et al. 1956). After a microscopic study of this enucleated eye, Christensen reported the following on the observed pupillary pigment nodules:

[a] "Several features of this specimen are particularly interesting. Until the present time these pupillary nodules have been considered as simple cysts that probably formed from secretion of fluid or mechanical irritation associated with severe miosis; however, it is evident from this globe and our patient with aniridia that extreme miosis cannot explain the phenomena adequately. In addition, most authors have been concerned with the least significant feature of the disturbance, that is, cyst formation. Cysts do occur, but most of the excrescences in this enucleated eye were solid nodules composed entirely of pigment epithelial cells. Furthermore, the cysts which were formed contained fluid permeated with pigment rather than clear fluid, as previously supposed. Of greater significance than the cysts was the new growth of the iris pigment epithelium beyond the borders of its normal limitations. This growth was highly selective, since there was no obvious effect on other structures of the iris or ciliary body. To our knowledge, extension of the epithelium beyond the limits of its supporting mesoderm into the anterior chamber has no parallel in response of the other ocular tissue to medicinal therapy. This proliferation of pigment epithelium is the most intriguing of the tissue changes observed and stimulates most thought, since it is a hyperplasia that borders on neoplasia. Finally,

when treatment is discontinued, these nodules recede. The mechanism of this recession is as much a mystery as their formation, but in all probability they undergo simple atrophy following cessation of stimulation."

(c) A more cautious and thoughtful approach has been advanced by Edwards (1958) when he states:

[1] "All miotics have a place in strabismus diagnosis and treatment. D.F.P. is by far the most powerful and consequently is much better for diagnostic use. However this great strength of D.F.P., and the consequent side effect of iris cysts, make it desirable to use other drugs wherever possible. The occurrence of the iris cysts and pigment epithelium metaplasia must be studied further before they can be dismissed as insignificant tags."

(d) Chin, Gold and Breinin (1964) have advised that a mydriatic (phenylephrine 2.5%) be added to phospholine iodide 0.125% and have observed no cyst formation in 20 cases treated in this manner. Wheeler and Moore (1964) however have found that the use of phenylepherine (Neo-synepherine) "is not quite an ideal solution because of the discomfort caused by Neo-synepherine." Knapp and Campobianco (1956) have reported that, "The danger of iris cysts is minimal if daily instillation is not continued longer than two weeks. In those cases in which the deviation was eliminated on daily instillation of the miotic or by glasses, D.F.P. is administered every other night or less frequently without producing iris cysts of significant size."

(2) *Allergic reactions* have been reported by several authors, Knapp and Capobianco (1956), Hill and Stromberg (1962), Miller (1960) and Records (1967) among others.

(a) These symptoms have taken the form of red eyes, eye pain, puffy lids and brow ache.

[1] Miller (1960) for example found that: "Intolerance to medication was more striking in older children and adolescents. The majority of patients over the age of 13 years refused to use any of the miotics because of intense headache and eyeache. Even the appearance-conscious girls preferred glasses to miotics."

[2] In addition, he reports two cases of superficial punctate keratitis in which the resulting lesions disappeared on the cessation of isoflurophate.

(3) *Blurred vision and micropsia*

(a) These are variously estimated to occur in 1 to 25% of the cases treated.

(4) *Cataract formation*

(a) Chamberlain (1968) reports:

[1] "The possibility of cataract formation following prolonged use of these miotics has been reported, particularly in glaucoma. A single paper in 1960 described transient anterior subcapsular lens opacities in a child on daily DFP for two months. No confirming publications have substantiated this finding in an accommodative strabismus patient. It would seem wise, however, to routinely check all individuals on miotic therapy with

dilation, and to include slit lamp biomicroscopy when feasible."

b. *Systemic side effects*

(1) Allergic Reactions

(a) These have taken various forms such as skin rashes, nausea, tantrums, coughs, yawning, hives, headaches and bed wetting which have all terminated on cessation of the miotic (Knapp and Campobianco, 1956; and Edwards, 1958).

(2) *Depression of blood and tissue cholinesterase* resulting from the use of phospholine iodide.

(a) The anticholinesterase effect at the ciliary motor end plates occurs as well at the myoneural junctions and synapses throughout the entire nervous system. Once this occurs:

[1] Hiscox and McCulloch (1965) find that: "Acetycholine accumulates then exerts its muscarinic action on the heart, smooth muscle and secretory glands, and its nicotinic action on skeletal muscle and autonomic ganglia." They then point out the occurrence of such symptoms as abdominal cramps, diarrhea, nausea and upper respiratory congestion which have been found in patients with glaucoma on prolonged 0.25% phospholine iodide therapy.

[2] Humphreys and Holmes (1963) found that 87% of glaucoma patients treated with phospholine seven months or longer measured blood cholinesterase levels below normal.

(b) Records (1967) points out:

[1] "Systemic absorption occurs via the conjunctival circulation or the mucosa of the nose, pharynx or gastrointestinal tract. Sufficient amount of medication must be absorbed into the general circulation before systemic signs and symptoms of toxicity will appear."

[2] "These include lacrimation, salivation, sweating, intestinal cramps with watery diarrhea, slow pulse, tightness in the chest with wheezing respiration, nausea, vomiting, urinary urgency and general fatigue. Severe intoxications, which are rarely seen may result in larynogospasm, a feeling of weakness and the involuntary twitching of skeletal muscles."

[3] In order to minimize the dangers to the young strabismic undergoing prolonged anticholinesterase therapy, Records advises:

[a] "The orthoptists should be aware of the signs and symptoms of anticholinesterase drug toxicity. Often children will be seen more frequently by the orthoptists during the course of orthoptic therapy than by the attending physician. Accurate observation and early reporting of suggestive signs and symptoms to the attending physician may prevent the development of serious toxic effects."

(c) Chamberlain (1968) warns that should emergency general anesthesia become necessary:

[1] "The possibility of a prolonged effect from succinyl choline can be

of importance. Parents of a child on phospholine iodide treatment should be made aware of this factor so that they may inform their anaesthesiologist in the event that surgery should be necessary. Miotics should be withheld for about six weeks before elective strabismus surgery. D.F.P. apparently does not depress the cholinesterase levels and may therefore be the medication of choice in the management of accommodative strabismus."

[2] Hiscox and McCulloch (1965) have reported a case of cardiac arrest in a glaucoma patient from just such a depression of blood cholinesterase level following prolonged topical use of phospholine iodide.

D. Dosage and Administration

1. *Pilocarpine* acting on the ciliary and iris sphincter muscles directly, is administered in the form of: "aqueous drops in strengths between 0.25 and 4 percent. The miosis lasts for from 8 to 24 hours but is very variable, and is often less marked with young children than with adults. The ciliary spasm lasts about 2 hours and again is usually less in young children than adults" (Whitwell, 1962).

a. Several authors observe that the intended dosage is often diluted by the tendency of children to secrete copious tears, and to spasmodically contract the orbicularis upon topical instillation of the medication. Since the effect on the ciliary lasts only 2 hours or so, it can be seen that frequent instillations are called for to maintain the desired effect on the accommodative mechanism, and through this, the strabismus deviation.

2. *Eserine,* which causes a reversible combination with cholinesterase, may be instilled in strengths of from 0.25 to 2% aqueous or oily solution. Its miotic effect lasts for from 1 to 3 days while the duration of the ciliary spasm is usually 3 hours.

a. Abraham (1949) reports a myopia of 5.00 D. one half hour after the instillation of the first of three drops of 0.25 eserine salicylate at 5 minute intervals. It is generally agreed that the "fierce" reaction to eserine and the need for its frequent instillation make it one of the less desirable miotics.

3. *D.F.P.,* one of the two commonly used long acting cholinesterase inhibitors, is topically instilled once a day or less. Since it hydrolyzes in water to become inactive it must be dissolved in an anhydrous oil base. It is used in strengths of 0.025 to 0.1% in drops or an ointment of 0.35%. Wheeler and Moore (1964) complain that: ". . . weaker solutions become increasingly unstable so that manufacturers have been unwilling to put it on the market as a drop weaker than 0.1 percent; most of us feel that this is too strong for strabismus cases."

a. Several authors warn that care must be taken to avoid picking up tears with the eye dropper on instillation, since their return to the bottle will weaken or inactivate the solution. The recommendation has been made by other writers that instillation be made at bedtime so that the symptoms frequently occurring shortly after the instillation will be masked by sleep. The importance of reducing the dosage and frequency of instillation as rapidly as possible in order to avoid iris cysts is generally conceded.

4. *Phospholine Iodide* is the second of the long acting cholinesterase inhibitors in general usage at this writing. It does not have the disadvantage of hydrolysis in aqueous solution and is much more stable than D.F.P. with the result that despite its tendency to lower the blood and tissue cholinesterase levels, as mentioned previously, "most ophthalmologists are using P.I. for strabismus in 0.125 percent, 0.06 percent or in even weaker dilution" (Wheeler and Moore, 1964).

IV. TRAINING

A. The modern history of scientific functional correction of concomitant strabismus dates from the publication in 1743 of the momentous discovery by the French naturalist, Buffon, that the visual acuity in the deviating eye of the unilateral strabismic is usually subnormal and is capable of improvement in many instances by the prolonged occlusion of the dominant or fixing eye. This was an attack on a monocular perceptual anomaly concomitant with one type of strabismus but did not deal with the motor or binocular perceptual aspects of strabismus. The further practical implementation of the rehabilitation of strabismus awaited first the intervention of the mirror stereoscope by Wheatstone (1838) and then the refracting stereoscope by Brewster shortly thereafter. The elucidation of the relationship between accommodation and convergence by Donders (1864) provided the theoretical framework for developing the first systematic method for the "re-education of binocular vision" by Javal (1864-65). Motivated by the "slaughter of the oculomotor muscles" as he referred to the results obtained by the strabismus surgery techniques then in vogue, Javal for the next thirty years devoted himself to applying the rapidly growing body of knowledge in experimental psychology, physiology, neurology and physiological optics to the problem of re-establishing single binocular vision in the manifest strabismic. Over this period he was able to report literally hundreds of cures obtained by non-surgical means (Javal, 1896).

B. Thus, the modern visual training for strabismus which is employed today is an advanced therapeutic discipline with a long and illustrious history. Orthoptics or orthoptic training has been formerly used as a synonym for visual training but this in some quarters, has come to mean largely or solely the stimulation of fusion reflexes and development of amplitude and quality of fusion, usually on instruments, either as a pre-operative or post-surgical regimen. The term visual training in strabismus, on the other hand, will be used here to embrace the non-surgical treatment of strabismus and includes: occlusion, accommodative-convergence training, the development or improvement of accommodative facility, ocular calisthenics, pleoptics, hand-eye coordination, speed and span of binocular perception and the coordination of visual perceptual and gross motor skills, as well as the more traditional fusion training given both with and without the use of instruments. In general, training procedures for strabismics are systematized in a regimen for eliminating the sensory, perceptual and motor anomalies discovered in the testing program described earlier in Chapter XXX. As has been mentioned previously for testing, the order of training techniques actually utilized may not follow exactly the order presented here which is arranged in a logical sequence for pedagogical reasons. As training proceeds, the order of improvement in skills will necessarily dictate the sequential progression of the actual training stages so that interaction is constantly occurring between areas of improvement and the next level of training undertaken.

C. **Monocular Perceptual and Motor Training**

1. *Perceptual and Sensory*

a. This area usually has to be trained *extensively* only in constant *unilateral strabismus accompanied by amblyopia.* Any attempt to train binocularity before an adequate monocular directional sense in each eye is developed may prove harmful to the long range efforts to achieve functional binocularity. It is helpful and preferable to obtain central fixation and normal or near-normal central acuity but in cases where a lack of neurological integrity of the macular or foveal pathways can be demonstrated, the development of peripheral or para-macular fusion may suffice to enable binocular function alignment to be obtained. The major tasks here are the acquisition of the ability to fixate centrally, i.e. to place the image of an object of interest on the viewing fovea, and the *fixation reflex,* i.e. the ability to maintain the image there over time for both stationary and moving targets. This is usually accomplished in several stages:

(1) Complete Direct Occlusion

(a) If the child is under 5 years of age, the preferred first step is complete monocular occlusion of the non-amblyopic eye, regardless of the fixation pattern. The fixation pattern is evaluated with a visuscope-type instrument and recorded. At biweekly intervals, the fixation pattern is again evaluated and recorded and the single letter and whole line acuity is recorded as well. Tracing, coloring, pointing and picking up small objects all help to enhance the tendency for central fixation.

(2) Use of macular "tags" or cues to the strabismic to indicate the projection line of his own macula.

(a) This may be done in the amblyopic eye itself by means of entoptic phenomena such as Haidinger's Brush or Maxwell's Spot, whose manifestation is restricted to the macular area.

(b) A "tag" may also be placed with the use of after-images. This may be effected homolaterally by an examiner who places the after-image on the amblyopic macula with an ophthalmoscope-euthyscope pleoptophore type of pleoptic instrument or it may be done contralaterally with an after-image which is "transferred" as by the Brock After-Image Transfer technique.

(c) In general the after-image approach has more utility in pursuit and saccadic training over a wide area while the Maxwell Spot and Haidinger Brush are better used for stationary tasks and hand-eye coordination. The transferred after-image has the additional advantage in that it can be used for home training since it does not necessitate a skilled examiner to "objectively" place a light on the amblyopic macula. It requires only a centrally fixing contralateral eye. Since the binocular pathways are being stimulated through the "transfer" process, preparation for the next stage, i.e., binocular interaction is being undertaken as well. It cannot be used on all patients however, especially in cases exhibiting Anomalous Retinal Correspondence, where transfer usually cannot be achieved.

(d) The macular "tags" literally "show" the strabismic where to place his amblyopic macula to fixate centrally. Skills are generally built up in the following order:

[1] Stationary monocular fixation

[a] The subject attempts to fixate letters or numbers, for example, on the face of an instrument capable of producing a Maxwell Spot or Haidinger Brush.

[b] If his fovea wanders from the desired fixation point, he is given immediate visual feedback indicating the direction and magnitude of the error of fixation.

[c] The task is usually easiest to perform at a close distance such as 12 inches, and when ability is somewhat developed at this distance, the distance to the target is gradually increased until accurate pointing is attained at 24 inches.

[2] Stationary monocular fixation with pointing

[a] Once some skill has been gained in fixation with the eye under training so that the target of interest can be placed and retained on the fovea, the next goal is to enhance accurate coordination in the art of visually directed pointing. This is accomplished by using letters or numbers on the face of the instrument producing the entoptic phenomena. Involvement of the hand helps to further stabilize central fixation.

[3] Monocular pursuit or tracking movements

[a] At this stage the patient is usually switched to procedures involving both direct and transferred after-image macular "tags." The patient is then asked to "project" the after-image to a swinging ball suspended on a string, the spot from a flashlight beam shining on the wall, letters on a chart across the room, and similar fixation locales. Once this can be carried out, the patient next "traces" the after-image around picture frames, corners of the room, and finally any object in the field of view.

[4] Monocular saccadic movements

[a] The amblyopic eye, now capable of fixation, pointing and pursuit movements is next trained to fixate one object, then release fixation and take up a new fixation object as directed.

[5] Monocular prism saccadic

[a] A perturbation is now introduced in the saccadic visual-motor task by placing a prism before the amblyopic eye with base-apex line successively oriented in different directions. In this case the figure and ground are both displaced so that visual information derived from an adequate monocular directional sense, must now more fully guide the successful saccadic movement. The training should now continue until the patient not only can re-establish fixation rapidly and with ease, but can also report the apparent movement of the fixated target and the ground for variously oriented prisms of power as small as 2^{Δ}. Flax (1963b) points out that by training this ability to perceive the resulting apparent movement, the integrity of the ocular muscle feed-back information is both enhanced and integrated with that of the visual.

[6] A repetition of [1] to [5] is now carried out still maintaining fixation with the amblyopic eye but at this time leaving the contralateral non-amblyopic eye uncovered.

[7] Again performing tasks [1] to [5] but alternating fixation from one eye to the other.

(e) The amblyopic eye generally by this time has shown a noticeable improvement in central fixation and both single letter and whole line acuity.

(3) Tasks in which the eye leads or directs the hand or foot.

(a) Macular "tags" or cues are no longer used or needed to point out to the patient the projection direction of the fovea. The patient is now asked to perform a variety of tasks in which kinesthetic feedback is matched to the newly learned visual direction of his macula. Such tasks are:

[1] tracing mazes
[2] coloring in or filling in open letters in the newspaper
[3] batting a swinging ball on a string
[4] picking up BB shot with tweezers
[5] bouncing a ball to hit a coin.
[6] darts, quoits, or bow and arrow
[7] kicking a ball

(4) Daily home training is assigned for periods of up to one hour. Occlusion is carried out between office and home training sessions in two modes (Kavner and Suchoff, 1966):

(a) *inverse,*

[1] in which the amblyopic eye is occluded. This mode is generally used until the eye is capable of sustaining central fixation.

(b) *direct,*

[1] once the amblyopic eye can sustain central fixation for a period of an hour the non-amblyopic eye is occluded between tracing sessions.

(c) Partial occlusion is sometimes continued in the form of binasal occluders until fusion can be maintained regularly at some distance.

(5) Pigassou and Toulouse (1967) present yet another approach to the treatment of eccentric fixation in children over 5 years of age with strabismus amblyopia:

(a) Along with complete occlusion of the sound eye, they prescribe an "inverse" prism to be worn in the prescription for the amblyopic eye.

[1] The orientation and power of the prism used are determined by the direction and amount of eccentric fixation. Thus, the orientation of the base is in the same direction as the eccentrically fixating macula, so that for example a nasal fixator would wear the base *in* (inverse).

[2] The power of the prism is determined by the degree of eccentricity and should be slightly greater than this amount, so that for 4° (8^{Δ}) eccentric fixation, a 10° prism should be used.

(b) This procedure is thought to weaken the habitual eccentric fixation response by setting up a kinesthetic-visual mismatch between the straight ahead position and the eccentric fovea. The presence of the prism forces the eye to "redress," e.g. in the example above, to diverge so that the physical position of the macula is in the "straight ahead position." To grasp an object, the patient now moves his hand along the line which the fovea points. The same holds for walking and other activities. Presumably this builds up a proprioceptive ego-centric localization match with the fovea.

[1] As the eccentric area loses the "principal visual direction" i.e. the line along which the hand is directed, there develops a large instability of fixation. The more the amount of eccentricity exhibited originally, the more the instability which is now revealed.

(c) When the fixation is foveal but the acuity is still poor, the prism is reduced, regardless of previous eccentricity to 6°, with the base located in the same inverse direction. Constant direct occlusion is maintained.

(d) The visual acuity then generally improves within a period of 3 weeks to 4 months to close to normal. They allow another month of occlusion to stabilize the result, and then proceed to binocular training.

2. *Motor Training*

a. Eliminate limitations of gaze

(1) These are usually found in the field of gaze opposite the direction of deviation in constant unilateral squints. Vigorous ocular calisthenics are called for to insure complete amplitude of movement in all monocular fields of gaze free from nystagmus and painful or pulling sensations.

b. Develop the quality of movements

(1) Here the tendency to compensate for poor oculomotor skills by head and body movements is eliminated and smooth and steady pursuit movements are instilled. Schrock (1965) points out that five types of extraocular pursuit movements should be trained: horizontal, vertical, oblique, rotary and vergence.

c. Facility of Accommodation

(1) In unilateral strabismics with amblyopia there is frequently found an inequality of direct accommodative response which can be reduced or eliminated with "accommodative rock" training.

(a) An accommodative stimulus target is maintained at a given distance and convex and concave spheres are alternately placed before the eye under training. The patient is asked to clear the target rapidly and sustain each accommodative level called for by the lens change. The power of the lenses is increased when satisfactory accommodative facility is demonstrated at a given dioptric level.

D. Binocular Perceptual and Motor Training

1. Following successful establishment of central monocular fixation and normal motility skills, a meaningful attempt to achieve binocular integration can be inaugerated.

a. It should be noted that equal "whole line" or single letter visual acuity in the two eyes need not be achieved before binocular training is undertaken. Usually, with amblyopes, both types of training may be carried on simultaneously once central fixation and adequate motility skills are achieved.

b. As pointed out earlier, in the chapter on strabismus testing, unless the patient can demonstrate a bona-fide binocular colorluster response at or near the centration point, caution is essential in attempting to break down deep seated strabismic adaptations. If these are disrupted and a masked underlying neurological impairment or deficit is present, intransigent constant diplopia or similar complications may result.

2. *Anomalous correspondence (ARC)*

a. Anomalous correspondence sometimes also called *ambiocularity,* is generally accepted to be an adaptation of the sensorial relationships of the two retinas in which areas that ordinarily project to disparate points in space demonstrate a common visual direction (Levinge, 1954).

b. Anomalous correspondence bears the same relationship in the sequence of binocular training that eccentric fixation does in monocular, i.e. it must be alleviated before further progress can be made toward functional binocularity.

(1) Flom (1963) lists studies by 6 different investigators reporting results in treating constant esotropia with anomalous correspondence, the total results being 17 cures of

305 patients for a cure rate of something slightly over 5%. Exotropes fare much better with 13 cures of 26 patients, a 50% cure rate. Flom estimates that: "anomalous correspondence is present in about 50% of esotropias and is a serious deterrent to functional correction of squint."

(2) It is felt that one of the reasons for the intransigence of the anomalous correspondence perceptual adaptation is that the patient functions so well with it. For example, a relatively full field of view binocularly with rudimentary peripheral stereopsis without diplopia or confusion is manifested under everyday seeing conditions by the strabismic with anomalous correspondence.

c. *Traditional methods of treatment are:*

(1) Occlusion

(a) The idea here is to attempt to weaken the anomalous space percept which requires two seeing eyes by preventing its manifestation through eliminating the stimulation of non-corresponding points in the two eyes.

(b) Practiced in its most rigorous form the occluder is only removed during closely controlled and supervised training sessions.

(c) The occlusion may be complete occlusion of one or alternate eyes or may be partial and accomplished with binasal or bitemporal occluders.

[1] In these latter instances it is felt that only the retinal areas with anomalous common visual directions need be prevented from seeing simultaneously.

(2) Training at the Angle of Deviation (Objective Angle)

(a) Targets are placed along the foveal lines of each eye in an instrument such as a major amblyoscope, mirror cheiroscope or stereoscope and through rapid blinking on the part of the patient, or flashing or oscillating the targets (where this is possible), or changing the levels of illumination between the two eyes, the targets are perceived by the patient to superimpose or fuse (Kramer, 1953).

(b) Lyle and Jackson (1953) recommend in addition a process which they term "Kinetic Biretinal Stimulation" in which the tubes of a major amblyoscope are locked at the patient's angle of squint, and with the patient looking straight ahead, the locked tubes are moved rapidly from side to side through an excursion which varies with the size of the patient's suppression area.

[1] They are of the opinion that the patient learns normal correspondence through this simultaneous stimulation of corresponding points.

(c) Stimulation of "monocular diplopia" (really binocular triplopia) (Walraven Technique) (Stobie, 1955).

[1] This is a program for calling attention to the three images, a fused composite and an extra image, frequently noticed by anomalous corresponders who have been in training for some time at the objective angle.

[a] After the patient has been taught alternate fixation, the angle of the major amblyoscope tubes is made divergent with respect to the patient's objective angle using fovea fusion targets. The patient is

asked to maintain fixation with his habitually nonfixing eye and the targets brought to the subjective angle. Flashing is generally necessary to maintain fixation, and at this point the patient often experiences binocular triplopia.

[b] Since the "true" image located on the nasal retina is dim, it is usually easily suppressed. The patient is asked to concentrate on this "dim" image while the tubes are brought closer to the objective angle. Flashing and blinking are usually necessary to keep the two images visible and to maintain the fixation of the habitually deviating eye.

[c] The "true image" becomes less dim and if all goes well fusion occurs. Concentration by the patient on the fused image causes the false or "extra" image to dim and eventually disappear.

(d) Use of vertical dissociation (Ludlam, 1962).

[1] With perimacular targets set at the patient's objective angle, 30° or 40$^{\Delta}$ of vertical dissociation is introduced. Whereas a horizontal separation of the two targets in agreement with the angle of anomaly is found with no vertical dissociation, the two targets usually are seen to line up vertically one above the other, with *no* horizontal displacement with the large vertical dissociation in place.

[2] The vertical displacement is then slowly reduced while the two targets remain one above the other. Usually, when the two targets approach to the point of just touching, they "spring apart" to the horizontal separation dictated by the angle of anomaly. The formerly B.U. prism is then placed B.D., and the process repeated.

[3] Placing a +12 D. sphere in the lens well before each eye, or a red glass before one and a target before the other, will frequently allow the targets to be superimposed from a vertical direction but still not from the horizontal.

[4] Once superimposition is achieved, some of the previous techniques listed are used to expand the range of normal correspondence.

(3) The Use of After-Images

(a) Tomlinson (1965) reports 60 to 75% of cases restored to normal retinal correspondence (N.R.C.) after use of the "after-image method." In this technique the patient has an annular after-image impressed on the macula of one eye with a euthyscope-pleoptophore type of ophthalmoscope. Para-foveal superimposition targets are then employed in a major amblyoscope and the subject is asked to attempt to superimpose the targets "in the center of the doughnut after-image."

[1] Reportedly, the subjective angle repeatedly coincides with the objective angle after several attempts in most cases.

(b) At this time the course of treatment proceeds with the use of fusion and stereo targets for the duration of the after-image which is reinforced upon fading.

(c) Tomlinson reports that even when "the subjective angle remains anomalous it is almost invariably closer to the objective angle than before the after-image was induced."

(d) Between treatments one eye is constantly occluded either unilaterally or alternately depending on fixation preferences to prevent simultaneous stimulation of non-corresponding points.

(4) Physiologic Diplopia

(a) Tibbs (1958) advocates the training of normal physiological diplopia in space. She notes the very frequent occurrence of the establishment of N.R.C. responses in an amblyoscope with the patient still demonstrating A.R.C. on a red-green test in space.

(b) A red filter before one eye is used to make it easier to identify normal physiological diplopia when it occurs. The patient, an esotrope, is directed to fixate a light at, or nearer than, his centration point with his left eye, with the red filter before his right. The examiner rapidly covers and uncovers the patients right eye (filter) and requests the patient to report the position of the "blinking red light" at distance. Once the patient consistently reports this blinking red light on the right of the near light, the covering and uncovering is stopped and the patient asked to note that the near light (or lights) appear(s) "framed" by (i.e. lies between) the red and white lights at distance.

[1] This procedure has now established a normal correspondence response in the periphery where it is usually easiest to demonstrate.

(c) In order to next establish normal physiological diplopia in the paramacular and macular areas, the patient, while fixating the near light along his midline, walks toward the distant light. The separation of these diplopic images decreases as he nears the distance light and suppression or reversion to ARC usually occurs.

[1] Rapid cover-uncover at a distance several steps back from the point where the "framing" was lost usually restores the previous NRC response and the advance continues until the two objects fall within Panum's fusional areas, and are fused.

(5) Luster Through The Closed Lid (Brock, 1941; Schrock, 1966)

(a) The patient is requested to view a gray card upon which is a black dot, with one eye closed, at a distance of 5 feet. Taking into account the angle of strabismus deviation, a lighted penlight is placed approximately on the visual axis against the lid of the closed eye.

(b) The patient is then asked if he is able to see the red glow resulting from the light shining through the closed lid at the same time as he sees the black dot on the gray card with the open eye.

[1] Blinking the open eye and rhythmically flashing the transilluminating light both help to achieve this objective.

(c) The next aim is to ascertain whether the light is seen in the same direction as the contralaterally viewed black spot.

[1] Moving the light before the closed lid in the direction necessary to achieve superimposition usually effects this goal.

(d) The third aspect of correct response in this test is to ascertain whether the red glow is perceived by the patient to lie directly in front of the closed eye or is "projected" "as a general red glow . . . . . . a luster effect over the gray cardboard" (Brock, 1941). This projection is often the most difficult of the three objectives to meet and may require time.

[1] When used as a home training exercise, the attempt to project the glow may be used with any number of familiar objects around the room, e.g., faces, lamp shades, venetian blinds, or pictures on the wall.

[2] Often the proper "projection effects" can be accomplished when one eye, for example, the right one, is open, but when attempted with the left eye open, the same results are not immediately achieved.

[3] Progress resulting from work with the recalcitrant eye, while slow, is usually successful in achieving luster and "projected glow."

(6) Newer Approaches

(a) *Vary the Squint Angle*

[1] It has been observed that anomalous corresponders with constant esotropia, which are generally held to constitute the most intractable group, almost always have in addition to their constant strabismus an invariant angle of anomaly at all times and fixation distances. It was hypothecated that this invariance of the difference between the objective and subjective angle of squint, called "co-variation" by Halldén (1952), provides the basic spatial and kinesthetic support for the anomalous perceptual system. Many cases were also observed to be either fully corrected hyperopes or to have no refractive error. Two approaches are therefore used to attempt to introduce some variation into the angle of anomaly. This is accomplished by the prescription of either a change of lens power (either isometropic or anisometropic) or introduction of prism, or both.

(b) *Prism*

[1] In this technique, similar to that first advocated by Peckham in the 1940s, the arbitrary inclusion of 8°BO in one lens and 8°BU in the other is made, in an attempt to "dissociate" the visual phenomena and the kinesthetic or proprioceptive feedback from the extraocular muscles maintaining the constant angle of anomaly. The patient usually responds by changing his deviation in several days, if not hours, in such manner as to maintain the same relative position of the retinal imagery in each eye. Once this happens the practitioner switches the left lens to the right eye and right to left. The anomalous corresponder, if he now wishes to keep the same relative retinal image positions must make the opposite vergence and supraduction movement.

(c) *Lens Power Change*

[1] At the same time that the prism is being varied, changes in spherical lens power are introduced. If the patient is an alternator this change is

frequently made in anisometropic form.

[a] Thus an isometropic hyperope wearing a full prescription of +3.00D might, for example, be started with the Rx:
R. +1.00D = 10° BI
L. +2.00 = 8° BO

[2] This would introduce variable accommodative as well as prismatic effects which would serve the purpose of "stressing" or introducing a mismatch into this "artificially contrived" system of binocular vision. These effects can be made opposite when the right and left lenses are switched. The exact lens power and prism values having maximal effect can be worked out empirically in a training session. The patient and parent are both warned that the onset of diplopia is a good sign, much sought after, and if it is too annoying for the child, a clip-on occluder is placed on one eye for at least part of each day.

(d) Ludlam (1961) has also reported that the peripheral fields frequently exhibit normal correspondence in the after-image test while demonstrating ARC when sampled at the macula. In addition, almost always, the *removal of contours or borders* from the binocular field will allow a normal binocular luster response to be exhibited. Utilizing both of these phenomena, the following training program has been introduced.

[1] The patient, wearing red-green anaglyph glasses, faces a smooth well-illuminated wall having no borders, shadows or contours at a distance corresponding to his centration point. Binocular color luster is experienced under these circumstances. This can best be identified as an integration or mixture of the two monocularly seen colors. Objects such as cloth felt animals, houses, trees, etc., which cling to the wall are introduced from the periphery into the patient's binocular field while the patient continues to fixate the "bare wall" and experience luster. When the objects approach the macula too closely a "split field" response i.e. half red-half green, is usually perceived.

[a] If this happens at the moment *any* object is introduced into the binocular field, the contrast of the borders is lowered by lowering the level of illumination and placing e.g. +15.00D spheres in clip-on form on the patient's glasses. These procedures are generally effective in enabling objects to be introduced into the periphery of the patient's binocular field. Moving the patient closer to and farther from the wall, while his head is moved laterally and vertically and he blinks his eyes will usually produce an initial split-field response, i.e., A.R.C., but with continued practice, the response can usually be converted to binocular luster (N.R.C.) under all of these conditions.

[2] The patient is next switched to anaglyph peripheral stereo responses e.g. the Keystone stereo motivator followed by the intermediate viewer with perimacular stereoptic targets, and the case completed with more traditional paramacular and macular fusion and stereoptic approach in and out of instruments.

(e) *Rapid Alternate Flash*

[1] It has been observed by clinicians for some time that rapid alternate

flash on a major amblyoscope and rapid blinking are effective means of securing N.R.C. responses at the objective angle at which A.R.C. is experienced under the same conditions without the blinking or flashing. Gibson and Meakin (1951) have described a therapy designed to convert A.R.C. to N.R.C. using a symmetrical binocular flashing technique. Allen (1966) has developed an instrument which makes use of the Bartley Brightness Enhancement Phenomenon and has claimed that application of the technique for as little as 15 minutes converted one patient from a previously anomalous response on the Bielschowsky after-image test to that of normal correspondence. He explains that by introducing rapid alternating flashes of light at approximately alpha rhythm frequency, the visual system does not have time "to build up normal inhibitory interactions, hence such frequencies are capable of penetrating 'functional' blocks and preventing the operation of 'defense mechanisms' and other inhibitory phenomena" (Allen, 1966).

(f) *After-Image Transfer Training (Ludlam)*

[1] An intense long lasting after-image of a vertical line is implanted on the fovea and macula of one eye by means of a xenon strobe lamp.

[2] The patient then covers that eye and attempts to project a transferred after-image to the contralateral eye, similar to the technique of macular after-image "tags" described earlier in this chapter under amblyopia treatment.

[a] Often it is found that the transfer can occur in one direction, as, for example, the direct after-image of the left eye is transferred to the right eye, but not the reverse. This is similar to the effect described previously for luster through the closed lid, wherein 'projection' of the glow can also only be effectuated in one direction, as with the left eye but not the right.

[3] Repeated flashing will usually bring about, first, intermittent "transfer," followed after further repetition by regular "transfer."

[4] The transferred after-image is then traced around the borders of objects at different distances to further integrate and reinforce the "correct" perceptual-motor relationships.

3. *Fusion Reflex*

a. Once ARC has been eliminated an attempt may be made to establish binocular integration. Constant strabismics who have not had an opportunity to bifixate for many years are generally unable to make a positive bifoveal motor fusion response in a contrived diplopia situation to eliminate the diplopia by fusion as the normal observer can, but frequently will either suppress or actually repel the two perceived images of the object so that their separation is increased. The development of the *fusion reflex,* thus, is as important to functional binocularity as the development of the *fixation reflex* is to monocular rehabilitation in amblyopia.

b. *In Instruments.*

(1) In using an amblyscope or stereoscope-type instrument, fusion targets are placed near the objective angle and the patient encouraged to blink, squint and exert effort to

reduce the separation and accomplish superimposition and fusion. It is important to eliminate any residual vertical displacement when the fusion reflex is being thus stimulated. Flashing lights, oscillating the targets, changing the relative level of illumination between the two eyes, and the introduction of lenses to stimulate accommodation are all helpful in bringing about a fusion movement.

c. *In Space*

(1) A 3° B.O. or B.I. prism is interposed at the centration point, with the patient viewing a target he is holding, e.g. a pencil. The same regimen as described above is carried out to stimulate a fusion reflex movement. Two advantages are:

(a) The patient has actual tactual and kinesthetic knowledge of the location of the object he is attempting to fuse, and

(b) he can move the object closer and further as well as transversely to provide still other cues and stimuli for fusion.

4. *Physiological Diplopia Training*

a. Once the subject can fuse at the centration point in space and can make small "jump" fusion recovery movements, a corresponding point horopter in the macular area has been established, in effect. This "small central horopter" can be expanded to the periphery by stimulating the awareness of physiological diplopia, i.e. the diplopic nature of extra-horopteral points.

(1) Employing the same space training situation described above for training the fusion reflex, a second object is held or placed about one foot behind the initially fixated object.

(a) At this stage diplopia is usually experienced.

(2) The second object is slowly brought closer and the diplopic awareness of the now more closely spaced images is maintained.

(3) Once this is accomplished without occurrence of suppressions, the second object is then placed nearer to the patient than the fixated object and diplopic awareness trained from this direction as the objects are brought closer together.

b. A third step in physiological diplopia training is the establishment of what Ludlam has termed *"Panoramic Physiological Diplopia."* Here the subject, while bi-fixing an object at his centration point, is asked to be aware of the diplopic nature of all the objects in his surround (near and far) which do not lie on the corresponding point horopter.

5. *Building Quality of Fusion and Stereopsis – Antisuppression Training*

a. With fusion developed at the objective angle in instruments and at the centration point in space, and the ability to recognize the diplopic nature of extra horopteral objects established, the next procedure is to reduce the effective size of Panum's Fusional areas, eliminate suppressions and enhance stereoptic awareness and stereo acuity.

(1) These objectives can largely be met by training upon instruments with controlled stereo targets, macular or paramacular fusion targets, and pointers, and cheiroscopic tracing, all at the objective angle.

6. *Fusion Amplitudes*

a. Fusional amplitudes of two varieties are developed, upon instruments and in space.

(1) Smooth

(a) In this type, appropriate vergence movements must be made by the patient to keep objects in space or targets in instruments fused while the vergence demand is *continuously* varied. In some instrument situations, where the accommodative demand level is kept constant, motor fusion (relative positive or relative negative vergence) is demanded. In space and other instrumentation, accommodation and convergence are allowed to vary simultaneously. The latter is generally considered the more primitive skill and easier to develop initially. The targets used in instruments may be flat fusion or stereo targets.

(2) Jump or Discrete

(a) In this form, an abrupt instantaneous change in vergence is demanded, usually by the introduction of B.O. or B.I. loose prism. The fixated object of interest should be perceived as double and a corrective or compensatory vergence or duction movement made to re-fuse the images. This sequence is then repeated at different fixation distances and in different fields of gaze. The prism is introduced with the base apex line slightly (5° to 15°) tilted away from the horizontal so that some supra and infra duction, as well, is demanded in the recovery movement.

[1] A variation of this technique is the covering and uncovering of one eye with prism in place. Fusion is interrupted and then regained after removal of the cover.

[a] The base of the prism may be initially oriented to aid fusion, (e.g., B.O. in esotropia) and the power reduced as the jump duction recovery amplitudes increase.

[b] After sufficient skill is developed, the base should be placed opposite to the direction which had abetted recovery of the original imbalance, (e.g., now B.I. for esotropia) and the power increased as rapidly as the acquired skill will allow.

[c] This can be used to expand the jump recovery ranges in various fields of gaze, where limitation of gaze, or incomitancy, is discovered.

[d] This cover-uncover-recovery technique has been found especially useful in cases of the so-called "A" and "V" syndrome discussed in Chapter XXIX "Non-Comitant Strabismus." Here the size of the horizontal imbalance is found to vary with the level of gaze in the vertical meridian. From the centration point where fusion has been established, the gaze is elevated and cover-uncover and jump-duction is then developed with loose prism. The procedure is repeated for ever increasing amounts of elevation and depression of gaze.

[e] Another version of the technique is to maintain a given object of fixation with prism in place and by means of head nods, swings

and rotations of the eyes move fixation to different affected areas of gaze where a variable angle or limited motility is found.

7. *Dissociation of Accommodation and Convergence*

a. In the previous methods which have attempted to bring about binocular integration, no specific effort was made to establish amplitudes of accommodation free of convergence, (relative accommodation) although when ranges of motor fusion are established, relative convergence free of accommodation is a result. Two methods of dissociating the accommodative function from convergence are in common usage.

(1) Stereoscope tromboning.

(a) By manipulating the separation of the targets to be fused, conditions can be created where a positive stimulus to accommodation with increasing amounts of divergence are demanded, i.e. when a wide separation (generally 9 cm or more depending on the P.D. and instrument optics) between the targets is presented and the card holder is brought nearer to the patient. When the card holder is pushed further out on the shaft, the demand for relaxation of accommodation and a decrease in divergence is made by use of this same target.

(b) By the use of narrow target separations, (e.g. 4 cm or less depending again on the P.D.) a requirement of ever increasing convergence and positive accommodative stimulus accompanies advancement of the slide toward the subject, while decreasing convergence demand accompanies relaxation of accommodation when the slide carrier is pushed away. Tromboning, i.e. the continuous movement of the slides of different separations in and out on the shaft with an attempt by the patient to maintain fusion and clarity, will assist in developing relative accommodation and convergence amplitudes.

(2) Binocular accommodative rock is also an effective means of building up relative accommodative amplitude.

(a) An adequate accommodative stimulus is maintained at a fixed distance (newsprint at 16″ for example) and a binocular convex dioptric stimulus is presented (e.g. +2.00). The patient is asked to clear the writing while keeping it single thus exerting negative relative accommodation. Paired concave lenses (e.g. −2.00 D) are next introduced requiring a positive relative accommodation response to clear it and yet maintain fusion.

E. Gross Motor and Perceptual Motor Training

1. As stated in the previous chapter on Testing, the present state of the art of formalized testing and training of perceptual motor and gross motor relationships in strabismus is not advanced and the following material is mostly derived from Ludlam (manuscript in preparation). It is an area however, that is furnishing techniques which enable training to be performed on younger children than ever before, and which is making it possible for "curved" strabismics to perform as binocular individuals rather than the "straight eyed squinters" referred to by Flax (1963a). It should be pointed out that it is very possible for a strabismic to build a relatively effective performance pattern despite moderate to serious deficiencies in one or more motor areas. Flax (1964) in this regard, points out, "This becomes very apparent in the treatment, for instance, of strabismus. Gross motor procedures are apt to have a favorable effect on ocular posture if properly applied in the formative years to an individual who has not adequately compensated to the ocular deviancy; they are not apt to change the eye position of a well adjusted strabismic who has managed to achieve good bodily coordination, good balance, good bi-lateral interweaving, and adequate spatial ability despite the ablation or serious distortion of one visual circuit."

a. *Bilateral Performance*

(1) Bissaillon in 1957, holding that strabismus is so frequently only a local manifestation of a general lack of coordination suggests the therapeutic utilization of directed play activities with emphasis placed on bilateral experiences such as:

(a) swinging while suspended by two hands
(b) trampoline
(c) bouncing hobby horse
(d) swings
(e) wheelbarrow
(f) jungle gym

as well as many of the more traditional orthoptics and visual training techniques.

(2) Additional activities found to be helpful in this same regard are:

(a) jumping rope
(b) swimming
(c) bicycle riding
(d) basketball throwing (two hands)
(e) drawing two circles simultaneously on the blackboard.

b. *Balance*

(1) Wearing anaglyph glasses and neutralizing prism over his habitual correction, the patient views a peripheral stereo target placed at the end of a 12 foot long walking board and mounts and starts across viewing the stereo target the entire time. It is hoped that the equalization of vestibular and postural innervations brought about to support the balancing task will allow better binocular performance. This device is frequently found to be helpful in this regard.

c. *Perturbation of the Strabismus Perceptual Adaptations*

(1) The following techniques have proven useful clinically not only by providing a faster breakdown of strabismic perceptual adaptations during the actual training period but also by apparently helping to integrate binocular pattern with the other sensory and motor systems to provide for a more lasting functional cure.

(2) The patient standing on one leg while leaning sideways and wearing anaglyph glasses, attempts to elicit physiological diplopia. Anti-suppression training and development of the fusion reflex at the spatial centration point are carried out while this posture is maintained. Some patients are able to manifest and sustain normal responses in the skewed or bent position, for weeks and even months during training before they can manifest these binocular fusion responses in the upright position. The probable reasons postulated for the success of these techniques have been offered under Gross Motor and Perceptual Motor Testing in Chapter XXIX.

(a) Ludlam has observed several patients who have been able to project a "transferred" after-image only when the body is leaning over to such an extent that both eyes are on one side of the body midline long after the eyes were straight and presumably "functionally binocular."

(b) Several additional patients have been able to increase binocular span of perception on the tachistoscope in a "leaned" (10° to 20° from vertical) position up to a level not achievable in the upright position even after aligned functional binocularity has been achieved.

(3) Development of various aspects of binocularity both while a child is dizzy from being spun on the examiner's stool and while bending over looking through his legs are training procedures previously mentioned in Chapter XXX on Testing and sometimes provide a breakthrough opportunity in difficult cases when none other is readily available.

d. *The Planned Introduction of Noise and Interference*

(1) It has been frequently noticed (Ludlam) that a former strabismic who has just recently regained binocularity is quite susceptible to loss of binocularity and a temporary return to a strabismic posture from such apparently unrelated stimuli as hunger, anger, sickness, fatigue, surprise, or a strong emotional feeling about something. The introduction of noise and interference during the training procedures by which the binocular skills are being learned has been found helpful (Ludlam) in shortening this period of susceptibility to loss of binocularity due to non-visual influences. Once some level of binocularity has been achieved both with and without instruments, the examiner, after explaining the intent of such actions to the patient should make it a practice to talk to the patient during the sessions, clap his hands, pound the table, stomp the floor, drop a book, slam the door, laugh, involve the patient in conversation and otherwise provide a continuous barrage of extraneous stimuli during the time in which the patient is building his functional binocularity.

F. Side Effects and Complications

1. Since visual training is the conservative "natural" or physiological method of treating strabismus, employing "nature's tools" (Lancaster, 1967), and allowing time for the visual system to adapt to the changed visual inputs and oculomotor innervation which have been coaxed rather than forced, it would seem *a priori* that serious complications would be non-existent. Workers in the field have found, however, that at the outset, some temporary discomforts frequently accompany training but that these generally disappear quickly with proper management. These untoward concomitants are:

a. headaches
b. diplopia and visual confusion
c. pulling or strain
d. perceived spatial distortion
e. dizziness and nausea
f. blurred vision
g. loss of balance
h. initial decrease in reading ability or school performance

V. SURGERY

A. This is one of the oldest methods of treatment of concomitant strabismus. The usual surgical program involves hospitalization of from two to five days, a general anesthetic for all children and for "nervous" adults, complete binocular occlusion with bandages for one to three days after the procedure has been performed, atropinization and avoidance of near work for a period of about a month, removal of the sutures a week after their implantation, the home instillation of medication to aid healing and to reduce swelling and redness, and regular after care visits to the surgeon for at least three months.

1. Alone it is usually not successful in securing a lasting functional binocular result. As Kennedy and McCarthy (1959) observe at the conclusion of their study of surgical results on 315 esotropes:

a. "With surgery, one can only *attempt* to align the eyes; it does not of itself purport to keep them where they were placed. Where they eventually stabilize depends on the particular idiosyncrasies of each individual patient, and one cannot always forecast the long term outcome."

2. Surgery does have the advantage however of usually producing *some* results *quickly*. In the case of large angles of deviation it is often necessary to include surgery along with refractive correction and training to effectuate a lasting result.

B. Strabismus Surgery At An Early Age

1. *A priori* it might seem that the greatest usefulness for the surgical approach to strabismus care would be in cases of very young infants where alignment of the visual axes could be "mechanically" effected and the opportunity offered for the establishment of normal optomotor reflexes, with prevention of the establishment of anomalous perceptual adaptations such as amblyopia and anomalous correspondence.

a. Based on a sample of 50 patients Ing, Costenbader, Parks and Albert (1961), have claimed that the earlier the operation, the better the fusion and alignment of the former esotropic deviation obtained. Thus they conclude: "Binocularity can be attained by the early surgery of the congenital esotropia. Surgical treatment before the age of one year gives the highest percentage of patients exhibiting binocularity."

b. Taylor, D. (1967) basing his views on a study of 117 patients, suggests that delaying surgery beyond twelve months of age will lessen the probability of converting a tropia to a phoria.

c. Fisher, Flom and Jampolsky (1968) subjected to statistical analysis the data upon which these claims were made and found neither claim to be justified. They found that fusion is no more likely to occur when surgery is performed between six and 12 months than between 12 and 18 months, and conversion of a tropia to a phoria is no more likely to occur between six and 12 months of age than between 12 and 24 months. When surgery is performed using Taylor's surgical technique and with no training, the results after 24 and 36 months are claimed to be significantly worse than those performed at an earlier age.

d. In a still further report stressing the need for early surgery, Nutt (1961) reported a series of 44 concomitant convergent strabismics operated upon before their 3rd birthday whose onset of the strabismus had occurred from birth to 18 months of age. He found that the results "are not encouraging" in that not one patient had achieved binocular single vision. The author nevertheless concludes, "Although the results are disappointing, I would still advocate early operation."

e. Fletcher and Silverman (1966) provide data on 96 cases of infantile esotropia which lends support to a skeptical outlook for the results of early surgery. They report that results in 40% of the cases operated upon under 18 months of age were found to be "unacceptable," whereas less than 10% of those operated between 18 months and seven years could be placed in this unsatisfactory category. They conclude: "The children operated on from the age of four to 18 months did *not* obtain better fusion than those in any other age group. There is, indeed, an alarming number of children in the young age group who are considered unacceptable."

(1) In addition to the alarmingly poorer results the authors found that "those children operated on at four to 18 months had a higher incidence of multiple surgeries (72%) and vertical muscle surgeries (35%)."

f. From the evidence presented by Folk (1956) there does not appear to be any advantage in early surgery of exotropia either.

g. Others, notably Bonsor (1959) and Illingworth (1959), point to the possible psychological trauma involved in the hospital stay and from the general anesthetic.

C. Surgical Objective

1. The usual objective of surgical procedures on the extraocular muscles in strabismus is to either weaken or strengthen the *action* of certain of these muscles (Simpson, 1956). This is true even though "the basic factors in the etiology of strabismus are rarely in the muscles themselves and thus the "surgical procedures are not directed at the primary pathogenesis" (Costenbader and Albert, 1962).

2. Surgery can be said to change the binocular alignment by altering the *action* of those muscles operated upon such that the mechanical forces which are brought to bear on the globe are changed.

3. "In addition things other than basic alignment may be purposely or inadvertently changed" e.g. proptosis, enophthalmos, torticollis, head positioning, the accommodative-convergence relationship, and the size of the palpebral aperture. Costenbader and Albert point out that:

a. "An incomitant deviation may be made more comitant by appropriate surgery. On the other hand, at times, asymmetrical surgery may result in incomitance."

D. Types of Surgical Procedure

1. Although there are various combinations of procedures advocated by many authors in the field, the basic isolated procedures on the horizontal muscles are as follows:

2. *Procedures intended to weaken the action of muscles*

a. Tenotomy

(1) The first surgical procedure, the tenotomy, employed in the treatment of strabismus was originally used by Dieffenback in 1839. This simply consisted of cutting the muscle at its insertion, and was referred to by Javal as "the slaughter of the oculomotor muscles." It is rarely performed today except in cases involving spasm of the inferior oblique which is either secondary to paresis or paralysis of the opposite superior rectus, or in rare primary cases: It is also performed on an eye afflicted with incurable paralysis of the superior oblique (Perera, 1949).

b. Recession

(1) The recession consists of a tenotomy followed by the reattachment of the tendon of the sectioned muscle by suturing it at a selected point back of its original attachment (Perera, 1949). It also reduces the action of the muscle on which it is performed but provides an "element of *precision and safety* lacking in tenotomy."

c. Tendon lengthening

(1) This is a procedure described by Hollwich (1966) as corresponding "to the orthopedic principle of restoration of the form and function of ocular motility by eliminating the shortening of the strabismic muscle." There have been many modifications of the original technique described by Gonin (1911) but all utilize the original insertion or part of it and effectuate the lengthening of the muscle tendon "by means of a tongue-shaped displacement and suture" Hollwich (1966).

3. *Procedures designed to strengthen or increase the action of a muscle*

a. Advancement

(1) In this procedure, the insertion of the muscle on the globe is moved forward (nearer the cornea) with resulting increase in leverage for a given amount of muscle contraction. Some degree of enophthalmos is an obvious concomitant.

b. Resection

(1) In this case a piece of the muscle or tendon is cut out and the ends of the remaining muscle are sutured together, resulting in a shortened muscle. Again, the associated enophthalmos must be considered.

c. Tendon or Muscle Tucking

(1) This is a method of effecting a permanent shortening of a muscle by means of a fold or tuck in the muscle or tendon.

E. General Considerations

1. *Procedures of choice*

a. Costenbader and Albert (1962) recommend the following procedures in concomitant strabismus.

b. For exotropia

(1) The choices lie between tightening the lateral recti and relaxing the medial recti muscles, whether bilateral or unilateral procedures should be undertaken; and if unilateral, whether more than one muscle should be included. Factors which control the decision are: the size of the deviation, the accommodative-convergence relationship, palpebral fissure abnormalities, and tendencies to incomitance.

(a) *Purely non-accommodative esotropia*

[1] The deviation should be fully corrected if the possibility of achieving binocular vision is thought to exist. If not, an undercorrection is recommended. If the deviation measures greater than 25°, "a bilateral medial rectus recession or a recession of the medial and resection of the lateral recti of the same eye are the procedures of choice."

(b) *Partly accommodative*

[1] The accommodative element should be estimated by the wearing of a full cycloplegic correction and miotics for at least six to eight weeks. Only the non-accommodative element should be operated. If the esotropic deviation is larger at near than distance, a relaxing procedure e.g. recession of the medial rectus is recommended since this has a greater effect at near than distance.

(c) *Purely accommodative esotropia*

[1] This condition is generally not ideally suited for surgery.

c. For exotropia

(1) Again the fundamental surgical choices lie between relaxing the lateral recti or tightening of the medial recti. The decision is again influenced by the accommodative-convergence relationship, size of the deviation and the status of the palpebral fissure.

(a) *Constant exotropia*

[1] A slight overcorrection which may induce temporary diplopia is advised. The combination of procedures utilized depends on whether the exotropia is greater for distance or near. If greater at distance, recession of the lateral recti is recommended as being most effective, while if the near deviation is larger, resection of the medial recti is the indicated choice.

(b) *Intermittent exotropia*

[1] The authors warn that undercorrection, overcorrection and recurrence of the deviation are not unusual, so that Costenbader and Albert recommend a conservative course as follows:

[a] "Thus it would seem wise to reserve surgery for those patients whose exotropia is moderate to large, frequent and annoying to them."

d. Hypertropia

(1) This is felt by Costenbader and Albert to be an unusual type of case since "comitant vertical deviations are rarely encountered." If they do occur, conservative surgery on the vertical recti is recommended. They recommend care from the additional point of view of adversely affecting the resultant lid position.

2. *Influence of Heredity*

a. Schlossman and Priestly (1952) after stating that: "The most important and controversial subject in strabimus is the correlation between the type and amount of squint and the type and amount of surgical correction" point out that the predictability of the result of a contemplated procedure is improved if the results obtained on another strabismic member of the family are observed. They present several examples to substantiate this thesis.

3. *The Relation Between Size of Original Deviation, Amount of Surgery and Results*

a. There have been many rules and formulas relating the linear change of muscle tendon or position of insertion produced by surgery to the change in the strabismic angle, such as those offered by Obrien (1951). However, it is now generally recognized that no predictable or meaningful relationship usually exists (Schlossman and Priestly, 1952), and rules for the purpose are without merit (Breinin, 1967).

(1) Little or no relationship has been found between the measuring prism and the amount of surgery performed as measured by calipers in millimeters (Scobee, 1951; Cashell, 1952; Schlossman and Priestley, 1952; Costenbader and Albert, 1962; and Breinin, 1967).

(a) Cashell (1952) reports that a combined movement of the medial and lateral recti of 10 mm. produced a change of angle from 14° to 68°.

(2) Scobee (1951) points out that the amount of surgical correction obtained in a

patient with esotropia is far more likely to be directly proportional to the extent of deviation present before the surgery than to the mm. measurement of the surgery.

(3) Multiple factors affect the surgical decision and result, so that purely mechanical concepts of surgery are inadequate (Breinin, 1967).

b. Strabismus surgical technique then, would seem to be largely an art, the success of which, in a given instance, depends upon the surgeon's personal experience in observing and considering a multiplicity of factors as well as the surgeon's assessment of the "particular idiosyncrasies" manifested in each individual case (Kennedy and McCarthy, 1959).

F. Complications

1. A traumatic approach such as surgery to the delicate tissues of the ocular adnexa made while the patient is under the effects of general anesthesia, not surprisingly, frequently causes multiple complications. Dunlap (1966) observes that:

a. "The great majority of complications occurring in the surgical treatment of strabismus are created by the surgeon. These complications result from sins of both omission and commission. They may be divided into three groups arising from (1) inadequate examination or knowledge, leading to incomplete or inaccurate diagnosis and evaluation; (2) errors in surgical judgement, leading to overcorrections, undercorrections or new forms of imbalance; (3) poor surgical techniques, leading to a wide variety of abnormal results in function or appearance, or to the creation of new pathology."

b. "Occasionally a complication may occur as an unforseeable accident that is not the fault of the surgeon."

2. The complications which may result have been classified here in six categories:

a. *Oculomotor*

(1) These usually result from errors in surgical technique or judgement such as rough handling of tissue, poor dissection, improper use of muscle hook to free adhesions, rough sponging, or failure of the surgeon to effect proper hemostasis, causing adhesions (Dunlap, 1966).

(2) Problems commonly observed to arise in the resulting post-surgical oculomotor performance, include:

(a) limitation of gaze
(b) induced incomitance
(c) overcorrection
(d) undercorrection
(e) induced cyclotropia
(f) induced vertical tropia
(g) pain on excursion

b. *Ocular*

(1) Serious ocular after effects have been reported and observed as follows:

(a) Amputation neuromas of the eye muscles (Wolter and Benz, 1964)
(b) Marginal keratitis and corneal ulceration (Nauheim, 1962)
(c) Unsightly redness and scar tissue

(d) Anisocoria
(e) Retinal tears (Dunlap, 1966)
(f) Postoperative infections
(g) Postoperative detachment of a muscle
(h) Sunken caruncle (Dunlap, 1966)
(i) Inclusion cysts

c. *Postural.*

(1) When cyclotorsional incomitancies have been induced by poor surgical technique and adhesions, the patient often compensates by a head tilt or turn and/or body torque. This enables him to utilize his remaining oculomotor function at maximum effectivity in order to maintain single binocular vision and comfort.

d. *Visual*

(1) Posner and Schlossman, (1951) point out that since the time of von Graefe, diplopia has been, on occasion, an annoying postoperative complication following the surgical treatment of strabismus.

e. *Psychological and Educational*

(1) Psychological

(a) The strabismic child tends to exhibit or manifest more psychological problems than does the non-strabismic control (Pollie, Hafner, and Krasnoff, 1964). Bonsor (1959) has observed that, the psychologic trauma produced by surgery, under general anesthesia, to so precious an organ as the eye, appears to be immense to such a child.

(2) Educational

(a) Ruedemann (1953), in reviewing over 20 years of experience in treating strabismus with resulting functional performance in only 10% of cases, finds himself repeatedly "embarrassed and chagrined" that the treated eyes tend to revert to their pre-operative deviation and that "the central vision of the operated eye is not maintained." He also notes: "Although the youngster is somewhat improved many are unable to carry on in school at an intelligence level equal to their age and normal social group."

[1] He further states: "It was my contention as long as 20 years ago that unless we carried these patients completely to 3rd grade fusion and unless they could hold this fusion over long enough periods of time with good fusional amplitude, we were developing our own group of neurotics, our own group of people who had nervous breakdowns, and people with inferior intellectual abilities."

(b) Flax (1963) agrees, noting that the relationship between visual space, auditory space, kinesthetic space, and verbal space exists even if the eyes are not aligned, and he does not wonder that strabismus surgery which causes enormous dislocations in these perceptual matchings has such dismal results. He concludes:

[1] "It is not surprising that so few postoperative patients ever manage to utilize their eyes as a team in normal binocular function and still fewer ever become fully efficient at matching their visual systems to the rest of their bodily motor-perceptual systems. Many 'cured' strabismics with

straight eyes and some degree of fusion perform in their daily activities as if their eyes still turned."

f. *Death*

(1) That a patient may have to forfeit life in undergoing *optional* strabismus surgery when other safe methods exist for strabismus remediation may seem shocking to some, but such occurrences have been regularly recorded for some time. The usual cause of death in strabismus surgery, as in other types of ocular surgery, is from cardiac arrest caused by the so-called oculocardiac reflex.

(a) Slowing of the hearbeat rhythm (bradycardia) which accompanies pressure on the eyeball was first described independently by Aschner and Dagnini in 1908. The afferent limb of the reflex is thought to be carried by the trigeminal nerve via the ciliary nerves, ciliary ganglion and nasociliary nerve. The efferent pathway is known to be mediated by the vagus nerve. In the unanesthetized subject, pressure on the eyeball generally produces only a slight response and is known to reduce the pulse rate in cases of racing heart (paroxysmal tachycardia) (Deacock and Oxer, 1962). General anesthesia, however, renders the heart vulnerable to relatively intensive vagal stimulation (Reid, Stephenson and Hinton, 1952).

[1] Bietti (1966) also stresses the import of the oculocardiac reflex and of its elicitation by surgical manipulation of the ocular muscles, to different degrees in various subjects. Sorenson and Gilmore (1956) also note that some degree of bradycardia is inevitable every time that the medial or lateral rectus is stretched, and that cases of fatalities following strabismus surgery might be due to this cause rather than, as often ascribed, to the anesthesia.

(b) Kirsch, et al., (1957) have estimated the incidence of "cardiac arrest" at one in 3,500 cases of ophthalmic surgery. Gartner and Billet (1958) have estimated that 45 Americans, most of them aged less than nine years, die each year in the course of eye operations.

[1] In contrast, Dunlap cites figures from New York Hospital showing not a single fatality from eye surgery in more than "3,600 muscle operations" over a period of 25 years.

[2] None the less, a recent report of cardiac arrest requiring open chest massage and resulting in brain damage is reported occurring in California, (N.Y. State Optom. Assn. J., 1963).

(c) There has been much activity aimed toward devising methods to avoid the untoward consequences of the oculocardiac reflex. Kirsch, et al. (1957), Mendelblatt, Kirsch and Lemberg (1962) and Berler (1963) all claim to be able to eliminate the oculocardiac reflex with a retrobulbar block.

[1] Bosomvoorth, Ziegler and Jocaby (1958) however, found that 12 of 17 patients on which this retrobulbar block was administered still evidenced heart rhythm variations. Subsequent work by Rhode, et al. (1958) and Reed and McCaughey (1962) agreed with Bosomvoorth, et al., concerning the relative ineffectiveness of this approach but strong claims are still being made for it.

[2] Bietti (1966) stresses the importance of having a defibillator and

pacemaker handy in "cases of surgical procedures involving either a pulling or stimulation exerted on the ocular muscles." To emphasize the importance of this suggestion he points out that: "... the use of drugs aiming to modify the circulatory effect of the O.C.R. can only be effective if cardiac fibrillation has not already taken place, since the slowing-down of the cardiac activity, and consequently of the circulation, make impossible a prompt and adequate distribution in the organism of the employed substances. We must therefore be always immediately ready for any maneuver of reanimation."

VI. UNTREATED STRABISMUS

A. While it would be most instructive to know what the expected natural history of untreated strabismus would be over a long period, no such study seems to have been reported. Two studies, however, have appeared which have dealt with long range trends in strabismus. The first is one in which long term follow-up has been carried out with minimal care (refractive correction and occlusion for amblyopia if present). The second is an epidemiological study.

1. Noordlow (1951) followed 122 convergent strabismics for an average period of 10.2 years with only refractive care and some amblyopia training.

a. His findings were that the "primary static angle" in constant, convergent, concomitant strabismus does not show any definite change before age seven but from this time until 15-16 years of age it changes in over 50% of the cases, decreasing in 41.7% by three to 24 arc degrees (over 50°) and increasing in 12.5% by amounts ranging from 5° to 22°. Functional recovery occurred in one percent of his sample.

b. In intermittent squints, the "primary static angle" is unchanged in 25% and decreased by nine to 18 arc degrees (i.e. as much as 40°) in 75% of the cases.

c. At the conclusion of his observations 42.3% had no squint, 42.3% had an intermittent squint and 15.4% had a constant strabismus.

d. He concluded that no definite relationship existed between change in refractive error and change in angle.

2. Weve (1954) on the basis of his study of 5,000 school children found that there was 50% less strabismus between the ages of 12 and 13 than at five and six. From these figures, Weve estimates that the strabismic child has a 50% chance of spontaneous improvement.

a. A similar epidemilogical study by Frandsen (1960) also found a reduction in the occurrence of strabismus in the population from ages 6-7 onward.

VII. RESULTS

A. An important factor in the assessment of the results for all of the methods of treatment previously described is the criteria utilized to differentiate successful cases from those adjudged to be unsuccessful. Thus, various studies have been reported which consider only immediate cosmetic effects, others which have been concerned with function and cosmesis at termination of treatment, and only a few which have considered appearance and binocular function over the long term. The five forms of treatment are analyzed in terms of both short and long term observations.

B. Refractive Correction

1. Since refractive correction is now viewed as only one step in the functional rehabilitation sequence of strabismus, there are very few recent studies in which *only* refractive care is given to

any sizable number of these patients. The few studies which have been found are usually only secondary observations from a large sample in which other types of therapy are featured.

2. *Short term*

a. Guibor (1936) states that, in his experience, refraction, atropine, and occlusion cure 30% of strabismics.

b. Law (1938) in analyzing the results of strabismus therapy at a British hospital, concludes that of 91 patients seen, 30 (33%) were cured with spectacles alone.

c. Kennedy (1954) reports on the results obtained using concave lenses to correct divergent strabismus. Of about 150 cases treated by this method he found 103 to be successful by "having met and maintained one of the following three criteria:

(1) eyes cosmetically straight with no fusion 28%;
(2) eyes straight and fusion present 54%;
(3) eyes straight, fusion constant 18%."

(a) The stated percentages cover only the successfully treated cases. These patients were reported not to have manifested "any symptoms attributable to the minus lenses."

d. Ludlam (1961) using criteria of functional binocularity as well as alignment, evaluated the results of strabismus training over a four year period at his institution. He found that although a large number of the 284 strabismics visiting the orthoptics clinic were cured by a combination of orthoptics and visual training and spectacles, only nine (3.7%) were fully corrected with spectacles alone.

C. Pharmacological

1. The major pharmacological treatment of strabismus at present is centered in the use of miotics.

2. *Short Term*

a. Abraham (1949)

(1) Of 50 of the 80 cases "available for report," 11 were cured by use of the miotic for an average of 15 months (range two to 32 months) i.e., functional binocularity and alignment was present without glasses.

(2) Thirty were helped, i.e., achieved "grossly normal function" and single binocular fixation while using the miotic (with glasses if necessary).

(3) Nine were ranked as failures with miotic therapy.

(4) The role of the miotic in the results obtained is not immediately clear since "surgery alone or in combination was done some time before the use of miotics in 18 cases."

b. Edwards (1958)

(1) Of 36 strabismic patients treated with pilocarpine, 27 continued treatment long enough to be reported on. Of these, nine improved and 18 showed no improvement.

c. Knapp and Capobianco (1956)

(1) Tabulation of their results with D.F.P. on 277 cases is as follows:

(a)	Still on glasses and D.F.P.	2
(b)	Developed exotropia	2
(c)	Back on essential glasses for school	5
(d)	Reaction to D.F.P.	20
(e)	Allergy to D.F.P. or peanut oil	3
(f)	Pigment cysts of pupillary seam	16
(g)	Failed to return	11
(h)	Preferred glasses	2
(i)	After treatment for amblyopia	38
(j)	Still esotropia	124
(k)	Still on D.F.P.	44
(l)	"Cured"	10

d. Koskinen (1957) of a total sample of 136 found:

(1) Accommodative strabismus

(a) Seventeen of 31 were cured.
(b) Average time of treatment was one year.

(2) Partially accommodative

(a) Eleven of 58 were cured and 14 improved.

(3) Non-accommodative esotropes whose "angle measurement was not influenced by glasses."

(a) Of a total of 47 none were cured but for 2, a permanent decrease in angle was achieved.

e. Miller (1960)

(1) In 38 cases of accommodative esotropia on which three different miotics were tried, a maximum of four were found to have measurable decreases in convergence of 5^{Δ} or more and five patients (with phospholine iodide) to have an increase in relative fusional divergence of 6^{Δ} or more although all showed "some improvement."

f. Abrahamson and Abrahamson (1964)

(1) Of a sample of 32 accommodative and eight non-accommodative esotropes, 23 were found to have been "benefitted" by the miotic (P.I. 0.06%). No estimate of functional binocularity was reported and 13 of the patients had surgery prior to miotics. Eyes were cosmetically straight in 17 patients during and after the miotic therapy.

2. *Long Term*

a. Although the method is relatively new and prolonged use of the medication is generally inadvisable, two large sample long term (three years or more) studies have been reported.

b. Wheeler and Moore (1964) in evaluating the use of D.F.P. for periods of from one to nine years in a sample of 155 esotropes, tabulated the comparative effects on the strabismus of refractive correction and miotics as follows:

(1) **Table XXXII-1**

Type Deviation	No. of Patients	D.F.P. Same As Rx	Rx Better Than D.F.P.	Rx and D.F.P. Both Needed
Accom. Esotrope Normal AC/A	25	16 (64%)	4 (16%)	5 (20%)
Accom. Esotrope Abnormal AC/A	45	23 (51%)		22 (49%)
Partial Accom. Esotropia	60	39 (65%)	21 (35%)	21 (35%)
Nonaccommodative Esotropia	25	25 (100%)		

(a) The AC/A ratio was considered normal by Parks' (1958) criterion, i.e. if the angle of deviation was the same or within 10^{Δ} at distance and near, the AC/A ratio was considered normal, if not, it was held to be abnormal.

(2) Concerning the part played by orthoptic training, these authors state: "Orthoptic training does not significantly improve the high cure rate in accommodative esotropia over that achieved by miotics and glasses, but it probably accelerates the elimination of all treatment."

c. Chamberlain and Caldwell (1965) report on the results of miotic therapy on 316 of a total of 580 esotropes seen over a three year period. Four different miotics were employed with the following results:

(1) **Table XXXII-2**

Drug	Cases	Improved	Not Improved	Inadequate Trial
D.F.P.	314	193 (61%)	103 (33%)	18 (6%)
P.I.	70	44 (62%)	20 (29%)	6 (9%)
Humorsol	22	8 (36%)	12 (55%)	2 (9%)
Pilocarpine	14	1 (7%)	10 (72%)	3 (21%)

(a) "Improved" meant either or both:

[1] The restoration of binocularity as evaluated on the Worth 4 dot test and Wirt test.

[2] A fifty percent reduction in the deviation, if this constituted a significant cosmetic improvement.

(2) Of the total of 316 patients, 314 were introduced to miotic therapy with D.F.P. while 2 were initially given P.I. The change to a second miotic was made for such reasons as redness, irritation, swollen lids, brow aches, significant iris cysts and blurred distant vision. It should be noted that 104 patients (33%) were switched to a second miotic.

d. In both of these long term studies it has not been made clear whether any of the cured convergent strabismics have been "weaned" from the drug, i.e. whether after cessation of the administration of the miotic, the patient maintained functional binocularity. This by any reasonable standard should be the definition of a "cure" by use of miotics.

3. *Summary*

a. Miotics administered with care and under close supervision have shown some usefulness in diagnosis and for a few selected cases, in treatment.

(1) These favorable treatment cases would seem to be infants where full alignment can be achieved and in strabismic children with high AC/A ratios.

(2) Usually used in combination with single vision glasses, "pharmacological training" with a long period of slow withdrawal of the drug, appears to both decrease the AC/A ratio and increase the fusional divergence ability to enable alignment to be secured without bifocals.

b. Miotics seem to have no place in the treatment of strabismus with normal AC/A ratios, where astigmatism of more than 1.00 D is present, and where complete alignment is not secured alone or in combination with glasses.

D. Visual Training

1. *Overall results*

a. Although training methods have varied as have the patient selection procedures and criteria for results, several studies give an idea of the variation in efficacy of orthoptics as a sole remediation measure in moderately sized samples of manifest strabismus. These are listed in chronological order.

b. *Short term*

(1) Hicks and Hosford (1935) after training 32 patients three to 13 years of age, for nine months, using the techniques recommended by the various instrument manufacturers, found that five (16%) were cures, and concluded that orthoptics was of little value except in conjunction with surgery.

(2) Feldman (1935) cites results of 87 cases after one year's work. Cures, or almost cures were obtained for 25 patients (29%), 25 showed little improvement or were dropped by the clinic, and 37 dropped out of their own accord.

(3) Law (1938), deprecating the work of the "orthoptic department presided over by a medically unqualified certified orthoptist" at the Paddington Green Hospital, states that of 91 patients seen, 30 were cured with spectacles alone, 27 (30%) patients were cured by orthoptics, occlusion, and spectacles; and the rest could not be cured.

(4) Burri (1940) reports on two samples of strabismus patients trained at once-weekly sessions with no homework assigned.

(a) The results in the first group of 115 patients were 25 cures (22%), 40 improved with orthoptics, one was cured with spectacles and 59 patients could not be helped orthoptically.

(b) The second sample, showing better results, had a total of 64 patients; 20

were orthoptics cures (31%), 22 improved with orthoptics alone, and 22 were orthoptic failures.

(5) Nugent (1940) referring to 43 orthoptic cures out of 81 patients trained, concludes that "about 50% of all cases of strabismus can be cured with refraction, occlusion, atropine and orthoptics."

(6) Gillan (1945) describing his orthoptic work with 63 children, five to twelve years of age, treated for periods ranging from one month to sixteen months, found 23 (37%) orthoptic cures, 25 almost straight (five degrees or less residual deviation) and 15 failures. Optimistic about his orthoptic results, he states that deviations of twenty-five degrees or less may be treated orthoptically with success.

(7) Giles (1949) reports on two studies.

(a) One by Hogg shows 82 percent success in a strictly selected sample of 50 patients, taken from an analysis of 116 orthoptic records.

(b) Gray and Hallmark show 92.7 percent success, in another sample, of 41 five to fourteen year olds, again strictly selected as to prognosis, from a larger group of 82 records.

(8) Douglas (1952), after a review of the literature and a denunciation of the work thus far published to support the efficacy of orthoptics as either a specific, or ancillary procedure in the treatment of strabismus, studied the results of two hospital orthoptic departments.

(a) On the basis of 203 patients, he deduces that only 42 (22%) were helped by orthoptic treatment. His conclusion is that an orthoptics department "can be profitably used for diagnosis, supervision of occlusion, and to maintain a closer liaison with the patient and his parents," all secondary to surgical treatment.

(9) Flom (1958) in an epidemiological study of strabismus and its treatment, analyzed the results obtained with 101 patients given orthoptic treatment from his total sample of 179. Making explicit the *criteria* (hereinafter called the *Flom Criteria*) by which the results are to be categorized, he uses functional and alignment criteria as follows (Flom, 1958):

(a) Functional cure

[1] Clear, comfortable, single binocular vision must be present at all distances up to the near point of convergence, which is normal itself;

[2] stereopsis and normal ranges of motor fusion present;

[3] occasional turning of the eyes may occur (up to 1% of the time) provided diplopia is experienced whenever this happens;

[4] "correction lenses" and small amounts of prism, (up to 5^{Δ}) may be worn if necessary.

(b) Almost cured

[1] All criteria of "Functional Cure" except,

[2] stereopsis may be lacking,

[3] strabismus may be exhibited up to 5% of the time,

[4] larger amounts of prism may be used to maintain comfortable binocular vision.

(c) Moderate Improvement

[1] Improvement in more than one defect of the strabismus.

(d) Slight Improvement

[1] Improvement in one of the defects of the strabismus.

(e) No Improvement

[1] No improvement in the strabismus or any of its associated defects.

(f) Using these criteria, he categorized the cases who had undergone training as follows:

TABLE XXXII-3

[1] **For the 61 esotropes:**

[a]

cured	*10 (16%)*
almost cured	*5 (8%)*
moderate improvement	*15 (25%)*
slight improvement	*15 (25%)*
no improvement	*16 (26%)*

[2] **For the 40 exotropes the comparable figures were:**

[a]

cured	*10 (25%)*
almost cured	*11 (27%)*
moderate improvement	*6 (15%)*
slight improvement	*5 (13%)*
no improvement	*8 (20%)*

(10) Ludlam (1961) also making use of the "Flom Criteria" analyzed the results of training 149 concomitant strabismics unselected as to prognosis or results and found:

(a) **Table XXXII-4**

	Eso	**Exo**	**Hyper Eso**	**Hyper Exo**
Functional Cure	10 (19%)	27 (47%)	4 (23%)	8 (40%)
Almost Cure	21 (40%)	22 (38%)	10 (59%)	7 (35%)
Moderate Improvement	11 (21%)	7 (11%)	0	4 (20%)
Slight Improvement	6 (10%)	2 (4%)	2 (12%)	0
No Improvement	6 (10%)	0	1 (6%)	1 (5%)

[1] The presence of a hyper component in the above was limited to those cases manifesting 2° or more of vertical imablance.

(b) Ludlam concluded: "The results of the study indicate that orthoptics including occlusion and in conjunction with refraction, yields results on a large number of unselected strabismics, in which the eyes are straight cosmetically, and binocularly functional 95% of the time or better in 76% of our sample (73% according to the Flom criteria), at dismissal from regular clinic training. These results were obtained under clinical conditions which were not optimal; (group therapy, poor control, different practitioners, etc.) and better results should be obtained where these unfavorable factors do not enter."

b. *Long Term Results* – defined here to mean results determined at least 3 years after dismissal from training.

(1) Ludlam and Kleinman (1965), re-examining 81 of the 113 cured patients in the Ludlam (1961) study cited previously, three to seven years after dismissal from training found:

(a) "By a strict Flom Criteria application, 89% of the samples were placed in one of the two "cure" categories. Thus, 72 of 81 former strabismics, brought to a "cure" status by orthoptic training, remained both cosmetically straight and functionally binocular through a period from three to seven years after completion of training."

(b) The change in the "Flom Criteria" classification between the short term and long range studies was found to be:

[1] 26 upgraded, 38 remained the same and 17 downgraded.

(c) These authors also observed that: "The 'Almost Cured' strabismics as judged by the Flom Criteria tended to either become full fledged 'Functional Cures' (22 of 41) or to drop to Flom Criteria 'Failures' (7 of 41). Relatively few (29%) were able to maintain their status as 'Almost Cures' over the intervening three to seven-year period. This would seem to indicate that there is a point beyond which training must establish normal ocular neuromuscular reflexes, in order to maintain long-range functional binocularity."

(d) An important observation by these authors was made on the long range change in imbalance direction:

[1] "Of extreme interest were the 14 strabismics who, upon re-examination seven years after dismissal from training, showed a direction of imbalance opposite to the direction of the original strabismus. Of these, 13 were found to be long-range Flom Criteria 'cures,' while one had switched from an original esotropia to an exotropia. This demonstration of the variation in direction of binocular imbalance, in addition to the several studies reviewed which showed spontaneous changes in strabismus angle of as large as 50° over a period of years, would seem to underscore the futility of any therapy based in large degree on the size of the 'static angle' of strabismus, and not including fusion training."

(2) Hawkins (1961) analyzing the results of 1,749 strabismics orthoptically treated at the London Refraction Hospital over an eleven year period (1948-58) notes that only two cases apparently produced a spontaneous cure. From this finding he observes: "Orthoptic success is no accident. It is due to the presence of the factors necessary for success."

(a) Using extraordinarily rigorous criteria, he defines his classifications as follows:

[1] Full Binocular Vision

[a] normal Snellon acuity
[b] no deviation at any distance with or without glasses on cover test
[c] good fusion and stereopsis
[d] normal convergence
[e] appreciation of physiological diplopia
[f] possession of normal fusional reserves
[g] absence of symptoms
[h] binocular single vision without any intermittent deviation

[2] Restricted Binocular Vision

[a] Any condition in which the above cannot be fully satisfied but where there is a measure of binocularity, e.g., large heterophorias or intermittent strabismus with suppression.

[3] Cosmetic Cure

[a] "No functional binocularity of fusion but the eyes appear satisfactorily straight with or without prisms in the primary position of regard."

(b) He found the cases considered to be divided as follows:

[1] 466 (26.6%) of the patients were found to fit the category "Full Binocular Vision"
[2] 133 (7.6%) were classed as "Restricted Binocular Vision"
[3] 35 (2%) were categorized as a "Cosmetic Cure"
[4] 991 (56.7%) ceased treatment
[5] 124 (7.1%) were still under treatment

(3) Other Reports or Comments Not Actually Studies

(a) Cantonnet and Filliozat (1934), in the introduction of their classic volume on orthoptic rehabilitation of strabismus, estimate that 70% of all strabismus can be "re-educated" usually in a period of from 6 to 15 months.

(b) Smith (1943) states that the efficacy of orthoptics as a specific sole remedy of strabismus in his clinical experience is about 70%. In 1954, he raised his estimate and stated that at least 75% of non-paralytic strabismus can be corrected entirely by orthoptic treatment and spectacles.

(4) Since there appear to be at present only two formal studies of the overall long range effects of orthoptics or visual training as the *sole* therapeutic technique utilized and these from different countries, it is obvious that additional investigations to substantiate these results are needed.

2. *Amblyopia*

a. Again, the criteria used to define the amblyopia initially, the idiosyncrasies of the individual amblyopes in the sample, the type of treatment rendered, the type of testing performed at the conclusion of treatment, and the criteria used to classify the results all influence the apparent efficacy of the therapy employed.

b. *Traditional direct occlusion of the non-amblyopic eye*

(1) Parks and Friendly (1966) over a 12 year span evaluated the efficacy of intensive complete direct occlusion on a sample of 117 eccentrically fixating strabismus amblyopes under the age of four years. The authors found that 116 (99%) of this number had central fixation restored and 100 (86%) of these successfully treated patients had 20/30 or better Snellen illiterate E acuity. Stress was placed on proper explanation to, and motivation of, the parents and "emphasis was put on the importance of successful therapy and the consequence of failure." The report concludes that strabismic amblyopes under four years of age respond well to direct total occlusion of the fixing or non-amblyopic eye.

(2) Gregersen and Rindziunski (1965) in a long term evaluation of cured amblyopes, remeasured 53 patients who had been treated by elastoplast occlusion more than 10 years previous. The average age of the sample at the time of treatment was between four and five years. At the follow-up the average age was 17 years.

(a) Expressing the acuity in decimals the *average* values were:

[1]

	Situation	*Acuity*
[a]	before treatment	.2 – (20/100)
[b]	after occlusion	.8 – (20/25)
[c]	at follow-up	.5 – (20/40)

[2] Thus, the 53 patients on average can be seen to have lost a substantial portion of their original improvement.

[3] Specifically:

[a] About one-sixth of the patients (9 of 53) lost the entire original visual improvement.

[b] Approximately sixty percent (31 of 53) lost half of their gain.

[c] About one quarter (13 of 53) suffered no visual loss over the 10 year period following treatment.

(b) The authors observe that the combination of alignment of the eyes and good binocular function tend to preserve or maintain the fixation and acuity improvement brought about by direct occlusion treatment.

[1] They conclude that in spite of the reduction in the original improvement in 75% of the cases: "occlusion therapy of the dominant eye, is still the most effective, cheapest, and easiest method for treating squint amblyopia, if only the treatment is consistent and early so that it can start before true eccentric fixation has had a chance to develop."

(3) Scully (1961) reports a group of 57 convergent strabismics with non-central fixation in which 51 had a "plastic type of fixation" and six had "rigid eccentric fixation." The group was treated by constant occlusion of the fixing eye for periods of two to 24 weeks and all but one achieved "bilateral central fixation" as determined by the visuscope. Of the 30 old enough to respond to acuity measurements with the E

test, 27 had equal acuity in each eye. Scully feels that the excellence of his results is due to: "...the fact that none had had any previous treatment, the majority attending for treatment at a relatively early stage after the onset of the squint and, perhaps even more important, to the intensive and rigorous nature of the occlusion used."

(4) Kupfer (1957) in a most interesting report of seven adult male amblyopes aged 18 to 22 whose amblyopia "resulted from a childhood squint" showed extraordinary improvement in acuity in five of the patients within a period of 24 weeks. The vision initially was hand movements for two patients which improved to 20/40 and 20/25 respectively, two others with initial acuity measured at 20/200 improved to 20/30 and in the final case, "a facultative amblyope" improved from 20/70 to 20/20 in two weeks. Complete total occlusion of the non-amblyopic eye was carried out under hospitalization during which regular intense foveal stimulation was undertaken in the amblyopic eye in order to bring about central fixation. This skill was usually learned in four to 10 days and the acuity improvement starting at near distances quickly spread to distance targets as well. It would thus appear from this report that positive differential stimulation of the macula with respect to the peripheral retina as well as the negative differential to be employed in conventional pleoptics is successful in recovering central fixation and acuity in squint amblyopia.

c. *Pleoptic Treatment*

(1) Girard, Fletcher, Tomlinson, and Smith (1962) present the results of "Cuppers technique" pleoptics for 72 amblyopes.

(a) In this technique, the peripheral retina is "dazzled" by means of a treatment ophthalmoscope which spares the macular area so that a doughnut shaped after-image allows the patient to visualize the position of his own macula. "Localization treatment" to restore steady central fixation by use of Haidinger Brush and other techniques in the amblyopic eye is undertaken to normalize fixation and acuity.

(b) Of the total sample, 20 originally had central fixation and 52 had eccentric fixation.

[1] Of the 20 with central fixation, 15 achieved 20/30 or better acuity.

[2] Of the 52 initially found to have eccentric fixation, however, only 27 attained a level of 20/30 acuity or better.

[3] Of the total, 69 patients (96%) were found to show some improvement.

(c) The amblyopia in 68 cases was felt to be related to strabismus or anisometropia or a combination of these.

(d) The number of treatments to obtain "maximum visual acuity" ranged from 3 treatments in one day, to 90 over a period of almost two years.

(2) Verlee and Iacobucci (1967) treated by different methods two matched samples containing 50 patients each, aged three to 12.

(a) The first group had been treated "with the pleoptic method of Cuppers" which featured eight weeks of occlusion of the amblyopic eye prior to the application of formal pleoptic techniques, and such inverse occlusion was continued between treatment sessions until central fixation was established. The range of treatment period was four to 16 weeks.

(b) The other group was treated by direct occlusion i.e. complete full time elastoplast occlusion of the non-amblyopic eye. The occlusion period ranged from 1.5 to 9.0 months with a mean of about 3.05 months. The patching was terminated when no further "improvement in fixation pattern and acuity" was measurable over a three to four week period.

(c) Once central fixation and acuity were attained the patient was encouraged by orthoptic methods to use the former amblyopic eye either through fusion, if this were possible, or through alternation.

(d) They reported a higher percentage of "good results," i.e. whole line 20/30 acuity or better and central fixation, for the direct occlusion method for age ranges three to six and six to nine years but about equal results for direct occlusion and pleoptics in the 9-12 year old group. They conclude that: ". . . full-time occlusion of the sound eye should be the initial step in the treatment of all patients having amblyopia with eccentric fixation."

(3) Von Noorden and Lipsius (1964) after carefully describing the fixation behavior of 58 strabismic amblyopes, aged five to 17, treated these patients by various pleoptic techniques after Bangerter and Cuppers.

(a) In evaluating the results of 46, they find that the fixation area moved closer to the fovea but was not made central in 12 (26%), fixation was "normalized in 22 (48%), while visual acuity was improved in 13 (28%)."

[1] The authors note pleoptics was more effective with regard to normalizing fixation than for improving visual acuity to normal and not a single patient achieved 20/20. They further observe: "in 30 instances vision was 6/21 (20/70) or less at the end of therapy and thus conditions for the development of binocular vision remained quite unfavorable."

(b) Six of the 24 patients showed whole line improvement of acuity at follow-up tests performed an average of 22 months later, while nine evidenced acuity at the pre-treatment level or worse. The remaining nine demonstrated linear acuity at the same level or at least better than pre-treatment measurements. Thus, 11 out of 24 patients in which a follow-up was carried out were found to have less demonstrable acuity than at the termination of therapy.

(c) The writers note: "Consequently, ocular alignment with full binocular functions and adequate fusional amplitudes or strabismus with true alternation are prerequisities for stabilization of visual acuity in a formerly amblyopic patient."

(d) Von Noorden and Lipsius conclude: "The introduction of pleoptics has rejuvenated interest in amblyopia, advanced our knowledge of its pathophysiology and improved our diagnostic armamentarium. As a practical therapeutic method, however, it has failed to produce significant improvement or permanent cure in the majority of our amblyopic patients."

(4) Gortz (1960) reported the results of treatment of 88 cases of amblyopia with eccentric fixation. Of this total sample he found that 71 (81%) developed central fixation after an average number of 17.5 half-hour sessions of Cuppers-Bangerter pleoptic treatments.

(a) Of these patients with acquired central fixation, the author made a further subdivision:

[1] 53.4% were designated as quiet central fixaters.
[2] 18.2% were held to have restless central fixation;
[3] 9.1% were labelled as marked fixation nystagmus.

(b) The final acuity measurements of this 81% converted to central fixation were:

[1] 35.3% measured 0.7 to 1.0 (20/30 to 20/20);
[2] 32.9% exhibited 0.4 to 0.6 (20/50 to 20/40) and
[3] 31.8% achieved less than 0.4 (20/50).

(c) The acuity classifications are not matched to the central fixation categories so the number coming from each group is not known. The author stresses the importance of binocular status for the final result and decries the practice of treating amblyopia as "an isolated phenomenon. The basic aims of eccentric fixation amblyopia treatment should be in the following sequence of importance: change of fixation, monocular localization and the improvement of visual acuity."

E. Surgical

1. Reports of the results reveal large variations, affected by both the vagaries of the sample cited, and, probably more important, by the previously noted fact that the method involves more art than science and is influenced markedly by the nature of the surgical technique used and the experience of the particular surgeon. The criteria for success, i.e. whether functional and visual criteria are employed, as well as cosmetic factors, to adjudge results, will also have a strong influence on the success rate reported. The reported results which follow are not meant to be exhaustive but have been selected to be illustrative. The results in this section will be presented under short and long term categories.

2. *Short term*

a. Bedrossian (1962) operated on 35 intermittent exotropes whose V.A. in each eye was equal or within two lines difference. 26 of them had no vertical deviation. The criteria for a functional cure were a residual distance deviation of 10 prism diopters or less, fusion indicated by the synoptophore or Worth four dot test at distance and near, and bifoveal fixation at distance and near as indicated by cover-uncover test.

(1) Of the 26 cases without a vertical element, 13 were cured by one operation; five cured by a second operation; seven needed further surgery, i.e. more than two procedures; one overcorrection was also overcome by further surgery.

(2) Four out of the nine cases with a vertical component were listed as cures.

b. Scobee (1951) in a study designed to show "what may be accomplished without orthoptics" presents the results of surgery on 171 patients. He utilized the identical surgical procedure on each patient regardless of the amount of deviation measured. Of the entire group of patients he found that 68 (40%) achieved fusion, (30% of the non-accommodative and 42% of the partly accommodative cases) and 88 (51%) of his sample had "anatomical anomalies" associated with the oculorotary muscles believed significant in the etiology of the esotropia. This proportion of anomalies was a revision downward from a previously published estimate of 90%.

c. Mulberger and McDonald (1954) in discussing results of surgery on 147 exotropes define excellent results as eyes straight and fusion present.

(1) The cases falling in this classification were: of 25 intermittent exotropes, eight obtained excellent; of 41 alternating exotropes, six were excellent; of 63 constant exotropes, one was excellent; of 18 postoperative exotropes (former esotropia), one was classified as excellent. Thus a total of 11% achieve cosmetically straight eyes and fusion.

(2) Good results were defined as: 10° or less residual esotropia or exotropia (36%).

(3) Improved results had a residual deviation of 11° to 20° (29%).

(4) Poor results were defined as a deviation of greater than 20° (24%).

d. Noordlow (1960) finds a simple mechanical relationship exists between the static angle of squint, the amount of surgery, and results, in 82.8% ± 7.9% of a sample of 345 constant convergent squints.

(1) In one type of operation: parallelism was obtained in 52.5% of 238 patients after one operation, and in an additional 19.8% after two operations.

(a) Cosmetically satisfactory results were obtained in 16.8% and unsatisfactory in 10.9%.

(2) In a second type of operation (107 cases) parallelism was obtained after one operation in 51.5%, and in an additional 18.5% after two operations.

(a) Cosmetically satisfactory results were 28%, and unsatisfactory 1.9%.

(3) No mention is made of any binocular testing in judging results. All the strabismic angles were measured by perimetry.

e. Dunnington and Wheeler (1942) reporting the results of surgery on 211 esotropias, define a "cure" as having no more residual angle than 10°. Of the 163 cases requiring only one operation, 43% achieved this "cure" status, 44% achieved an under-correction of greater than 10° (average 20°) and 13% resulted in overcorrection (post-operative exotropia). The initial angle of deviation was taken as the larger of the distance or near cover test angles. No mention was made as to whether glasses were worn when these measurements were taken. The authors state their belief that surgical results "are still a long way from the goal of achieving binocular single vision and fusion in a large percentage of cases."

3. *Long Term Results*

a. Kennedy and McCarthy (1959) in one of the best executed and complete studies of the results of esotropia surgery reviewed by the present author, evaluate the results of 315 patients. The range of follow-up visits was 1.8 to 4.5 years with an average of 2.6 years.

(1) In only 32 patients (10%) could some degree of fusion be elicited at the follow-up examination. The authors state their belief that 1/3 of this group owed their functional cure status to formal post-operative orthoptics.

(2) In 13% or 42 cases the esotropia reverted to the pre-operative deviation or greater.

(3) In 28 cases (9%) post-operative exotropia developed.

b. Lyle (1959) presented his results with 142 cases of constant concomitant convergent strabismus. Of 42 cases operated on from 1½ to two years of age, six (14%) developed binocular single vision. Of 100 operated on from ages five to 10 years, 14 (14%) obtained binocular single vision. All patients were seen three years or more after operation.

(1) The results of 128 cases of non-accommodative convergent strabismus according to age of onset were: of 96 patients, onset two to four years – 22 (23%) obtained binocular single vision; of 32 patients, onset four to eight years – 120 (62.5%) developed binocular single vision.

(2) Results of 131 cases of primary divergent concomitant strabismus treated by surgery were as follows: of 94 intermittent cases, 80 had no deviation and full binocular single vision, 14 remained intermittent. In 37 cases that were constant prior to surgery, 13 (35%) obtained full binocular single vision and 24 (65%) obtained no binocular vision. The last surgical treatment of the above cases was two years or more previous to recheck.

(3) Lyle feels that the prognosis as far as establishment of binocular single vision is concerned varies according to age of onset or according to the stage of normal development which had been reached by the binocular reflexes when the squint became constant.

c. Morgan and Arstikaitis (1954) in a review of 1,000 post-operative cases of strabismus (500 private and 500 clinic), found that the type of operation did not seem to influence results as long as "the proper operation was done." Most of the patients had not had orthoptic training and the authors state that: "The results varied tremendously depending on when muscle findings were taken after the operation. Some cases, where there appeared to have been good results one or two months after operation, became over-corrected in a year or so."

(1) Cover Test and "excursion" (version) tests were employed in examining the children. The age range of the sample was from birth to 15 years of age. They noted that the cosmetic results obtained in the older age group were best and the poorest were for the group 2-4 years of age. They observe: "It would appear that early operation does not necessarily give a better immediate result."

(2) Since functional binocularity was not considered in the evaluation, the results were discussed in terms of residual deviation. According to the authors 69% of the private patients had a residual deviation of 10^{Δ} or less while 56.5% of the clinic patients achieved a similar result.

(3) They conclude that the experience of the surgeon "plays a large part in obtaining good results" and state:

(a) "It is hoped that this brief survey will give some encouragement to those who also have trouble in straightening crossed eyes. It is not until you have had many years of experience that you realize how little you know about strabismus. Most of the patients come back for yearly examination so we have a good opportunity to observe our failures. Fortunately most of the parents and children are not very critical. If the parents are happy we do not point out that the eyes are a few degrees off, and we do not mention binocular vision. Our impression is still that the ideal time to treat these cases is as early as possible."

d. Dunlap, E. (1963) in operating on 100 unselected patients with intermittent exotropia, none having had orthoptics and observed for from one to five years, found the results were: 12% excellent, 21% good, 24% fair, 43% poor.

(1) The categories of results were defined as follows:

(a) Excellent – Phoria on cover test, ductions of 20° base-out distance and near, and 7° base-in distance and near, minimal suppression. Diplopia elicited when eye deviates.

(b) Good – Large exophoria (up to 20°), 10° base-out and base-in, intermittent exotropia 10° at distance.

(c) Fair – Intermittent exotropia less than 20° distance but good recovery. Intermittent exotropia less than pre-operative angle but no more than 20° residual.

(d) Poor – Residual exotropia larger than 20°. Residual esotropia 10° or more distance and near.

(2) Influential factors were: size of turn, presence of a vertical component, subnormal vision or anisometropia. Not influencing the results were: age of stated onset of turn, age of patient at time of surgical correction, time interval between onset and surgical correction, refractive error and amount of deviation ratio at 6M and 1/3 M. The author noted that a factor of possible long term significance is the development of progressive myopia; 14 patients in the series developed it after originally having a hyperopic error.

(3) Hardesty (1965), commenting on the grim surgical outlook for intermittent exotropia as pointed up by these results of Dunlap, states:

(a) "Few problems in ophthalmology are more frustrating than surgical treatment of intermittent exotropia. To correct an exotropic child for a few months or a few years only to watch his eyes return to their intermittent divergent state is an unpleasant experience for both the child's parents and the ophthalmologist. It is especially distressing to observe such a failure after a second surgical procedure which has involved the remaining two horizontal muscles. Here we must face the fact that, if further operative intervention is permitted by parents, the result will be even more unpredictable as we are now forced to operate on scarred muscles."

e. Bridgeman (1963) reviewed his results of surgical treatment on non-accommodative constant convergent squints whose age of onset was before two years. "Straight" is defined as having a residual deviation of less than 14° esotropia, 10° of exotropia or 2° vertical. Eight (4%) achieved binocular single vision. Nine other cases were placed in this group at one time but failed to maintain it. Thirty-seven (18%) were classed under the term "partial binocular vision." These patients had some fusion at some distances but were still strabismic under some conditions. One-hundred forty-seven others (78%) had no fusion under any conditions.

(1) The author concludes from his results:

(a) "It does not appear essential to success that the visual axes should be rendered absolutely parallel and the eyes orthophoric. There would be no guarantee that such a perfect result, seldom actually attained in squint surgery, would persist indefinitely, and in any case in those instances in the series where binocular single vision was achieved . . . such perfection was not necessary."

f. Fletcher and Silverman (1966) analyzed the surgical results of 260 partially accommodative and non-accommodative esotropes after a two to seven year follow-up.

(1) They observe that 94 (64%) of the 146 partially accommodative convergent strabismics and 33 (29%) of the 114 non-accommodative esotropes "retain some grade of fusion." While finding that the results of asymmetrical and symmetrical procedures were similar, they note that: ". . . 69% of the children treated by symmetrical surgery required multiple surgical procedures whereas only 43% of those treated asymmetrically required further surgery."

(a) It should be observed that for their group labelled "infantile esotropia," those operated on at ages four to 18 months had an incidence of multiple surgery of 72%.

(2) Discussing these problems they observe: ". . . it becomes apparent that the surgical treatment of non-accommodative esotropia is for cosmetic purposes primarily and the avoidance of poor cosmetic results, under or over correction, is of prime importance. In the presence of poor fusional potential, early and repeated surgeries on the non-accommodative esotropia patient who is cosmetically acceptable are not justified."

(3) They continue: "The presence of prior fusion in the patient with non-accommodative esotropia enhances the probability of obtaining fusion after surgical treatment. On the other hand, the presence of prior fusion does not enhance this probability in the child with partially accommodative esotropia until after age seven years. Early surgery, in partially accommodative esotropia is still primarily for cosmetic purposes and not to obtain better fusion results."

F. Surgery and Orthoptics Combined

1. Reading the surgical results cited in the previous section gives the impression that surgical precision in alignment is of the order of magnitude of 10^{Δ} to 15^{Δ}. Since orthoptics and refractive therapy alone cannot usually be counted on solely to bring about binocular alignment of non-accommodative deviations above 50^{Δ}, it can be seen that a combination of the two methods is helpful and in fact necessary in at least those cases having large angles of deviation or where surgery has been applied prior to training. In some quarters where the surgical approach has been assumed to be primary and especially where application of training methods has been inept and restricted (so that sole use of training to effect strabismus cures has not even been attempted) orthoptic training has largely been utilized post-surgically to correct "residual deviations." In such cases the remark of Davis (1941) that orthoptic training "does not cure squint but squint cannot be cured without it" seems to apply. The reports of several such evaluations follow:

2. Costenbader (1961) in studying results of treatment of 500 cases of infantile esotropia, by surgery, spectacles, orthoptics, miotics and occlusion; classified the results as to both alignment and fusion. No mention of the time required in treatment, the observation period, or the specific methods of treatment utilized, was made. Alignment was measured with prism and alternate cover test, and fusion with the Wirt stereo tests and Worth four dot tests.

a. The author's results can be summarized as:

(1) Fifty-six of the 80 not subjected to surgery (76%) attained both fusion and alignment.

(2) Of the 228 patients undergoing one surgical procedure, 87 (38%) also achieved these results.

(3) Of those requiring two or three surgical procedures, 52 of 145 (36%) and 13 of 41 (32%) respectively were judged as possessing both alignment and fusion.

(4) The six patients requiring more than four surgical procedures were regarded as failures.

b. Those factors identified by Costenbader as of little consequence in the cure of infantile esotropia are:

(1) Age of onset within the first year of life.
(2) The duration of the squint.
(3) The age at first alignment.
(4) The refractive error.

c. He concludes that esotropia of very early onset can be cured, but only if all factors are favorable.

3. Cashell (1952) analyzing the results of surgical and orthoptic treatment of 1,119 esotropes, three years previous, finds that 374 possessed single binocular vision.

a. Of this number, half possessed some fusion in instruments, prior to treatment.

(1) Of those that were binocular before treatment 83.7% had no change or showed improvement on the reanalysis, the rest were worse or unknown.

b. Of those exhibiting no binocular ability 67.9% remained the same or showed improvement, the rest were worse or changed in an unknown manner.

c. The author notes the introduction of a vertical deviation occurring in 25% of the cases from the surgery. He feels post-operative cases invariably present difficulties. Torsional effects and limitations of motility seem an inevitable aftermath of surgical treatment in many of the cases seen.

4. Berens, Elliot and Sobacke (1941) analyzed the results of treatment of 324 strabismics over a two year period. This sample was divided into three groups. Group one consisted of 144 patients who underwent strabismus surgery but received no orthoptic training. Group two included 83 patients who received orthoptic training only after surgery. Group three consisted of 97 patients to whom both pre- and post-surgical orthoptics were administered.

a. An analysis of group one, treated solely by surgical means, showed 32 (27%) to be phoric. In group two, treated post-surgically with orthoptics, the results were 42 (50%) hetero or orthophoric. In group three, 63% achieved a phoric status after pre-and post-surgical orthoptic regimen.

(1) Thus, as the authors note: " . . . the post-operative results were almost 300% better in the patients receiving orthoptic training before and after operation (group III) as compared with the group on which only surgery was performed (group I)."

(2) And they conclude:

(a) "In our opinion orthoptic training is an indispensable adjunct to the surgical treatment of strabismus; that is, in overcoming anomalous retinal correspondence and amblyopia, and in developing fusion with increased amplitude. Most of the actual reduction of the deviation in strabismus usually must be obtained by operation and the correction of ametropia."

5. Douglas (1952) reviewed 100 concomitant convergent squints treated by orthoptics and surgery.

a. Thirty-six, when originally discharged, were reported as cured and with single binocular vision. At the time of follow-up exam, eight to 16 years after dismissal, 35 of the 100 had single binocular vision.

(1) The tests used for evaluation were: Cover test (distance and near), case history, cosmetic appearance and a depth test.

b. Of the 36 patients discharged as cured, 14 were found to have a manifest deviation. Of these the author suspects six never had been cured and the remaining eight relapsed. Twenty-two of the original 36 cures remained with straight eyes, but in only two of these, were the findings similar to those of normal individuals.

(1) In seven, binocularity was poor, duction ranges averaging 3^{Δ} to 50^{Δ}, with none showing stereopsis on small targets.

(2) Fair binocularity was possessed by 13 of the 22.

c. Of the 64 patients who were considered cosmetically satisfactory on discharge, 13 at the follow-up exam were found to have binocular vision. Douglas feels the most important single factor to be the age of onset. He also expresses doubt that orthoptic training has any value in the treatment of squint and asks rhetorically whether the absence of simultaneous binocular vision is such a very great deprivation.

6. Engel (1962) re-examined 125 patients seven years or more after treatment. Of these, 28 had no surgery, 97 had surgery, 33 had more than one procedure, 16 had exotropia and 109 had esotropia.

a. After re-examination, of the 38 who were considered completely cured (functional and cosmetic), 24 had surgical correction (of which seven underwent more than one procedure); of the 44 rated as practically cured, 35 had undergone surgery (seven more than once). Ten of these patients, at the time of re-examination, revealed small amounts of exotropia when originally they had exhibited esotropia. Combining the cured and practically cured, of the 82 (65%) who achieved single binocular vision, 23 had been given orthoptics only, while 59 had received orthoptics plus one or more surgical operations.

b. She concludes that those who obtain good fusion with good amplitudes and stereopsis and equal vision in both eyes do maintain single binocular vision through the years (only four did not). The 125 patients were all not cured at the time of initial dismissal.

(1) A cure is defined as cosmetically straight eyes under cover test, normal motility and ranges, normal V.A., good stereo and fusion under all circumstances.

(2) Practically cured was described as good V.A. in both eyes, moderately large heterophoria, good fusion and stereo in instruments and intermittent diplopia in anaglyph situations. Acceptable ranges varied with the test situation.

VIII. PROGNOSIS

A. The forecast in an individual case of the course of any affliction or condition as complicated and multifaceted as strabismus with a usually idiopathic etiology, is a hazardous and speculative undertaking. There are however, certain generalities which emerge from the foregoing description and discussion of the methods and results of treatment. Using the general strabismus parameter classification format of Ludlam and Kleinman (1965) we have:

B. Motor Aspects of the Original Strabismus Condition

1. *Size of the deviation*

a. A squint angle after neutralization of the accommodative components larger than 35^{Δ} or habitually smaller than 5^{Δ} can usually be said to present a more difficult outlook than deviations which fall within this range.

2. *Frequency of occurrence of the original deviation*

a. Except for the poor surgical results reported for intermittent exotropia and divergence excess, the prognosis for functional and cosmetic results are better in the intermittent and periodic squinter than in those manifesting a constant strabismus.

3. *Direction of deviation*

a. This factor is closely associated with frequency where Flom (1954), Schlossman and Boruchoff (1955) and Ludlam (1961) all have found statistically significant relationships between non-constancy and exotropia and Flom (1954) and Ludlam (1961) between esotropia and constancy so that much of the confusion surrounding direction of squint is caused by "failure to compare constant esotropia results with constant exotropia results and occasional eso's with occasional exo's" (Ludlam and Kleinman, 1965). The generally poorer surgical results in intermittent exotropia are again probably representative of the failure of the surgeons to take proper note of the different mechanism and chronology of the etiology in divergence excess and esotropia.

4. *Hyper, cyclorotory and "A" and "V" manifestations*

a. Hypertropia was not found to be an impediment to achieving functional cures either as a handicap or prognostic indicator by Ludlam (1961) or Ludlam and Kleinman (1965). Scobee (1951) on the other hand, holds the presence of a hypertropic component to be indicative of an incomitant condition and hence to be a factor indicating poor surgical outlook.

b. Cyclorotary or cyclotorsional deviations are almost always, in the experience of the present writer, secondary to surgery or associated with a non-comitant strabismus. While some success in building fusional cycloductions has been reported, a cyclotorsional component involving more than 5°, if it is to be eliminated, almost always calls for surgical intervention.

c. "A" and "V" components, at least of moderate degree, are not as handicapping to a successful non-surgical result as they seem to be to a surgical one. Vigorous calisthenic jump duction and accommodative rock training slowly working into the affected area seem at this writing to show promise in alleviating this condition.

5. *Variety of squint fixation*

a. Flom (1954), Ludlam (1961) and Ludlam and Kleinman (1965) have all found that the prognosis and results for alternating and unilaterally fixating strabismics are about the same. Giles (1949) on the other hand, holds the unilateral fixator to have a better prognosis than the alternator.

6. *Non-concomitancy*

a. Non-comitancy in strabismus, especially where a major limitation of gaze is involved, caused by either neurological or mechanical-anatomic factors as reviewed in Chapter XXX, is generally held to be a poor prognostic factor for functional cure with almost any type of treatment rendered.

C. Sensory Anomalies in the Strabismus Condition

1. *Amblyopia*

a. The inability to fixate centrally and steadily in the amblyopic eye appears at the present writing to be a greater handicap to obtaining a functional binocular cure of strabismus than is poor resolution.

b. With no clear cut decision in sight, the field of amblyopia remediation is presently in great ferment as to the form of treatment which might yield best long term results for lasting acuity.

(1) The best course of action at present seems to be conventional occlusion of the non-amblyopic eye in pre-school children combined with feedback producing tasks.

(2) If the eccentric fixation cannot be converted to a steady-central form within four to six months by this technique, the placement of macular tags by pleoptic approaches and inverse occlusion should be tried.

c. The present outlook is that results in improving acuity in amblyopia are erratic and unpredictable, but that the ability to fixate centrally can usually be restored. Strabismic amblyopia is no longer the block, in treating strabismus, to functional binocularity that it was in former times. Achieving high quality fusion assures the long-range stability of the improved central acuity.

d. Investigators such as Alpern, et al. (1967) feel that all of the factors involved in the strabismus amblyopia condition may not yet be recognized.

2. *Anomalous Correspondence (A.R.C.)*

a. This has traditionally stood as one of the major impediments to successful strabismus rehabilitation attempts. The most optimistic reports in the literature show better than three out of four functional *failures* in esotropes with ARC, over the short term (Flom, 1963). Exotropes have not fared as badly with claims of 38% and 62% cure being reported (Flom, 1963). Newer methods described earlier seem to be yielding closer to 50% rates of conversion to N.R.C. for esotropes over the short term (Ludlam, manuscript in preparation). Whether these methods will maintain long term normal correspondence in functionally cured esotropes is at present unknown.

b. This sensory anomaly, variously estimated as occurring in from 20 to 60% of the convergent strabismic population, still stands as the major obstacle to a functional cure in concomitant esotropia.

3. *Suppression* preferably with periods of intermittent diplopia is the least onerous perceptual adaptation to strabismus and offers the highest level prognosis for functional cure, 64 of 86 (74%) (Ludlam and Kleinman, 1965).

4. *Constant Intractable Diplopia (horror fusionis)* while thankfully very rare, has been discovered usually as a post-surgical artifact where proper sensorial workup has not been performed prior to the surgery. Bielschowsky (1935) Knauber (1944), Treleaven and Bannon (1948), von Herzau (1960) and Fisher and Ludlam (1963) all have found large amounts of aniseikonia to be responsible in individual cases which have responded to correction with proper iseikonic lenses.

D. Time as a Factor in Strabismus

1. *Age of Onset*

a. An early age of onset is deemed to make a functional cure more difficult but not impossible. Ludlam (1961) found a 50% cure rate for strabismics with an age of onset under one year of age. Others such as Douglas (1952) feel age of onset to be the single most important factor in prognosis. Early therapy especially for amblyopia, anomalous correspondence and limitations of gaze is undoubtedly important and should be stressed.

2. *Age at the Start of Treatment*

a. This area is related closely to age of onset and the consensus is that treatment should be begun as soon as is practicable after the first appearance of strabismus. The practical results of early surgery do not substantiate this intuitive feeling for early mechanical alignment of the squint (Fletcher and Silverman, 1966; Nutt, 1961; Fisher, Flom and Jampolsky, 1968). Early institution of amblyopia therapy, however, seems to bear fruit, (Parks, 1966) and early training seems to be important in achieving functional cures judged by initial short-term training results. Once a cure has been achieved, however, such therapy has only a slight relationship to the long term outcome of results accomplished through training (Ludlam and Kleinman, 1965). Miotic therapy appears to be more effective in bringing about a permanent change in AC/A ratio in children over the age of seven years (Parks, 1958; Hill, and Stromberg, 1962).

3. *Time Elapsed Since Dismissal*

a. When functional binocularity has been achieved, there appears to be no linear relationship between time elapsed since dismissal and long term results (Ludlam and Kleinman, 1965).

b. When non-functional cosmetic alignment has been achieved, the long term results are not predictable (Kennedy and McCarthy, 1959; and Morgan and Arstikaitis, 1954).

c. The results of retention of acuity in a cured amblyopic eye is related to the level of functional binocularity achieved (Gregersen and Rindziunski, 1965).

d. The long range result of untreated strabismus is toward less esotropia in terms of large drift after the age of seven.

E. Refractive and Accommodative Convergence Aspects

1. *Ametropia*

a. In accord with Donders' original observations, a correction for a hyperopic error aids in the alignment of esotropia, and correction of myopia helps correct an exotropic deviation. The opposite types of corrections, that is hyperopic in exotropia and myopic in esotropia or anisometropia tend to reduce the chances for a functional cure. Miotic drops have been reported to help in anisometropia and low hyperopic cases of esotropia and convergence excess esotropia. Bifocals also aid in this latter condition.

2. *AC/A Ratio*

a. This ratio is utilized in prescribing lenses to correct a strabismus. The higher the ratio, the more change in deviation is accomplished for a given dioptric unit of lens accepted. Miotics have been employed with mixed reports of long range results, i.e. a permanent change in AC/A brought about after withdrawal of the medication. Ludlam and Kleinman

(1965) observe that the further from an expected 4/1 ratio the more likely is the occurrence of orthoptic failure. Surgery also can bring about a change in AC/A ratio.

3. *Relative Accommodation*

a. This degree of freedom in the synkinetic linkage between accommodation and convergence is essential to the comfortable maintenance of clear binocular vision. Rankin (1963) feels it is a major factor in the spontaneous development of binocular vision in a sample of 88 esotropes she observed. Ludlam and Kleinman (1965) found that 28 of 80 cured strabismus patients being re-evaluated 3-7 years after their original dismissal from training, manifested "breaks" rather than "blur" findings on the positive and negative relative accommodation tests. They question whether these findings were a function of the type of training given or whether it is "related to the etiology of the original strabismus condition."

(1) It should be noted that the "break" rather than the "blur" in duction tests is also manifested by a large number of non-squinters, although the exact proportion for comparison is unknown.

F. Methods of Treatment

1. *Refractive Correction*

a. Although this is a useful adjunct to the other forms of strabismus therapy, it generally alone can produce between 20 and 30% cures in an unselected strabismus population. This mode of therapy includes single vision prescriptions, bifocals, prismatic corrections, and size lens prescriptions for aniseikonia, and contact lenses.

2. *Pharmacological Method*

a. This mode of therapy will temporarily help many of the 20 to 30% of strabismics capable of help by spectacles and contact lenses. The long range sole effectiveness of this "opticians nightmare" (Knapp, 1956) is still debatable, but in combination with refractive correction, it can sometimes produce results which drops alone and spectacles alone cannot produce. It holds out hope as a method by which babies with accommodative esotropia and convergence excess can be aligned until they can make use of refractive corrections and cooperate in training procedures which will refine and peak their deficient optomotor reflexes. The miotic medications, of course, cannot supply a prismatic correction or the differential magnification needed to correct aniseikonia. The numerous potential systemic and ocular side effects limit the effectiveness of long range uses of the medication.

3. *Training*

a. Almost no matter what the cause, classification, age of onset, size of deviation, refractive problem, sensory anomaly and previous therapy (radical or conservative), training is necessary to bring about functional binocularity and normalization of the optomotor reflexes. Training in conjunction with refractive correction can be used as a sole remediation measure for the majority of concomitant strabismics with a high percentage of success and almost no discomfort and no danger. It is generally unsuccessful as a sole remediation procedure only in the areas of large strabismus angles (50^Δ and more of deviation with no accommodative components); cyclotorsions; extreme "A" and "V" components; where one eye is sightless or mostly so; or where ocular or systemic pathology prevents binocular vision.

b. It has a single drawback in that its course is sometimes slow and difficult. In answer,

Cantonnet and Filliozat (1934) rebut: "That, of course cannot be denied, but it is certainly better to untie a knot than cut the string."

(1) They continue: "... re-education obtains binocular equilibrium and the subject recovers a lost function. That is surely worth persevering six or eight or even twelve months. Can a foreign language or the piano be learned in fifteen days?".

4. *Surgery*

a. This is the oldest, traditional, potentially dangerous, but fastest method of changing a strabismic deviation. That it does not deal with basic causes even its most prolific proponents readily admit. The one theoretically strong argument for its indescriminate use is in the very young strabismic where mechanical alignment might prevent serious sensory or perceptual observations. As previously stated, its use in this regard leaves much to be desired. Its present application is an art developed by trial and error through experience of the individual surgeon, with no valid mathematical relationship between the surgical caliper and ocular deviation. Its other necessary uses are in large-angle strabismus, non-comitancies, cyclotorsions and marked mechanical-anatomical anomalies in the extraocular musculature. Its use as a sole remediation procedure results in reports of functional cures ranging between 10% and 40%, depending on the individual surgeon, the characteristics of the sample reported, and the criteria used to judge results.

REFERENCES

Abraham, S. (1949): The Use of Miotics in the Treatment of Convergent Strabismus and Anisometropia. A.J. Oph., 32: 233.

Abraham, S. (1961): Present Status of Miotic Therapy in Nonparalytic Convergent Strabismus. A.J. Oph., 51: 1249.

Abraham, S.V. (1954): Intra-Epithelial Cysts of the Iris. Their Production in Young Persons and Possible Significance. A.J. Oph. 37: 327.

Abrahamsom, I. and Abrahamson, I. (1964): Preliminary Report on 0.06 Percent Phospholine Iodide in the Management of Esotropia. A.J. Oph., 57: 290.

Allen, M.J. (1966): The Bartley Phenomenon and Visual Rehabilitation – A Home Training Technique. Opt. Weekly, 57 (30): 21.

**Alpern, M.; Petrauskas, R.; Sandall, G. and Vorenkamp, R. (1967): Recent Experiments on the Physiology of Strabismus Amblyopia. Am. Orth. J., 17: 62.*

**Alpern, M.A. and Hofstetter, H.W. (1948): The Effect of Prism on Esotopia – A Case Report. A.A.A.O., 25: 80.*

Apel, R. & Lowry, (1959): Preschool Vision published by American Optometric Association, St. Louis.

Aschner, B. (1908): Uber einen bisher noch nicht beschreibenen reflex vom auge auf kreislauf und atmung. Wien Klin Wschr, 21.

Bedrossian, E.H. (1962): Surgical Results Following the Recession – Resection Operation for Intermittent Exotropia. A.J. Oph., 53: 351.

Berens, C.; Elliot, A.; Sobacke, L. (1941): Orthoptic Training and the Surgical Correction of Strabismus. A.J. Oph., 24: 1418.

Berler, D. (1963): The Oculocardiac Reflex. A.J. Oph., 56: 954.

**Bielschowsky, A. (1935): Congenital and Acquired Deficiencies of Fusion, A.J. Oph., 18: 925.*

Bietti, G. (1966): Problems of Anesthesia in Strabismus Surgery, IOC, 6: 3.

Birnbaum, M. (1963): The Use of Miotics in the Treatment of Esotropia. O.J.R.O., 100 (19): 29.

Bissaillon, A. (1957): Fifty Cases of Squint – Visual Training at Work – Optometric Extension Program Papers, 30, Series 7, Duncan, Oklahoma.

Bonsor, A. (1959): Some Comments on the Question of Early Operation. Br. Orth. J., 16: 114.

Bosomvoorth, P.; Ziegler, C. and Jocaby, S. (1958): The Oculocardiac Reflex in Eye Muscle Surgery, Anesthesiology, 19.

Breinin, G. (1967): Research in Strabismus, Chapter 5, in Vision and Its Disorders, Monograph 4, National Institutes of Neurological Diseases, Bethesda, Maryland 20014, p. 50.

Breinin, G.; Chin, N. and Ripps, H. (1966): A Rationale for Therapy of Accommodative Strabismus. A.J. Oph., 61: 90.

**Brewster, D. (1856): The Stereoscope, its History, Theory and Construction. J. Murray, London.*

Bridgeman, G.J.O. (1963): Convergent Squint of Early Onset – Results of Treatment. Br. Orth. J., 20: 45.

Brock, F. (1941): Conditioning the Squinter to Normal Visual Habits. Opt. Weekly, 32: 819.

**Brock, F. (1953): Visual Training – Part II. The Problems of Subnormal Vision and Amblyopia Monograph, reprinted from the Opt. Weekly, Chicago, Illinois.*

*de Buffon, F. (1743): Bull et Mem de L'Academie de Science, Suppl. III.

Cantonnet, A. and Filliozat, J. (1934): Le Strabisme, English Translation published by M. Wiseman and Company, London.

Cashell, G. (1952): Long Term Results of Treatment of Concomitant Convergent Strabismus in Terms of Binocular Function. Trans. Ophth. Soc. U.K., 72: 367.

Chamberlain, W. (1968): Judicious Use of Miotcs. A. Orth. J., 18: 125.

Chamberlain W. and Caldwell, E. (1965): Miotics in the Management of Strabismus. A. Orth. J., 15: 32.

Chin, N.; Gold, A. and Breinin, G. (1964): Iris Cysts and Miotics. Arch. Oph., 71: 611.

Christensen, L.; Swan, K. and Huggins, H. (1956): The Histopathology of Iris Pigment Changes Induced by Miotics. Arch. Oph. 55: 666.

Cooper, E. (1963): Accommodative Esotropia in Clinical Practice. A. Orth. J., 13: 42.

Costenbader, F. (1961): Infantile Esotropia. Trans. Amer. Oph. Soc. 59: 397.

Costenbader, F. and Albert, D. (1962): Surgery of Strabismus, IOC, 2 (4): 939.

Cushman, B. & Burri, C. (1941): Convergence Insufficiency. A.J. Oph., 24: 1044.

Dagnini, G. (1968): Analisi di alcune forme di allaritmia Cardiaca, Bull Sci med Dologna 8, series Vo. 8.

*Darwin, D. (1801): Zoonomia. Quoted from Duke-Elder, W., Textbook of Ophthalmology, Vol. 4, Mosby, St. Louis, Mo., 1949.

Davis, W. (1941): Physiotherapy in Ophthalmology, North Carolina Medical Journal, 2: 1.

Deacock, A. and Oxer, H. (1962): The Prevention of Reflex Bradycardia During Ophthalmic Surgery. Br.J. of Anaesthesia, 34: 451.

Dieffenback, J. (1839): Uber die Heilung des angeborenen Schielens mittels Durchschneidung des inneren geraden Augenmuskel, Med F, Vol. 8 Jgg, No. 46.

Donders, F. (1864): Accommodation and Refraction of the Eye, New Sydenham Society, London.

Douglas, A. (1952): Treatment of Concomitant Convergent Strabismus in Terms of Binocular Function. Trans. Ophth. Soc. U.K., 72: 383.

Dunlap, E. (1963): Surgical Management of Intermittent Exotropia. A. Orth. J., 13: 20.

Dunlap, E. (1966): Complications in Strabismus Surgery in Strabismus IOC, 6: 609.

Dunnington, J. and Wheeler, M. (1942): Operative Results in Two Hundred Eleven Cases of Convergent Strabismus. Arch. Oph., 28: 1.

Edwards, T. (1958): The Use of Miotics in Strabismus With Emphasis on Pilocarpine. A. Orth. J., 8: 142.

Engel, D. (1962): An Evaluation of 125 Orthoptic Cases Over a Period of Years. A. Orth. J., 12: 125.

Feldman, J.B. (1935): Orthoptic Treatment of Concentric Squint. Arch. Oph., 13: 419.

Fisher, N.; Flom, M. and Jampolsky, A. (1968): Early Surgery of Congenital Esotropia. A.J. of Oph., 65: 439.

Fisher, H. and Ludlam, W. (1963): An Approach to Measuring Aniseikonia in Non-Fusing Strabismus – A Preliminary Report. A.A.A.O., 40: 653.

Flax, N. (1963a): New Concepts on the Control of Binocular Deviations. J.A.O.A., 34: 451.

Flax, N. (1963b): Prism Saccadic Training, O.J.R.O., 100: 31.

Flax, N. (1964): The Use of Gross Motor Procedures in Optometric Practice. Unpublished Paper Presented, April 1964, at Optometric Extension Program Meeting on Kinesiology, Cincinnati, Ohio.

Fletcher, M. and Silverman, S. (1966): Strabismus, A. Study of 1,110 Consecutive Cases. A.J. Oph., 61: 255.

*Flom, M.C. (1958): The Prognosis in Strabismus. A.A.A.O., 36: 509.

Flom, M. (1963): Treatment of Binocular Anomalies of Vision, in Vision of Children, edited by Hirsch, M. and Wick, R. Chilton, Philadelphia. p. 197.

Folk, E. (1956): Surgical Results in Intermittent Exotropia, Arch. Oph., 55: 484.

Frandsen, A. (1960): Occurrence of Squint; A Clinical Statistical Study, in Different Groups and Ages in the Danish Population. Munksgaard, Copenhagen Acta Ophthalmologica, (Kbh.) Suppl. 62, 38: 158.

Gartner, S. and Billet, E. (1958): A Study on Mortality Rates During General Anesthesia for Ophthalmic Surgery. A.J. Oph., 45: 847.

Gibson, H. and Meakin, W. (1951): Symmetrical Binocular Flicher in the Treatment of Abnormal Retinal Correspondence Trans. of the Inter. Opt. Congress, p. 315.

Giles, G. (1949): The Practice of Orthoptics, 2nd edition, Hammond and Hammond, London.

Gillan, R.U. (1945): An Analysis of 100 Cases of Strabismus Treated Orthoptically. B. Orth. J. 29: 420.

Girard, L.; Fletcher, M.; Tomlinson, E. and Smith, B. (1962): Results of Pleoptic Treatment of Suppression Amblyopia. A. Orth. J., 12: 12.

Gonin, J. (1911): Des Procedes apte a replacer la tonotomie dan l'operation du strabismex. Ann Oculiste, 145.

Gortz, H. (1960): The Corrective Treatment of Amblyopia with Eccentric Fixation. A.J. Oph. 49: 1315.

Gregersen, E. and Rindziunski, E. (1965): Conventional Occlusion in the Treatment of Squint Amblyopia. Acta Ophthalmological, 43: 462.

Guibor, G. (1936): Early Diagnosis and Non-Surgical Treatment of Strabismus. A.J. Diseases of Children, 52.

Guibor, G. (1959): Squint and Allied Conditions. Grune and Stratton, New York, 1959.

Hallden, U. (1952): Fusional Phenomena in Anomalous Correspondence. Copenhagen Munksgaard, Acta Ophthalmologica, Supplementum 37.

Hardesty, H. (1965): Treatment of Recurrent Intermittent Exotropia. A.J. Oph., 60: 1026.

Hawkins, E. (1961): An Analysis of Strabismus Cases. Br.J. Phys. Opt., 18: 139.

Hermann, J. (1966): The Specific Role of Contact Lenses in Sensorimotor Anomalies. A. Orth. J., 16: 30.

Hicks, A.M. & Hosford, G.N. (1935): Orthoptic Treatment of Squint. Arch. Oph., 13: 1026.

Hill, K. and Stromberg, A. (1962): Echothioplate Iodide in the Management of Esotropia. A.J. Oph., 53: 488.

Hiscox, P. and McCulloch, C. (1965): Cardiac Arrest Occurring in a Patient on Echothioplate Iodide Therapy. A.J. Oph., 60: 425.

Hollwich, F. (1966): Technique and Indication of Tendon – Lengthening by Gonin Strabismus. IOC, 6: (3): 591.

Humphreys, J. and Holmes, J. (1963): Systemic Effects Produced by Echothioplate Iodide in the Treatment of Glaucoma. Arch. Oph., 69: 737.

Illingworth, R.S. (1959): The Pediatrician and the Eye. Trans. Oph. Soc. U.K., 79: 335.

Ing, M.; Costenbader, F.; Parks, M. and Albert, D. (1966): Surgery for Congenital Esotropia. A.J. Oph., 61: 1419.

Javal, E. (1896): Manuel de Strabisme Paris, Maisson and Cie, 45 and 79.

Johnson, D. and Antuna, J. (1965): Atropine and Miotics for Treatment of Amblyopia. A.J. Oph., 60: 889.

*Journal of the New York State Optometric Association (1963) 31: 6.

Kavner, R. and Suchoff, I. (1966): Pleoptics Handbook. Published by the Optometric Center of New York, New York.

Kennedy, J. (1954): The Correction of Divergent Strabismus with Concave Lenses, A.A.A.O., 31: 605.

Kennedy, R. and McCarthy (1959): Surgical Treatment of Esotropia. A.J.

Oph., 50: 508.

Kirsch, R.; Somet, P.; Kugel, V. and Axelrod, S. (1957): Electrocardiographic Changes During Ocular Surgery and Their Prevention by Retrobulbar Injection. Arch. Oph. 58: 348.

Knapp, P. and Capobianco, N. (1956): Use of Miotics in Esotropia. A. Orth. J., 6: 40.

*Knauber, E. (1944): Anomalies of Fusion Associated With Aniseikonia: A Preliminary Report. Arch. Oph., 31: 265.

Koskinen, I.K. (1957): Experiments with the Use of Miotics in Convergent Strabismus. Acta Ophthal. (Kbh.) 35: 521.

Kramer, M. (1953): Clinical Orthoptics, (2nd ed.), C.V. Mosby and Co., St. Louis.

Kupfer, C. (1957): Treatment of Amblyopia Ex Anopsia in Adults, A.J. Oph., 43: 918.

Lancaster, J. (1967): The use of Natures Tools in Orthoptics. A. Orth. J., 17: 27.

Law, F. (1938): On the Value of Orthoptic Training, Br. J. Oph., 22: 192.

Levinge, M. (1954): Value of Abnormal Retinal Correspondence in Binocular Vision. Br. J. Oph., 38: 332.

Ludlam, W. (1961): Orthoptic Treatment of Strabismus. A.A.A.O., 38: 369.

Ludlam, W. (1962): Lecture Notes, Summer Residency Program, Strabismic Orthoptics, Optometric Center of New York.

Ludlam, W. and Kleinman, B. (1965): The Long Range Results of Orthoptic Treatment of Strabismus. A.A.A.O., 42: 647.

*Ludlam, W. and Pierce, J. (1968, in press): Clinical Techniques for Strabismus Training, Professional Press, Chicago.

*Lyle, D. (1959): Neuro-ophthalmology. Arch. Oph. 60: 950.

Lyle, T. and Jackson, S. (1953): Practical Orthoptics in the Treatment of Squint. H.K. Lewis, London.

*McLaughlin, (1967): Oculomotor Adaptation to Wedge Prisms, Perception and Psychophysics.

Mendelblatt, F.I.; Kirsch, R.E. & Lemberg, L. (1962): A Study Comparing Methods of Preventing the Oculo Cardiac Reflex. A.J. Oph., 53: 506.

Miller, J. (1960): A Comparison of Miotics in Accommodative Esotropia. A.J. Oph., 49: 1350.

Morgan, A. and Arstikaitis, M. (1954): A Review of 1,000 Postoperative Cases of Strabismus. Trans. Canadian Oph. Soc., 7: 46.

Morgan, M.W. (1961): Anomalous Correspondence Interpreted as a Motor Phenomenon. A.A.A.O., 38: 131.

Mulberger, R. and McDonald P. (1954): Exotropia Surgery. Arch. Oph., 52: 664.

Nauheim, J. (1962): Marginal Keratitis and Corneal Ulceration After Surgery on the Extra Ocular Muscles. Arch. Oph. 67: 46.

Noordlow, W. (1951): Spontaneous Changes in Refraction and Angle of Squint, Together with the State of Retinal Correspondence and Visual Acuity in Concomitant Convergent. Strabismus During the Years of Growth. Acta. Ophthalmologica, 29: 383.

Noordlow, W. (1960): The Angle of Squint, Amount of Surgery and Results of Operation in Constant Convergent Strabismus. Acta Ophthal. 38.

Nugent, O. (1940): Functional Training, An Aid in the Surgical Correction of Strabismus. A.J. Oph., 23: 68.

Nutt, A. (1961): Surgery in the Treatment of Concomitant Strabismus, Trans. Oph. Soc. U.K., 81: 757.

Obrien, C. (1951): Strabismus Ophthalmic Symposium, ed. James H. Allen, C.V. Mosby, St. Louis.

Parks, M. (1958): Abnormal Accommodative Convergence in Squint. Arch. Oph., 59: 364.

Parks, M. and Friendly, D. (1966): Treatment of Eccentric Fixation in Children Under Four Years of Age. A.J. Oph., 61: 395.

Perera, C. (1949): May's Manual of the Diseases of the Eye, 2nd ed. Williams and Wilkins, Baltimore.

Pigassou, R. and Toulouse, J. (1967): Treatment of Eccentric Fixation. J. Pediatric Oph., 4 (2): 35.

Pollie, D.; Hafner, A. and Krasnoff, J. (1964): The Strabismic Child and his Psychological Adjustment. J. Pediatric Oph., 1 (2).

*Posner, A. and Schlossman, A. (1951): Relation of Diplopia to Binocular Vision in Concomitant Strabismus. Arch. Oph. 45: 615.

Rankin, D. (1963): Incidence of Spontaneous Improvement in Convergent Strabismus. Br. Orth. J., 20: 54.

Records, R. (1967): Side Reactions to Anticholinesterase Therapy for Strabismus. A. Orth. J., 17: 44.

Reed, H. and McCaughey, T. (1962): Cardiac Slowing During Strabismus. Surgery, B.J. Oph., 46: 112.

Reid, L.; Stephenson, H. and Hinton, J. (1952): Cardiac Arrest. Arch. Surgery, 64.

Rhode, J,; Grom, E.; Bajares, C.; Anselmi, A.; Capriles, M. and Rivas, C. (1958): A Study of the Electrocardiographic Alterations Occurring During Operations on the Extraocular Muscles. A.J. Oph. 46: 367.

Ripps, H.; Breinin, G. Baum (1961): Accommodation in the Cat. Trans. A. Oph. society, 59: 176.

*Ripps, H.; Chin, N.; Siegel, I. and Breinin, G. (1962): The Effect of Pupil Size on Accommodation Convergence and the AC/A Ratio. Investigative Ophthal., 1: 127.

*Rubin, W. (1966): Reverse Prism in the Treatment of Strabismus and Amblyopia. A. Orth. J., 16: 62.

Ruedemann, A. (1953): Foveal Coordination. A.J. Oph., 36: 1220.

Schlossman, A. and Priestly, B. (1952): Role of Heredity in Etiology and Treatment of Strabismus. Arch. Oph. 47: 1.

Schlossman, A. and Boruchoff, S. (1955): Correlation between Physiologic and Clinical Aspects of Exotropia. A.J. Oph., 40: 53.

Schrock, R. (1965): Introduction to Visual Training. Optometric Extension Program, Postgraduate Courses, Vol. 38, Series 1N1, Duncan, Oklahoma.

Schrock, R. and Heinsen, A. (1966): The Schur-Mark Out Office Vision Training System, 3rd edition., Published and distributed by Keystone View Co. Meadville, Pa. Development of Binocularity B1-1.

Scobee, R. (1951): Esotropia – Incidence Etiology and Results of Therapy. A.J. Oph., Series 3, 34: 817.

Scully, J. (1961): Early Intensive Occlusion in Strabismus with Non-Central Fixation. Br. Medical J., Dec. 16., p. 1610.

Simpson, D. (1956): Surgery for Strabismus. A. Orth. J., 6: 130.

Sloan, L.; Sears, M. and Jablonski, (1960): Convergence – Accommodation Relationship, Arch. Oph., 63: 283.

Smith, W. (1943): Orthoptics as a Remedial Procedure in Squint and Amblyopia ex-anopsia. A.A.A.O., 20: 165.

*Smith, W. (1954): Clinical Orthoptic Procedure, 2nd edition, (C.V. Mosby), St. Louis, Mo.

Sorenson, W. and Gilmore, J. (1956): Cardiac Arrest During Strabismus Surgery. A.J. Oph., 41: 748.

Stobie, D. (1955): Congenital Strabismus, The Common Sense Approach. Arch. Oph., 77.

Taylor, D.M. (1967): Congenital Strabismus. The Common Sense Approach. Arch. Oph. 77: 478.

Tibbs, A. (1958): A Short Method for Treating Anomalous Retinal Correspondence. A. Orth. J., 8: 37.

Tomlinson, E. (1965): Treatment of Anomalous Retinal Correspondence

Employing Retinal Afterimage. A. Orth. J., 15: 59.

**Treleaven, C. and Bannon, R. (1948): Obstacles to Binocular Vision. O.J.R.O., 85 (16): 35.*

Verlee, D. and Iacobucci, I. (1967): Pleoptics Versus Occlusion of the Sound Eye, A.J. Oph., 63: 224.

**Von Herzau, W.: Horror Fusionis und Konvergenzeszess bei Anisometropia and Aniseekonie, Klinische Monats fur Augenheilk, 137: 781.*

Von Noorden, G. and Lipsius (1964): Experiences with Pleoptics in 58 Patients with Strabismus Amblyopia. A.J. Oph., 59: 41.

**Walter, J. and Benz, C. (1964): Bilateral Amputation Neuromas of Eye Muscles. A.J. Oph., 57: 287.*

Weve, H. (1954): The Operative Treatment of Strabismus, Docum. Ophtha. Vol. 7-8., p. 495.

**Wheatstone, C. (1838): Philsophical Transactions, Royal Society of London.*

Wheeler, M. and Moore, S. (1964): DFP in the Handling of Esotropia. A. Orth. J., 14: 178.

Whitwell, J. (1962): Miotics and Strabismus, Br. Orth. J. 19.

Addendum 33

On page 212 under (3) is this addition:

(4) Depth perception may also be influenced by cyclotorsional movements (see below) by virtue of "inclination angle" (the angle through which an object leans forward or behind the parallel plane vertical). This is in turn introduced by the "declination angle" between the corresponding angular deviations of the vertical retinal meridian and the meridian along which the retinal images fall. (Adams & Levene, 1967)

On page 226 under 6b is this addition:

7. A slight excyclophoria is common for distance targets (zero convergence) but the amount of excylophoria increases when the eyes are converged or elevated, and may become encylophoric when the eyes are depressed and looking at a distance object. (cit. by Adams & Levene, 1967)

a. The effect of convergence and of accommodative-convergence upon cyclophorias has also been studied by Allen (1942). As noted earlier, an increase in excylophoria accommodative convergences were found to be more influential in four others. Two subjects showed little effect from either type of convergence innervation while in one subject, the entire change was associated with accommodative-convergence alone. Hyperphorias produced little effect, but an increase in the direction of the excyclophoria occurred slowly during dissociation of the eyes up to a period of as long as one hour. Cyclophoria also varied cyclically with the amplitude of the phoria up to 2° and for a period of two minutes.

On page 450 under D 1 e is this correction:

e. Goldmann in 1932 used a split ocular similar to the Lobeck eyepiece (a double prism in the plane of the image of the ocular) and a diaphragm at the site of the exit pupil. Two half images of the cornea, contiguous to each other, are observed. A micrimeter screw moves the halves towards each other until the anterior border of one part just touches the posterior one of the other. The hairlines must be kept clear and the observor's refractive error must be fully corrected.

On page 559 the term "Ainsler Test" occuring in section 5 should correctly be "Amsler Test."

On page 824 under 5 is this addition:

a. Tubis (1954) however, in comparing a polaroid test of disparity with the dissociated vertical phoria test, concludes that the dissociated phoria test if reduced by 20 to 25% of its value, is a reliable measure of imbalance.

INDEX

A

B

C

D

E

F

I

J

K

L

M

N

Q

R

S

T

W

X

Y

Z